Bioethical Prescriptions

OXFORD ETHICS SERIES

Series Editor: Derek Parfit, All Souls College, Oxford

Bioethical Prescriptions

TO CREATE, END, CHOOSE, AND IMPROVE LIVES

F. M. Kamm

OXFORD
UNIVERSITY PRESS

OXFORD
UNIVERSITY PRESS

Oxford University Press is a department of the University of Oxford.
It furthers the University's objective of excellence in research,
scholarship, and education by publishing worldwide.

Oxford   New York
Auckland   Cape Town   Dar es Salaam   Hong Kong   Karachi
Kuala Lumpur   Madrid   Melbourne   Mexico City   Nairobi
New Delhi   Shanghai   Taipei   Toronto

With offices in
Argentina   Austria   Brazil   Chile   Czech Republic   France   Greece
Guatemala   Hungary   Italy   Japan   Poland   Portugal   Singapore
South Korea   Switzerland   Thailand   Turkey   Ukraine   Vietnam

Oxford is a registered trade mark of Oxford University Press
in the UK and certain other countries.

Published in the United States of America by
Oxford University Press
198 Madison Avenue, New York, NY 10016

© Oxford University Press 2013

First issued as an Oxford University Press paperback, 2016

Library of Congress Cataloging-in-Publication Data
Kamm, F. M. (Frances Myrna)
Bioethical prescriptions : to create, end, choose, and improve lives / F. M. Kamm.
pages   cm.—(Oxford ethics series)
Includes index.
ISBN 978-0-19-997198-5 (hardback : alk. paper)—ISBN 978-0-19-064961-6 (paperback : alk. paper)
ISBN 978-0-19-997199-2 (updf)
1. Medical ethics. 2. Bioethics. 3. Medicine—Philosophy.
4. Human experimentation in medicine—Moral and ethical aspects. I. Title.
R724.K25   2013
174.2—dc23   2012047872

For Derek Parfit and Thomas Scanlon
With gratitude for their kindness and continuing support

CONTENTS

ACKNOWLEDGMENTS

This collection of essays has been in preparation over several years, longer than I had originally expected. This was due to my inability to refrain from making revisions, and also to other projects whose deadlines intervened. I am indebted to many sources of support during these years.

I worked on the manuscript in 2007–8, as a Senior Fellow at the Petrie-Flom Center for Health Law Policy, Biotechnology, and Bioethics at Harvard Law School. I thank Professor Einer Elhauge for his support, as well as Professor Glenn Cohen, who was a fellow at that time and is now co-head of the Center. The kindness and efficiency of Kathy Parras, the Center's administrator at the time, was much appreciated. I am grateful to the Harvard Kennedy School for their support of a half-year sabbatical during that time, as well as in Fall 2010, when I continued work on the book (among other projects).

In Spring 2011, I was a Fellow at the Department of Clinical Bioethics at the National Institutes of Health. I am grateful to Dr. Ezekiel Emmanuel, who first invited me to the department, to Dr. Christine Grady, who is its current director, and to Dr. Marion Danis for their support. The lively intellectual environment at the Center that also allows for focused individual work was wonderful. I am grateful to Theo and Vann Ooms for providing me with wonderful living quarters during my NIH visits.

Since I arrived at Harvard University in 2003, my colleagues in the University-wide Program in Ethics and Health—including Dan Brock, Norman Daniels, Nir Eyal, and Dan Wikler—have helped create an atmosphere hospitable to philosophical work in bioethics from which I have benefited. Additionally, the directors and faculty of the Edmond J. Safra Center—including Dennis Thompson, Larry Lessig, Arthur Applbaum, and Eric Beerbohm—have supported the work of analytic philosophers on practical ethics. I am grateful to them and indebted to Mrs. Lily Safra for her support of the Center.

For help in the typing, editing, proofreading, and puzzle-solving that made possible creating the final manuscript, I am greatly indebted to Olivia Bailey, Margaret Collins, Lynne Meyer-Gay, Paul Julian, Jean Valois, and the staff at Oxford University Press. The index was constructed by Olivia Bailey, Paul Julian, and Douglas Kremm. My Harvard Kennedy School assistants, Camiliakumari Wankaner and Lisa MacPhee, have done excellent work in helping me with my teaching responsibilities and faculty finances during this period. Maria Twarog, Agnes Mosejczuk, and Hubert Mosejczuk have helped in many practical ways. The memory of my dear parents, Mala and Solomon Kamm, has sustained me.

Acknowledgments of those from whom I received comments on the chapters in this book are included in each chapter. For the most part, these were individuals who commented on the articles on which the chapters are based. Johann Frick, however, read all the chapters once I had made revisions and gave me extremely helpful suggestions with respect to substance, style, and organization, for which I am very grateful. Since some material in this book goes back to projects I first engaged in as a graduate student and junior faculty member, my thanks extend to Barbara Herman, Thomas Nagel, and the late Robert Nozick. I am grateful to Rosamond Rhodes for including me in the bioethics projects she organized during those times. I am grateful to Shelly Kagan, Jeff McMahan, and Larry Temkin, with whom I have regularly discussed my work more recently. I am especially grateful to my colleague Thomas Scanlon for his support and to Derek Parfit, whose encouragement and reflections on my work have made it possible for this book to be part of the wonderful Oxford Ethics Series that he edits.

INTRODUCTION

This book presents revised versions of published articles, mostly subsequent to 1990.[1] There would have been much repetition had I not sometimes excised and rearranged parts of the original articles, so some chapters involve structural changes from the originals. However, I have tried to keep the substance of the original articles mostly intact.[2] Hence, the chapters do not necessarily represent my current views.

This book's title plays with the concept of a doctor's prescription only with regard to bioethical content. This may suggest that bioethical prescriptions are something like "Transplant the organ into person A, not person B, and call me in the morning" or "Remember two moral distinctions and take plenty of fluids." The essays collected here do not provide such simple directives. However, the second suggested "prescription" is an alert that what may be prescribed is to take account of certain factors rather than to adopt a specific act or policy (consider this the book's warning label). Nevertheless, after fairly intricate examination of an issue, I believe it often becomes clear that one course of action or one type of policy is morally superior to another and why this is so.

This book begins with our end insofar as its first part, "Death and Dying," deals not with our creation but our cessation.[3] This is partly because later discussions of other topics make frequent reference to death. The first chapter is a philosophical analysis of Tolstoy's novella *The Death of Ivan Ilych*. The analysis considers whether the way we live affects how we die by examining why Ivan fears death and how this connects with general factors that make death bad. Chapter 2 presents and explains many of the distinctions thought to be of moral relevance in discussion of suicide, physician-assisted suicide, termination of life-saving treatment, and euthanasia. In chapter 3, I critically examine the arguments for physician-assisted suicide in the so-called Philosophers' Brief on the topic. In chapter 4, there follows an alternative Four-Step Argument for the moral permissibility of physician-assisted suicide and objections to the argument. This chapter also raises the issue of whether doctors might have a duty, not merely a permission, to assist suicide. Chapter 5 considers some of David Velleman's objections to physician-assisted suicide, and chapter 6 deals with Baruch Brody's views on assisted suicide and euthanasia. Chapter 7 is concerned with the moral permissibility of relying on advance directives when dealing with demented patients. Chapter 8 concludes the part with a critical examination of arguments that have been given for and against the brain-death criterion of death.[4]

Part II, "Early Life," addresses some moral issues that arise at the beginning and in early years of life in connection with the destruction or harming of that life.

Chapters 9 and 10 deal with the moral significance of destroying human embryos for research and of other means used to acquire human stem cells for research purposes. There follow several chapters that deal with destruction of embryos and fetuses in abortion. Chapter 11 examines Ronald Dworkin's position on abortion as presented in his *Life's Dominion*.[5] Chapter 12 presents a condensed version of arguments I first presented in *Creation and Abortion* concerning whether and when abortion would be permissible if the fetus were assumed (for the sake of argument) to be a person.[6] This discussion broaches the topic of the ethics of creating people and what creators owe the people they create (taken up again in chapter 15). Chapter 13 discusses the views of Jeff McMahan for the most part as they bear on the moral status of life in its earliest stage, its connections with later stages of life, and how this bears on the morality of abortion.[7] Chapter 14 deals with Munchausen Syndrome, a clear case of abuse by parents of young children within a medical context, examining conceptual issues that arise in characterizing it and ethical issues that arise in trying to stop it.

Part III, "Genetic and Other Enhancements," concerns ethical issues related to genetic modification, cloning, and more generally, creating people with worthwhile lives. It begins in chapter 15 with a discussion of issues raised in *From Chance to Choice*,[8] and also in "Justice and Nature" by Thomas Nagel;[9] in "Wrongful Life, Procreative Responsibility, and the Significance of Harm" by Seana Shiffrin;[10] and in "Shopping at the Genetic Supermarket" by Peter Singer.[11] Among the issues are whether and to what degree social justice requires genetic modification for purposes of treatment and/or enhancement, what duties parents have to control the genetic makeup of, and more generally to benefit and not harm, their offspring, and how genetic modification would affect the disabled. Chapter 16 is concerned with distinguishing different types of moral status (in a broad sense) and the relation of moral status to the permissibility and impermissibility of doing harm to some entities to prevent harm to, or promote the good of, other entities. In this regard, it compares uncloned persons with clones and embryos and also shows the bearing of these issues on the Non-Identity Problem and on treatment of future generations. Chapter 17 considers in detail Michael Sandel's arguments against certain types of human enhancement in order to determine what is and is not morally wrong with the pursuit of enhancement of the human species.

Part IV, "Allocating Scarce Resources," deals with the allocation of scarce lifesaving and health-promoting resources. Chapter 18 is an overview of issues concerning equity and health, including an introduction to possible principles for allocation at micro and macro levels. Chapter 19 deals with certain views of Norman Daniels about the relation between health and equal opportunity. The following three chapters deal with specific allocation problems. Chapter 20 deals with whether it is morally permissible to stop the use of a drug in a population where it is doing good in order to do more good in another population. Chapter 21 concerns whether someone's disability status is morally relevant to his receiving a scarce medical resource; it includes discussion of QALYs and DALYs and the views of Peter Singer. Chapter 22 compares some of my views on the relevance of disability in allocation decisions with some more recent views of Peter Singer and Dan Brock. Chapter 23 attempts to describe in more detail some principles for allocating scarce resources and to extend their use from medical contexts to nonmedical contexts (such as education and legal services).

Part V, "Methodology," concludes the book with chapters on the relations between moral theory, theorizing about practical moral problems, and the actual application of moral solutions to practical problems. So far as possible, material from published articles on these topics has been chosen that bears directly on bioethics. Chapter 24 is a discussion of the philosopher's role in advising government (or other institutional) bodies where compromise between conflicting parties may be necessary in order to achieve any good outcomes. One section of this chapter presents the view of some that argument by analogy rather than by moral theory is most useful in affecting public policy. On account of this, chapter 25 discusses Ronald Dworkin's opposite view that theory and not analogy is what is needed, at least in Supreme Court legal reasoning. Chapter 26 deals more generally with the relations between normative ethical theory, discussions of practical ethics, and the actual application of moral solutions to practical problems. Chapter 27 concludes by briefly describing and defending the use of hypothetical cases in moral reasoning as employed throughout this book.[12]

Notes

1. Prior to that, my articles on bioethics were the basis of some sections of *Creation and Abortion* (New York: Oxford University Press, 1992) and *Morality, Mortality*, Vol. I (New York: Oxford University Press, 1993).

2. Exceptions are new sections in chapters 12 and 15.

3. It thus echoes T. S. Eliot's thought, "In my beginning is my end" (in his *Four Quartets*, Part II, "East Coker" (New York: Harcourt Brace, 1943).

4. Excerpts from "On Death, without Exaggeration," from Poems New and Colllected 1957–1997 by Wislawa Szymborksa and translated from the Polish by Stanislaw Baranczak and Clare Cavanagh, which appear on page 1, are reprinted by permission of Houghton Mifflin Harcourt Publishing Company (English translation copyright(c) 1998).

5. Ronald Dworkin, *Life's Dominion: An Argument about Abortion, Euthanasia, and Individual Freedom* (New York: Knopf, 1993).

6. Kamm, *Creation and Abortion.*

7. In his *The Ethics of Killing: Problems at the Margins of Life* (New York: Oxford University Press, 2002).

8. Alan Buchanan, Daniel W. Brock, Norman Daniels, and Daniel Wikler, *From Chance to Choice: Genetics and Justice* (Cambridge: Cambridge University Press, 2000).

9. Thomas Nagel, "Justice and Nature," *Oxford Journal of Legal Theory* 17(2) (1997).

10. Seana Shiffrin, "Wrongful Life, Procreative Responsibility, and the Significance of Harm," *Legal Theory* 5 (1999).

11. In S. Y. Song, Y. M. Koo, and D. R. J. Macer (eds.), *Asian Bioethics in the 21st Century* (Tsukuba: Eubios Ethics Institute, 2003), pp. 143–56.

12. Chapters 8, 12, and 21 are, I believe, the most difficult. If one finds them daunting, this should not at all discourage one from reading other chapters.

PART ONE

Death and Dying

On Death, without Exaggeration

Whoever claims that it's omnipotent
is himself living proof
that it's not.

There's no life
that couldn't be immortal
if only for a moment.

Death
always arrives by that very moment too late.

In vain it tugs at the knob
of the invisible door.
As far as you've come
can't be undone.
—Wislawa Szymborska

1

Rescuing Ivan Ilych

HOW WE LIVE AND HOW WE DIE

We are all likely to agree that Ivan Ilych did not live as he should have.[1, 2, 3] The question is, what does this have to do with the sort of death he had? That is, would someone who had lived differently necessarily have had a different sort of death, in the sense that his process of dying and also what his death itself signified would be different? And would everyone who lived as Ivan lived have Ivan's sort of death? Tolstoy exhibits a critical attitude toward Ivan, his wife, and doctors when they think that there is a way for him to avoid death on this occasion by doing something different (for example, taking medicines regularly). Their need for control is taken to exemplify their failure to understand what is going on. When Ivan asks himself why he has to suffer physically and die if not because he has done something wrong for which he is being punished, our first impulse is to disagree; this is not the explanation of what is happening to him.[4] However, I wish to consider the possibility that Tolstoy's story reveals how we can have some control over our deaths—the process of dying and what death itself signifies—by how we choose to live. I shall consider several characteristics of Ivan's death and dying process and see whether their presence could vary with how we live.

I

One of the characteristics of Ivan's death is that he does not believe that it could possibly happen to him.[5] Ivan says that he knew the syllogism "Caius is a man, men are mortal, therefore Caius is mortal," and he believed it to be true of Caius and of man in the abstract—but what did that have to do with him, Ivan? He was not a man in the abstract but someone with particular characteristics and a rich subjectivity.[6] Perhaps Ivan's logical difficulty may be described as follows: he thinks that the universal premise "All men are mortal" does not apply when a man has particular characteristics and especially an active subjective life. So, in a sense, he is raising an objection to the correctness of the universal premise. Of course, he is wrong to think that having particular characteristics and an active subjective life are defenses against death. However, he also makes another mistake. He treats Caius, who would be a particular person with a particular history and rich subjectivity, as a man in the abstract and therefore not in possession of characteristics that would protect him from mortality as much as Ivan's version of those characteristics are supposed to protect Ivan.

Ivan's reason for failing to see that the syllogism applies to him though he believes that it applies to Caius connects up with the way he has lived his life: he has not taken seriously the nonabstract reality of other persons (which is not to say that he has taken his reality as seriously as he should have either). So, when something bad happens to them, he finds no reason to think that it will happen to him. In his professional role as a judge, he has never taken seriously what their fates mean to the people whose lives depend on his decisions. He has focused on the law and its outcome, not on its impact on the persons at trial. In his personal relations, he has developed standard responses to his wife that will prevent his life from being upset by having to engage with her problems. It would be easier for him to accept the universal premise in the syllogism and its application to him if he took seriously—given his knowledge that others die—that others have the same special reality to themselves that he has to himself.

Ivan's failure to seriously accept a universal premise also shows itself in his inability to accept that he can come to be treated by others as he has treated others. The "turning of the tables" motif is strong in the story. Doctors treat him as a set of organs rather than as a person whose life is at stake, in the way he has treated defendants as interesting cases rather than as persons whose lives were at stake.[7] His wife takes up a standard line to help her cope with his illness as he took up a standard line with her. (Her line fails to deal seriously with him as a dying person; she claims that he is to blame for not following doctors' orders and if he followed them, he need not die.) In sum, Ivan believed that it was all right to act on a maxim toward others that he would not be willing to universalize, including to have applied to himself.

However, if Ivan were treated *only* as he has treated others, he would not have received the honest and sympathetic concern of Gerasim, his servant. Possibly, Gerasim's help may be seen as a cosmic return for Ivan's own better impulses, which are described as being repressed after childhood.

Despite his difficulties with including himself in universals and his mistaking why others are susceptible to them, there is one logical move with which Ivan has no problems. One way of thinking of this move is from the singular case involving something bad happening to himself to the *universal* of something bad happening to everyone. Once he realizes that he will die, he reflects on the coming deaths of others who are as foolish as he was in not realizing that they will die. Instead of pitying them as he wishes to be pitied, he takes satisfaction in their susceptibility to the universality of death. Similarly, once he realizes that he has not lived as he should have, he becomes aware of how almost everybody around him is repeating the mistakes he made. Again, instead of pitying them the errors of their ways, he hates them for it. (This hatred may stem from the fact that living as they have, they were co-conspirators in his wasting his life. He could not have done it so well without them.)

The move from one's own case to the universal is not an error if one's fate is caused by a property that others also have, and the cause of mortality is such a property. So, the syllogism he grasps is: (1) I am mortal in virtue of being human; (2) they are all human; therefore, (3) they are all mortal. Similarly, if doing x is the wrong way for Ivan to live because it is the wrong way for human persons in general to live, it will be wrong for everyone as well.

If he makes this move from his own case to the universal, the universal has more reality for him than it had when he believed its content only applied to some others, because he now applies it to his inner circle of family and friends who have also (in his thoughts) previously been exempt from death.[8] He also applies it to people to whom (unlike Caius) he attributes a subjectivity, for, in calling them fools, he recognizes their beliefs about themselves that they will not die.

However, there is a slightly different way of interpreting the logical move with which Ivan has no problems. He moves from his own case to the cases of those who he thinks are *like him*—that is, his friends and their deaths become as nonabstract for him as his own. This does not yet generate a true universal from the subjectively real personal and so it does not transmit the force of the personal in order to *de*abstract even the death of Caius. This version of his syllogism is: (1) I, even with my special characteristics, am mortal in virtue of being human; (2) others who share my special characteristics are human; therefore, (3) they are mortal.

Going from his own case to the case of those he can see as like him in many ways (rather than transforming the still too abstract universal) mirrors what happens to his so-called friend, Peter Ivanovich, at the very beginning of the story. Even if Peter, like Ivan, cannot move from Caius and all men to his own case, he can move from Ivan's death to his own. He becomes aware that someone very much like him has died and it could happen to him. Tolstoy implies that this is how death becomes subjectively real to someone who is not yet dying, rather than through the universal syllogism. The death of someone like oneself makes clear that many of the characteristics that one has and Caius lacks cannot save one, since they did not save one's friend who also had them. But there is still a route of escape for someone like Peter, who is not the one dying—he can just rely on his bare particularity to save him, at least for the time being. He says, "I am not Ivan, so he is dead and I am not." The further implicit thought is, "Possibly I won't have to be dead."[9]

A true friend (let alone a clearheaded thinker), however, might not be able to latch onto this separating mechanism. On the one hand, true sympathy draws a friend closer to the person who died so that he thinks more about the bad thing that has happened to his friend and his own loss of that friend rather than about what all this implies about his own mortality. But, on the other hand, identification with one's friend also reinforces a sense of equality (or perhaps even personal subordination to the friend), so one is more likely to accept a shared fate with one's friend. The thought comes, if it was possible for death to happen even to my beloved friend, why *should* it not be possible that it happen to me?[10]

In addition to his failure to be convinced by the syllogism concerning Caius, Ivan believes that if something as important as his being mortal were true, there would have been some clue to it arising from his own subjectivity, independent of empirical evidence and logical implications from universals. He thinks there would have been an instinctive awareness of his own mortality in the way, we are told, he had instinctive awareness of the right way to live (as evidenced by his initial revulsion at socially approved norms). But as he repressed and ignored these intimations of how to live, he no doubt would have repressed and ignored intimations of mortality had they existed.

Hence, I believe we can agree that the way Ivan lived does explain one characteristic of his death, namely his shock at the fact that it will occur. Tolstoy contrasts Ivan's ignorance on this matter with the open-eyed awareness of death that common folk like Gerasim have, an awareness that they do not repress. Presumably, it is part of their goodness to recognize the reality of others and not think of themselves as remarkable exceptions; this, more than mere logical abilities in dealing with a universal premise, helps explain their knowledge of their own mortality.

II

Closely related to Ivan's shock at the fact that he can die is the second characteristic of his death, namely his shock at how something as important as death can come about at a time of no particular consequence. It need not come from fighting in a battle for some important cause but, rather, from something as trivial as a misstep on a ladder while decorating. It is this that adds one element of the absurd. It also helps explain his disbelief that he will die now—after all, nothing important enough has happened to merit being the cause of his death. Of course, Tolstoy arranges his story so that Ivan's death results from his greed and concern with appearance and trivialities: he hits himself while arranging a curtain in his new home.[11] Would a person who did not live as Ivan had avoid such an absurd end? Good people may also die of missteps, even if not from those produced by (habitual) greed. But, presumably, they realize that an absurd end is possible, and so are not shocked by it. (And they may be continually grateful that something of this sort has not yet happened, given that it always might.) Again, how one lives seems to have some impact on how one dies.[12]

III

Once he knows that he will die, what are the sources of Ivan's fear of death? (I am now speaking only of fear of death, not fear of the process of dying.) There are three: (1) death means no more of the goods of life (*a*) of the type he has been having and (*b*) of new types he might have; (2) it means extinction of himself; and (3) it means that (*a*) he has wasted all the life he had and (*b*) there will be no more chances to rectify that. He first focuses on how he will have no more of the types of goods he has been having (1*a*), then he focuses on extinction (2), but ultimately it is the waste of life and no chance of rectifying this (3) that are his preeminent concerns with death. These are characteristics that Ivan believes his death will have. Ultimately, I am concerned to see if he is right about his own death and whether these characteristics attach to everyone's death. But to begin with, I shall consider the relation between these three characteristics.

Can we really distinguish the badness of having no more goods (1) from the badness of extinction (2)? I believe we can. One common philosophical view of why death is bad is that it interferes with having more goods of life.[13] (These goods might come to us if we lived, even if we have no plans for the future with which death would interfere. The completion of plans is just one sort of good with which death can interfere.) This is certainly one reason why death is bad, and it is involved in (1) and also in no rectification (3*b*). But Ivan is also concerned that *he will be nothing*. (Although he exhibits the inability to grasp the very idea of his own extinction by confusingly asking, "Then where shall I be when I am no more?" [p. 42].)

We can try to distinguish concern for one's extinction from concern that one will not have more goods of life by imagining the Limbo Man.[14] He is someone who could ensure that his life is longer or even never over without thereby increasing the amount of goods (or ills) that he has in his life. He merely selects to spread out his conscious life over an indefinite future, going into unconscious limbo (a coma state) in the intervening times. If this were possible, God could grant someone a much longer life or even immortality without granting him any more goods of life than a mortal being would have. Those whose concern with death is focused only on its limiting total goods will not find the Limbo Man's strategy helpful; those who are concerned with extinction—a conscious self not being all over—should find it helpful.

What leads Ivan to eventually focus on waste and no rectification (3) is really his recognition that avoiding the end of the sort of "goods" he has been having (1*a*) would not be worthwhile in his case.[15] He has been living a bad life—a living death, some have called it[16]—and more of the so-called goods he has been having would just be more of the bad. So, in his case, death is not bad because it prevents a continuation of goods he has been having; if it did only this, it would just prevent more bad things. One way to understand what Ivan realizes as he is dying physically is that he died morally, emotionally, and spiritually a long time ago. (The most remarkable passages conveying this insight are as follows: "And the longer it lasted the more deadly it became. 'It is as if I had been going downhill while I imagined I was going up. . . . life was ebbing away from me'"; "There is one bright spot there at the back, at the beginning of life, and afterwards all becomes blacker and blacker and proceeds more and more rapidly—in inverse ratio to the square of the distance from death.'")[17] This shows us that moral, emotional, and spiritual death can happen to someone without his knowing that it has happened. When Ivan is uncertain whether he is dying physically and no one in his own circle tells him the truth, his brother-in-law comes from outside and says, "Why, he's a dead man! Look at his eyes—there's no light in them" (p. 41). But there was no one in his life who remarked in this way on Ivan's earlier (moral, emotional, and spiritual) death, since this was considered the normal course of events in his circle. This latter type of death and dying process can go undiagnosed for far longer than the physical death, and it is very dangerous for that reason.[18]

If no more of the goods that one has been having (1a) were the only reason death is bad, death would not be bad for Ivan. Indeed, if only the *prospect* of death could make someone like Ivan reconsider the life he had been leading in order to see that it had not been right, and the prospect was inseparable from the actual occurrence of death, then the occurrence of death could be at least instrumentally good. That is, in Ivan's case, it is not just that death will rob him of life but that the prospect of death and the process of dying are robbing him of pleasant illusions about his life. This is something we may dread about the process of dying, but it may have good aspects. Still, death would interfere with true goods of life that Ivan could now recognize and might seek if he lived on. So death is bad for reason (1b). However, there might be a new type of good with which death need not interfere (and which the prospect of death helps cause): Ivan's final insight or some conversion or rebirth before death. (I shall investigate this possibility in more detail below in discussing the process of dying.)[19] Some people like Ivan may only have good in their lives by dying in the right way, in Tolstoy's view. If they went on living (again, assuming that the prospect of death that might reform a person cannot be separated from death's occurrence), they would only live bad lives, and that would be worse than a good death.

It is because Ivan comes to believe (let us assume correctly) that his life has been trivial and nasty that he thinks death would not interfere with any *goods he has been having*. Nevertheless, death coming now would still imply, if it interferes with his having some future life with real goods, that his whole life had been wasted. Further, as he sees it at one point, it interferes with his *rectifying* his so-far wasted life. (This is the waste and no rectification of [3a] and [3b].) Indeed, merely not having more future (real) goods seems to take a back seat in Ivan's case to not being able (in having them) to rectify the past or at least rescue his life from being a total waste. If he could have had those future goods, his (extended) life would not have been as much of a waste, and if he could have done certain things in the future, that might have made up for the past or even redeemed the errors of the past. (*How* future good could make up for the past or even redeem the past is an important question that I shall discuss only briefly below.)

The desire that his life not have been a waste becomes stronger than the desire that he not be extinct or even that he have a future with real goods per se. (One's life not being a waste is a second-order property that supervenes on some of the real goods in it, presumably.)[20] Given that his strongest desire is that his life not have been a waste, *immortality* per se (the absence of death) would not necessarily be a solution to what Ivan fears will be the consequence of death in his case. That is, what he comes to be afraid of most need not go away if he were immortal (and knew this about himself). For one could live immortally a trivial and nasty life. Though there would always be time to make one's life not be a total waste, such a rescue need not necessarily take place. And it would be peculiar to think that if one has only a little bit of life, it matters if one wastes it, but if one has an infinite amount of life, it does not matter if one wastes it. Just because one can never waste it all (there is always more to waste), this does not mean that waste would not matter.

Still, focusing on "waste" can be deceptive. To waste something (e.g., time) is, ordinarily, not to make good use of it. If one thinks of a good life as a product—a fixed amount of good—one could produce that product with more or less waste. For example, if one had a long time in which to produce the fixed amount of good, one might waste a lot of time and still produce the good. If one had a short time in which to produce the fixed amount of good, one could do it if there were less waste. But if it was the product that was important, it might not matter that there was more waste of time in one life than in the other. If one immortally lives badly, there will be not only inefficient squandering of "resources" but also no good product, and it is the absence of the good product that would be the import of saying that someone's life is or was a waste in the sense that he wasted his life. That is, the resources were not used to produce the product.[21]

On the product view of waste, the problem is that you did not produce a product (your life was a waste). On the resource view of waste, the focus is on how many opportunities were squandered. Your life need not have been a waste even though you wasted a lot of it. But neither the "product" nor the "resource" view of waste is completely adequate. This is because it is important how we live each moment—not just that we produce a fixed product. Nor is it true that if we waste a moment of time of which we are to have an infinite number, its loss as a resource is what matters. What is important is that we should have been *living* differently at that point in time. It is important how we live each moment because it is important *that we respond correctly*, all the time, to the value or disvalue of persons, things, and events that surround us and are in us. This is the real reason why the person who lives immortally must still worry about whether his life at each moment is worthwhile.

Hence, it is not true that if there is no death, and one will not be extinguished, and there is no end to the possibility of future real goods, that one need not care, even continually, about the content of one's life. It is not just that in the absence of immortality one must focus on the secondary, partially compensating good of having lived a mortal life well. It is not correct to think either, "I'm going to live forever; it does not matter how I live," or "So what if it is a waste, *as long as* it will last forever."[22] The latter thought suggests that extinction (2) is the worst part of death and most to be avoided, even at the expense of having a life full of bad things. But Tolstoy's view, I think, is that it would be better to exchange an immortal bad life for a mortal one that has good in it.

The temptation is to read "Ivan Ilych" as though the prospect of death is necessary to make one think about the worth of one's life and the possibility (or necessity) of death is what makes it necessary to live a good life.[23] Such a reading implies that people like Ivan, who do not believe that they will die, will not properly evaluate or take seriously the worth of their lives. But, I have argued, it is not true that it is only if we can die that we should be concerned with the way we are living. It is not because of death that we *need* to be rescued from a worthless life. Nor, I believe, is it true that only if we face the prospect of death will we be concerned with the way we live. There are many events and relationships in life that alert us to the importance of how we live. It is true that Ivan might have needed the prospect of death and (on the supposition that the prospect and reality could not be separated) the reality of death in order to be concerned with the real worth of his life; *he* needs death, on Tolstoy's view, for the opportunity it gives him to be rescued.[24] (How it might do this is investigated in more detail below.) Nevertheless, at the risk of failing to appropriately generalize from Ivan's case, I think that not all who have been living as Ivan has need death or even its prospect in order to be rescued.

It must be admitted, however, that Ivan's case makes one think of an asymmetry in the relation between the worth of one's life and, on the one hand, living and, on the other hand, dying. If one believes that one will be living a trivial life (when one could live a good one), one does not necessarily feel the need to leave life. That is, if one is to *go on living life*, one need not believe that one is going to be living something good. But if we are to leave life, we think that we should *have* lived something good. We may stay on in life without having had, and even without the prospect of having, a justified life (though we should try for a justified life). But we should not leave—we should be locked into life—until we can make something worthwhile of our life (when this is a possibility). So long as we do not close the production, there is not the same need to make a tally of what we have or will produce, in order to go on. But if we are closing the production, we should make a tally. We should not bring the production to an end, eliminating any possibility of future improvement, until there is something sufficiently good left behind. So if we have not had a certain amount of good in our life by t_{10} and even never will, this does not mean that we are not justified in *going on* beyond t_{10}, but not having a certain amount of good might interfere with being reconciled to *not going o.n* beyond t_{10} if goods are possible beyond t_{10}. This asymmetry focuses on the *instrumental role* of living a worthwhile life: that is, whether we must live it in order to be reconciled to doing something else—either to live on or leave life. Hence, I shall call it the Instrumental Asymmetry.[25]

I have been speaking of Ivan's concern with wasting his life and how waste comes about if one lives a worthless life. In concluding this part of the discussion, I want to emphasize that we should still distinguish the concern with waste (in any of the senses distinguished above) from a concern with the mere worthlessness of one's life for at least one reason: Suppose that one has been living a worthless life but it is the only life possible for human beings. Then there is no wasted life because there was nothing else better to have been done. The idea of a wasted life depends on the possibility of a worthwhile life. If there is no such possibility, rather than fear that death now will make a worthwhile life impossible, the thought of suicide (putting an end to a life that can only be worthless) might be understandable. (This is so, even if suicide is not morally required.) By contrast, if one has been living a worthless life and there is and always was a better alternative, one should at least now try to live that alternative, and death may interfere with doing this. (Just possibly, one might punish oneself for having wasted life so far by committing suicide, rather than altering one's life. This would be the attitude of someone who thought that he did not deserve another chance after what he had wasted so far. Ivan never exhibits this frame of mind.)

Now we come to our continuing question: Would the things that I have said Ivan fears about death be present in the death of a person who had lived as he should (assuming he has lived as long as Ivan)? (I am still speaking only of fear of death, not fear of the process of dying.) Let us consider (1), (2), and (3) from page 7, above. In the death of the person who lived as he should, no more continuation of the sorts of goods he had been having (1a) as well as no more new sorts of goods (1b) would be present. (This assumes the person would continue to live well.) Indeed, aspect (1a) of death would actually be worse in the case of a good person than in Ivan's, since death would prevent the continuation of *real* goods he had been having in the past, not trivial and nasty pursuits. However, the additional real goods to be gotten from living on are not needed as much by the good person as by Ivan, given that the good person will have had many of them already but Ivan will not. This is consistent with the person who has lived as he should deserving the future real goods more than Ivan does. Waste (3) would not be present because the life of a person who lived as he should would not have been a wasted one, nor will rectification be needed. Extinction (2) will be present (or absent) both for those who lived as they should and for those who did not, depending on whether there is a type of life after death for both types of people. Even without life after death, Tolstoy may believe that extinction does not really occur, or at least will not be a bad thing to happen, for someone who lives correctly. This could be partially true if living correctly means investing oneself in others or in values and projects outside oneself. For then extinction could correctly be a minor matter to the person who dies, if he correctly cares most about something other than himself. If what he correctly cares about most goes on, nothing very important happens to him when he dies. The view that physical death would not involve extinction at all, even if there were no afterlife, is most clearly conveyed in the death of the master in Tolstoy's "Master and Man." The master comes to identify so completely with Nikita his servant that the master thinks that he will live (and so not be extinct) so long as Nikita lives.[26] (Presumably, by transitivity, the master will also live so long as those through whom Nikita lives continue to live.)[27]

It should be noted that focusing on identification with others who go on living ignores another form of detachment from self: identification with those who have already died. Such identification cannot work to correctly reduce one's concern with death by attaching one to continuing life. Rather, it shows that any form of intense identification that makes one think less about oneself and that also makes one willing to share a fate because it has befallen loved ones can reduce to some degree the importance to oneself of one's extinction, perhaps correctly so. Furthermore, identification with those who have died or will die, without identification with others in the future, means one is not hostage to life continuing on. If all life is extinguished, it is enough that there once was worthwhile life. But then, that would be true even if one did not identify with anyone, as it could be enough that there once was a worthwhile life and it was one's own.

As I see it, Tolstoy's view of how to live correctly is meant to eliminate or diminish the importance of extinction (2) and waste and no rectification (3) as characteristics of death even if there were no afterlife, and to diminish the significance of no more goods (1).

IV

What of the process of dying that Ivan lives through, aside from death itself? Ivan is a judge by profession and my interpretation of the penultimate part of the story is that in his process of dying, Ivan is putting himself on trial. (From a religious perspective, God will be one's ultimate judge. But it may be that until one believes in that judgment, one's own judgment of oneself is especially crucial.) However, as I see it, there are two trials that Ivan puts himself through which should be distinguished (though Tolstoy never explicitly says this). The initial trial begins when an inner voice that seems separate from Ivan questions him, and he responds. ("'What is it you want?' . . . 'To live . . .' 'How?' . . . 'as I used to . . .'"[28]) The inner voice is like an impartial judge who prompts Ivan to testify in his own case and leads him to see truths about his life (that I have discussed in section III).

Suppose that a trial shows that one has not lived as one should have, one comes to realize it, and one is dying. What should one do? At one point, as we have seen, Ivan believes that he is in this situation, that he has lost out on everything worth having and there is no possibility of rectification. This is when he suffers extreme mental agony. If he were to die, the agony would end. So perhaps suicide or at least wishing for death is what he ought to do. After all, his belief that his life has been wrong and that there is no rectification possible cause him agony. So why should he still fear death, as it will end this agony? Why does he not see death as a release from agony? This is the question with which I shall be concerned here.

For one thing, Ivan still fears extinction (2), which he envisions as "the black hole." When he is in a position to see the truth about his past life and suffer from it, he is also in a position to see other truths—for example, that extinction is really coming. Rather than accept these two truths, he struggles against them both. But, Tolstoy says, Ivan resists death at this point *because* he tries again to justify his past life, rather than because he is concerned with extinction per se. Hence there are two patterns that are candidates to represent what is going on after the first trial ends in a verdict that he has lived badly. In pattern 1, Ivan is in agony from his awareness of the truth about his life. He could avoid this agony by dying, but he fears the black hole. This leads him to find another route to avoid the agony: reexamine his verdict about his life in the hope that it is wrong. In pattern 2, though he is afraid of the black hole in itself, he is primarily afraid of dying without being able to justify and find the worth of his life. In pattern 2, changing his beliefs about his life is not a necessary alternative if he is to be able to stay alive without agony instead of going into the hole. Rather, changing his beliefs about his life is necessary if he is to be able to reconcile himself *to going* into the dreaded hole.

Pattern 2 is a more accurate representation of Ivan's state of mind, I think. Ivan resists death totally because he feels he cannot die until he knows that his life was good. Ivan is a judge by profession, but possibly everyone will put himself on trial and resist leaving until he knows that his life has been good. *Tolstoy is warning us that when someone must die, his primary concern will not be with death per se but with how he has lived his life.* (I shall consider below whether a trial is necessarily a part of the dying process of a person who has lived as he should.) If Tolstoy is right, then if one is offered an ignoble means of avoiding death on one occasion, one should remember that so long as one remains mortal, one will eventually come to be concerned more with having used those ignoble means than with the temporary continuation of life that their use made possible.

However, according to Tolstoy, Ivan's double *resistance*—to the truth about his death and to the truth about his life—actually causes more suffering than the *awareness* of the two truths. The most suffering now is caused by not getting into the black hole in the right way, and what impedes getting in the right way is the attempt to justify his past life. Ivan has a device in him (the inner voice) that has gotten him to the truth but he lacks, as yet, anything that helps stabilize him in the face of the truth. If we interpret all this in the light of the trial metaphor, we can see that Ivan is now in a second trial in an Appeals Court. He is appealing the initial verdict that his life was no good. The problem is that at this second stage he is no longer responsive to an impartial element inside himself. He is trying to bend the truth so that he gets a result more pleasing to himself. The defense, not an impartial judge, is running the appeals trial.

What someone in Ivan's situation should be doing, according to Tolstoy, is at least dying right if he could not live right. But Ivan is not doing this either, and that becomes a further source of his suffering. The problem is not that his dying process includes the first trial, it is how he reacts to its verdict. We should, I think, be more precise about the two trials. Consider figure 1.1.

| | | Belief about Life | |
		Good	Not Good
Life	Good	Knowledge	Deception
	Not Good	Deception	Knowledge

FIGURE 1.1

This figure shows that there are two dimensions: what one's life was actually like and what one believes about it. To *know* that one's life was good, it must actually have been good and one must have something like a justified belief that it was good. (Figure 1.1 cuts corners as it does not represent the element of justification of one's belief.) But one's life could be good without one knowing this. There is a difference between (*a*) refusing to leave life because one's life has not been good (and one knows it), (*b*) refusing to leave life because one does not know whether it has been good or bad, and (*c*) refusing to leave life until one knows that one's life has been good. Let me try to make the significance of these distinctions clearer.

The Instrumental Asymmetry discussed earlier (page 11) says that one's life should have amounted to something worthwhile before one is ready to leave (or to be reconciled to leaving). But according to the Instrumental Asymmetry, if the life was good, it will be acceptable to leave and to be reconciled to leaving, whether one knows that it was good or not. One's life will have either been good or not been good, independent of one's beliefs or knowledge of it. Knowing that one's life has been good can arguably make one's life better.[29] But resisting death in order to evaluate one's life (by having a first trial) will not, by itself, make it have been a good life. In particular, if the life was not good, resistance to its ending in order to know that it was not good will not make it be a good life. So, it might be said, why not end the agony of worrying about whether one's life was good, skip the trials, and just die?

The answer to this may be that even a bad life has a good component added to it if one knows the truth about oneself, at least if one has an appropriate reaction to this truth, for example, not joy but sadness or even agony. On this view, Ivan's life is more worthwhile because he responds with agony to the verdict. That his life becomes more worthwhile does not, of course, mean that it is necessarily an experientially better life for him to live. (This is one reason why, though it could be wrong to interfere with painful personal growth when it is spontaneously in progress, one would not necessarily encourage it when it is not spontaneous.) Further, the Instrumental Asymmetry says that it makes sense to resist the ending of a production when it has been bad, even though one may go on living if the production has been and will be bad. But in order to know whether one should resist in this way, one needs to know whether one's life really was bad (and might still be good). This is one reason to hold the first trial and not just let death come, letting the chips fall where they may based on the actual merit of one's life, independent of one's knowledge of its merit. So the strategy suggested by the Instrumental Asymmetry is to resist death to gain knowledge about one's life, in order to know whether one should resist further so as not to leave before making one's life worthwhile.

However, at the Appeals Stage, Ivan is not resisting death for these reasons. In particular, he is not resisting because he has not yet done a tally or because he knows that his life has been bad and it must not end in this state. Rather, he is resisting death because he is busy appealing the initial verdict. He wants to be able to prove that his life was good, even though if it were good it would not really matter very much for the acceptability of his leaving that he know it. (So he is not thinking that he must know whether his life was bad in order to resist death if his life was bad.)

Why is it important to him to know that his life was good? His most important concern is that his life actually have been good. If the knowledge that the life was good were not only a component of a good life but a necessary component, he would have to know that it is good in order for his life to be good. But such knowledge does not seem necessary for the life to be good. Still, it seems quite understandable to want to know if what one most wanted to happen did happen, and it can also make the good life better to know it was good. So Ivan's case shows that we not only want our life to have been good, but in the end we will want to know that it was good before we can leave in peace. (Yet, the desire to know is still a separable desire, as shown by the fact that one could want to know even if one did not care to make one's life better by knowing. This is also shown by the fact that if someone wants to know whether x is so, primarily because he is concerned that x be so, he should be willing to make the following bargain: decrease the probability of his knowing that x is so, if this will increase the probability that x is so.)

Ivan's case has another element in it, however. If he does not get the knowledge that his life was good, he will not just be without any beliefs about his life. He has already had a verdict in the first court, and this verdict says that his life was bad. He is in agony. He wants the agony to end. He might end it by thinking, "The verdict could be wrong. What I most want is that it be wrong, not that I know that it is wrong. My knowing will not affect whether it was wrong or not, so I'll forget about knowing." But if Ivan has done a careful tally the first time, he needs more than the possibility that it might be wrong to end the agony. He needs evidence that it was wrong in order to end the agony. Or alternatively, as mentioned above, if he died, the agony would end as well. But he—and presumably we all—would want agony from our doubts about our life to be relieved by knowledge of the worth of our lives, not just by death that terminates our ability to agonize. If Ivan were to know that his life is good, the state of affairs (i.e., the goodness of his life) with whose existence he is concerned would be a cause of his knowledge of it, and through this knowledge be a cause of his agony stopping. By contrast, if his agony stops because he dies, this has nothing to do with that which he most wants to be true—that he had a good life—being true. So the primary reason why death is not an appropriate escape from his agony about his life is not that he fears the black hole. It is that he primarily wants his agony to be *unjustified* by the facts about his life, and dying cannot make that be the case. He wants the agony to go away because he comes to know that his life has been worthwhile, and dying cannot make this so.

However, if we want to have the good news on Appeal, we also risk getting bad news instead, namely that one's life was not any good. And according to the Instrumental Asymmetry, this should set up a resistance to dying. But this is not what happens to Ivan, in part because in his case resistance is useless; he must die now. What actually happens after Appeal shows that there is another way to react to the knowledge of the badness of one's life besides resisting death, and another reason—besides resisting death (if the life is bad), quenching curiosity, or ending agony—to try to get the knowledge about the goodness or badness of one's life before dying. This additional reason is related to what has already been said about self-knowledge adding a worthwhile component to a bad life, but it goes beyond it. For those who do not have the option of not leaving life, knowledge can make some rectification possible when it seemed too late for rectification. Here we are also broaching the issue of how Ivan can be rescued.

What happens to Ivan is that something outside of his will pushes him closer to death, and death turns out to involve meeting not a black hole but a light of revelation.[30] The revelation involves a permanent commitment to the truth that his life was not lived correctly. It also involves the correction of a *mistaken* belief that caused a great measure of his suffering: that there was no more possibility of rectifying the waste of his life. If he does not resist two truths—about the lack of worth of his past life and about death being irresistible—the third belief (no possibility of rectification) turns out not to be true at all. So if he had not come to know and accept that his life was bad, there could not have been this possibility of rectification.

The rectification comes not merely in dying without resistance to the truth about himself. For him to accept without any backsliding that his life was wrong is for him to permanently accept a new set of values according to which his life fails. So it involves leaving behind the values of the old Ivan. One sign of this is his showing pity and love for others; indeed, dying for their sake. "He was sorry for them, he must act so as not to hurt them: release them and free himself from these sufferings."[31] So if one has lived badly, and one comes to realize both this and that one is dying, the thing to do is to immediately do whatever it is right to do *now*, for example, ask forgiveness, care for the welfare of others, and so on. When he says, "Yes, it was all not the right thing . . . but that's no matter,"[32] one thing he presumably means is that it does not matter now, since it does not stand in the way of doing what it is right to do now.[33] It is correct to focus on whether one's life is right when one can still make one's life (including one's death) better by doing that, or perhaps even to just have the knowledge. After this, continuing to focus on it is self-indulgent. The importance of Ivan's coming to know the truth about himself may seem connected to a version of the view that the unexamined life is not worth living, namely that the unexamined life is not worth dying. But the unexamined life can be well worth living or dying, as it can be life full of good thoughts and good deeds. And, in the end, I think Ivan's story shows instead that commitment to and action on correct values is a higher good than self-knowledge.[34]

Indeed, on Tolstoy's view, the good person's dying process may include a far more cursory "trial" than the bad person's, suggesting that reflecting on one's good life is not as necessary as ferreting out faults, and that being good allows one to forget about self-knowledge. There is an interesting comparison to be made between the trial Ivan puts himself through and its resolution, and a much shorter trial that a Tolstoyean good person, Nikita, puts himself through when he thinks that he is dying.[35] He too reviews his life. When he finds a fault, he does not torture himself with it—he says that God will forgive him as he made him to be the way he is. We might say that this is letting oneself off too easily, but it is very similar to the attitude Ivan eventually takes toward the deeper faults of his own life, which is the other aspect of his saying, "Yes, it was all not the right thing . . . but that's no matter."[36]

When Ivan commits himself to his new values, he still feels physical pain but loses his fear of death. He claims that this is because death does not exist. How may we interpret this? One interpretation is that when he shows pity for his son and wife and thinks about their welfare rather than his own, he is able to identify with others and forget about himself. Then personal extinction is not significant enough to give rise to fear. Indeed, identification can be so complete that one believes that one lives through others who remain. If this belief were literally true, there would be no death.

A somewhat different interpretation of why he says that there is no death is that by becoming someone with different values who casts off his past self, he does not die when his old self dies. From his point of view, he has just passed through a "death" already. It may be because he has self-transcended in this way that he also says that death is over. But also keep in mind what was said above: Ivan discovers that he died morally, emotionally, and spiritually a long time ago, so when he shakes off his old self, he is also shaking off his living death. In this sense, too, death is over.

Tolstoy emphasizes how short the period of time is in which Ivan is aware of an important positive truth about life, and also that he never again is unaware of that truth. He latches on to it and is held, as if mesmerized. The duration is of less importance than the completeness of absorption and its permanence while he lives. Wittgenstein said that if by eternity is understood not endless temporal duration but timelessness, then he lives eternally who lives in the present. Because Ivan comes to live so completely in the moment, he may think that there is no death. For if our *sense* of time moving on (to death) is a function of felt changes taking place, then constancy gives rise to the sense that time is not passing and that this moment will never end. Hence, looked at secularly, Ivan may say that there is no death because he is so engrossed in the experience of his new insight and new nature that he is subject to a new illusion, namely that he in his new state will not die. (Of course, if part of the white light experience is being privy to the truths of Christianity, that God exists and there is everlasting spiritual life, then there would be no illusion.)

We can conclude, I think, that there are really three deaths of Ivan Ilych: his moral, emotional, and spiritual death that happened long ago; the death of his old self (accompanied by a rebirth); and his physical death.

V

Is Ivan's struggle worthwhile? He has the time to minimally act as his new self—pitying his child and wife, trying to ask for forgiveness (which is important, even though he does not successfully communicate with those he intends to reach). But since there is not much time to act as his new self, the joy he feels may come from simply *being* the new type of person. (Of course, it may also come from the new relationship he [believes that he] begins in his new identity, that with God whose understanding he comes to believe in.)[37] He dies in triumph. Unlike the trials he has presided over in his life, a firm self-imposed judgment of "guilty as charged" does not lead to punishment. (Ivan's is a triumph that none of those who hear of his agony knows about or would understand. His friend fears that he will have an end like Ivan's, but of course, there could be endings that are much worse. This is a point to which I shall return below.)

If we abstract from the issue of entering into a life after death, the story can be taken to imply that it is worth a great struggle to come to have a good will or to know an important truth about the meaning of life, even if one does not have the opportunity to live in accord with that will or truth. This change allows one to reject and detach from the bad life one leaves behind as a new person. But looked at in one way, the change at the end of Ivan's life amounted to only a few good thoughts taking place in a brief minute. How could this be worth a great struggle? Suppose that such thoughts in one minute occurred somewhere in the course of his life, not at its end, and then were followed by his old way of being. Would they count for much? If such knowledge occurs at the end of one's life, does it have greater importance? I believe that where in a life story some event occurs can be important because the pattern of one's life can be important. (This pattern, how-ever, is something that should come about because of what one does for reasons other than trying to achieve a pattern.) For example, it is better to start off badly in life and head toward improvement than to start off well and head toward decline, even when we hold constant all the nonpattern goods and bads that are distributed in the two different patterns.[38]

Why might this be? Among the factors that could be at work[39] are, first, that our ideal of rational change involves not moving from a current position unless we move somewhere as good or better. Given this, if one wants to keep on living, and in that sense move somewhere, we should move to an equally good or better state. Second, decline within life suggests vulnerability, of both a higher state and of retention of what one has. Ending on a high point within life means that only death, not change in life itself, ends a better state. I think that these two factors are plausible components of an explanation of the importance of incline versus decline within life. Less plausible is a third suggestion: you most likely are what you end up being. (This seems to conflict with the fact that someone's identity as a genius is secure even if he ends senile.) However, if Ivan's true nature were what he is at the end, the question would arise of why it is more important to end as one's true self than to have been it at some earlier point. The first two factors could provide answers.

David Velleman suggests that a life on an incline is better than one on a decline only if the good is caused by, and so in some way redeems, the bad. For example, he thinks that a bad start in a marriage is redeemed by what one learns from it to make the marriage better later. By contrast, a bad marriage followed by winning the lottery is not preferable, he thinks, to winning the lottery followed by a bad marriage.[40] I disagree with Velleman. First, it seems to me that the incline is preferable even when there is no causal relation between the bad and the good, as when one wins a lottery after a bad marriage. Second, I do not think that the redemption of the bad by the good could be the explanation of the importance of the upward trajectory of a life. For imagine that one had a crystal ball that allowed one to see the bad mistakes that one will commit in the future as one goes into a decline (Crystal Ball Case). One could, at present, redeem the future decline by acting on one's foreknowledge so as to improve one's present from what it would otherwise have been, to the same extent as one could redeem one's bad past by using it for future good. But the fact that in the Crystal Ball Case the bad future is at least partially redeemed does not alter the relative badness of a declining rather than an inclining life, I think. Hence, inclines are better than declines even when redeeming the bad is held constant.

The Crystal Ball Case could also be used to criticize another hypothesis about why an incline toward a good character is better than a decline from a good character, holding all other events in the life constant. The proposal is that good at the end happens in response to everything else in the life, whereas an early peak cannot have the same significance because it is not a response to everything in the life. But if someone at the beginning of his life looked into the crystal ball and responded to this by becoming good, that good stage would be a response to everything else in the life. Yet the inclining life is still, I think, preferable to the declining one.

The pattern of Ivan's life (according to his description of it, plus our sense of its end) is illustrated in figure 1.2.

Good

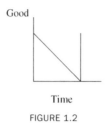

Time

FIGURE 1.2

Notice that figure 1.2 not only describes a life that ended on an upturn but also describes a life in which there is a radical reversal—from a relative and absolute low point to a great peak. (Indeed, the figure might be more accurate if the end point were the highest point in his life.) Hence, Ivan's life is not on an incline in the standard sense. This may raise problems for the ideal-of-rational-change explanation of the good of inclines that I have offered. For consider figure 1.3. At least quantitatively, there seems to be more rational change in a life represented by it than in a life represented by figure 1.2. It is only the last part of the life in figure 1.3 that is radically inconsistent with rationally justified change (given that the decline is from a great high to a great low) and only the last part in figure 1.2 that is consistent with rationally justified change (given that the rise is from a great low to a great high).

Good

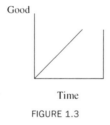

Time

FIGURE 1.3

Suppose figure 1.2 is still preferable to figure 1.3, or at least that more weight is given to how one ends up (while one is still a competent individual) than to other parts of one's life. This would suggest that an explanation of the significance of how one ends must involve more than the ideal-of-rational-change explanation suggests. The second factor, which focuses on what happens prior to nonexistence brought about by death, emphasizing that a great good is not being diminished within life but only by the end of life, should play a greater role in an explanation.[41]

However, I do not think that the mere fact that the life ends on an up note, even as the effect of a big reversal, would always be important enough to merit Ivan's struggle. It is when the brief-lived upturn represents a *stable* change of character or heart, rather than merely an event in someone's life story with whose reversal death interferes, that the brief upturn is worth the struggle. It would amount to achieving the good will that Kant said had incomparable value even if circumstances prevented any actions from being undertaken with it.[42] The worth of Ivan's struggle might then depend on the intrinsic, nonconsequentialist value of being a certain sort of person. By contrast, if a change had occurred earlier in his life's trajectory, but his character or values then declined again, the change would not have been stable. Stability goes beyond the genuineness of a new insight on how to live. If his altered views on the value of his life were merely genuine, they would not necessarily be more stable than the genuine feelings of sympathy for him that Ivan's wife has when he dies, feelings that do not last even until his funeral. If the few seconds at the end of his life represent a stable turning toward the good, they are more than just good components in a bad life; they could be called salvation, even if they do not make his life as a whole a good one.[43]

Stability, however, implies that if Ivan *had* lived on, he would not have reverted to his old views and way of life. But can we really believe that when placed back in his ordinary family and professional life, he would have thought, felt, and acted differently? And if we cannot believe this, are we left with only the first two proposed explanations—rational change and no reversal within life—of the importance of his brief understanding being at the end rather than somewhere in the middle of his life?

To answer this last question, perhaps it will help to consider the case of someone who foresees that in the future he will change his values and behave *for the worse* (while still being a competent agent). He might take steps now while he still can to prevent that change in himself, even taking the extreme of ending his life in order to prevent the downturn. In this case, the hold on him of his higher values is unstable, but they are nevertheless controlling in that they determine whether he lives on to live by worse values. In this case, even without stability of the good values, the fact that the worse values were prevented from coming on the scene makes the life better. In Ivan's case, of course, his new values were not employed to help halt his life; he just dies in the midst of his conversion. But suppose one believes that Ivan *would* have, while in his converted state, turned his back on future life if he knew that he would revert to his old ways. Achieving such a set of controlling values in his conversion makes his struggle worthwhile, even if we cannot believe that he achieves stable new values. In addition, there is the element of the actual trajectory. Unlike the person who in his midlife conversion *would have* interfered with his reversion had he foreseen it coming, but did not foresee it, Ivan has the luck to end without a decline within life.

A somewhat different way of understanding conversions that it is reasonable to think would not last is to think of them as stable in some but not all circumstances. Some people may be capable of being aware of what is really important only in a certain narrow range of conditions—for example, in a hermit's retreat. (If they will forget when they leave that circumstance, perhaps they should not leave.) Some people may only achieve the awareness when they are completely detached from daily life, and forget and act badly in daily life. If you will behave badly in every circumstance but one, arguably you should stay in that one circumstance. If being at the point of death—however long one stays there—is the only circumstance in which someone has it in him to realize what is worthwhile and act from that knowledge, then struggling to get there, not struggling to get away from there (and even struggling to not get away), may be right. We can say that Ivan found the place in which he could instantiate his better nature, and while it would be a shame if he could not go back to ordinary life retaining his insights, it is also a shame that he cannot stay in his special place longer.

Of course, a change in a person need not be all or nothing. Few can take back to daily life the perspective they have on a "high mount," but the experience can nevertheless color ordinary life. And it is not so hard to believe that such a partial stable change might have happened to Ivan had he lived. Prince Andrei, in *War and Peace*, feels very much that the sort of love he finds when dying detaches one from life, even though it solves the mystery of life. It is not the sort of love for a particular person (Natasha) that would take him over again if he lived on. Yet, even in his case, when he temporarily "returns" to life, his most detached perspective has its effect on his relations with particular people. For example, it makes possible his forgiveness of Natasha.

Hence, Ivan's life is saved, if he has become the sort of person (in the product sense described earlier, page 9) that one should be in life, or has achieved good controlling values, even if he cannot live his life as this sort of person or with these values because death cuts short his life. Less plausibly, Ivan's life is saved merely because he sees a truth and never again fails not to see it because it is placed at the end of a trajectory. His life may also be saved in the sense that something happens in it that is important enough to compensate for the bad that is also in it (and this could be true even of someone who sees the truth in midlife but forgets it). Ivan has wasted much of his life, but his life is not therefore a waste.

However, seeing the light, a stable or partial transformation of character, or commitment to good controlling values would still not imply that Ivan's life as a whole was good. Indeed, just as we can correctly punish a criminal who has reformed from his past crimes, Ivan remains accountable for his past mistakes (unless his past mistakes are forgiven by God). Possibly, his past is partially redeemed because it serves as the opportunity for reflection that transforms his values. Ivan's new insights, after all, do not come from reading a book but from learning from his mistakes.[44] And because of his change, he is able to detach from and disown much of his past life, even if he is responsible for it. In this sense, he is rescued *from* his past life.[45]

VI

How does the way Ivan lived relate to other bad things in his process of dying besides the trials? Is it true that these would be different for someone who had lived as he should have? One of the bad things for Ivan is his experiencing fear of death, a reasonable response to awareness of the bad properties of death itself (described in section III above). (Had Ivan died in a coma, his death would still have these bad properties, but he would have no fear of them during the dying process.) In addition, there is his loneliness that results from those around him not being honest with him about his impending death and the pretense that he must act out in their presence. (The story is remarkably modern in its view that honesty with the dying is important.) He desperately misses honesty, understanding, and pity.[46]

If he had lived as he should have, he would not have feared death in the same way he does because, I have argued, death would not have had all the same bad properties. If he had lived as he should have *and* others had lived as they should have—an important second condition—he would not have lived a superficial life in which knowledge was repressed and honest feelings were not expressed between *equals*. Then his family, friends, and colleagues could more freely have given what he desires when he is dying. Furthermore, he could accept these things from them. As it is, when his friends and wife do show him pity, he rejects it. He can only accept pity from Gerasim, not a social equal and not a "citified" servant but someone who readily admits that Ivan is dying and accepts that everyone—including himself—will die.

There are at least three possible qualifications to this answer. First, Tolstoy's description of the death of people who lived (as he thought) correctly does not involve their asking for pity or needing much support through a difficult dying process. For them, Tolstoy thinks, the process is not difficult. They neither pity themselves nor desire to be pitied, though they may need physical help and wish not to be abandoned.[47] Hence, living the sort of life that made honesty and deep feelings possible and expressible would not necessarily give Ivan what he now wants (to be babied and pitied), since he might then not want this. Indeed, it seems that it is Tolstoy's ideal that someone who has lived as he should quickly resigns himself to impending death and only wants to continue as long as he can to do the things that gave value to his life.[48]

Second, Tolstoy says that Gerasim treated Ivan as Gerasim hoped that he would be treated when his time came. He wills a certain sort of treatment universally, a form of Kantian or Golden Rule universalization. But the story also describes another form of concern for a dying person, and the question arises whether this other type of concern is even more laudable. It comes from those who do not openly recognize that they will die—for example, Ivan's son and even his wife who also represses awareness of her mortality. Both of these people, at Ivan's end, pity him from love. Is this inferior to or does it surpass Gerasim's universalizable maxim? The problem with concern from love is that it can be unstable. Tolstoy shows us at the very beginning of the story that once Ivan is dead, his wife recalls only how his agony interrupted her peace of mind and how his death mars her financial future.

Yet, there are two different ways to interpret the alternations in Ivan's wife. (1) Even someone who can have such a genuine feeling as sympathy from love is capable of the deepest hatred and self-absorption. (The former leads her to wish for her husband's death long before he is ill. The latter leads her to think only of herself immediately after his death.) She will act on these negative impulses in the absence of a steadying principle. This is the Kantian side of Tolstoy, insofar as he thinks that reliance on emotions is insufficient for appropriate behavior. But seen in reverse, all this becomes: (2) Even someone who is bad enough to wish from hatred that her husband die and to think only of herself after his death can still have an honest feeling of sympathy from love in response to his death. In this sense, Ivan's death also brings his wife back to emotional (and some might say even moral) life in relation to him. There is a power in the good emotion (even in the absence of a principle that guides it) that can overcome the bad emotions.[49]

Third, it is true that we all die, but we do not all die at the same time. If we are not synchronized in this way, this makes it possible for some to help others in need; but it also means that some will be engaged in living while others are dying. Perhaps those who are dying and know what the dying are going through can make the end of their lives more worthwhile by consoling and supporting each other as well.

VII

So far, I have tried to contrast death and dying in those who have and have not lived correctly (at least as Tolstoy sees it, given his substantive view about what correctness is). I have done this by considering cases of individuals who go through what might be called a "complete" dying process, fully conscious, competent, and so on. In Ivan's case, there is, let us suppose, justifiable agony (an appropriate reaction to reality), followed by a (let us suppose) real triumph. In the case of the person who lived right, we may have justifiable peace all the way through. The life is a triumph, but there is no dramatic return of the lost sheep to the fold.

However, not everybody who lived correctly or incorrectly will go through a complete dying process. Indeed, many people would prefer their deaths to be sudden and unexpected. (This assumes that they have taken care of practical matters and that a sudden death does not deprive them of much quality time alive that they would have had in a prolonged dying.) There is a modern school of thought, however, that speaks of the dying process as an important stage in life. This suggests that no one should skip it if he can, going straight from normal activity to death. But is it necessary to be aware of and cope with all impending bad things, such as death, that will happen to one? Suppose that we find someone on the point of a sudden death and there are two ways to save him: either so that he has his dying process (decline, awareness of a bad that will happen, and coping with it) or so that he continues for the same period of time to live well without any indication of impending death, followed by a sudden death. I do not think that it would always be wrong to choose the second option. If so, a dying process is not a stage that no one should skip. The smaller the amount of ordinary life that one should give up in order to go through the dying process, the less important the process is shown to be.

Still, these judgments are consistent with a dying process being a good thing that one gives up in order to get something even better. The dying process would be shown to have actual negative value if people would be reasonable to give up time alive with knowledge of impending death but with no other negatives in it (e.g., pain) in order to die suddenly sooner. That is, they are imagined to reasonably say "no, thank you" to more time alive, just because it is accompanied by this knowledge of, and need to cope with, impending death. This negative value might be overridden, however, if coping would lead to self-knowledge or good moral change. After all, if sudden death had happened to Ivan, he would never have experienced his self-understanding and conversion. On this assumption, let us consider which sort of dying—sudden or prolonged—is really preferable for the two types of people, those who have lived wrong (Wrong) and those who have lived right (Right).[50] I shall argue that prolonged dying is more important for Wrong than for Right, and also that what Right stands to lose if he has a prolonged dying is less important than what Wrong stands to lose if he has a sudden death. So if we are not sure whether we are Wrong or Right, it might be reasonable to opt for a prolonged dying, though we are not required to.

Consider Nonconscious Ivan who either dies or goes into a coma immediately after he bangs himself while decorating. There is no agony but also no truth and no triumph. Ex post (i.e., once one knows how things will turn out for Ivan), one can think that Ivan is better off than Nonconscious Ivan. Now imagine Totally Agonized Ivan, who will go through agony at the realization of the truth about himself but will never have a triumph, dying in agony. (For example, he dies before or during what I have described as his Appeal.) If we should pity even people who lived wrongly, we should prefer that someone have Nonconscious Ivan's fate rather than Agonized Ivan's. Yet Agonized Ivan's life seems a more worthwhile one; it involves coming to recognize both what has value and an important truth about his life. It is just that the more worthwhile life (seen from outside that life) may be worse for the person to live through.[51] Ex ante, when we know that Ivan is in mental agony but do not know whether Ivan will triumph or just be Totally Agonized, we may be tempted to cut short the spontaneous process of awakening that he is going through, giving precedence to avoiding the pain the person is going through.[52] We could do this by letting him die or by giving him drug-induced artificial relief. (Untruthfully trying to convince him that he really had a wonderful, meaningful life is problematic for many reasons.) We would be trying to prevent the worst experience for the person (represented by Totally Agonized Ivan) rather than taking a chance that a triumph will happen. However, it might be wrong to do this so long as there is a chance for triumph, though the probability of triumph could be relevant. Indeed, if Totally Agonized Ivan were about to expire naturally, we might appropriately try to keep him alive longer (if this were not contrary to his wishes), if there is a good chance that he will reach the final resolution that Ivan does.

A third alternative character, Miserable Ivan, would die in agony not through realization of a truth about *his life* but by coming to know the truth about the death of a loved one or from a purely physical pain. Here, shielding the person from the truth or providing drug-induced relief seems appropriate, for it is not a matter of forestalling a positive resolution to his own life. Finally, consider Deceived Ivan, who has a dying process in which he never realizes the sad truth about himself, and dies happy with the life he has led, though unhappy with death. Unless it is very important that someone live through the awareness that he is dying per se, Nonconscious Ivan's fate might be preferable to Deceived Ivan's, for the latter's happiness is just the product of a mistaken considered judgment and continued self-deception.

What about someone who has lived as he should—Right? If he dies immediately or goes into a coma, he loses the opportunity to live with an awareness of dying and he is unable to evaluate his life. Suppose that he would evaluate it correctly. We think that he then misses at least something good due to the immediate death or coma. But the good is not the important good of correcting one's values and then transcending one's bad past. And what if he misevaluates his life? That is, he will, for the first time, think that he had a bad life when it was really good and he will die in unrelieved agony from this.[53] This seems worse than the immediate death. Indeed, it seems more of a bad thing that someone who lived correctly should die thinking he failed than it is a good thing that someone who lived correctly should come to know this truth through the dying process. If we are uncertain which would happen, therefore, it seems reasonable to prefer the immediate death in the case of the person who lived as he should.

There is also the possibility that a "good" person might, while still mentally competent, undergo a sincere reversal of values—bemoaning the fact that he did not live in what is in fact a bad way.[54] Should we prefer sudden death for someone who at least seems to be good because it forecloses this possibility? Above, we considered the person who knows that his character or values will deteriorate and he prefers to end his life before this happens. It seems better that such a deterioration *not* take place even if it means that some important flaw in the character of the "good" person is never revealed.

It turns out that those who did not live correctly can need a full dying process more than those who lived as they should. But there is a catch: What if we do not know whether someone has lived correctly or incorrectly? (If it is the principle that lies behind one's conduct that determines the answer, it will be especially hard to know the answer.) Using figure 1.1 and repeating a bit of what was said above can help us decide whether going through the dying process stage is better when we are uncertain about our life and character. It is important that Wrong come to know the truth and rise above it. It may be worth risking his dying while deceived or agonized if there is a real possibility (or sufficiently high probability) of a good change. It is important that Right not die deceived that his life was bad, and even more important that he not make a sincere reversal to evil. It is not as important that he die knowing about the goodness of his life. But it is much more important that Wrong know the truth and rise above it than that Right avoid deception. Deception may be painful but it will not turn Right's life into a failure, while Wrong's transformation can prevent a disaster.

We are left with the relative weights of Right turning toward evil and Wrong turning toward good. If each of these turnings would be due to the free choice of the person, then it seems wrong for someone who is uncertain of his own character to direct that there be an interference with his free choice, a choice that might lead to good if he is Wrong, in order to protect himself from a bad choice if he is Right. (This is consistent with his preferring an interference with his future choice for bad when there is nothing good to be weighed against this interference.)[55]

Hence, if we are unsure whether we (or the people we are dealing with) are Right or Wrong, a prolonged conscious dying seems better than sudden death after all.

Notes

1. An earlier version of this chapter was published in *Ethics* 113 (January 2003): 202–33.

2. For comments on earlier versions of this chapter, I am grateful to Richard Arneson, Derek Parfit, John Richardson, Thomas Scanlon, members of the Stanford Ethics Group, the Department of Philosophy, University of California at San Diego, students in my graduate class at Harvard University, and the editors of *Ethics*. This chapter was written while I was a fellow at the Center for Advanced Study in the Behavioral Sciences, supported by Mellon grant 2986639 and AHRQ/NEH Fellowship grant FA-36625-01.

3. Leo Tolstoy, "The Death of Ivan Ilych," trans. Louise Maude and Aylmer Maude, in *The Kreutzer Sonata and Other Short Stories* (New York: Dover, 1993). In brief, this is the way Ivan lived. He conformed to the social code, having a profession, a wife, and a family, but he was driven by concern for social and professional climbing, had no deep feelings for others, enjoyed having power over them, and got pleasure from superficial pursuits. We may not agree that everything was *all* wrong with his mature years. For example, he was an incorruptible judge. This should count for something positive, at least if the laws he applied had any justice in them. One may even argue that the real pleasure he took in his last interior decoration project can be defended. However, when Tolstoy has Ivan say that his life was *all* not right, Tolstoy may have in mind that the *reasons* why Ivan did even the useful acts in his life were wrong. That is, the principle (or maxim) of his conduct was competitive social climbing. Tolstoy would then be suggesting that when we judge our lives, we focus on the maxim at the root of it, rather than on mere behavior. But surely it would be correct to feel better about a life in which we did not kill someone (due to an accidental intervention) than one in which we did, even if the deep maxim in each life that led us to act as we did was equally wrong. This is the problem of moral luck. Even if this were true, we should remember that Tolstoy's point is that someone who was not a bad person in the most obvious

criminal way can still have a remarkably worthless life. Since most people are not criminals, this makes Ivan's story of greater relevance to us.

4. Perhaps a Christian would not have the first impulse. After all, original sin is thought to account for why we all die.

5. Not in the sense that Epicurus thought that death could not happen to him—i.e., when death was present, he was not, and when he was present, death was not.

6. Tolstoy, "Ivan Ilych," p. 44.

7. "Ivan Ilych" can be read, in part, as a primer on professional ethics.

8. It is bizarre that Ivan thinks that they all were immune from death, given that Tolstoy says that several of Ivan's children had already died. However, this may also be an indication of how distant he was from his own children; for if they were as abstract for him as Caius, it is no surprise that he does not include them in the circle of those who cannot die. (Perhaps the frequency of death in pre-antibiotic times required one to put it out of one's mind?) The fact that others in his circle were taken by him also to be exempt from death reduces the plausibility of the view that he believes he cannot die because the end of his subjectivity is the very end of the world, although something like this may be going on (p. 42) when he says "when I am not, what will there be? There will be nothing."

9. Peter Ivanovich is by no means the worst of the characters Tolstoy portrays. He is vulnerable to truth and capable of horror at the report of Ivan's agony. The character who represents the devil is Schwartz. He maintains an air of amusement at the funeral and seduces Peter away from serious thoughts to a card game. (Might the choice of the name "Peter" be intended to remind us of Saint Peter, who also tried to be faithful to his friend but was not completely successful?)

10. That is, there is a crucial difference in attitude between (*a*) simply drawing a conclusion about yourself from the fact that something has happened to someone with traits you share and (*b*) being unwilling to attribute traits to yourself that might make you fare better than someone else. The latter, however, is still not the same as being as appalled at someone else's death as one is at the idea of one's own death. The more one is appalled by the idea of one's own death by comparison to the death of a friend, the more one thinks the worst has not yet happened when a friend dies but one still remains alive, the less one cares about the deceased by comparison to oneself. By contrast, in a case of extreme attachment, one's own death becomes anticlimactic, not because one no longer values one's life after the friend's death, but because one truly believes that one's death does not mean more to one than the death that has already happened. This should imply that one would have been willing to give one's own life to save the friend. (That the deaths are equal implies randomizing the chance of death, but to this must be added the desire that one's friend not suffer it.)

11. Even more harshly, the landowner in "Master and Man" (in *Tolstoy's Short Fiction*, ed. Michael R. Katz [New York: Norton, 1991]) dies when he does because he goes out in pursuit of more land, as does the character in "How Much Land Does A Man Need?" (in Tolstoy, *The Kreutzer Sonata*).

12. Perhaps, however, in Tolstoy's worldview, there is always a hidden meaning to what seems an absurd end, so that it is really a fitting end.

13. See Thomas Nagel's "Death," in his *Mortal Questions* (New York: Cambridge University Press, 1979).

14. For more on the Limbo Man and the distinction between (1) and (2), see F. M. Kamm, "Why Is Death Bad and Worse than Pre-natal Nonexistence?" *Pacific Philo-*

sophical Quarterly 69 (1988): 161–64, and F. M. Kamm, *Morality, Mortality*, Vol. 1 (New York: Oxford University Press, 1993).

15. See especially Tolstoy, "Ivan Ilych," p. 56: "'What is it you want?' . . . 'To live . . .' 'How?' . . . 'as I used to' The nearer he came to the present, the more worthless and doubtful were the joys."

16. See John Bayley's excerpt from his *Tolstoy and the Novel* (London: Chatto, 1966), reprinted in Katz, *Tolstoy's Short Fiction*, pp. 420–23.

17. Tolstoy, "Ivan Ilych," pp. 56–58. This is a striking parody of the aim to quantify, creating a Newtonian formula for diminishing value in life.

18. In the movie *The Sixth Sense*, the physically dead who survive in some nonphysical state do not realize that they are dead. Tolstoy asks us to believe that something similar is true of Ivan and those in his social circle: they do not realize how "dead" they are.

19. See James Olney, "Experience, Metaphor, and Meaning: The Death of Ivan Ilych," *Journal of Aesthetics and Art Criticism* 31 (1972): 101–14.

20. We can show that (i) desire for goods that might make one's life not be a waste is separate from (ii) desire for more goods per se, by considering someone who knows that his life will not have been a waste and who still wants more goods. He does not want them for the purpose of rescuing his life from being a waste.

21. I am, of course, focusing on a sense of "a wasted life" that involves someone wasting his life. Hence, the life's having good effects on others through their own efforts or by natural processes does not imply that the life was not a waste. If someone's wasted life serves as a useful lesson to many people, this does not mean that his life was not a waste in the relevant sense.

22. When Woody Allen complains that life is full of misery, suffering, and pain, and, furthermore, it's all over too soon, he may seem to gesture at a view behind the second thought. But Allen's quip merely suggests extinction is worse than endless bad stuff. His quip leaves it open that one might court extinction in exchange for some good stuff, even though death could then become bad both because we would have no more goods of life (1) and because of extinction (2).

23. I mean "possibility" in the sense that one is uncertain whether one will have to die.

24. Tolstoy's anger toward people like Ivan increases in his later stories—e.g., in "How Much Land Does a Man Need?" For these people, unlike Ivan, death brings no conversion. These people, Tolstoy seems to think, deserve death rather than need it for the good its prospect can produce.

25. Does the asymmetry involve two sides of the same coin? For if one had to leave if one's life would never be worthwhile, it could not be true that one should *not* leave if one's life had not yet been worthwhile. But it is possible that one could appropriately go on living without living a worthwhile life, even if one did not need such a life in order for it to be appropriate to leave. Hence, the asymmetry does not involve two sides of the same coin.

26. Tolstoy, "Master and Man," p. 268.

27. An oddity in the ending to "Master and Man" is that while the master believes that he will live if Nikita does, he also believes that in dying he is going to meet God. He then would be in two different places at the same time, if we take things literally. In "Master and Man," both Nikita and the master think that it is only the master who has something big to lose if he loses his life. In truth, the master's life is not (on Tolstoy's view) worth living, so he would not lose much in losing that life, but his life can be saved from worthlessness if he dies in a certain way (e.g., by saving Nikita).

28. Tolstoy, "Ivan Ilyich," p. 56.

29. Alan Wood emphasized this point.

30. The light may be due to nothing more than (what we now know is) some increase in a brain chemical before death. But in the story Ivan does not just bask in serotonin bliss. And in any case, if the transmission of a spiritual message requires a physical process, this only makes it like any meaningful message that requires a physical script.

31. In "Master and Man," the Master dies for his servant (although it is not clear that he knew this is what he was doing) when he might possibly have lived instead. Ivan could not live instead, but he dedicates his death to his family's welfare. So (related to n. 1) his outward behavior in dying is the same as it would otherwise be, but the principle (maxim) behind it is different.

32. Tolstoy, "Ivan Ilych," p. 62.

33. From a religious point of view, it may not matter because of divine forgiveness. More on this below.

34. Similarly, in Tolstoy's *War and Peace*, when Prince Andrei is first at a point close to death, this awakens him to "divine love"—love for friend and foe—that is different from love for any particular person. But this sort of love also allows him to respond differently to particular people—e.g., forgiving a particular enemy and also Natasha, his unfaithful fiancée. Still, there is a noticeable difference between Ivan's death and Prince Andrei's eventual actual death scene (when the oscillation between his passing away and his returning to ordinary life is over). Prince Andrei dies in a completely detached frame of mind; when his son is brought to him in tears (like Ivan's son), Andrei takes leave of him in a disengaged and perfunctory manner. By contrast, Ivan connects emotionally with particular people around him. Interestingly, the contrast reminds us again of the relation between commitment to a universal syllogism and to its particular implications. At the end, Prince Andrei is focused on the universal and is beyond its implications for particular people, but Ivan connects some universal truth with its implications for relations to particular people.

35. See Tolstoy, "Master and Man," p. 262.

36. It is a mistake, however, to think that even if God forgives one's faults, it is not important to be fault-free or for Ivan to achieve correct values after all. Being forgiven is not the same as becoming a good person or having a better life. These are good in themselves, not just means to avoid needing to be forgiven. It might be said, further, that it is only if one comes to have the correct values that one can fully believe that there is a God who will forgive one whether one was good or not, and so Ivan must first transform himself before he can be open to the good news. Still, this would just mean that his struggle is necessary in order for him to *know* that he will be forgiven, not that the struggle is necessary in order for him to be forgiven. By contrast, the view that only those who are repentant—not everyone—will be forgiven would imply that Ivan must struggle to achieve new values, and go through the agony of rejecting his past values and most of his past life in order to be forgiven. (Nikita just has to recognize occasional failures to live up to values he already holds.) There is another connection between trying to be good and the existence of a forgiving God. An appropriate response to a supernatural person who is forgiving and so exhibits a form of goodness is to be good oneself and avoid giving cause for forgiveness. By contrast, if the impersonal universe simply does not register our faults, there is no appropriate response to this, per se, other than perhaps relief that one will suffer no punishment.

37. In "Master and Man," the Master is presented as dying in joy because he believes that he hears a supernatural voice of one to whom he is coming (p. 268).

38. Michael Slote discusses the issue of inclines and declines in life in "Good and Lives," in his *Goods and Virtues* (Oxford: Clarendon, 1983). I first discussed views I had developed independently on this topic as the commentator on Slote's paper at the 1982 New Jersey Regional Philosophical Association meeting. Subsequently, I discussed inclines and declines in life and between nonexistence and life in "Why Is Death Bad and Worse than Pre-natal Nonexistence?" and then in *Morality, Mortality*, Vol. 1. David Velleman discusses the issue of patterns in life in his "Well-Being and Time," *Pacific Philosophical Quarterly* 72 (1991): 48–77. When Ivan notices the downward pattern of his life (as quoted in sec. III), he does not mean to imply that the total of goods and bads in his life would have been no different if he had had an upward pattern instead. Rather, he sees his upward alternative life as starting from the same point at which he did start, but going up; this would have entailed more overall nonpattern goods in his upward rather than downward life.

39. Discussed, along with others, in *Morality, Mortality*, Vol. 1, pp. 67–71.

40. See Velleman's "Well-Being and Time." This, of course, need not mean that one may produce the bad just so that good may come of it.

41. Figures A1 and A2 solidify this result by testing for whether a dramatic reversal to good or a dramatic reversal to bad, placed elsewhere than at the end, has as much significance.

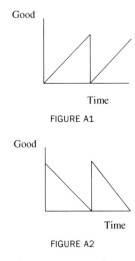

FIGURE A1

FIGURE A2

42. Jay Wallace pointed out the connection with Kantian good will.

43. I expand on this in the text below.

44. As noted earlier, David Velleman's "Well-Being and Time" argues that the past can be redeemed by such a role in producing future events.

45. I am grateful to Richard Arneson for his questions concerning the value of a change at the end of life that prompted the discussion in sec. V.

46. We should keep in mind that even though Ivan died at home, not in an impersonal hospital, he was surrounded by coldness.

47. Again, see Nikita's almost death and real death in "Master and Man."

48. This is important to remember in connection with discussions (e.g., Y. J. Dayananda, "The Death of Ivan Ilych: A Psychological Study on Death and Dying," reprinted in Katz, *Tolstoy's Short Fiction*) that interpret Ivan Ilych as an imaginative "confirmation" of Elizabeth Kubler-Ross's empirical description of the stages most people go through in the dying process (see her *On Death and Dying* [New York: Macmillan, 1969]). These stages are denial, anger, bargaining, depression, and resignation. On the one hand, such an interpretation will completely miss the point of Ivan's case, since Kubler-Ross does not describe as a typical stage individuals' rejecting the worth of their lives as Ivan does. Her patients' anger and depression do not arise from such a rejection. So Ivan has characteristics that they lack. On the other hand, Tolstoy's descriptions of the dying process of people whom he thinks have lived as they ought do not involve denial, anger, bargaining, or depression. Tolstoy and Kubler-Ross are not superimposable.

49. What of Ivan's son's honest feelings? We are told that he is at an age when he is beginning to be corrupted, and we can expect that in the normal course of events he would become like Ivan. But, sad to say, with his father dead, he may have a better chance to avoid emotional and moral corruption. For his father was the embodiment of social values and as such would have played a large role in his warping. (According to these values, Ivan judged that his daughter was a success but not his son. And, of course, it is his son and not his daughter who feels deeply about his death. She is absorbed in starting a new married life. Like Lear, Ivan has misunderstood the relative worth of his children's characteristics.)

50. Obviously, these are simplified extreme types. Most people fall in between.

51. I discuss the two points of view on a life, from within and without, in *Morality, Mortality*, Vol. 1. They seem to correspond to what Ronald Dworkin calls the critical versus experiential values. See his *Life's Dominion* (New York: Knopf, 1993).

52. Again, I am distinguishing how we should respond to the spontaneous awakening. I am not recommending that we should induce the awakening. While it is worthwhile, it is painful, so it seems that only the (inner needs of the) person himself should determine whether it starts.

53. This could happen because impulses that the right-living person repressed, or emotions he did not indulge, get the upper hand when he is in a weakened state. Then "their" view of his life is dominant. Someone who approved of Ivan's life will say that this is just what happened to him.

54. This case is different from changes due to dementia, which do not reflect on the true moral character of the person.

55. Admittedly, this conflicts with the possibility that those who have been good deserve more consideration of their interests than do those who have been bad. It also assumes that a sudden death does not involve a very rapid version of what happens in a prolonged dying.

2

Conceptual Issues Related to Ending Life

In order to discuss the morality of ending life, it is necessary to understand a range of concepts and distinctions that may have moral significance.[1] This chapter is intended to introduce those concepts and distinctions. Later chapters will deal with the moral issues.

Suicide involves someone ending his life, intending his death either as an end itself or as a means to some further end. Assisted suicide involves someone helping another person commit suicide. Sometimes, we can help people accomplish their goals without sharing their goals. Hence, it remains open that someone who assists a suicide does not intend that the person end his life; perhaps he intends only that the person be able to do whatever he wants to do.[2] Often, it is physician-assisted suicide in which people are most interested.[3]

Euthanasia involves someone doing something to bring about another's death—in particular, killing or letting die—with the intention that the person die because the death is in the best interests of the person who will die. It differs from physician-assisted suicide undertaken in the interest of the person who dies partly in that it involves killing or letting die by someone other than the patient (e.g., the doctor) in order to end the patient's life. (Unlike suicide and assisted suicide, death being in the person's interests is involved in the definition of euthanasia. One can commit suicide when this is against one's interests. One cannot succeed in euthanizing someone if the death is not in that person's interests.)

How can death be overall in someone's interest?[4] Some have argued that the idea of euthanasia makes no sense because it is logically impossible to seek to benefit someone by bringing about his death, given that death eliminates the person. We cannot produce a benefit if we eliminate the potential beneficiary, it is argued. But someone can be benefited by death even if it involves his nonexistence, just as someone can be made worse off by death even though it involves his nonexistence. To be benefited or made worse off, one need not continue on in a state of good experience or bad experience. For example, if one's life would have included goods if it had continued, then at least *one* of the ways in which one is made worse off by death is that it interferes with those goods; as a result of death, one has had a less good life, a life that is seriously worse overall than one would have had. The shorter **33** life is not worse because it contains an additional intrinsic evil (e.g., pain). Rather, it is comparatively worse than it might have been.[5]

Similarly, if one's life would have gone on containing only misery and pain with no compensating goods, then, it might be argued, one will be benefited by having had a shorter life containing fewer such bad things rather than a longer one containing more such uncompensated bad things. The shorter life is not better because it contains more goods. It is better because it has fewer evils and so is comparatively better than the longer life. For example, we could imagine, independently of any question of active termination, that someone could prefer that he was created to a life of 60 years with no pain in it than to be created to a life of 61 years where the last year was full of pain. He could prefer this because the shorter life would be better for him.

But we said that *one* of the ways death is bad for us is by depriving us of goods of life. If there is *another way* in which death is bad for us, then even if death eliminates uncompensated misery, it may still not benefit us. Suppose the *end of the person*, independent of its causing the end of more goods of life, is a separate harm that death causes to the person. Then it is possible that this harm could outweigh the elimination of life's miseries.[6] But it is also possible that the elimination of the miseries is such an important good that it overrides the harm of the end of the person. Prolonging our life as persons may not be worth every misery, especially since we cannot be immortal in any case.

Deciding whether death would be best for someone may not involve just weighing the forthcoming goods and bads. That is, the mere fact that bads would outnumber goods in the future does not show that the shorter life would be better. The longer life may be better for the person if the future would have certain significant goods, regardless of what bad will also be present.[7] But, in addition, it may be that some near future event will be so bad that even if it would eventually be followed by an outweighing degree of good, one should not have to go through the bad event. There is a nonconsequentialist quality to this reasoning—for just as the nonconsequentialist says that there are some things one need not do to promote best consequences in general, this reasoning claims that there are some things a person might reasonably decline to go through even to promote the best consequences for himself.

Some also insist that we must consider how the future goods and bads connect psychologically with the interests of the person at the time his death would occur in determining whether death is good or bad for someone. (These are known as time-relative interests.) For, it is argued, even if future goods would belong to the person in question if he continued living, the fact that he now would not have even an indirect psychological connectedness to himself in the future makes the person now have no stake in remaining alive to get those future goods. (For example, consider a case in which someone would undergo radical dementia and experience goods as the demented person.)[8] It might also be suggested that we must consider how what will happen from now on completes the life the person has already had—the same future attached to different pasts might render one life, but not another, bad overall.

Not all actions that bring about death involve suicide, assisted suicide, or euthanasia. For example, if we disconnect a patient from life support simply because he does not want invasive treatment or if we give pain relief via morphine that as a side effect kills the patient, our acts will bring about death but will not involve suicide, assisted suicide, or euthanasia.

Discussions of suicide, assisted suicide, euthanasia, and terminating treatment for other reasons are complicated by the fact that many subtle distinctions in how these might be brought about are often thought to have moral relevance. In this section, I shall describe some of these distinctions without judging how they affect moral permissibility.

Intending and Foreseeing

Suicide and euthanasia involve intending death by some party. This is to be distinguished conceptually both from doing something foreseeing, even with certainty, that death will come about as a side effect (as in giving morphine for pain), and from doing something because (that is, on condition that) it will cause death. For example, one might give a drug to reduce a patient's pain only because (i.e., on condition that) the drug also unavoidably eventually has a side effect of causing his death. This is because death is the only thing that will interfere with another eventual side effect of the drug that is worse for the patient than either pain or death. Giving the drug only if it has death as an eventual side effect, and refusing to give it if it does not, still would not imply that one intended the death, I think.

Consider this in more detail. Suppose a doctor wants to give her patient the only drug that will alleviate his pain. Unfortunately, one eventual side effect of the drug is convulsions. Because a life with convulsions is more unbearable for this patient than a life of pain, the doctor and patient decide to use the drug *only* because in the presence of convulsions, the drug also has the side effect of unavoidably and quickly ending the patient's life. They do this because while the patient finds pain preferable to convulsions, he finds death preferable to pain (and to convulsions). If the drug would not also cause death when it produces convulsions, the doctor would not give the painkiller and, if she gives it, it is in part *because* death will be *the cause of* there being no convulsions. Nevertheless, I believe the doctor's acting in this way need not mean that she *intends* the death of her patient. A sign that she does not intend the death of the patient is that she *would not do anything additional, by act or omission, to bring it about that the painkiller can result in death*. If it does not result in death, she simply will not use it. And if she uses it, it is because she intends its painkilling properties. Similarly, a doctor may give a painkiller that helps only temporarily and that would leave the patient in more pain than he was in to begin with when it wears off, when ending the pain is more important to the patient than that he remain alive, only *because* the drug also causes death before the painkiller wears off. Here this doctor also need not intend the death in giving the painkiller. That we use the drug only because it has an effect does not mean that we intend this effect. Call these the Painkiller Cases.[9]

The causal structure of these Painkiller Cases is that the means (painkiller) to the greater good (no more pain) causes a lesser evil relative to pain (death) and this lesser evil sustains a greater good (no more pain) that would otherwise end (by interfering with the return of pain or convulsions). These cases seem to involve acting with an intention *under a condition* but *not intending the condition*. That is, *if* death occurs (the condition), one will act intending no more pain, but one does not intend that death occur.

One common test for whether we intend rather than merely foresee an effect is that we would not continue to act if the effect did not come about. This is known as the Counterfactual Test. But that test turns out not to be discriminating enough to test for intention, since the doctor in the Painkiller Cases would not give the painkiller if it did not also cause death but she need not intend the death. Is it possible that it is correct to describe the doctor's *intention* as giving pain relief free of convulsions? *If so, then bringing about death is the means to that end*, where "means" is used in the sense of "what a person must do to bring about his end." Yet it seems the doctor need *not* intend the means (so conceived) to her end when the means will occur without her intending that it does.[10]

Active and Passive

Suicide, assisted suicide, and euthanasia may each have what are called passive and active versions. Active suicide involves one inducing one's own death—for example, by shooting oneself. Active assisted suicide could involve a doctor giving a patient death-inducing pills for the patient to use. (Here the doctor makes possible an active suicide.) Active euthanasia involves someone inducing another's death— for example, by injecting a death-causing drug. However, passive versions of suicide, assisted suicide, and euthanasia may involve acts or omissions. Hence, in this discussion, the distinction between passive and active is *not* the same as the distinction between omission and act. For example, a doctor could commit passive euthanasia by performing the *act* of pulling a plug on the lifesaving treatment he was providing to a patient because death was in the patient's interest. Even though he performs an act, pulling the plug does not introduce a cause of death: it removes a barrier to death that he was providing and allows an underlying problem to kill the patient. These factors, I believe, help make what he does passive euthanasia. (Perhaps he could perform passive physician-assisted suicide by pulling the plug on sedation of a patient so that sleepiness does not interfere with a patient's killing himself. Here, he acts to remove a barrier to the patient's committing suicide; he does not provide the means of inducing death.) Passive euthanasia, passive assisted suicide, and passive suicide could take place by omission as well. For example, in passive suicide, a patient may omit taking his lifesaving drug with the intention that death occurs.

Killing and Letting Die

The active/passive distinction drawn in this way and the intending/foreseeing distinction are different from the killing/letting die distinction. Which of the behaviors I have described so far is killing and which is letting die? This question is not settled by considering the agent's intentions. One can omit lifesaving aid intending death without this being a killing. And one can kill by injecting a person with a painkilling drug that has a side effect of causing his death, even though one did not intend to kill him but only to relieve his pain.

It seems that all active (vs. passive) suicide and euthanasia involve killings because they induce death. (This does not mean that all killings must involve inducing death.) A doctor actively terminating treatment he provides could also be a killing if, for example, it triggers an electrical discharge that induces the patient's death. (Active assisted suicide does not involve a killing by the agent who is the provider of the death-inducing substance.) Passive euthanasia that involves someone acting to terminate treatment that is lifesaving and that neither he (nor an agent he represents) is providing can be a killing, even though it removes a barrier to death and does not induce it. For example, this happens when such a person has the consent of neither the person who will die nor of the person who provides the treatment. This is true even though there is no inducement of death. By contrast a doctor who terminates aid she is providing, or removes that over which she has a right, lets die (perhaps wrongfully) rather than kills when she just removes a barrier to the cause of death, even if the patient objects to terminating treatment. Consider the following analogy: I am saving someone from drowning and I decide to stop. Even if I must actively push a button to make myself stop, I am still letting the person die rather than killing him. (If a patient acquired rights over a treatment machine once attached to it, this could change a letting die into a killing. Hence it is important to decide that, sometimes at least, temporary use involves no such transfer of rights.)[11]

Still, even when a doctor pulls the plug on aid he is giving, the fact that he acts makes him a partial *cause* of death, the underlying problem being the other partial cause. So, there is the following difference between not beginning treatment and terminating treatment that one or one's device provides: only in the latter case does *letting die cause a death*, at least in part. Still, only a killing *introduces a cause* which induces death, rather than merely removing the barrier to a cause of death that is or will be present.[12]

Consent

Why does consent of the patient sometimes matter and sometimes not matter to whether terminating treatment is a killing? If one removes what one is providing (or what one has a right over) that helps make lifesaving treatment possible, then one either lets another or oneself die. One lets oneself die, for example, when one removes one's body from the treatment, or denies consent to another's interference with one's body. The doctor lets die when she removes her (hospital) resources and the patient dies through lack of support. If one is a representative of those who either provide treatment or provide their own bodies to the treatment process, in terminating treatment one will let die. One becomes a representative of someone who provides his body for treatment, and then decides not to provide it, if one receives the latter's consent to terminate treatment. Hence, a doctor who removes treatment she is providing (or that she has a right over) may not require patient consent in order (as a conceptual matter) to perform a letting die in terminating treatment, though it may still be an impermissible letting die. However, some other agent may require patient (or doctor) consent in order to perform a letting die rather than a killing in terminating treatment. (None of this speaks to the permissibility of any of these acts of letting die or killing.)

To summarize a bit, active euthanasia is killing. Passive euthanasia by omission is letting die. Passive euthanasia by action can be a killing or it can be a letting die (that helps cause death), depending on such factors as who owns the life-support machine and who is running it. Once a patient forms an intention to commit suicide, he can do so actively, which involves killing himself, or passively (either by an omission or an act which terminates his life support), which involves letting himself die. If a doctor actively assists an active suicide (either by, for example, giving lethal drugs or giving drugs to facilitate a patient's suicidal act), he assists in killing; if he actively assists a passive suicide (for example, by giving drugs to keep a patient awake so that he can pull his own plug on a life-support machine), he assists a letting die. If a doctor passively assists an active suicide (either by, for example, omitting sedation or terminating it), he assists a killing; if he passively assists a passive suicide, he assists a letting die.

Voluntariness

The role of consent leads us to the next distinctions: that between the voluntary, the involuntary, and the nonvoluntary in the context of suicide, assisted suicide, and euthanasia. "Voluntary" means willed by the party who is either killed or let die; "involuntary" means against the will of the party killed or let die; and "nonvoluntary" means killing or letting die takes place when the person who is killed or let die has not willed it, but also has not ruled it out. (It might also refer to acting without knowledge of the will of the person killed or left to die. However, this "agent-subjective" use is consistent with the person in fact actually being against or for being killed or left to die.) Suppose someone has designated a surrogate decision-maker to decide about killing or letting die. Then while he may not have willed his death under that description, he could have willed his death under the description "the surrogate's choice." In the case of assisted suicide, the question of voluntariness is about whether the person who wills to die also wills the assistance of another.

That someone's act or choice is voluntary does not ensure that it is a fully autonomous choice of a rational agent. Someone could be irrational, uninformed, or (possibly) coerced when he makes a voluntary choice. Suicide seems by definition to be voluntary, but it is not necessarily always a fully autonomous choice. Terminating treatment, euthanasia, and assisted suicide could be voluntary, involuntary, or nonvoluntary. While someone may choose against euthanasia, assisted suicide, or terminating treatment, thus making it involuntary were it to occur, this choice too may not be fully autonomous or rational.

Permissibility

The last distinctions to which I shall point are among the morally permissible, impermissible, or dutiful. None of the previous distinctions we have discussed has been assumed to be equivalent to, or to serve as conclusive evidence for, the permissibility or impermissibility of conduct. So, the fact that some behavior would be a killing or an involuntary withholding or termination of treatment should not be assumed to settle the question of whether the behavior is permissible or impermissible. For example, it might sometimes be permissible for a doctor to refuse, against the will of the patient, to provide lifesaving treatment when not providing treatment is in the patient's best interests. On the other hand, a doctor's terminating treatment that constitutes a letting die against the will of the patient may sometimes be impermissible, even if it is not a killing. Killing someone who autonomously chooses to be killed might sometimes be permissible. *Not* refusing treatment to a patient or *not* killing him could sometimes be *im*permissible, for all that has been said so far, and then one would have a *duty* to not treat or to kill.[13]

Notes

    1. This chapter combines revised parts of my "Ending Life," in *The Blackwell Guide to Medical Ethics*, eds. R. Rhodes, L. Frances, and A. Silvers (Oxford: Wiley-Blackwell, 2007), pp. 142–61, and revised parts of "Physician-Assisted Suicide, Euthanasia, and Intending Death," in *Physician-Assisted Suicide: Expanding the Debate*, eds. Margaret P. Battin, Rosamond Rhodes, and Anita Silvers (New York and London: Routledge, 1998), pp. 8–62.

2. This analysis disagrees with that presented by the majority of Supreme Court justices in *Vacco et al.* v. *Quill et al.* and *State of Washington et al.* v. *Glucksberg et al.*, where they claim that a physician who assists in suicide necessarily intends the death of the patient, whereas one who terminates treatment may only possibly intend the death.

3. Some doctors, such as Dr. Timothy Quill, claim that they only intend to give their patients an option to end their lives; *New England Journal of Medicine* 329 (14) (September 20, 1993): 1039. Doctors may even give the option because they think having the option will reduce a patient's eagerness to commit suicide. So, some doctors may give the option to commit suicide, intending to prevent the intention to commit suicide. I believe that a doctor will not be, strictly speaking, assisting in suicide if he gives a prescription for lethal drugs prior to the patient's forming an intention to use them. If the patient does not subsequently attempt suicide, the doctor certainly does not assist in it, though he did make possible the choice between doing it and not doing it. If the patient takes the drug, having formed the intention to do so after the doctor gave her the drug, the doctor has helped her kill herself, but this is not quite the same as assisting in suicide. If he gave drugs to give a choice (i.e., before he knew an intention was formed), then even if he is present at the time she takes the drug, this is also not strictly assistance in suicide, even if he does not stop the suicide. However, if a doctor gives the lethal drug knowing the patient has formed the settled intention to use it and she uses it, he assisted in suicide. However, he may still do this only intending to help a patient do what she wants. If he gives a medicine that keeps the patient alert in order that she can commit suicide, then strictly speaking he also assists in suicide, but not in a way that gives rise to legal concerns (by contrast to giving lethal drugs).

4. Death is distinct from the process of dying which leads to it.

5. A comparative analysis of the badness of death is offered by Thomas Nagel in "Death," reprinted in *Mortal Questions* (Cambridge: Cambridge University Press, 1979). I discuss it in *Morality, Mortality*, Vol. 1 (New York: Oxford University Press, 1993).

6. In *Morality, Mortality*, Vol. 1, pp. 19–22, I argued that the simple coming to an end of the person was itself an evil to the person.

7. Philippa Foot takes this view in "Euthanasia," in her *Virtues and Vices* (New York: Oxford University Press, 2002).

8. On this suggestion, see Jeff McMahan, *The Ethics of Killing* (New York: Oxford University Press, 2003).

9. I discussed them in my *Intricate Ethics* (New York: Oxford University Press, 2007), chapter 4.

10. For more detailed discussion of the distinction between intending and acting on condition of, and also discussion of and intending the means to one's end, see chapter 4 of my *Intricate Ethics*.

11. Notice that my analysis of terminating aid differs from Dan Brock's analysis in "Voluntary Active Euthanasia," reprinted in *Life and Death* (New York: Cambridge University Press, 1993). Brock believes that if a greedy nephew, in order to get his aunt's inheritance, pulls out the plug on her life-support machine without her consent or anyone else's, he kills. Brock notes that a doctor who pulls a plug at the request of the patient in the patient's interest may make the same exact physical movements as the nephew. Brock concludes from this that if the nephew kills, the doctor does. Their motives and intentions are not the same and the permissibility of their behavior may differ, but they both kill. I disagree that they both kill. It might be thought that an explanation for this is that one must

extend one's *temporal perspective* in order to determine who kills and who lets die. That is, one cannot just look at the behavior at the time of terminating treatment; one must check to see what the person did earlier—e.g., did he set up the machine to help the aunt and is he now disconnecting it? But this is not correct, as the following cases show. Suppose the nephew set up the machine to help his aunt, but the machine does not belong to him and he goes away, leaving it running on its own. If he returns and turns off the machine without permission of his aunt or the owner of the machine, he kills. On the other hand, suppose someone else takes a machine that belongs to the nephew (with or without his permission) and sets it up to give life support. If the nephew stops it, he will have let his aunt die, not killed her. (I owe the last two cases and the emphasis on the importance of ownership of the means of support to Timothy Hall.) Suppose a life-support machine is not the nephew's and he did not start it, but he remains running it. If he pushes a button to stop his doing so, he lets die. In sum, if one stops aid that one is providing or that one's means provide, one lets die, permissibly or impermissibly. For a more detailed presentation of this analysis, see my *Morality, Mortality*, Vol. 2 (New York: Oxford University Press, 1996) and unpublished work by Timothy Hall.

12. Though, as the Nephew Case shows, not all killing induces death. See my *Morality, Mortality*, Vol. 2.

13. Chapters 3–6 that follow discuss the substantive issue of whether and when euthanasia, suicide, and assisted suicide are permissible.

3

Problems with "Assisted Suicide: The Philosophers' Brief"

I. Summary of the Brief's Argument

In "Assisted Suicide: The Philosophers' Brief"[1, 2] (henceforth "The Philosophers' Brief"), Ronald Dworkin et al. argue that if it is permissible to omit or terminate medical treatment with the intention that the patient die, it is permissible to assist in killing with the intention that the patient die, at least when the patient consents. One reason they give for this is that there is no intrinsic moral difference between killing and letting die. Another reason is that they think that people have a right to make important, intimate choices about their own lives, and to be killed or let die could equally be a means to facilitate these choices.

One part of their argument builds on the U.S. Supreme Court's 1990 decision in *Cruzan* v. *Missouri*, in which the Court majority assumed (if only for the sake of argument) that competent patients have a constitutional right to refuse life-preserving treatment. Dworkin et al. say that the existence of a right to refuse treatment also implies a right to assistance in suicide from a willing physician. If, as *Cruzan* indicates, it is permissible for doctors to let a patient die even when the patient and the doctor intend the patient's death, then, Dworkin et al. think, it is permissible for doctors to assist in killing. In the preface to "The Philosophers' Brief," written after the U.S. Supreme Court heard oral arguments on the case, Dworkin notes that several justices rejected this link between *Cruzan* and the assisted-suicide cases. These justices sought to distinguish them by reference to a "common-sense distinction" between the moral significance of acts and omissions: assisting suicide is an act and thus requires a compelling moral justification; in contrast, not providing treatment is an omission, a matter of "letting nature take its course," and can be justified more easily.

Dworkin says in the preface that "the brief insists that such suggestions wholly misunderstand the 'common-sense' distinction, which is not between acts and omissions, but between acts or omissions that are designed to cause death and those that are not." This means that Dworkin et al. believe that common sense denies that there is ever a moral difference between action and omission per se, and affirms only a moral difference between intending and not intending (even while foreseeing) death. Presumably, the latter *moral* distinction will only matter sometimes, since, they think, intending death is sometimes justified when the patient consents.

II. Counterarguments

A. ACTION/OMISSION VERSUS KILLING/LETTING DIE

Dworkin et al. do not construct their argument on the assumption that when a doctor assists patients in committing suicide by giving them potentially lethal pills, the doctor always intends the patients' deaths. They recognize that it need not be true that the doctor has this intention; in giving the patients potentially lethal pills, the doctor may only *intend* to give them a choice of whether to live or die. Hence, even if it were wrong to intend patients' deaths in combination with acting to help them attain this end, this need not be what is involved in assisting a suicide. However, since Dworkin et al. try to defend assisted suicide even on the assumption that the doctor does intend the patient's death, I shall focus on cases in which this intention is present.

I agree that the act/omission distinction will not bear much moral weight in this setting, but this does not mean that if intending versus foreseeing death matters, nothing else does; killing versus letting die, which is not the same as act versus omission, may also matter. When doctors remove life-sustaining treatment by pulling a plug at time t, they act (though they do not necessarily kill) and their act could be as permissible as not starting treatment at time t (an omission). I have tried to argue elsewhere that if doctors are terminating aid at time t that they (or the organization whose agent they are) have been providing, then in certain cases they *let die* rather than kill, and their act is as permissible (or as impermissible) as not starting treatment at time t would be.[3] The doctors *let die* even though they act because (1) the patient dies of some underlying cause whose effects the life support was counteracting,[4] and (2) the patient loses out only on life he or she would have had with the support the doctors (or organization whose agent they are) are providing.[5] Consider the following analogy: I am saving a man from drowning and I decide to stop. Even if I must actively push a button to make myself stop, I still let the person die rather than kill him, and my act is as permissible (or impermissible) as not beginning to provide aid. By contrast, suppose that (1) were true but (2) were not, because some stranger who was neither providing the life support nor owned the machine that was providing it pulled the plug. This would be a killing (whether it was permissible or not).

Is there always a moral difference between instances of letting die (by act or omission) and killing, holding other factors constant? I do not think so. Some terminations of treatment could be killings that would be no more difficult to justify than cases of letting die (that involve omissions or acts). Hence, if killing versus letting die sometimes matters morally, this does not mean it must always matter. For example, suppose that one particular hospital in a community has faulty electrical wiring. If the doctors at that hospital accede to a patient's request to discontinue lifesaving treatment by pulling the plug on the life-support machine, she will get an electric shock and die (Faulty Wiring Case I). In another hospital, if the same patient stopped getting the treatment at her request, she would die immediately of her underlying condition. I think that in these cases, it is no harder to justify discontinuing treatment when this kills than to justify discontinuing treatment that just lets the patient die; it is not true that if the patient is in the first hospital, she may not have aid terminated, but if she is in the other hospital, she may. In Faulty Wiring Case I, the patient is killed by the shock; she does not die because of her underlying medical condition (that is, condition 1 is not satisfied). However, the patient loses out only on life she would have had with the doctor's aid (condition 2). This factor, which is always present in letting die cases, is present in this particular killing case and helps render the particular killing on a moral par with letting die.

Indeed, we might go even further: suppose that a patient requests termination of lifesaving treatment but due to faulty wiring, we are physically unable to end his connection to a machine by just pulling the plug or turning off the machine. Instead, we would have to first give the patient an electric shock (which would kill him) in order to be able to disconnect the machine from him (Faulty Wiring Case II). In Faulty Wiring Case I, the shocking that leads to death is foreseen, not intended. In Faulty Wiring Case II, the shocking is intended as a means to remove a patient from the machine. I do not believe that the patient must continue to get unwanted lifesaving treatment just because we would have to kill him as an intended means in order to stop his getting treatment, at least if he would have died of an underlying cause if he simply had not gotten the treatment.

There are also other commonly accepted instances in which doctors kill their patients, and doing so is morally and legally permissible. When a doctor gives morphine to ease pain, foreseeing that it will also cause death, the doctor also acts, and kills (though without intending to kill). Yet it is permissible to do this, at least if the patient permits it.

B. KILLING/LETTING DIE VERSUS INTENDING/FORESEEING DEATH

However, I part company with Dworkin et al. when they argue that once patients have consented, we can *always* move from the permissibility of letting the patients die, intending their death, to the permissibility of physician-assisted suicide (assumed here to involve intending death) that involves patients killing themselves. Killing and assisted killing are not always on a moral par with letting die. Let me explain by reference to some types of cases, considering physician killings as well as assisted killings.

(a)

In all cases of the first type, doctors act *against* their patients' wishes to live. Dworkin et al. agree that doctors may permissibly deny a lifesaving organ to a patient who wants it in order to give it to another, but *not* kill a nonconsenting patient in order to get that patient's organ for another. They say that this is not because of a moral difference between letting patients die and killing them, but because the doctors merely foresee death in the first case but intend it in the second. Intending patients' deaths against their wishes makes the behavior impermissible, according to the authors of "The Philosophers' Brief." I shall now try to show (i) that intending patients' deaths against their wishes does not alone make not-aiding impermissible, and (ii) that whether in the presence or absence of intending patients' deaths against their wishes, killing can be impermissible while letting die is not impermissible.

(i) Suppose that a doctor denied an organ to a patient and gave it to another person who needed it more only because the person who was denied the organ was the doctor's enemy whose death he intended; giving the organ to the needier person was only a pretext. (Call this the Enemy Case.)[6] Though we can conclude that the doctor has a bad character, I do not think that his giving the organ to the needier patient was impermissible.[7] This shows that intending patients' deaths when it is against their wishes does not necessarily make not aiding them impermissible.[8]

(ii) Now, I shall defend the claim that killing versus letting die can make a moral difference in the absence of intending death against a patient's wishes, though one still acts against his wishes. Suppose it were intending death and not killing that makes a moral difference in the case where doctors kill a patient against his will in order to get his organs for others. Then it should be as permissible to kill a patient when his death is not intended as it is to let him die when his death is not intended. Suppose that a doctor, in order to transplant organs (innocently obtained) into several patients, uses a gas that he foresees will seep into the next room where another patient lies, killing that patient who wishes not to die (call this the Gas Case). In this case, the doctor does not intend the death of the patient in the other room, but only foresees that patient's death as a side effect of the needed gas.[9] Presumably, transplanting when this effect will occur is wrong, even if it cannot be done otherwise, because using the gas will kill someone. Yet letting the patient next door die against his wishes simply because one is busy transplanting organs into several needy patients is permissible. So in cases in which we merely foresee death, killing may be wrong even if letting die is not. This suggests that there is a per se moral difference between killing and letting die that can lead to different moral judgments in at least some cases. Another way to show that the difference between killing and letting die can matter is to show that when a patient wishes not to die, letting die with the intention that death occur might be permissible—though killing with such an intention is not. I have already said that sometimes letting die would not be wrong (as in the Enemy Case discussed above) when the bad doctor chooses to aid a needier person only because she intends the death of someone else. Compare this with a killing in which the bad doctor would use the only way of saving a needier person only because that way of saving him will kill the doctor's enemy as a side effect (as in the Gas Case), and he intends to kill his enemy. This killing is impermissible.

Dworkin et al. claim that a doctor who lets a patient die of easily treatable pneumonia against the patient's wishes, intending that the patient die so that his organs are available for use in others, has done something wrong, as has a doctor who kills the same sort of patient, intending that he die. I agree. When the letting die and the killing are both wrong, I would say that this is because both doctors do what is against the welfare of the patient and violate his rights. The first doctor would do this if he violates the positive right to treatment, *not* because not treating is a side effect of doing something more important, such as saving two other people (by innocent means that do not involve getting the first patient's organs). The second doctor violates the negative right against being killed. But this does not always imply, as Dworkin et al. think, that a "doctor violates his patient's rights whether the doctor acts or refrains from acting *against the patient's wishes* in a way that is designed to cause death."[10] This was already shown by the Enemy Case. But there are other types of cases in which one does *not* act against a patient's interests that show this as well. For example, suppose that a patient wishes not to die, but it would be in his interest to die. If a treatment is experimental, or in general something to which the patient has no positive right, it may be permissible to deny it to him because death would be in his own best interest.[11] I do not believe that the patient acquires a right to have the experimental therapy merely because the doctor's reason for refusing it is that he aims at the patient's death, which is in the patient's interests but which the patient does not want. But killing the patient if he wishes not to die would violate his rights and be morally wrong, even if it were in his best interests to die and the doctor acted for his best interests. Once again, we see a case where a moral difference between killing and letting die surfaces.[12]

(b)

Next, consider the second type of case, in which the patient consents to death. These are the cases that bear directly on whether the killing/letting die distinction is morally relevant in the assisted-suicide contexts. Does the distinction between killing and letting die make a moral difference to the scope of permissible refusal of lifesaving treatment versus the scope of permissible assistance to killing? Dworkin et al. seem to suggest that the scope of permissible refusal of treatment and permissible assistance to killing should be the same. They say that if doctors can turn off a respirator intending death, then they can prescribe lethal pills intending death. Prescribing pills is a way to assist patients to kill themselves, even when they are not currently receiving life support, and it is this sort of assisted killing that Dworkin et al. think is permissible. In addition, by turning off a respirator, they have in mind cases where the patient is then left to die. It is these sorts of cases of killing and letting die that I shall compare first with respect to scope.

Mentally competent patients may legally refuse treatment, intending to die, even when it is *against their best interests* to do so (as it would be if their treatment process will not be experientially bad and might cure them) and, on many occasions, even when they would be cured. Presumably, in many of these cases they would also be within their rights to insist on the doctor terminating treatment, even if their intention is to die and they would thus be committing suicide. Furthermore, even if the doctors in these cases improperly intend that the patients die, the treatment must be terminated at the patient's request. *This is because the alternative to letting the patients die is forcing treatment on them.* We think that the right of mentally competent patients not to be physically invaded against their will is typically stronger than our interest in the patients' well-being (even if the right could be overridden for considerations of public safety). But if such patients ask for assistance in killing themselves when it is against their medical interest to die, it might well be morally impermissible for doctors to assist them in killing themselves. This is, at least in part, because the alternative is not forcing treatment on them. Certainly, if someone's reason for wanting to die is to sacrifice himself as a martyr in a political protest, it would be ludicrous to go to a doctor for assistance in suicide, though he could have a doctor terminate treatment. Even if his own nonmedical best interests were at stake—for example, he must die in order to ensure his glorious postmortem reputation—it would be inappropriate for a physician to assist in his killing. So, contrary to what Dworkin et al. say, doctors might in some cases be permitted and even required to turn off a respirator, even when they intend death, but not be permitted to prescribe lethal pills.[13]

Why is judgment about the best interests of the patient only determinative when we give him something that will cause his death but not when we allow him to die (by nontreatment or by terminating treatment)? Philippa Foot argued that when we actively interfere with people, we must be concerned not only with whether they want our interference but also with whether we harm them.[14] Both their right to autonomy and our duty not to harm apply. (This implies that the latter duty does not entirely stem from a right not to be harmed that others can waive.) If we give patients a death-producing drug, even when they ask for it and take it themselves, and even if we just foresee and do not intend their deaths, I think that the same dual condition applies (even though such active involvement does not amount to actual interference).[15]

When we let patients die by disconnecting life support, not interfering with autonomy is shown to override patient welfare as the dominant consideration. If we do *not* let the patients die, we will be interfering with them against their wishes, violating their right to autonomy by forcing treatment on them. Not doing this takes precedence over acting in their interests. By contrast, if we do not help patients carry out suicides they will for themselves when (by assumption) these suicides are not good for them, we do not interfere with them against their will.

We respect their right to autonomy, which is essentially a negative right to not be interfered with. It is true that we may not be promoting their autonomy considered as a value (i.e., we may not be seeing to it that their own values determine how their lives go). But it is a mistake to assimilate autonomy as a value to autonomy as a right. Promoting others' autonomy may interfere with our own autonomous choice or duty to not do them harm, or otherwise require involving ourselves with their lives. In sum, we can insist on acting for competent patients' good against their will only when in doing so we do not violate their right to noninterference.

So the alternative to letting die has such a morally objectionable feature—forcing treatment, which a patient has a right we not do—that even if we think that both the competent patient's and the doctor's intentions are wrong, we must permit termination of aid. In contrast, the alternative to assisted suicide may simply be leaving patients alone; this often does not violate any of their rights against us, and so we may permissibly, and sometimes we should be required to, refuse to help them because we disapprove of their goals. Many people—including Supreme Court justices whom Dworkin cites—might, then, reasonably distinguish terminating treatment from assisting in a suicide. The move from *Cruzan's* (assumed) right to refuse treatment to the permissibility of assisted suicide is, therefore, not generally available.[16]

The argument against the *general* moral equivalence of assisting suicide and terminating aid, even when the competent patient consents to these, has also helped us see that sometimes killing or assisting in killing *will* have the same moral standing as terminating aid. For example, in Faulty Wiring Case I, if we terminate treatment we will kill a patient (or assist in killing her when we help the patient disconnect herself). This is because she dies of the electric shock from disconnection. But since the patient will continue to be interfered with against her will if we do not do this, we should disconnect her or assist her in disconnecting herself from life support, even if this is not in her interest, if she competently requests this.

In sum, I have argued that the approach of "The Philosophers' Brief"—which claims that when terminating treatment while intending death is permissible, assisting suicide while intending death is also permissible—does not succeed. In particular, I argued that it is not always permissible to assist killing while intending death when it is permissible to let die or terminate support while intending death. Even if it is sometimes permissible to assist killing while intending death, as it is permissible to let die intending death, this would not be because there is never a moral difference between killing or assisting killing and letting die (including terminating life support). I argued that such a difference shows up in several cases involving suicide.

III. A Theoretical Argument

I have examined the case-based arguments in "The Philosophers' Brief" for Dworkin et al.'s conclusion that the distinction between killing and letting die does not matter per se. I shall now very briefly consider a second, more theoretical, argument that Dworkin et al. make in favor of physician-assisted suicide. They adopt the principle proposed in *Planned Parenthood* v. *Casey*: one has a right to self-determination in the most intimate and important matters in one's life. From that principle, they deduce a right to determine the time and manner of one's death, and by implication, whether to achieve death by being left to die or by having help in killing oneself.

Does this principle also imply that people have a right to assisted suicide from a willing physician if they decide that their medical treatment is consuming too much of their families' finances, or if they wish to give up their life for some noble cause, given that they would have a right to refuse treatment for these reasons? I suggest that this principle is too broad if it yields these conclusions.[17]

IV. A Close Alternative

There is a somewhat different type of case-based argument that might be constructed to show that if we may let people die while intending their death, it is also permissible to assist in a killing while intending the death. When *death is (at least) the least evil* of the options for the person who dies,[18] the greater good is a medically appropriate aim (e.g., having no pain or great suffering rather than gaining postmortem glory), and the patient consents, then assisting in the killing with the intention to bring about death will be permissible, if letting die with the intention to bring about death is permissible. This is, I believe, a different argument from those presented in the brief. It does not imply that if patients consent, we may always assist in their suicide, even when it is against their interest to die (because death is not then a lesser evil by comparison with continuing on in their lives). It is only when we add the qualifier "when death is (at least) the least evil of the options" (as well as patient consent) that we get a certain moral equivalence of assisting in a killing and letting die.

The first premise in "The Philosophers' Brief" argument, that it is permissible to terminate treatment with the intention to bring about death, is available without assuming that death is (at least) the least evil of the patient's options. This is because it is often permissible to terminate treatment at the wishes of a competent patient even when death is a greater evil than living on and so not in a patient's interest. Because the first premise can be true without "the least evil" clause, we cannot move easily from the first premise to the conclusion that assisting in a killing is also permissible, for the plausibility of that conclusion is often dependent on the truth of the clause.[19] It may be true that when death is "the least evil," the greater good is a medically appropriate aim, and the patient consents, it will also be true that killing or assisting in a killing is as acceptable a means to death as letting die. I have not denied this.

Yet I do not necessarily recommend relying on this alternative argument. My sense is that showing that intending the patient's death need not be a bad intention—there need not be anything wrong with having this intention per se—is a crucial moral issue. Not in the sense that a bad intention would make an act impermissible—I have already argued against this in the Enemy Case—but in the sense that the ending of a life that is bad for someone is a factor that helps make action permissible. (That is, the act is not permissible merely despite this happening.) Intending a factor that speaks in favor of permissibility is to have an unobjectionable intention. When we allow that it is permissible to let die intending death, we can do so without inquiring in this way into the value of intending death per se, since (as argued above) the alternative to allowing termination of treatment is forcing treatment on someone, and this we may not do despite someone's ending treatment with a bad intention. But when we want to kill or assist in killing someone, forcing treatment is not the alternative, so then it is more important to show *why* intending death on account of its being "the least evil" is morally acceptable. This is what we are forced to do by another type of argument, called the Four-Step Argument, that I discuss elsewhere.[20] The alternative argument I have presented here threatens to conceal the importance of doing this: it deceives us into thinking that we have already argued for the moral acceptability of intending death per se when we conclude that letting die while intending death is permissible.[21]

Notes

1. This chapter is a revised part of my "Dworkin on Abortion and Assisted Suicide," in *Dworkin and His Critics*, ed. J. Burley (Oxford: Wiley-Blackwell, 2004). That chapter was a revised version of my "Ronald Dworkin on Abortion and Assisted Suicide," *Journal of Ethics* 5 (2001): 200, 221–40. I thank Ronald Dworkin for his response to that article in his "Replies to Endicott, Kamm, and Altman" in the same issue, pp. 265–66. Parts of this chapter also appeared in "A Right to Death," *The Boston Review* 22 (1997).

2. See Ronald Dworkin, Thomas Nagel, Robert Nozick, John Rawls, Thomas Scanlon, and Judith Thomson, "Assisted Suicide: The Philosophers' Brief," *New York Review of Books* 44 (March 27, 1997): 23. The brief was submitted to the U.S. Supreme Court as it decided *State of Washington et al. v. Glucksberg et al.*

3. See F. M. Kamm, *Morality, Mortality*, Vol. II (New York: Oxford University Press, 1996); *Intricate Ethics* (New York: Oxford University Press, 2007); and chapter 2 this volume.

4. Note that this underlying cause need not be the original illness from which the patient suffered. It could be some condition that developed subsequent to his beginning life support, and even caused by having life support, that also makes him dependent on life support.

5. I should add, where their support does not merely counteract a threat they present to what the patient would have had independently of their support.

6. Even though either patient will die without the organ, one can be needier than the other; for example, because one would die at a much younger age than the other if not helped.

7. However, if we care about the doctor (for example, he is our child), we may wish that he had been prevented from acting permissibly in accord with his bad character. For

example, we may wish he had overslept and never had the opportunity to act out his bad intention.

8. Surprisingly, given that she is one of the coauthors of the brief, Judith Thomson argued similarly in "Physician-Assisted Suicide: Two Moral Arguments," *Ethics* 109 (1999): 497–518.

9. Philippa Foot first discussed this case in "The Problem of Abortion and the Doctrine of Double Effect," *Oxford Review* 5 (1967): 5–15.

10. Dworkin et al., "Assisted Suicide: The Philosophers' Brief," p. 45.

11. It would not *violate his rights* even if death were not in his interest, since the treatment (by hypothesis) is not one to which he has a right. Still, refusing this treatment when it is in the patients' interest to live could be impermissible for reasons other than that it violates a right.

12. However, it is worth noting that it might sometimes be permissible to kill patients when it is against their interests to die, they do not want to die, and the doctor intends their death. Recall the Faulty Wiring Case I, where it was as permissible (or impermissible) to detach a patient from a life-support machine when this killed him (by shocking him) as when it let him die. Suppose that a patient who is on life support in the hospital with faulty wiring does not want to die and it is not in his interest to die. But ten other patients come into the hospital and they can be saved if and only if they, instead of the single patient, are hooked up to this one life-support system. Perhaps it is permissible to detach him to help the others, though the shock produced will kill him against his wishes when it is not in his interest to die. Furthermore, suppose that the only person who can detach him and attach the ten others is a doctor who does so only because she intends the single person's death as he hates him. I do not think that this alone would make detaching him impermissible (Faulty Wiring Case III). Killing in this case may be permissible because it involves terminating life support by those who have jurisdiction over providing the life support and terminating produces better consequences. This does not show that killings or assisting in killings that do not involve terminating life support would be permissible when patients do not want to die and it is not in their interest to die. Again, showing that killing sometimes makes a moral difference does not show that it always does, and showing that it sometimes does not make a moral difference does not show that it never does.

13. In *Compassion in Dying* v. *Washington*, the majority of the Court suggested that they could not distinguish morally or legally between what is already permitted—that is, both terminating treatment intending death and giving morphine foreseeing that this will cause death—and assisting in a killing intending death (see 79 F.3d 790, 823 [9th Cir. 1996], *rev'd nom. Washington* v. *Glucksberg*, 117 S.Ct. 2258 [1997]). Yet the *Compassion in Dying* Court was concerned to limit the doctor's right to assist in killing patients to cases where the patients' lives are going to end shortly anyway and death is not against their interests. Suppose, however, that the distinction between giving lethal pills to a person who is not on life support *and* terminating life support when this allows the patient to die makes no moral or legal difference (as claimed by the justices). Then terminating treatment should be permitted *no more broadly* than assisting killing. For example, treatment should be required for a competent *non*terminal patient who will die without it (as giving lethal pills to such a patient would be ruled out). But such treatment is not required. The justices may have mistakenly thought that if intending death does not rule out terminating lifesaving treatment and killing does not rule out giving morphine for pain relief when it will also cause death, the combination of intentionally killing or assisting killing intending death must be permitted,

even when what kills serves no other purpose (such as pain relief). But the premises do not imply the conclusion, I think.

In his response to the original version of this article (which did not differ in substance on the issue of assisted suicide from this chapter), Dworkin said: "Kamm agrees that the distinction between act and omission is not morally relevant in the context of the assisted suicide cases and I agree with her the distinction is sometimes morally important in other, very different, cases" (Dworkin, "Replies to Endicott, Kamm, and Altman," pp. 263–67). But we can now see that while I argued above that the distinction between acts and omissions is inadequate, I have also now argued that the different distinction, between killing and letting die, can be morally relevant in the context of the assisted-suicide cases, not just in "very different" cases. The fact that a doctor may permissibly terminate lifesaving aid for competent patients when it is against their interest to die, but may not give pills to assist competent patients to die when it is against their interest to die, is meant to show this. (Furthermore, I did not say that the distinction between acts and omissions "is morally important in other, very different, cases." In his response, Dworkin seems not to distinguish the acts/omissions distinction from the killing/letting die distinction, yet I argued that it was important to do so.)

14. Philippa Foot, "Euthanasia," *Philosophy & Public Affairs* 6 (1977): 85–112.

15. However, I also think that on at least one model of doctoring, if patients will a doctor's interference or involvement, the doctor may help them if it is merely not clear whether what they do will be harmful. For more on this, see chapter 4 this volume.

16. This is especially true because the *Cruzan* Court did not base its view that patients have a right to direct termination of their treatment on the view that sometimes death is not against the patient's interest.

17. In fact, Sandra Day O'Connor's separate concurrence in the Supreme Court decision in Glucksberg seemed to argue that the principle recognized in Casey only implies that the government could not require a person to die in certain abhorrent conditions, but if there were means other than assisted suicide to avoid the conditions (for example, means such as terminal sedation or painkillers), there could not be said to be a right to use one means in particular (i.e., assisted suicide).

18. "Evil" is used as equivalent to "bad," in this context. I add "at least" since some may think that death can sometimes be a positive good. I also assume that death is not only at least *a* lesser evil, but *the* least evil of the patient's options. (I owe the latter point to Seana Shiffrin.)

19. Dworkin et al. argue that the State may regulate assisted killing to make sure it is done with the patient's consent and is in his interest (given his own values). In keeping with the view that there is no difference between killing and letting die for the patient, Dworkin suggests that the same regulations should apply to decisions to let patients die. But I have already suggested that the reason for allowing letting die may be different from the reason for allowing killing or assisting in killing.

20. See chapter 4 this volume.

21. I am grateful to Joshua Cohen, Seana Shiffrin, and Timothy Hall for their comments on an earlier version of this chapter.

4

Four-Step Arguments for Physician-Assisted Suicide and Euthanasia

In this chapter, I shall present three arguments for the permissibility of physician-assisted suicide.[1] I shall focus on *active* physician-assisted suicide (e.g., when a physician gives a lethal drug to a patient and the patient takes it, in which case both the physician and patient are active).[2] I shall assume the patient is a competent, responsible agent, who gives his being in physical discomfort (pain, nausea, etc.) as the reason for intending his death.[3] I am assuming, therefore, that though the pain is a source of suffering, it does not undermine his rational agency in a way that threatens responsibility for choice. Current legal proposals for permitting physician-assisted suicide focus on procedures that determine the patient to be competent; hence they are concerned with showing that when (and only when) one knows that a still-reasonable being would die is physician-assisted suicide permissible. (This insistence that we may only aid in the destruction of a being once we have certified its high status may strike many as perverse.)

Furthermore, in the cases of physician-assisted suicide I shall consider, I assume death is in the patient's interest given his alternatives. In this respect, the cases are like euthanasia, though in general, physician-assisted suicide is unlike euthanasia in that it does not conceptually require that death be in the patient's interest. How can death be overall in someone's interest? Suppose death shortens a person's life so that the life has fewer bad things in it and does not deprive him of any significant good things because there would not have been any. Then death might be in someone's interest because his shorter life is a better thing than his longer life would have been. For example, we could imagine, independently of any question of active termination, that someone could reasonably prefer, for his own sake, to be created to a life of sixty years with no pain in it than to be created to a life of sixty-one years where the last year was full of pain. This could be so even if death is bad not only when it deprives us of goods but because it puts an end to us.[4] Putting off our being all over may not be worth every misery, especially since we cannot be immortal in any case. Someone does not have to continue on after death experiencing good things (e.g., pain-free postmortem conscious life) in order for the shorter life to be better for him. In any case, I shall assume this is so.[5]

Dworkin et al., in "Assisted Suicide: The Philosophers' Brief,"[6] try to argue that if we may let die (including terminating treatment) while intending death, then we may assist killing while intending death.[7] By contrast, we shall here try to argue that if we may treat patients when they consent though we *foresee* that this treatment will rapidly kill them, then we may kill or assist in killing patients when they consent, though we *intend* their death.

Prequel to the Arguments for Physician-Assisted Suicide and Euthanasia

It is morally (and legally) permissible for doctors, at least with the consent of a terminally ill patient, to give morphine for pain relief where pain is severe and otherwise not manageable, even if they foresee *with 100 percent certainty* that death would thereby soon occur (and sooner than it would without morphine) due to the morphine.[8] (Call this the Morphine for Pain Relief Case, or MPR.) Notice that this could be true even if the morphine put the patient in a deep unconscious state from which he never awoke before he died from it, so that he did not experience conscious, pain-free, worthwhile time alive. (It is important to emphasize this, since suicide or euthanasia will not produce pain-free life prior to death. If we want to hold factors constant between cases, we should not imagine a case where we foresee death that also has an additional good experience in it that is absent in the case in which death is intended.) Why may doctors act in MPR? One reason given is that, in this particular type of case involving a terminal patient, the *greater good is relief of pain* and the *lesser evil (indeed, the least evil possible in the circumstances) is the loss of life* (in the very same person), given that life would end soon anyway and is of bad quality. This means the patient is overall benefited by a shorter pain-free life rather than by a longer, painful life. In addition, in a nonterminal patient, it may be that some pain is so bad that even if it would eventually be followed by an outweighing degree of good, one should not have to go through it. (There is a nonconsequentialist quality to this reasoning, for just as the nonconsequentialist says that there are some things one need not do to promote best consequences in general, this reasoning claims that there are some things a person might reasonably decline to go through, even to promote the best consequences for himself.[9]) Giving morphine for pain relief might also be permissible in this nonterminal case, though death will result.

The absence of pain is a comparative good; that is, it is better than pain. Although it is not an intrinsic good (like pleasure), this does not stop it from outweighing an evil. (Similarly, relief of pain could outweigh brief nausea that is a side effect of a painkiller.) In the MPR Case, the lesser evil of death is only a foreseen side effect. It is not intended, hence this is not a case of euthanasia. (The fact that death will occur with certainty does not mean it is intended. If someone has a drink to soothe his nerves and foresees that it will certainly cause a hangover tomorrow, that does not mean that he intends the hangover.) Still, in the MPR Case, the doctor gives a drug which is inducing death, so I see no reason not to call this a case of killing, even though the doctor does not intend the death. (It is quite possible to kill without intending death, as when one accidentally runs over someone while driving a car.)

However, it might be argued that there is another reason why giving the morphine in MPR is permissible. This reason does not require one to accept the view that death sometimes involves a lesser evil while pain relief is a greater good. (Hence, while this view is sufficient to explain the permissibility of MPR, it is not necessary.) Another reason is that doctors may give MPR foreseeing death because death will occur soon anyway if the patient is terminal.[10] Therefore, even if death were always a greater evil than pain, when it will occur imminently no matter what we do, it is permissible to produce an overall better state of affairs by giving morphine for pain relief to at least eliminate the pain, which is avoidable.

The two premises—death involves a lesser evil and imminence of death anyway—have different implications in cases in which the patient is not terminal. Only if death involves no more than the (least) lesser evil would we permit a doctor to give a painkiller that will hasten death if the patient would not otherwise die soon anyway, but would live on in great pain for a long time.

Now suppose the morphine has lost its pain-relieving effects on the patient. It can still be used to kill the patient as a means to ending his pain, and the patient requests its use to kill him in order to end his pain. Call this the Morphine for Death Case (MD). It is said by some that we may not give the morphine in this case. This is so even if relief of pain is still the greater good and death the (least) lesser evil, and though the consequences of killing him are *essentially* the same as in MPR. It is said to be impermissible to *intend the lesser evil* as a means to a greater good. Those who say this may support what is called the Doctrine of Double Effect (DDE), according to which it may be permissible to act for some greater good with the foresight that one's conduct will have some lesser evil as a consequence but impermissible to act with the intent to produce that same evil as a means to a greater good. (Though not all supporters of some version of DDE would rule out killing in MD.)

I said the consequences in MPR and MD were *essentially* the same. It is worth pointing out a way in which the cases differ somewhat. When morphine is a pain-killer, it produces at least a short span of life without pain. The death that is the side effect might be the effect of (a) the morphine itself—that is, a side effect of our means to the greater good of no pain; or (b) it might be the result of the greater good itself (being pain-free) produced by morphine. The former is what actually occurs. The latter would occur (though it does not in fact occur) if pain relief, rather than morphine, altered the body's chemistry in such a way as to lower the heart rate and lead to death. In both these scenarios, the death is clearly a causal effect of either the morphine or the pain relief, and the pain relief is caused by the morphine. In MD, where death is the means to pain relief, the pain relief does not involve a span of life without pain. Furthermore, the good of absence of pain does not follow as a *causal effect* of the death, even though the death is intended as a means to pain relief.[11] The nonexistence of pain is best described as a part of the whole which consists of nonexistence of the person; that is, pain relief is a part of death. The elimination of life has as one of its parts, not as its causal after-effect, the absence of any experience and hence the absence of bad experience (e.g., pain).

Given this, in what sense do we intend the lesser evil in MD? If an evil of death is the absence of a few more of the good experiences of life, and this is also a part of nonexistence, we need not necessarily be intending *it* if we aim at death in order to achieve its other part, namely the absence of the bad experiences. If we nevertheless are intending a lesser evil in MD—as is commonly thought—and not just foreseeing it, this must be because future nonexistence of the person (or end of life) is itself an evil, in addition to the loss of further goods that would have been made possible by life. Hence, we intend an evil in intending death only if there is an evil to death aside from the loss of goods of life. (It is surprising, I believe, that this view about what is bad about death is implied by the view that to intend death is not merely to foresee an evil.) By contrast, if we thought that the only thing that makes death bad is the absence of more goods of life, then we would not be able to say that in intending death and foreseeing the absence of these goods, we would be intending an evil. And the DDE then could not be used as an objection to killing in MD.

One alternative is to say that if we intend the whole (nonexistence), then we do intend all its parts, including the lesser evil of losing out on some good experiences. I do not think this is correct. Another alternative is to say that intending death is not per se to intend an evil. I suspect this is not right either. But, to repeat, if it were, the DDE could not be used to argue against the administration of morphine in MD.[12]

Let us assume that we do intend an evil in MD. Without denying that sometimes the distinction between intending and foreseeing death makes a moral difference, I believe there is an argument to show that it provides no reason against performing euthanasia or physician-assisted suicide when death is the lesser evil (and indeed the least evil of alternatives available). The first step is to show that on many other occasions already, doctors (with the patient's consent) *intend the lesser evil* to a person in order *to produce his own greater good*. For example, it is permissible for a doctor to intentionally amputate a healthy leg (the lesser evil) in order to get at and remove a cancerous tumor, thereby saving the patient's life (the greater good).[13] It would be permissible for her to intentionally cause blindness in a patient if seeing would somehow destroy the patient's brain. It would be permissible for her to intentionally cause an hour of nausea if this were necessary to stop unbearable pain. Furthermore, it is permissible for her to intentionally cause someone pain, thereby acting contrary to a doctor's duty to relieve physical suffering, if this is a means to saving the person's life. For example, she might permissibly cause pain if this alone keeps a patient awake during lifesaving surgery that requires his responsiveness for success. The duty to save life sometimes just takes precedence over the other duty. Blindness, nausea, and pain are presumably intrinsic evils, so intending them is clearly intending lesser evil.

The Principle of Totality, a part of natural law theory (which also contains the DDE), permits us to destroy a part to save the whole and so seems to account for some of the above cases. But it also seems to conflict with, or override, the DDE. For insofar as the DDE is at issue, there should be a moral distinction not only between intending death and merely foreseeing it but also between intending to destroy sight and merely foreseeing its destruction. Insofar as we are not anymore dealing with a doctrine that denies the permissibility of intending all lesser evils for a person's own sake, *we are not really concerned with the DDE.* Rather, we shall find ourselves focusing on the specialness of intending death, for it is only then that we do not intend the destruction of a part of a person to preserve the whole of that person.

Now, we come to the next step in the argument for euthanasia and physician-assisted suicide: Why is it not permissible for doctors likewise to intend death when *it* is the lesser evil in order to produce the greater good of no pain, thereby benefiting the patient by giving her a shorter, less painful life rather than her enduring a longer, more painful one? Recall that one defense of MPR assumed that death would be the lesser evil and pain relief the greater good. That was one reason it was permissible to give the morphine. Indeed, one important reason we use the MPR case in this argument is to establish in a less controversial case the possible *relative values* of pain relief and death. Why may doctors not sometimes permissibly act against a duty to preserve life in order to relieve pain when death is the lesser evil and pain relief is the greater good, just as they can sometimes act against a duty to relieve pain in order to save a life when pain is the lesser evil and life the greater good? It is true that when we intend the destruction of the leg or cause blindness, we save the whole person, and in aiming at death, we destroy the whole person. But, as argued above, this may still overall benefit the whole person.

The Four-Step Arguments

A

The following Four-Step Argument is the result of our discussion so far. Assuming patient consent:

1. Doctors may permissibly relieve pain in a patient (e.g., by giving morphine), even if they know with certainty that this will cause the death of the patient as a foreseen side effect, when death is a lesser evil and pain relief is a greater good for the same person and only the morphine can stop the pain.[14] This is the Morphine for Pain Relief (MPR) Case.
2. Doctors may permissibly intentionally cause other lesser evils to patients when these are the necessary means to their medically relevant greater good (e.g., a doctor might permissibly intentionally cause a patient pain temporarily if only this would keep the patient from falling into a permanent coma).[15]

3. When death is a lesser evil for a person, it is not morally different from other lesser evils.[16]

4. Therefore, when death is a lesser evil and pain relief is a greater good for the same person (just as it is in Step 1), it is also permissible to intentionally cause death, or assist in its being intentionally caused, when it alone can stop pain. (For example, we could give morphine, which itself no longer relieves pain, in order to induce death. This is the Morphine for Death (MD) Case.)[17]

This argument applies to terminal and nonterminal cases. Recall that we also considered the possibility that death might always be a greater evil, and yet it would be permissible to act in MPR because of the unavoidable imminence of death. Using this premise, we could construct the following Alternative Four-Step Argument for terminal cases only.

Assuming patient consent:

1a. Doctors may permissibly relieve pain (e.g., by giving morphine), even if they know with certainty that this will cause the death of the patient as a foreseen side effect (*and even if death is a greater evil than pain*), when death is unavoidably imminent in any case (e.g., in a terminal patient) and the morphine alone can stop pain.

2a. Doctors may permissibly intentionally cause other (greater) evils that are unavoidably imminent anyway when these are the means to producing (lesser) goods in the same patient. (For example, suppose that it is worse to be blind than to be deaf. If a patient will shortly be blind anyway, it would be permissible to intentionally cause the blindness, if only this would prevent the patient from also going deaf.)

3a. When death is an imminent evil for a person, it is not morally different from other imminent evils.

4a. Therefore, doctors may permissibly intentionally cause death, or assist in its being intentionally caused, when death is imminent anyway and intentionally causing death alone can stop pain in the same patient (even if death is a greater evil and relief of pain is a lesser good).

In the Alternative Four-Step Argument, we need not assume that a shorter life with less suffering can be better for someone than a much longer one with more suffering, only that it is in one's interest to die somewhat sooner when death would come soon anyway and only dying sooner can reduce suffering.

The general structure of the two Four-Step Arguments is to show that in some carefully circumscribed cases, if we may permissibly kill people or assist in causing their death where we foresee the death as a side effect, we may also kill them intending the death, or assist them in intentionally causing their own death, when the death is the means to their (greater) good. Note that the arguments do not *merely* say that the doctors who permissibly give the morphine when it relieves pain may do so even if they intend their patients' deaths, though I believe this is true. In such a case, the morphine they give would relieve the patients' pain and even if that is not the doctors' aim in giving them the morphine, the fact that relief occurs can make the act permissible. In this way, the pain relief provides a pretext because it could justify the act of giving morphine, even when a doctor does not care to relieve pain but only intends death. Rather, the Four-Step Arguments are concerned in their conclusion with more than this; they are concerned with a doctor who (it is reasonable to think) could have no other reason for giving morphine besides killing since the morphine itself no longer relieves pain but only causes the death that is the means to pain relief. (Furthermore, even a bad doctor who does not intend that the patient not be in pain, but only wants to have the experience of intentionally killing or assisting in suicide, may permissibly proceed if the killing will in fact relieve the pain and pain relief can justify the killing or assisted suicide.)

The Four-Step Arguments are directed against the common use of the Doctrine of Double Effect (DDE) to rule out suicide, assisted suicide, and euthanasia. One need not agree with the more radical claim that the distinction between intending and foreseeing evil never makes a moral difference to permissibility in order to hold that it makes no difference when the lesser evil is A's pain, when we have A's consent, and when the greater good is saving A's life. We may act merely foreseeing the pain or intending it, as premise (2) in the first Four-Step Argument claims. The intention to cause something bad (the lesser evil) need not be a bad intention in itself, when the same person who suffers pain benefits more. The Four-Step Argument says, in part, that the same is true when death is a lesser evil and not going on living is the greater good.[18]

B

The structure of the Four-Step Arguments can be contrasted with that employed by the Philosophers' Brief.[19] Dworkin et al. argue that if we may let someone die (e.g., omit or terminate medical treatment) when he and we intend his death, then we may assist him by giving him lethal medication which he takes when he and we intend his death. I criticized this alternative argument on the following ground (among others): It is often permissible to let someone die when the person intends his death and we also intend his death, even when death is against the patient's overall best interest (and does not prevent an event which he could reasonably want to avoid regardless of future good). This is because the alternative is forcing treatment on him, and this we must not do if he competently refuses it. But it is not necessarily permissible to give a lethal substance to someone that he will take when death is neither in his overall best interest nor helping him avoid an event that he could reasonably wish to avoid regardless of future good. However, in medical contexts, if we are permitted to give someone a painkiller to stop pain though we foresee that the painkiller will also kill him, this will only be because the scenario in which he dies sooner is either overall better for him or helps him avoid an event one could reasonably wish to avoid regardless of future good. This crucial factor—that death is in his overall best interest—must be already present in the first premise of each Four-Step Argument, while it is not present in the let-die-hence-assist-to-kill argument. And the role of this factor in making action permissible is already endorsed by those (e.g., Catholic moral theologians) who can support MPR.

It may be permissible to go directly from the permissibility of letting die while intending death to the permissibility of killing or assisting killing while intending death *if death is a lesser evil* (relative to relief of pain, for example). This qualifier is not necessary in a Four-Step Argument because, in a Four-Step Argument, we *cannot get to the first step* without death being at least the lesser evil (or imminent). Hence we can move more easily from the first step to the conclusion that killing is permissible.

Still (as I claimed in chapter 3), it is true that when death is a lesser (and least) evil, the greater good is a medically appropriate aim, and there is patient consent, it will also be true that killing or assisting in a killing is as acceptable a means to death as letting die. I have not denied this. Why, then, focus on the Four-Step Arguments rather than on the let-die-hence-assist-to-kill-when-death-is-a-lesser-evil argument? As I have said before, my sense is that it is helpful to show that it is not bad to intend (i.e., someone could exhibit a good character in intending) the patient's death when the only reasonable justification for doing what kills or assists killing is that it kills or assists killing. I am here trying to distinguish (1) cases in which someone intends a death, but the properties and effects of the act are such that another agent could reasonably justify doing the act without intending the death (because, for example, the morphine stops pain directly), from (2) cases in which someone intends a death and the properties of the act are such that another agent could not reasonably justify doing the act without intending the death (because only death stops the pain).

We can imagine cases of type (1) where doing an act is permissible, even though the intention of the agent for the death of the patient is bad. This is true when we imagine a malicious doctor terminating treatment at a patient's request, though doing this is against a patient's interest, only because the doctor intends a patient's death against his interest. It is also true when we imagine a doctor terminating treatment at a patient's request when doing so *is* in the patient's interest, but only because the doctor wants to have ultimate power over a person's death. In such a case, the properties of the act could give another agent who did not intend the death good reason to act in the same way—that is, so as not to force treatment on someone or to act in someone's best interests. Similarly, when a doctor gives morphine that will relieve pain because he intends the act's other, death-causing properties, another doctor would have reason to do the same act intending only the morphine-caused pain relief while merely foreseeing the death. But if morphine no longer relieves pain, yet can still induce death, it is reasonable to think that only a doctor who intends death would have a reason to give the morphine and so this is a type (2) case.[20]

When we allow that it is permissible to *let die* while intending death, we can do so without inquiring into the morality of intending death or having death be a means to an end, as such, since (as argued above) the alternative to allowing termination of treatment is forcing treatment on someone, and not doing this could provide a justifying reason for termination. Hence even someone who incorrectly intends the death of patients might permissibly unplug them from life support at their request. But when we want to kill or assist in killing someone, forcing treatment is not the alternative; so then what we must do is show *why*, when death is a lesser evil or imminent, doing what could only be explained by someone's intending death is morally acceptable. This is what we are forced to do by the Four-Step Arguments. By contrast, the argument in "Assisted Suicide: The Philosophers' Brief" even modified as above threatens to conceal the importance of doing this by leading us to think that we have already argued for the permissibility of doing what could only be explained by intending death when we conclude that letting die while intending death is permissible.

However, as noted above, the fact that the Four-Step Arguments show that there is a morally acceptable intention to cause death is compatible with any particular doctor having a morally unacceptable intention to cause death while still acting permissibly in intentionally causing death. For example, suppose that the doctor knows that the only means to stop the patient's pain (the greater good) is to cause the patient's death (the lesser evil). However, this doctor does not intend that the patient not be in pain; she only wants to have the experience of intentionally killing someone as an end in itself. She differs from another doctor who has (it has been argued) the morally acceptable intention to produce death as a means to stopping pain. Yet the bad doctor may permissibly proceed. One argument we have considered so far says that this is because the facts of the case make it possible for some other agent to reasonably have a good intention for the same behavior. But an alternative explanation drops reference to intention altogether. It says that the doctor may proceed because the morally relevant objective features of the act—regardless of anyone's intention—remain the same: the death is a lesser evil to a person that causes greater good to that same person, and the person consents to the lesser evil. It is these constant objective features that make it true that there is a possible intention that focuses on them, and it is these objective features of the act that justify the act that make the possible intention morally acceptable (rather than vice versa). This alternative explanation is not concerned with showing that it is the fact that a possible agent could have a good intention when he intends an evil as a means that makes an actual agent's act permissible.

This point is the basis for the more radical critique of the Doctrine of Double Effect, namely that intention (actual or possible) per se rarely accounts for the moral permissibility or impermissibility of an act.[21] If this radical claim is true, then, I believe, Dworkin et al. are wrong in holding that what accounts for the impermissibility of a physician's act is intention to act against the best interests of a patient. It would be other facts of the case (that happen to also be possible objects of an intention) that account for impermissibility of an act.[22]

A Doctor's Duty?

A

Dworkin et al. claim that patients have a right to assisted suicide only from a willing physician. They do not claim that a doctor has a duty to assist suicide. Indeed, while they argue that the distinction between terminating treatment and assisting killing does not make a moral difference with respect to how we should treat the patient, they think the distinction makes a difference with respect to how we should treat the doctor. It affects whether he has a duty to act for a patient. They say that a doctor sometimes must terminate treatment because the alternative is forcing treatment, but because this is not the alternative if he does not assist killing, he can decide for himself whether to assist killing.[23] I have argued that it is just this distinction between the alternatives to terminating treatment and assisting killing that makes some factors—like patients' best interests, medically appropriate good a patient seeks, and possibly intentions—have a less significant role in terminating treatment than in assisting killing.[24]

I believe that yet another Four-Step Argument for a doctor's duty to assist suicide or to perform euthanasia may be available, as puzzling as the existence of such a duty seems. Assuming patient consent:

1b. Doctors have a *duty* to treat pain (e.g., with morphine), even if they foresee with certainty that it will make them cause the patient's death soon, because death is a lesser evil (including least evil alternative) and pain relief is a greater good, or because death is unavoidably imminent (even if it is a greater evil) and only morphine can stop the pain.

2b. Doctors have a *duty* to intentionally cause evils (e.g., pain, blindness) for a patient's own medical good when the evils are (least) lesser and the goods to be achieved by them greater, or when the evils are unavoidably imminent anyway (even if greater) and the evils are each the only way to achieve a medically relevant good.

3b. When death is a lesser or imminent evil for a person, it is not morally different from other lesser or imminent evils.

4b. Therefore, doctors have a *duty* to intentionally cause the patient's death or assist in its being intentionally caused when death is a (least) lesser evil and pain relief is a greater good, or when death is imminent anyway and pain relief is a good for the patient and only death can bring it about.[25]

Call this last Four-Step Argument the Doctor's Duty Argument. This argument, as well as arguments showing that it is morally permissible for a doctor to perform assisted suicide or euthanasia, is limited to the achievement of medically relevant goods, whatever they are. By contrast, suppose it would be in a patient's best interest to be killed in order to achieve posthumous glory. The good of posthumous glory is not a good a doctor is called upon to help patients achieve.

The Doctor's Duty Argument is important because some have claimed that doctors' *professional ethic*, in particular, implies that they may not engage in physician-assisted suicide. By contrast, this argument suggests that doctors' professional ethic sometimes calls for them to perform assisted suicide or even euthanasia. It is also important because it shows that while a doctor might, for example, permissibly raise a conscientious objection to killing a fetus in abortion, such an objection to assisted suicide or euthanasia is not similarly permissible. This is because harming people for their own greater good is morally different from harming one being for the sake of the greater good of another being. Hence, even if a doctor might conscientiously refuse to intentionally cause such evils as blindness in a fetus for the sake of helping a woman in whose body the fetus grows, he could be required to blind a person to save that person's life, with the person's consent. If one continues to believe that doctors may conscientiously refuse to assist in suicide in the cases I have described, one will have to show what is wrong with the Doctor's Duty Argument for the opposite conclusion.[26]

B

The Doctor's Duty Argument says that it can be a doctor's duty to participate in assisted suicide or euthanasia, because sometimes these behaviors are analogous to other interventions that are obligatory for doctors to perform. But this argument does not tell us the ground of doctor's duties and is compatible with several grounds. The degree of moral responsibility that a doctor has for the patient's death may vary depending on what is the ground of the doctor's duty to intervene. Consider two possible grounds.

The first takes the view that doctors have a duty of medical beneficence. That is, one of the projects to which they commit themselves is the good of patients, including relief of the misery of their patients so long as this is not against their patient's wishes. The second view emphasizes the patient's autonomy. In certain contexts, it is said, patients may decide for themselves what should be done for them. It is then a doctor's duty to serve the patient's will (given that it falls within a medically appropriate end), at least when it is not obviously against the patient's medical interests to do so. Hence, on the second view, the doctor should act as a patient's agent in carrying out her wishes when doing so is not obviously against her interests.

On the second view, the doctor commits himself to the project of being the patient's agent, at least so long as this is not obviously against the patient's interests, rather than to the project of doing what is best for the patient, so long as this is not against the patient's wishes. There is a reversal of emphasis in these two accounts. Only the second view *need not imply* in physician-assisted suicide either that the doctor agrees with the patient's decision to die or that the doctor is fulfilling his own project to do what is best for the patient, either in seeking the patient's death or by giving him the option to choose death. It can be argued that in prescribing a lethal drug, the doctor's intention is to either give the patient a choice about ending her life or to help the patient die simply because this serves the patient's will.

Intending in this way that the patient have what he wants can also lead a doctor to actively kill a patient when the patient decides that he wants to die but is unable to kill himself. Yet if the doctor does not in this case kill for the patient's good, but only to carry out the patient's wishes when it is not obviously against the patient's interests, then this active killing is *not* appropriately called euthanasia. (This is not a judgment of its moral permissibility, only of its type.) This is because euthanasia involves killing the patient intending his good. Hence, there is a form of active killing of the patient to which the patient consents that may be permissible even though it is not euthanasia. In this form of killing, unlike physician-assisted suicide by provision of lethal drugs to be used by the patient, the doctor causes the patient's death and does the patient's bidding, when it is not obviously against the patient's interests that she do so.

I suggest that on the agent model of the doctor, positive moral responsibility and accountability for all positive and negative consequences of killing the patient or providing lethal substances lie at the patient's doorstep. What is true about moral responsibility and accountability on the beneficence model of the doctor when the doctor performs either voluntary euthanasia or assisted suicide? On the beneficence model, seeking the death because it is good for the patient is at least a project of the doctor's. Let us assume the patient also seeks his good (though he could seek his death for some other reason, even when it is good for him). Then both decide the patient's death best fulfills their individual projects. But the doctor cannot fulfill his project without the patient's consent. Even though this is true, it seems to me that the doctor is more than the patient's agent once he gets the consent. Doctor and patient are like two people who build something together on land only one of them owns and whose permission is necessary. For this reason, doctor and patient may share positive moral responsibility and accountability for negative and positive consequences.

I suggest that if complete positive moral responsibility for any negative consequences of assisted suicide or voluntary euthanasia would be at the patient's doorstep in the agent model, this might be a reason for the doctor to feel free to act as an agent when she would otherwise be reluctant to act from beneficence. This includes cases where she thinks that the patient is doing the overall right thing in choosing death, but the doctor herself does not act in order to bring about death as a good.

The distinction I have drawn between two ways of conceiving the doctor's behavior is sometimes not recognized in discussions of these topics. For example, Dan Brock says: "Both physician and family members can instead be helped to understand that it is the patient's decision and consent to stopping treatment that limits their responsibility for the patient's death and that shifts responsibility to the patient."[27] Brock, however, also says in discussing assisted suicide: "Seeking a physician's assistance, or what can almost seem a physician's blessing, may be a way of trying to remove that stigma and show others that . . . the decision for suicide was . . . justified under the circumstances. The physician's involvement provides a kind of social approval." But I believe what makes the first claim true may make the second claim false. For it seems that only when the doctor is merely an agent does moral responsibility for the killing lie completely with the patient, and then helping the patient or killing him does not imply that the doctor has blessed the patient's decision or shown that it is justified under the circumstances.

Could it also be that what would make Brock's second claim true would make his first claim false? For if a doctor acts only because he approves of the patient's choices, then he may also be acting for the sake of his own goal to do good for the patient, as the patient acts for her goal. His acting for his own goal, rather than just as the patient's agent, could give the doctor a share in moral responsibility for both the negative and the positive aspects of the death. But it is also possible that Brock's particular scenario allows one to imagine that the doctor is still only an agent whose own views about the patient's good are fortuitously achieved without his committing himself to a goal of beneficence. If this were so, then the truth of the second claim need not make the first claim false.

Variants

Can variants of the Four-Step Arguments be applied to cases not involving pain relief? Perhaps so, but we must be careful how we argue. The danger that we will extend ourselves beyond what we are allowed is, I think, exemplified in Peter Singer's discussion of euthanasia. He describes the rules governing the practice in the Netherlands, as follows:

- Only a medical practitioner should carry out euthanasia.
- There should be an explicit request from the patient that leaves no room for doubt about the patient's desire to die.
- The patient's decision should be well-informed, free, and persistent.
- The patient must be in a situation of unbearable pain and suffering without hope of improvement.
- There must be no other measures available to make the patient's suffering bearable.
- The doctor must be very careful in reaching the decision and should seek a second opinion from another independent doctor.[28]

Singer then gives the following case as an example of a real-life instance of this practice:

> In the case of Carla, too, though she had a continuous infusion of morphine, she did not want to die by a gradually increasing dose, which would most likely have put her into a state of drowsy confusion for some days before death came. She preferred to die at a time of her own choosing, with her family around her.[29]

But this very case which he gives to illustrate the practice does not clearly fall under the rules he cites. The rules say that lethal medicine is to be administered only if there is unbearable pain and suffering. Apparently the Dutch take this to include psychological suffering and the sense that one's dignity will be lost. Assume they are correct. Carla could have had her pain relieved by morphine; she received a lethal injection because she did not want to die from an increased dosage of morphine in drowsy confusion. Is dying in drowsy confusion a threat to one's dignity? Did the thought of it cause Carla unbearable psychological suffering? If not, then Carla just had a preference for one way of dying and the rules do not imply this is sufficient to trigger physician-assisted suicide or euthanasia. It is striking that Singer himself does not notice—was not on the lookout for?—a possible transgression of the supposed rules. Even if the rules should be changed to allow that such a case is permissible, what worries many people is that violations of extant rules suggest that there will be insufficient attention paid to *any* rules.

Now consider a variant of the Four-Step Argument in which some of the steps may not be satisfied, even when death is a lesser (least) evil. Suppose a person will rapidly produce great paintings if he is given a drug that will, as a foreseen side effect, soon cause his death. Let us assume that producing great paintings is a greater good for him and death is a lesser evil. Still, it may not be appropriate for a doctor to give drugs to increase creativity if death is a rapid side effect of the drug. This is because the Four-Step Argument is made on the assumption that the greater good is a medically appropriate goal, and it is a problem in the philosophy of medicine (which I cannot here discuss) whether this patient's goal is medically appropriate. If we cannot assume the permissibility of doing what we merely foresee will cause death, we cannot use the Four-Step Argument to justify giving someone lethal pills if, for example, he intends to kill himself because only the onset of death will prompt last-minute brilliant painting. So I suggest what I shall call The Test: See if you can get the first step in a Four-Step Argument (involving causing only foreseen death) in order to see if eliminating some condition in someone's life or pursuing a goal permits one to help kill or assist in killing another as an intended means to the same goal.

How about death to end psychological suffering? The Test says: Could we permissibly give a drug that puts someone into a restful sleep in order to stop such psychological suffering if we foresaw that the drug would rapidly kill him as a side effect with no improved quality of life first? If not, then giving pills to a patient who intends to kill himself in order to end such psychological suffering would not be sanctioned by the Four-Step Argument.[30] How about incontinence? Would a doctor correctly give a drug to cure incontinence when she foresees that the drug will rapidly kill a patient as a side effect? If not, then physician-assisted suicide to end a life only because it involves incontinence will not be endorsed by the Four-Step Argument. Would we give a patient a cheaper drug whose side effect will soon cause death rather than give him a safer, more expensive drug, because the expensive drug would be a financial burden for his family? If not, then the Four-Step

Argument does not imply that we may perform physician-assisted suicide because his treatment is a burden on the family's finances.[31] Of course, the application of the (rough) test I have suggested—see if you can get the first step in a Four-Step Argument—may yield positive, rather than negative, responses to these questions.

However, now it is important to show that if we fail to get the first premise *for certain special reasons*, it is still possible to use a Four-Step Argument. These two reasons are: (1) giving the drug that has death as a side effect makes things worse than they would be if the patient simply died, and (2) giving the drug that has death as a side effect makes no positive difference for the patient, aside from that produced by death. Let us consider cases that illustrate these points.

A case that exhibits the first reason could arise if a drug that ended pain also left the patient in a totally dependent, subrational condition for a time before causing death. In the opinion of some, his being in this state could be a reason for not giving the drug that could not be raised against killing or assisting in killing him. So we could get the first premise needed for a Four-Step Argument—showing that we may do what foreseeably causes death—by subtracting what makes the case of foreseen death worse than the case of intended death. Then the Four-Step Argument will still be successful in justifying killing or assisted killing while intending death.

A case that exhibits the second reason for not getting the first premise—the drug that has death as a side effect makes no positive difference for the patient, aside from producing death—could arise if a drug that cures dementia in a very demented but calm patient would put him in an unconscious state and will soon kill him. If one refused to give the drug, this may be because, in giving the drug, one would not be making any positive difference to a patient's quality of life, since the undemented unconscious state is no better than the conscious demented state. That is, even if it had no fatal side effect, one would seem to lack a positive reason for giving the drug to a calm, demented person, knowing that he will only then go into a coma.[32] But just because a rational agent cannot act to give a drug that has death as an unintended side effect unless the drug produces some positive change that gives him a reason to act, this does not mean that seeking to *end a life* of a certain sort is not sufficient justification for action, when death is a lesser evil and avoiding what is in the life is a greater good. For example, suppose being calm and demented is no better and no worse than being undemented and in a coma, so one would not give a drug to produce the latter state. Still, the elimination of either one of these states might be a permissible goal in itself.[33] For, both of these states, because they involve a period of dependence in a subrational state before death, might be greater evils, given some patients' values, than death.

In sum, sometimes to get the first premise for a Four-Step Argument, we must *subtract* what makes giving a drug with foreseen death *worse* than death and also *compensate* for the absence of any positive reason for acting aside from seeking the benefit from death per se.

Some Objections to the Four-Step Arguments

Objections may be raised to the Four-Step Arguments for assisted suicide or voluntary euthanasia.[34] Almost all are based on the view that premises 3, 3a, and 3b are not true; that is, eliminating the person as a means to the person's own greater good is not morally the same as eliminating some part of him as a means to his greater good while he survives. In considering some of the objections, I shall keep in mind two issues that I believe are critical. (1) Does the objection show that physician-assisted suicide or euthanasia is morally wrong? (2) If it does, must it also rule out giving the morphine for pain relief when it is foreseen with certainty that it will soon cause death? It will be a big problem for any objection if it also requires us to give up the permissibility of MPR when this foreseeably causes death soon. The Supreme Court decisions in *Vacco et al.* v. *Quill et al.* and *State of Washington et al.* v. *Glucksberg et al.* concluded that such death-hastening, palliative care was *legally* permissible at least in terminal cases—premise 1a in the Alternative Four-Step Argument—and two justices (Sandra Day O'Connor and Stephen Breyer) emphasized that one important reason why they did not find laws against assisted suicide unconstitutional was that palliative care, even if it caused death sooner (and soon), was legally permitted.[35] If moral objections cannot be raised to physician-assisted suicide without also morally undermining morphine for pain relief which causes death soon, the legal distinction may be undermined as well; both will be justified, or neither. One general point of my discussion will be that many objections to physician-assisted suicide and euthanasia also rule out MPR, and objections based on the Doctrine of Double Effect (DDE) will rule out other procedures that seem morally and legally acceptable.

A. KILLING

It may be objected that the doctor who intends the death of his patient in physician-assisted suicide or active euthanasia is involved in a *killing* or actually doing the killing. Even if intending a lesser evil for a greater good is permissible when this does not involve killing, when it does involve killing it is impermissible. One way of understanding this objection is that the killing is what makes things wrong. But how can one object to the conclusion of the Four-Step Arguments solely on grounds that they permit killing when giving the lethal injection in MPR also involves killing, and we approve of giving the morphine in that case?

A patient's right to life includes a right not to be killed but, some have argued, the right to life is a discretionary right—that is, it gives one a protected option whether to live or die, an option with which others may not interfere; it does not give one a duty to live. If a patient decides to take morphine for pain though he knows it will kill him, he is waiving his right to live, as someone may waive her right to speak on a given occasion. By waiving his right, he releases others (or specific others) from their duty not to do what will kill him, *insofar as their duty not to do what will kill him stems from his right to live.*[36] More particularly, he may exercise a power that his discretionary right to life gives him to license another person to assist him or kill him. This gives the other person a permission, with which others may not interfere, to assist in a killing or to kill. Does this power stem from a right the patient has to kill himself so that if he had no right to kill himself, he could not give to another a right to kill him? Not necessarily, for someone might be prohibited from killing himself on his own (because he could not do it correctly, for example), but still have the moral power to designate someone else to kill him or to help him perform the act. So the power to give someone the right (a permission with which others may not interfere) to perform euthanasia or to assist in suicide need not be based on a general right to suicide, although it might be.

Furthermore, a person's right to life might be discretionary only in certain conditions—for example, when life gets bad enough—and the power to give others the right to kill him may be limited to those conditions. Those others may also be limited in what they may permissibly do because their duty not to kill or assist in killing someone *stems* not only from another's right not to be killed, but from their *duty not to harm him*, even if he wishes them to do what harms him. This may be a duty from which he has no power to release them, even if he waives his right not to be killed. But I have stipulated that the doctor is to assist in killing or kill only when death is the least evil alternative for the patient and no harm overall is done to the patient.

Suppose a patient may permissibly waive his right to life insofar as it protects him from others giving him morphine as a painkiller when it is known that it will kill him as a side effect. Then it is not the inability to waive this right (nor the duty others have not to harm) that stands in the way of others intentionally killing him or assisting in his intentionally killing himself.[37]

Notice that I have emphasized that this waiver is morally necessary even when the doctor wishes to give morphine that will kill as a side effect. This means doctors should get permission for giving the morphine as a painkiller if it will kill as a side effect, as well as for giving it to intentionally kill. I do not believe they generally do so.[38]

B. INTENDING DEATH AS A MEANS AND TREATING ONESELF AS A MERE MEANS

What other reason could there be for the impermissibility of intentionally killing a patient as a means to end his pain? Rather than pointing to the killing alone, we might point to the distinctiveness of intending death rather than intending other lesser evils, or perhaps the combination of intending death and killing rather than letting die.[39]

In one revisionist proposal for distinguishing morally between intending and foreseeing harm to people *other than ourselves, without those others' consent*, Warren Quinn distinguishes between (1) not treating people as ends, and (2) treating them as mere means.[40] We do the former, he says, when we pursue our projects without constraining our behavior in light of the foreseen harm to others. We do the latter when we treat people as being available for our purposes, as something we can take charge of and use to meet our goals, even when this involves harm to them and is against their will. This is true when the harm is life-destroying and also when it is not. He thinks treating them as a mere means is a more serious wrong than just not treating them as ends, when the harm is equal. (Here he divides the Kantian injunction to treat persons as ends in themselves and not merely as means into two components.) On Quinn's analysis, *intending the involvement or use* of a person in a way which we *foresee* will lead to uncompensated harm to him without his consent is taken to be as wrong as *intending the uncompensated harm* to him without his consent (and hence, treating such *harm* to him as available for our purposes). The traditional DDE would distinguish these two, ruling out only the latter, since the DDE claims that it is aiming at such harm (harm being an evil) which makes action impermissible.

(The traditional DDE, but not necessarily Quinn, also seems to rule out intending the harm when it leads to overall good for the person himself as well, even when he consents to it. It does not distinguish between *intrapersonal* harm for benefit when one intends lesser harm to the same person who will greatly benefit from it and *interpersonal* harm for benefit when one intends harm to someone for another's benefit.[41] Hence, the DDE seems to rule out steps 2, 2a, and 2b as well in the Four-Step Arguments. Ruling these steps out is clearly incorrect. Hence, let us suppose that it limits its objection to death alone.)

Suppose it is permissible for a person to take, or to direct another to help him take, his own life as a means to stopping his pain. This implies that the whole of his person is not off limits to be used to stop his pain. Quinn does not object to such intended use of a person for his own good. But suppose morality had a special interest in people not seeing themselves as under their control to be used even for their own purposes in this way. This would be consistent with its not having as much interest in their refusing to preserve their lives, especially when death is merely foreseen. For it is possible that taking control of one's life can only be done actively. If one intends one's death and so *omits* to stop a deadly natural event that one has not set in motion (or one *removes a barrier* to the natural event), the element of control of self may be less. This is one reason (it may be said) why the *combination* of killing and intending death is often more significant than the combination of omitting or terminating treatment and intending death. (We shall consider two other reasons to morally distinguish killing and terminating treatment below.[42])

Obviously, people can take control of their whole lives and devote their beings to the pursuit of certain goals within the living of their lives. But, it is claimed, when this is appropriate, they do not aim to destroy their persons but rather set their persons in one direction or another. So, in physician-assisted suicide or euthanasia, we treat the *destruction of a person* as available for purposes of achieving her good. (We move from merely taking control of the person to taking control of the person in order to cause an evil, the destruction of the person. We intend not only involvement of the person but her destruction.) The Four-Step Arguments say that we may intend death if it is a lesser evil and if we may intend other lesser evils for a person's own good. Part of the objection to these arguments suggested here is that acting with the intention to bring about the lesser evil of death is different because it involves treating our whole selves (or another person, if we are doctors) as something we may take control of to destroy, in order to achieve the same person's good. We do not have such an intention when we intend such other lesser evils as blindness.

Furthermore, in voluntary euthanasia and physician-assisted suicide, we use a rational being in this way—a being who judges, aims at goals, and evaluates how to act. One of the things that seems odd about killing or helping to kill only some-one who is capable of competently deciding to be killed—this is the point of com-plicated controls on euthanasia and physician-assisted suicide—is that one is *making sure* that one is destroying a being who has worth in virtue of its capacity for reasoning, who is still capable of exercising that capacity. This will not be so if the person is permanently unconscious or vegetative or otherwise no longer func-tioning as a rational being.[43]

The idea that there are limits on what we may do to ourselves as persons is Kantian. Kant thought that rational humanity in ourselves and in others is (and should be treated as) *an end in itself, and not merely as means*.[44] Even if bads out-weigh what in our life is *good for us*, the fact that one is a rational agent in life—judging, aiming, evaluating—gives one worth. Thus, I (and, in that sense, my life) may have worth, even if my life does not provide benefits to me that outweigh bads to me. The worth *of me* as a person is not measured solely by my life's worth *to me* in satisfying my interests and desires, or its worth to others in satisfying theirs.[45]

This means that whether our life is a benefit to us (or death instead would benefit us) is a different question from whether we have worth (or death would end something of worth). Still, it seems possible that being a creature that has this worth *may be part of what makes my life worth living*, even if the bads *to me* out-weigh the goods to me in my life. Or, put another way, even if the bads outweigh goods *other than the good of being a person*, my life may be worth living because I am a person. Perhaps, then, if my life is *worth living* (in part because I am a being of a certain sort), then death will not be a lesser evil, even though it *would* remove things that are in important ways bad *for* me and not eliminate things that are in important ways good *for* me.

However, if it were possible for my life *not* to be worth living, and indeed worth not living, despite the fact that I continue to be someone of worth, then death could be a lesser evil and it could benefit me.[46] This could be so when negatives in the life are very great. So actively destroying someone could be a benefit for him consistent with its eliminating a creature of worth. The apparent oddity of making sure one only kills a being of worth who has reasonably chosen to die might thus be explained away. This analysis would also show that when one says someone's life is not worth living or worth not living, one is not necessarily saying that they have no worth as persons or are mere disposable entities.

According to Kant it is wrong for others to treat me as a mere means to their ends. They will not do so if they treat me as a means when it is a condition of their action that this is also beneficial to me. It is said to be possible, and equally wrong, for me to treat myself as a mere means even for my own ends such as eliminating pain. As others should respect my worth as a person by not using me merely as a means for their purposes, I should have proper regard for my own worth as a person, and not simply treat myself as a mere means to achieving goods and avoiding harms. But, it is said, that is precisely what I do when I aim at my own death as a way to eliminate pain. So I ought not to pursue that aim, and therefore ought not to consent to a morphine injection aiming at death, or give one to a patient who has consented. The Kantian objection to the Four-Step Arguments, as it is construed here, is that, in physician-assisted suicide, but not in MPR, a person is treated as a mere means, and this violates the Categorical Imperative of morality to always treat persons also as ends-in-themselves.

The question is how suicide or physician-assisted suicide can treat a person as a mere means if (a) the person himself consents to death, and (b) he seeks death because it is (assumed to be) overall in his best interest, there being only great misery in his future? Ordinarily, we think that (for example, in the interpersonal case) if we seek someone's overall good, we cannot be treating him as a mere means, but must be treating him also as an end-in-himself, at least if he consents. I believe it is useful to distinguish *three* different ways in which one might treat a person as a mere means.

1. Calculating the worth of living on in a way which gives insufficient (even no) weight to the worth of the person *in himself*, rather than as a means to other goods;
2. Treating the death of a person as a mere means to a goal (e.g., ending pain);
3. Using a person in order to bring about his own end.

The first idea is that a person has worth in himself and is not merely a means to what is good for him as a sentient being. On this interpretation, we treat persons as a mere means if we give no weight in our decisions to the independent worth of the person (or rational agents). But when does this occur? It occurs in one way if we see rational humanity in ourselves as merely an instrument for getting a positive balance of sentient good over evil in our life, and we are willing to eliminate rational humanity when the balance is sentient evil over good. Then we do not attribute intrinsic worth to ourselves as persons.[47] This analysis implies that the fact that one treats one's rational humanity (in one view, what makes one a person) as a way to achieve a good for *oneself* (and when being a person only leads to pain, we subordinate it to getting rid of pain) is not enough to constitute treating one's person as other than a *mere* means. One may still fail to respect oneself, to take oneself seriously as a person. That we are satisfying our interests as sentient beings rather than those of others is not enough to rebut the charge of treating our rational humanity as a mere means if we do not give *enough* weight to it.

Though I do not doubt that this idea has force, it can equally well be an objection to terminating a course of life-saving treatment or to MPR, when one merely foresees one's death. This raises the second issue I said I would keep in mind—namely, is MPR also ruled out by the objection to MD? This is because if we give too little weight to the worth of the person or to the value of being a rational agent in itself, the evil of pain will too quickly serve as a justification for taking morphine even when it causes death as a side effect. Hence, this sense in which we could see rational humanity as a mere means does not distinguish between intending death (a necessary condition for suicide) and causing pain relief with mere foresight of death. Likewise, if we take the worth of the person seriously so that only a great deal of pain could override the importance of his continuing, we will not have treated rational humanity in ourselves and others as a mere means (in the sense we are now examining) in either physician-assisted suicide or MPR.[48]

It might be said that this observation should prompt us to rethink the permissibility of ever killing in the case of morphine for pain relief, where death is foreseen but not intended. For, it might be said, if we allow stopping pain ever to override continued existence of rational humanity in a particular person, we do not give *unconditional and incomparable value* to rational humanity. And not treating a person as a mere means, it may be said, requires that we attribute such a type of value to him. (To have unconditional value is to have value always, but that does not yet mean to have overriding value, which is transmitted by "incomparable."[49]) This willingness to disallow MPR seems unjustified, though there are different ways to argue this point. Consider one way. Suppose life involves such great pain that one's whole life is focused on that pain. Some may claim that when this happens, one's status as a rational being is compromised,[50] and so when we kill in MPR, we no longer destroy rational humanity or even kill in order to end an insult to rational humanity. The point here is to argue that rational humanity is overriding, not merely a value that can be outweighed; whenever it seems to be outweighed, it has already been undermined or would be put in a condition unworthy of it if life continues and killing is impermissible. But, we may ask, if the person who asks for morphine as pain relief is still able to rationally weigh considerations and is in control of his faculties, has his rational nature truly been undermined or violated by pain?

Suppose one thought that the *diminished opportunity* to exercise one's rationality (because one is always focusing on one's pain) counts as the relevant sort of compromise of rationality. In these circumstances, it might be said, we can act to eliminate pain by MPR. But then shall we condone a drug that causes death as a side effect for someone who sleeps most of the time? This is an odd view, and certainly not one that can be justified on the ground that rational humanity itself no longer exists. A final thought experiment may help in this regard: Suppose someone's life alternates between days when someone is fully rational and able to exercise his rationality and days of intense pain when he is still rational but limited in his ability to do anything but focus on the pain.[51] In this case, one cannot argue that death by painkiller is tolerated because rational activity is already extremely limited, since every other day the person can engage in rational activities. Yet the pain may still reasonably drive the person to take medication that foreseeably causes death, I believe.

I conclude that when pain justifies MPR with death as a side effect, it need not be a matter of the deterioration or humiliation of rational nature, just the burden of living. Hence, one must instead argue that in such circumstances, one does not lack self-respect if one does what will cause one's end, for in so doing we do not treat our life as a *mere* means to a balance of goods over bads for us. We might acknowledge the great (and normally overriding) importance of *being* a person and believe it is right in many cases to go on in life even if it has more bads than other goods besides rational agency. Though we reject the thought that the person is merely a means to happiness (even his own), we allow that some very bad conditions may overshadow the value of the person's continuation.[52]

The key to making this argument, I think, is distinguishing between the value of something and the value of its continuing to exist. It can be that a person's being out of pain does not have greater value than the person does, but it has greater value than the *continuing existence of the person* (i.e., *being* a person). In the light of the non-overshadowed, incomparable value of a person, because a person continues to have worth, we might decide that it is not only important that a person be out of pain but that it would be permissible for the person not to live on in pain. In this sense, killing or helping to kill the person or letting him die can respect the incomparable worth of the person, even if it eliminates him. Hence, contrary to what was suggested above, the permissibility of eliminating the person for the sake of his good does not show that he lacks overriding worth, only that his continued existence lacks overriding value. Nor does it show that we are not acting in response to a person's worth by responding to his autonomous request to end his pain by death.

What, then, about the second and third interpretations I offered of the idea of using a person as a mere means (page 73)? Can they justify the distinction between engaging in MPR though we foresee it will result in our deaths, and aiming at our deaths? To see the difference between the second and the third interpretations, consider an analogy: My radio is a device for getting good sounds and filtering out bad sounds. It is a mere means to a balance of good sounds over bad ones. Suppose it stops performing well, that it only produces static, but cannot be turned off. I can wait until its batteries run down and not replace them, or I can smash it now, thus using the radio itself to stop the noise it produces. Either way, I would see its termination as I saw its existence, as a mere means to a better balance of good over bad sounds. While I have always seen my radio as a mere means to an end, if I smash it, I use it as a mere means to its end (termination). This is sense 3 of "treating as a mere means." (If I see someone else destroy the radio and do not interfere, I may be intending its use as a mere means to its own end, although I do not use it.) If I let the radio run down, intending its demise, but do not smash it—I see it wasting away and do not replace its parts—then I do not necessarily see it as a mere means to its own end, but I do *see its end (termination) as a mere means* to a better balance of sounds. This is sense 2 of "treating as a mere means." (Sense 3 incorporates Quinn's concern with using something as a way to cause it harm or damage. Sense 2 is close to the concern of the traditional DDE.)

The sort of use of the person as a means that takes place in active suicide or euthanasia is analogous to the smashing of the radio: The person uses himself, or another uses him, as a mere means to his own death. Some people find this complete taking control of a life particularly morally inappropriate, perhaps because they think that our bodies belong to God and that we have no right to achieve the goal of our own death by manipulating a "tool" that is not ours (or intending that others manipulate it). This objection is not present if—here we have sense 2—we terminate medical assistance with the intention that the system run down, aiming at its death, for then we achieve the goal of death by taking control of what is arguably ours (the medication), not what is God's. This is another reason why someone may not object to terminating treatment, even when intending death as a means in sense 2 is present, but may object to killing: Terminating treatment, unlike intentional killing, does not involve using as a means in sense 3. As we have seen though, some hold that sense 2 is also more objectionable than merely foreseeing the death. They say that if we terminate medical assistance, intending death, then though we may not treat *our person* merely as a means to a balance of greater good for us over bads for us (sense 1), we do treat *our death (the end of our life, destruction of our person)* as a mere means to greater good over bad.

How much weight, then, should be placed on the second and third senses of "use a person as a means?" Should they really stand in the way of physician-assisted suicide or euthanasia? Here are some reasons for saying no. It cannot be argued, at least with secular moral arguments, that one's body belongs to someone else and that one cannot, therefore, use it as a means to achieve death. Notice also that if your body belonged to someone else, it isn't clear why you should be permitted to use it in order to administer morphine as a painkiller when you foresee that this will destroy the body. We aren't usually permitted to treat other people's property, even property they have loaned to us for our use, in ways that certainly lead to its destruction. Hence, an objection based on sense 3 also does not distinguish between morphine in MPR and MD. This eliminates sense 3 as an objection, if MPR is permissible.

That leaves us with the question of whether treating one's death as available for one's purposes (sense 2) is necessarily a morally inappropriate attitude to take to oneself if one has not undervalued the importance of one's personhood and of continuing to be a person (not violating sense 1). I must admit that when I consider all we may permissibly intend (destruction of parts of persons) and all we may permissibly cause with mere foresight (destruction of the whole person), I find it hard to see why we may not treat one's death as available for one's greater good (including avoidance of greater evils), as the Four-Step Arguments hold. If this is so, then at least sometimes a patient would do no wrong and have no inappropriate intention in intentionally causing his death. At least sometimes, a doctor who helped him by giving pills would also do no wrong and have no inappropriate intention merely because she killed, or assisted killing, aiming at death.

Notes

1. This chapter is a revised version of parts of my "Physician Assisted Suicide, the Doctrine of Double Effect, and the Ground of Value," *Ethics* 109 (1999). That article built on my "A Right to Death," *The Boston Review* 22 (1997); parts of my "Physician-Assisted Suicide, Euthanasia, and Intending Death" (henceforth "PAS, E, and ID"), in *Physician-Assisted Suicide: Expanding the Debate*, eds. Margaret P. Battin, Rosamond Rhodes, and Anita Silvers (New York: Routledge, 1998), pp. 26–49); and parts of "Ending Life," in *The Blackwell Guide to Medical Ethics*, eds. R. Rhodes, L. Frances, and A. Silvers (Oxford: Wiley-Blackwell, 2007).

2. The arguments I present would also apply to passive physician-assisted suicide (in which the doctor's role is passive). Such a case may involve a doctor stopping sedation so that a patient can take a lethal drug the doctor did not provide. (The active/passive distinction does not overlap with the action/omission distinction. For discussion of why this is so, see my "PAS, E, and ID," and chapter 2 this volume.) Passive euthanasia can be distinguished from passive physician-assisted suicide: in the former, the doctor either does not start or stops lifesaving treatment. In the latter, he stops or does not start *non*-lifesaving aid, and this enables the patient to end his life either actively (e.g., by taking lethal drugs) or passively (e.g., by refraining from nutrition). Active voluntary euthanasia can be distinguished from physician-assisted suicide by the fact that in active euthanasia (a) the doctor does the act which finally causes death, (b) the doctor intends death, and (c) the death is in the patient's interest. In physician-assisted suicide, the doctor only *may* intend death (while the patient must intend death for it to be a suicide), the doctor does not do an act that causes death, and the death may not be in the patient's interest. Some would say the doctor need not intend death in physician-assisted suicide because the doctor may only wish to give the patient a choice whether to die, assisting the possibility of suicide. But I think that a doctor who gives a patient a lethal drug for his use is only assisting suicide (rather than assisting the possibility of suicide) if she gives it once the patient has formed the intention to commit suicide himself. Here, the doctor is not merely making possible a choice, since the choice has been made. Still, she may only intend to facilitate the patient's doing whatever he chooses and not herself intend that the patient die. (For more on this, see "PAS, E, and ID" and chapter 2 this

volume). This analysis disagrees with that presented by the majority of U.S. Supreme Court justices in *Vacco et al.* v. *Quill et al.* and *State of Washington et al.* v. *Glucksberg et al.*, where they claim that a physician who assists in suicide necessarily intends the death of the patient, whereas one who terminates treatment may only possibly intend the death. (See the Court's decisions reprinted in Battin et al., *Physician-Assisted Suicide.*)

3. Studies done subsequent to publication of the article on which this chapter is based suggest that autonomy-based reasons rather than the discomfort-based reasons prompt most requests for physician-assisted suicide in Oregon, at least.

4. On this distinction, see my *Morality, Mortality*, Vol. 1 (New York: Oxford University Press, 1993) and chapter 2 this volume.

5. For more on death as a benefit, see my "PAS, E, and ID" and chapter 2 this volume.

6. Ronald Dworkin, Thomas Nagel, Robert Nozick, John Rawls, Thomas Scanlon, and Judith Thomson, "Assisted Suicide: The Philosophers' Brief," *New York Review of Books* 44 (March 27, 1997): 23.

7. See chapter 3 this volume for my discussion of the brief.

8. There is some question about whether high doses of morphine do actually kill the patient. Hence, our question is whether, if they do, giving morphine would be permissible.

9. I discuss the so-called Texas Burn Victim case in this way in my *Morality, Mortality*, Vol. 2 (New York: Oxford University Press, 1996).

10. I owe this point to Rivka Weinberg.

11. This point was emphasized to me by Timothy Hall.

12. Judith Thomson (in "Physician-Assisted Suicide: Two Moral Arguments," *Ethics* 109 [April 1999]: 497–518) argues that death (1) is no evil at all if one's future will contain only bad things in it, and (2) is, on balance, no evil if a few goods in one's life will be outweighed by great bads. By contrast, I am willing to say that death is an evil in (1) and (2). This is because I think that the elimination of the person is something bad in itself, even if it has as a part the elimination of the person's pain (whether or not it also eliminates some goods the person would have had, had he lived on). And it is the elimination of the person that is being intended (as a means) in MD; it is not just a side effect, by hypothesis. (Note also that in the MPR Case where the morphine relieves the pain, the death is more clearly an evil, since the elimination of the person does not involve as a part of itself elimination of pain, the pain already having been eliminated by morphine.)

13. Is the loss of a limb itself a lesser evil, or is it merely the absence of the good effects of having a limb that is a lesser evil? If only the latter, then this would not be a case of intending a lesser evil. But I do think loss of a limb is itself a lesser evil. However, notice that if death *only led to evil* and loss of a leg *only led to evil*, so each was not itself an evil, intending each might still be analogous behaviors. Hence, the permissibility of intending one might imply the permissibility of intending the other.

14. Again, I assume that death is not only a lesser evil but the least evil of the alternatives to pain in the circumstances. Saying that death is the lesser evil suggests that it must not deprive the person of so many future goods that the loss of them is a greater evil than the pain would be. However, as noted above, it may be that some pain will be so bad that even if it would eventually be followed by an outweighing degree of good, one should not have to go through it. To repeat, there is a nonconsequentialist quality to this reasoning— for just as the nonconsequentialist says that there are some things one need not do to promote the best consequences in general, this reasoning claims that there are some things

people might reasonably not go through even to promote the best consequences for themselves. Hence, when I say that death could be the least lesser evil, and so overall in a person's best interests, I should be understood to include the possibility that it instead prevents an event that one could reasonably wish to avoid regardless of an outweighing future good.

15. Here we might also imagine a case in which a doctor only assists the patient by giving him or her the means of causing the lesser evil of pain to himself, and the patient intentionally causes it. Notice that it would be permissible for a doctor to do this, even if he and the patient have the bad intention of bringing about the pain as an end in itself, for the pain does still lead to a greater good whether anyone intends that or not.

16. I thank Michael Otsuka for suggesting that I bring out this suppressed premise in the three-step argument presented in my "A Right to Choose Death," *Boston Review* 22 (1997): 21–23.

17. I first presented an argument like this in my *Creation and Abortion* (New York: Oxford University Press, 1992), and then in *Morality, Mortality*, Vol. 2 (New York: Oxford University Press, 1996), in addition to the articles cited in note 1.

18. These intrapersonal cases cast doubt on Thomas Nagel's explanation of why it is wrong to intend pain to one person to stop harm to others (the interpersonal case). He suggests it is because one is going "against the grain" of value, taking an increase in pain as a reason to act. But that will be true in the intrapersonal case as well and not make action wrong. See his *The View from Nowhere* (New York: Oxford University Press, 1989).

19. Dworkin et al., "Assisted Suicide: The Philosophers' Brief"; also discussed in chapter 3 this volume.

20. When Thomson criticizes the DDE (in "Physician-Assisted Suicide: Two Moral Arguments"), she focuses on cases of kind (1), claiming that the DDE is shown to be wrong because acts done by an agent who intends an evil are not therefore impermissible. This strategy is, I believe, effective against the DDE as usually presented. This is what I would call its "token version." That is, when it declares an act wrong on the basis of the intention of the particular agent who does it. But one might try to offer a "type version" of the DDE, which declares an act wrong on the basis of the intentions it is reasonable to attribute to *any* agent who would do that type of act. Thomson's examples are not, I think, effective against the type version of the DDE. By contrast, the Four-Step Arguments are intended to be effective even against the type version of the DDE, since it claims that even if no agent could reasonably justify doing the act without intending death, it is permissible to do the act because there is nothing wrong with intending and causing the death per se.

21. For which Thomson argues in her "Physician-Assisted Suicide: Two Moral Arguments." See also Thomas Scanlon, "Intention and Permissibility I," *Proceedings of the Aristotelian Society* 74 (Suppl.) (2000): 301–17, and his *Moral Dimensions* (Cambridge, MA: Harvard University Press, 2007).

22. For more on these issues, see my *Intricate Ethics* (New York: Oxford University Press, 2007), and chapter 3 this volume.

23. Recall, however, the Faulty Wiring Case I (discussed in chapter 3 this volume), where terminating treatment does involve killing. It is not clear what Dworkin et al. would say about a doctor's duty in this case.

24. See also chapter 3 this volume.

25. Are 1b and 2b true even when the patient does not care about the greater good that will occur? For example, in 1b, suppose he intends to die and that is the only reason he

consents to the MPR that will also kill him. (I owe this case to Tim Hall.) Or in 2b, suppose the patient simply intends to experience blindness and does not care if this will save his life. Consider if the doctor could permissibly refuse to give the morphine for pain relief once he finds out that his patient does not care about pain relief and only intends his death, on the following grounds: "I would like to avoid killing a person, but am willing to do so if death is the side effect of eliminating pain that the patient wants eliminated even at the cost of death. But when the patient does not care about the greater good, I refuse to produce the greater good if it means I will kill." If the doctor does not give the comparable argument against causing blindness to save a life, is this because causing death in giving morphine, even when it is the lesser evil and not intended by the doctor, plays a different role from causing blindness? Or is it because the removal of pain that the patient does not care about is not a greater good; that is, does his not caring about pain significantly change the weight of the positive value of its removal in a way that his not caring about life does *not* significantly change the weight of its positive value? In any case, suppose the doctor could permissibly refuse to give the MPR when the patient intends his death as his only end. This would show that the patient's not caring about the greater good does affect whether he has a right to be given pain relievers. It would also show that a doctor could point to the fact that he will be a killer as a reason for not acting (even when he would not intend death) *when this fact* is conjoined with another fact, namely the patient's not caring about relief from pain.

26. Notice that the Doctor's Duty Argument differs from the following one: "Suppose the Four-Step Argument is correct. Then, with patient consent, it is at least permissible for a doctor to intend a patient's death when it is a lesser evil for the sake of the patient's greater good. But if the doctor has a duty to relieve physical suffering, then she has a duty to do whatever is permissible in order to fulfill her duty. Hence, she has a duty to kill the patient, if death is the lesser evil, in order to produce the greater good of pain relief." This argument is unsatisfactory, since one does not have a duty to do whatever it would be permissible to do in order to carry out another duty. Sometimes, the permissible is still supererogatory. For example, it is permissible for a doctor to give up all his money to save his patient's life, and he has a duty to save his patient's life, but that does not mean he has a duty to give up all his money to save his patient's life. The Duty Argument is a better argument because it begins by pointing to giving morphine when one foresees it will cause death. This is an act that is, in some important respects, like the one that the Four-Step Argument says is permissible, namely giving morphine intending to cause death. The Duty Argument then points out that a doctor has a *duty* to do the analogous act of intentionally causing other lesser evils (such as pain when it keeps someone from falling into a coma) and shifts the burden of proof to showing why the doctor does *not* also have a duty to intend the death if it is permissible to intend it.

27. This and the subsequent quote are from Dan Brock, "Voluntary Active Euthanasia," *The Hastings Center Report*, March 1 (1992), Vol. 22, Issue 2, pp. 10–22.

28. Peter Singer, *Rethinking Life and Death* (New York: St. Martin's Press, 1994), p. 146. Note that rules may have changed since the time of Singer's discussion.

29. Singer, *Rethinking Life and Death*, pp. 147–48.

30. Some psychological suffering is a reaction to one's beliefs about a state of affairs (what I call propositional attitude suffering). There is another type of *nonpropositional* attitude psychological suffering—e.g., clinical depression or schizophrenia. Here the primary

cause of depression is not an evaluation of one's life but a chemical imbalance. I believe it can more clearly occupy the same role as physical suffering in the argument for physician-assisted suicide or euthanasia. The Solicitor General's brief in the Supreme Court review of two lower-court judgments permitting physician-assisted suicide argued that we have a right to avoid physical pain and also psychological suffering brought on by awareness of our life condition. This is a liberal position. By contrast, Daniel Callahan insists that there is a moral distinction between seeking means to avoid physical pain and to avoid psychological suffering. But he seems not to separate propositional from nonpropositional psychological suffering, and so treats clinical depression the same as inability to cope with life. See his "When Self-Determination Runs Amok," *The Hastings Center Report*, March–April (1992): 52–55.

31. The distinction between cases in which we may and may not give the drug that foreseeably causes death may bear on the different reasons that philosophers have isolated for wanting to die or to help someone die. One consideration is said to be mercy or charity, concerned with the patient's well-being. A broader consideration is referred to as the patient's critical interests. These essentially relate to his commitments, projects, and, in general, what he thinks is truly valuable in his life. (See Ronald Dworkin, *Life's Dominion: An Argument about Abortion, Euthanasia, and Individual Freedom* [New York: Alfred A. Knopf, 1993].) A patient may think the welfare of his family is more valuable than his own well-being. (The satisfaction of his desires for them is not followed by his own well-being if he dies for their sake.) Those who think it is permissible to be killed in order to preserve the finances of one's family may be giving much weight to critical interests. Nevertheless, if one thinks it is wrong to give the cheaper medicine in the case I described, one is denying that medical policy will be determined by the weight of the patient's critical interests. One may still think it is permissible to terminate the more expensive treatment at the patient's request, so as not to force treatment on him. But notice that a consequence of both not giving the cheaper drug that will shortly kill him *and* terminating the more expensive one is that, without *any* medication, the patient may die even sooner than if he were given the cheap medicine.

32. A doctor might well give the patient the drug if it had the side effect of causing death after a few moments of conscious, undemented life, because the patient's directive described a few moments of conscious, undemented life as a greater good and death a lesser evil. This leads us to consider how large a benefit, *besides any producible by death itself*, might be needed in order to make giving the drug permissible when it kills as a side effect. Suppose very little besides what is provided by death is needed—for example, a few undemented minutes with friends and family in addition to the end of dementia. This would show that the value of living on in the demented state is rated very low indeed. This in turn means that death, intended or not, does not deprive someone of very much (even taking into account any value introduced by the drug actually curing dementia but not leading to active consciousness).

33. The Finances Case is different: The cheaper treatment still provides some improvement and so gives some reason for action. The question is whether we should achieve this good if the drug causes death of the patient when another drug that causes the good for the patient without death causes financial drain on the family.

34. This part, in particular, presents revised versions of the last two articles mentioned in note 1.

35. See their separate concurring statements.

36. To waive one's right to life and give a right to another (a) to do what will kill one as a side effect, as well as (b) to deliberately kill one, is not the same as alienating or giving up one's right to life. Joel Feinberg makes this point in "Voluntary Euthanasia and the Inalienable Right to Life," *Philosophy & Public Affairs* 7(2) (Winter 1978): 93–123. The latter would occur if slavery were permitted. For then, one cedes one's right over one's life to another, and one may be forever under another's power to decide whether one lives or dies. It is true that if one successfully waives one's right to live and is killed, one will never again exercise one's right to live, and this is also a consequence of alienating one's right. But only in the case of alienating does one give one's right away and live on under the control of another person.

37. For discussion of waivers, see Philippa Foot in "Euthanasia," *Philosophy & Public Affairs* 6(2) (Winter 1977): 85–112; and Feinberg, "Voluntary Euthanasia and the Inalienable Right to Life." It is important to point out that when Foot argues for the permission to kill because a patient has waived his right to life and it is in his interest to die, she does not think there is any point in arguing separately for the permissibility of intending death rather than doing what one foresees will cause the death. She seems to think that the waiver plus its being in the interest of the person to die give another person permission to intend death; there is then no other reason why it is impermissible for him to do so. It is possible, however, that a patient could only give permission for someone to do what foreseeably kills him but not what intentionally kills him, for reasons having nothing to do with an inability to waive his right to life or with his being unable to release others from a duty not to do what kills him. That is why I say (in text) only that it is neither the inability to waive a right nor a duty not to harm that interferes with *intended* killing; this leaves it open that something else could interfere.

38. A religious version of the killing objection just considered is that a person does not have a right to dispose of himself because he belongs to God. But then why is it permissible for someone to take MPR to relieve his pain when it is known that it will destroy what belongs to God? To reject the Four-Step Arguments because we belong to God seems to require us to reject MPR, which is commonly thought to be morally permissible.

39. Suppose that one is convinced by arguments (such as those discussed in chapter 3 this volume) that an agent's intention cannot often account for the impermissibility of an act. Then one might just substitute throughout for "intending" the simple fact that someone's death is causally required to stop pain.

40. Warren Quinn, "Actions, Intentions, and Consequences: The Doctrine of Double Effect," reprinted in his *Morality and Action* (New York: Cambridge University Press, 1993). For a critical discussion of his views, see chapter 3 of my *Intricate Ethics* (New York: Oxford University Press, 2007).

41. Some may think it important to distinguish harming someone to help him avoid greater harm from harming someone to help him benefit in some other way. If one thinks death interferes with future benefits but it is also a harm, and in cases we are dealing with we are avoiding greater harms, the cases we deal with will satisfy the distinction. One might also simply speak of causing bad things to happen to someone (avoiding use of the term "harm") to benefit him or (more narrowly) prevent worse things happening to him. Our cases satisfy this description, too.

42. Considering another case in which the lesser evil may permissibly be foreseen but not permissibly intended may help strengthen the case against intending death. It is

permissible for me to lecture a class to give new knowledge, foreseeing that as an unavoidable side effect, a few false beliefs will be formed by the students (e.g., by misunderstanding my lecture). I tolerate this as a lesser evil to the greater good. But suppose I had to deliberately instill a few false beliefs to transmit more knowledge. I might lie to do this, but I need not. Rather I might turn in a certain direction while lecturing, knowing that this will confuse students and lead to a false belief. It might be wrong to do either this or lie. Similarly, it might be said, it is not always permissible to intend the lesser evil for a person's own greater good though one may bring it about with mere foresight. (Notice that in the classroom case, this need not mean that it becomes impermissible to give a lecture that will transmit new knowledge and also *unavoidably* lead to some false beliefs just because one actually intends that those false beliefs come about.) In this classroom case, it could be said that were I to lie, I would be insulting the students by manipulating them as a tool to their own greater good. If taking control over and destroying someone's life were like telling a lie or manipulating someone for his own good, rather than like amputating a leg for his own good, then perhaps it could be a constraint on performing assisted suicide or euthanasia even if the person consented.

43. However, a person who no longer functions as a rational being might still retain worth in virtue of having once exercised these capacities. Of course, in euthanasia and physician-assisted suicide, we might also terminate human life considered independently of whether it is the life of a rational being. Note also that some may think an entity is a "person," even if it is not a rational being but is more than mere human life (e.g., it has the capacity for self-consciousness). I wish the Four-Step Arguments to also apply to such a person, though my use of "person" in this chapter equates person with rational being. For purposes of my discussion, I do not think it is necessary to deny that preserving human life per se is as important as preserving persons or rational humanity. However, we must also not ignore the fact that there is more than one way in which to destroy a person. Hypothetically, one might lobotomize or drug someone so that he is permanently demented in order to eliminate pain. Then human life remains, but the person as rational being is destroyed. One might argue that killing the person is not as morally offensive a way to end pain as is destroying the person so that "he" lives on in these other ways. A complete argument for the permissibility of intentionally killing in physician-assisted suicide or euthanasia might have to distinguish these cases, and this will probably involve taking a stand on the worth of various forms of human life.

44. I have already noted that Quinn suggests we distinguish the idea of not treating persons as ends and treating them as mere means. I am focusing on the latter.

45. Because we have worth in ourselves, it can be important that our lives also be good for us. A Kantian might go so far as to claim that there is no value in pleasure or the absence of pain unless these occur in the life of a being that has worth. It is not that pain is not as unpleasant for a mouse as for a person; it is that the nature of the negative qualia alone does not provide a reason why it should not exist.

46. Or death would at least not harm (or be bad for) me. A life can be not worth living even if there are no intrinsic evils in the life from which death would be a release as when someone is permanently unconscious. When a life is worth *not* living, the intrinsic evils in it may be very great. (The concept of a life worth not living is due to Derek Parfit.)

47. This is how I understand Thomas Hill, Jr.'s version of the Kantian objection to suicide to his "Self-Regarding Suicide: A Modified Kantian View," in his *Autonomy and Self-Respect* (Cambridge: Cambridge University Press, 1991), pp. 85–103.

48. It is a problem with the account of Kantian objections to suicide given by Hill in "Self-Regarding Suicide" that none of the objections he raises really aim at suicide per se; i.e., they do not distinguish between intending death and doing what we foresee leads to death. He provides Kantian objections to some types of suicide by focusing on the claim that rational agency has worth in itself rather than being a mere means to other goods. But he fails to notice that we can lack the appropriate attitude to our lives, even when we merely do what we foresee will lead to our deaths, and therefore this inappropriate attitude does not suffice to distinguish between, for example, suicide and taking morphine to knock out pain when we foresee fatal results.

49. On the distinction, see Thomas Hill, Jr., "The Formula of the End-in-Itself," in his *Dignity and Practical Person* (Ithaca, NY: Cornell University Press, 1993). I thank Richard Arneson for calling this discussion to my attention.

50. For example, Tyler Burge, in conversation; and J. David Velleman, in "A Right of Self-Termination?" *Ethics* 109 (April 1999): 606–28. For my discussion of Velleman, see chapter 5 this volume.

51. Suggested by David Kaplan.

52. Suppose acting with the intention to bring about, or only with foresight to, one's death in order to stop pain does not always indicate a failure of self-respect or a failure to accord sufficient weight to personhood in itself. (This need not imply that such action is a duty or the only rational step to take.) Still, we can learn something from the arguments that focus on rationality being severely undermined or a person being put in a condition unworthy of him. Suppose that to relieve intense pain, there are two drugs. One has the side effect of eliminating personhood irreversibly by causing brain damage but not killing the patient. The other has the side effect of certainly killing the patient. It is possible that one should prefer the second drug. Likewise, if the only two ways to eliminate pain were (i) to intentionally eliminate personhood (because, hypothetically, neurons responsible for it control pain) without killing or (ii) to intentionally kill, it is possible that one should prefer the second way. Living on in a severely subrational state might be insulting to what was once a rational being in a way that having his life end is not. It is even possible that it would be *wrong* (not only less good) to intentionally destroy rationality in a still-living human being, or do what destroys rationality in a still-living human being as a side effect, in order to end pain. If so, this would indicate that death has specific virtues as a way of eliminating a person that can play a role in our allowing that ending pain may outweigh the value of the continuation of personhood.

5

Some Arguments by Velleman Concerning Suicide and Assisted Suicide

I wish to examine in some detail David Velleman's arguments concerning suicide and assisted suicide as presented in his "A Right of Self-Termination?"[1,2] Throughout my discussion, I shall keep in mind two issues that I believe are critical.[3] Issue (1): Does any objection to physician-assisted suicide that his account raises show that physician-assisted suicide for pain relief in particular is wrong? Issue (2): If it does, must it also rule out giving morphine for pain relief (MPR) when it is foreseen with certainty that the morphine will soon cause death? It will be a big problem for any objection if it also requires us to give up the moral permissibility of MPR when this foreseeably causes death soon. The Supreme Court decisions in *Vacco et al.* v. *Quill et al.* and *State of Washington et al.* v. *Glucksberg et al.* concluded that such death-hastening, palliative care was *legally* permissible, at least in terminal cases, and two justices (Sandra Day O'Connor and Stephen Breyer) emphasized that one important reason why they did not find laws against assisted suicide unconstitutional was that palliative care, even if it caused death sooner (and soon), was legally permitted.[4] If moral objections cannot be raised to physician-assisted suicide without also raising such objections to morphine for pain relief that causes death soon, the legal distinction may be undermined as well.

I

Velleman agrees that pain relief and sometimes even death might be best for a person.[5] He then argues (p. 611) that someone is rationally obligated to care about what is good (and best) for a person only if he cares about the person. This claim by itself, I believe, would create no problem for the permissibility of physician-assisted suicide, since one way of showing that one cares for someone is to seek what is good for him, and this, Velleman agrees, may be death.

However, Velleman moves from discussing mere caring about a person, which could occur even if the person is not worth caring for. He goes on to discuss the claim that bringing about something good for a person is important only if the person is important (i.e., is really worth caring for). If the person had importance merely as a means to some end, something else which had true importance in itself would be necessary to make doing good for the person important. But, he says, we assume that people do have importance in themselves.

The form of this argument is quite general: It matters that something good for some entity happens only if the entity matters. The value of what happens to him depends (in a certain way) on his value. Velleman says (p. 614): "But what would it matter how much I lost or gained if I myself would be no loss?" On the basis of these remarks, I interpret Velleman to be constructing a reductio argument whose general structure is as follows:

1. Suppose it matters that person X not be in pain (i.e., that X has one of the things that is good for him), simply because this would be good for him.
2. That X not be in pain (i.e., have one of the things that is good for him) could matter in this way only if X matters in himself.
3. If it is permissible to dispose of X (independent of concern for any other worthwhile thing, while X retains the characteristics that supposedly ground the importance of his having what is good for him for no other reason than that it would be good for him) just because his continuing existence is against his interests, X does not matter in himself (as he is a mere means to his interests being satisfied).
4. If X does not matter in himself, that X gets what is good for him because it is good for him does not matter.
5. Suppose it is permissible to dispose of X (independent of concern for any other worthwhile thing, while X retains the characteristics that supposedly ground the importance of his having what is good for him for no other reason than that it would be good for him) just because his continuing existence is against his interests.
6. Then, it does not matter that X not be in pain simply because this would be good for him. (The denial of no.1.)

This argument is supposed to show that there is no justification for physician-assisted suicide to end pain for the sake of X. The choice to destroy oneself (and seek a physician's assistance) for the sake of one's interest is said to be an irrational choice. I shall refer to this as the *Reductio Argument*. (Notice that this reductio argument applies equally to killing oneself and killing and assisting in killing another. But it might be said that, in the Kantian view, there is a particular incoherence in making use of one's agency to destroy one's *own* agency. If so, there is a self/other-asymmetry for which the Reductio Argument does not account.)

The Reductio Argument is distinct from other reductio-style arguments in Velleman's article. For example, he quotes (p. 612) my description of the right to life as a protected option to choose whether to live or to die that does not imply a duty to live. (I borrow this view from Joel Feinberg.[6]) But, he asks, why is it important to

protect people's options if it is not important to protect people? And if it is important to protect people, this means that they have no option to kill themselves so long
as they have the property that makes it important to protect them (e.g., they are
rational beings). This is a reductio of there being a right to life as a protected option
to live or to die. Call it *Reductio 2*. A slightly different *Reductio 3* involves the view
that in choosing to end his life for the sake of his interests, the person treats himself
as having no value in himself. But then how can he demand that we respect this
choice when the choice itself is based on the view that he is not worthy of respect
(i.e., does not matter)?

One possible problem with Reductio 2 is that the importance of protecting
people is not the presupposition of the importance of protecting people's option to live or to die. Rather, the presupposition of the importance of protecting
the option is the importance of *respecting* people, and respecting them does
not, on its face, rule out their retaining the option not to live.[7] Hence, if
choosing not to live because life is against one's interests does not imply that
one believes that one is not worthy of respect, it will still make sense to respect
the person's choice. (My reason for speaking of a right to life as a protected
option was only to show that from the idea of a right to life alone, one could not
derive a duty to live. This leaves it open that one does have a duty to live for
some other reason.)

One concern about the Reductio Argument is raised by considering its implication for cases: It seems to imply that we would not be morally justified in
euthanizing a cat to stop its pain. This is because it seems reasonable to say that
my cat's being out of pain matters just because it would be good for my cat.[8]
According to Velleman, this can be true only if my cat matters. I suggest my cat
matters in itself, not just because it matters to me. According to step 3 of the Reductio Argument, the permissibility of destroying the cat to stop its pain would
imply that it does not matter. Hence, it is not true that its being out of pain matters simply because it is good for the cat. According to the Reductio Argument,
there is a dilemma: If the cat's being out of pain matters just because it would be
good for it, the cat matters and hence it would be wrong to kill it to put it out of
pain. If it is not wrong to kill the cat to put it out of pain, then it does not really
matter for the cat's sake if the cat is out of pain (for the cat does not matter). So
why kill it?[9] But this seems wrong; it is not impermissible to euthanize cats when
we are trying to achieve what is good for them because we think they matter in
themselves to some degree. And because pain to them matters, it could even be
wrong not to euthanize them.[10]

This Cat Example suggests several possible grounds for objecting to step 3 in
the Reductio Argument:

(a) That it is permissible to destroy X for its own interests (independent of
concern for other worthwhile things) does not necessarily imply that X does not
matter.[11] Someone may matter, and the loss of her may matter, but less than getting

rid of her pain matters. This could be true because though the value of X being out of pain is dependent on the value of X, this is not enough for us to conclude that the value of X's being out of pain is *less* than the value of X. That is, something's having value may be necessary in order for it to give rise to something that has *more* value than it. For example, a beautiful scene in nature may give rise to even more valuable reflection on it only because it has value.[12] While I think this objection raises a possibility, I do not think it captures what is actually true in the use of suicide for pain relief.

(b) We should distinguish between (i) the value of something, and (ii) the value of *being that thing*, or put another way, the value of there being that thing or its continuing to exist. It may be that a person's not being in pain does not have greater value than the person has (contrary to what [a] suggests), but it has greater value than the continuing existence of the person. I think this objection gets to the heart of the matter.[13] We certainly might choose not to *create* a person in the first place because he would be in pain. (Velleman agrees that the appropriate response to the sort of value a person has does not necessarily involve creating more of them.) Also, in the light of the non-overshadowed value of a person, because a person is so important, we might decide that it is not only important that a person be out of pain but that it would be permissible for the person not to live on in pain. In this connection, consider again Reductio 2. Velleman says the presupposition of the importance of protecting the person's options is the importance of protecting the person. The sense of "protecting the person" that would make it an appropriate presupposition is probably "protecting the integrity or character of the person" rather than "protecting the continued existence of the person," for why would the continued existence of the person be a ground of the value of his current options?[14] Similarly, it is the value of the person rather than the value of the continuing existence of the person that makes sense as a presupposition of the value of what is good for the person. Hence, physician-assisted suicide may protect the person, even if it eliminates him, for it protects the integrity and character of the person by protecting the fulfillment of his reasoned choices. His choice of physician-assisted suicide would not be shown to be unreasonable because it depends on the value of his interests outweighing his value. Rather, his interests are held to outweigh the value of his continuing existence.

A passage from my earlier work on assisted suicide, which Velleman criticizes, is relevant to this. I said: "Suppose life involves such unbearable pain that one's whole life is focused on that pain. In such circumstances, one could, I believe, decline the honor of being a person, as we might acknowledge the great (and normally overriding) value of being a person ... [and yet] allow that some bad conditions may overshadow its very great value."[15] Velleman objects to this on Kantian grounds. (The quote he finds objectionable comes from a passage in which I was defending the right to take morphine for pain relief, not the right to commit suicide in certain situations. Hence, I assume he objects to it as a reason for taking pain medication, too.) He says: "Kamm says that the value of a person normally 'overrides' the value of other goods, but can be 'overshadowed' by conditions that are exceptionally bad . . . But . . . value *for* a person stands to value *in* the person roughly as the value of means stands to that of the end: in each case, the former merits concern only on the basis of concern for the latter. And conditional values cannot be weighed against the unconditional value on which they depend" (p. 613). He says this rules out suicide when done for the reason that life is not good enough for the person.

Notice that in the passage Velleman quotes, I say that the "value of *being* a person" (emphasis added) may be overshadowed, but when Velleman comments on the passage, he says, "Kamm says that the value of a person . . . can be 'overshadowed.'" But, I have argued, these values may be worth distinguishing.

One could also say that if one eliminates the person to avoid future deterioration of rational humanity—not just to avoid things that are no good for the person as a sentient being—elimination of the person does not indicate that his value is being overridden. Rather, one is acting appropriately in the light of his value, preventing a state that is unworthy of him. This is something Velleman might agree with, though (as we shall see below) he actually only discusses justifying pursuit of one's own or another's death in cases where the person is "coming undone" already at the time of assisting his death. These are supposed to be cases in which a property that grounds the importance of good things happening to someone is already diminished.

(c) Velleman tries to support the Reductio Argument by reference to an analogy to the means–end relation (as in the previous quoted passage): The value of what is good for a person stands to the value in a person as the value of the means stands to the value of the end to which it is a means. In the means–end case, it is clear that the value of the means cannot overshadow the value of the end; for example, it would make no sense to get rid of the end for the sake of the means. And the value of the end cannot overshadow the value of the means, for as long as the end has value, so do the means, at least if they are necessary means to the end. But I think the analogy is imperfect and does not support the Reductio Argument. In the means–end case, the value of the end is to be identified with the value of the existence of the end, since an end is here understood as something we try to bring about. I have suggested in (b) above that this may not be true in the case of the person. It is clear that Kant not only did *not* think that persons are ends in the sense that we must bring them into existence, he also did not think they are ends in the sense that we must do everything to keep them in existence. What is good for the person (pain relief) may take precedence over the continuing existence of the person without taking precedence over the value of the person, in the way that means cannot take precedence over existence of the end. Furthermore, even Velleman seems committed to denying the relevance of the second prong of his analogy, namely that the value of the end cannot overshadow the value of the means. This is because he believes that the continuing existence of the person *can* take precedence over doing what is good for the person, since he admits that what is good for the person may be his death. By contrast, the end, he says, cannot take precedence over the means to it. (I assume he is thinking of necessary means.) The problem with the analogy is that what is good for a person does not necessarily involve commitment to his existence, but what is a means to an end does involve commitment to the existence of the end.[16]

Just as he moved beyond an argument based on caring to the Reductio Argument, Velleman seems to move beyond the general Reductio Argument (which, I have argued, can also be applied to cats). He claims (pp. 611–12) that the particular value people have in themselves is dignity and this makes them worthy of respect. (This dignity is, presumably, not present in cats.) Often, respecting a person (unlike caring for him) will conflict with doing what is good for him (e.g., paternalistic action may be ruled out), and it can rule out doing what is good for him when it comes to assisting suicide. This is a special argument which may make the Reductio Argument unnecessary.[17] Unlike the Reductio, it need not deny that seeking someone's death because doing this is good for him has no value (because if the person could be eliminated for this reason, he would have no value and so what is good for him would have no value). That is, the question is, directly, whether the permissibility of eliminating a person in order to eliminate his pain indicates lack of respect for him qua person, even if the permissibility of doing so would not drain all value from doing what is good for the person for his sake, as the Reductio Argument claims.

We now need another argument to support the claim that suicide or physician-assisted suicide for pain relief shows lack of respect. Before considering this argument in section II, let us take stock of where we are. The Reductio Argument was intended to show that the value of relieving pain for the person's sake cannot override the value of the continued existence of the person. If it does not succeed in showing this, it is still possible that both physician-assisted suicide for pain relief (and MPR) are compatible with treating (rational humanity in) a person as an end and not as a mere means. They need not involve one sense of treating as a mere means, namely giving no intrinsic weight to rational humanity, and they also need not involve a second sense, namely not treating rational humanity as having unconditional and incomparable value.[18] This is because, for all that has been said so far, at least, giving unconditional and incomparable weight to the continued *existence* of rational humanity does not seem to be a necessary part of treating rational humanity as having unconditional and incomparable weight. But notice that if the Reductio Argument had succeeded in its criticism of physician-assisted suicide for pain relief, it should also rule out MPR. This is because in MPR, we would be doing what foreseeably causes the death of a person for the sake of

what is good for him as a sentient being (pain relief). We do this by using something that is essentially a lethal agent (i.e., certainly death-inducing as well as pain-
relieving in the circumstances), even if we do not intend its lethal properties.
Ruling out MPR will raise the problems associated with issue (2), described at the
beginning of this chapter.

II

The additional argument one finds in Velleman to support the claim that one
cannot respect a person if one eliminates her to stop her pain is what I shall refer
to as the *Exchange Argument*. It also supports the second sense of treating a person
as a mere means—that is, not giving her unconditional and incomparable value. If
it succeeds, it will also show that MPR is impermissible. Velleman claims that suicide is immoral when committed on the ground that life is not worth living and it
is in one's interest to die, for then one is trading one's life for benefits or for relief
from harms. He says: "I think Kant was right to say that trading one's person in
exchange for benefits, or relief from harms, denigrates the value of personhood"
(p. 614) and "[t]he Kantian objection to suicide, then, is not that it destroys something of value. The objection is not even to suicide per se, but to suicide committed
for a particular kind of reason—that is, in order to obtain benefits or escape harms.
And the objection to suicide committed for this reason is that it denigrates the
person's dignity by trading his person for interest-relative goods, as if it were one
of them" (p. 616).

Let me reconstruct and extend the Exchange Argument.

1. To exchange rational humanity for things that have interest-relative value
   (i.e., things that have value only because they are in the interest of
   persons) implies that rational humanity has only interest-relative value.
2. Things that have interest-relative value have a price.
3. Rational humanity would then have a price rather than dignity.

Indeed, on the Kantian view, to have a price just means that something is exchange-
able for something else. Consider some objections to the Exchange Argument:

(i) According to Kant, beautiful things (e.g., some art) have a value beyond
price, though not the dignity that persons have. Most would say (though perhaps
Kant would not, given his theory of beauty) that beautiful things have value in
themselves, even if no one cares about them and they satisfy no human interests.
Yet we may permissibly exchange beautiful things for money or food. The permissibility of exchanging them for things that have interest-relative value and a market price does not imply, I believe, that they only have interest-relative value. That
we can exchange one thing for another does not mean that they share the same
essential nature or type of value. The same might be true of persons.[19]

(ii) More importantly, I think that an exchange that puts a price on something in a pernicious sense, sometimes referred to as commodification if the price is monetary in nature, does not arise in the context of physician-assisted suicide for pain relief or MPR. Consider the following scenarios: (1) I will take away your severe pain by giving you a pill that does not kill you, only if you will then let me take out one of your kidneys so that I can use it. (2) I will take away your severe pain by taking out one of your kidneys, because this alone acts as a cure for the pain. (3) I will take away your severe pain by giving you a pill that does not kill you, only if you will then let me help you kill yourself because this is useful to me. (4) I will take away your severe pain by helping you to kill yourself, because death alone eliminates the pain.

In (1), we would say that we have placed a price on a kidney: someone has been paid something (a pill for pain relief) in return for giving up a kidney. But in (2), an ordinary case of doing what gets rid of pain, it does not seem appropriate to say—even Kant would not say—that we have placed a price on a kidney. Nevertheless, the kidney has been exchanged for pain relief. We removed it because it caused pain relief, without intermediate exchanges of it for something else (e.g., a pill) that causes pain relief. Kant thought it was inappropriate to sell one's hair. (Perhaps he would have said this even if one sold it to get money for pain relief.) However, he would not have objected to cutting off one's hair when this would directly relieve one's pain.

Similarly, it could be said that in (3) we place a price on life. (Someone arranges for his life to end in order to get the pill that stops his pain.) Perhaps we thereby treat life as less than it is worth, though not necessarily because any exchange signals the intrinsic equivalence of whatever is exchanged, which was the point of objection (i). But in (4), we do not place a price on life, even though we eliminate a rational human being to get rid of his pain and, hence, exchange a life for pain relief. If there is no price placed on a kidney in (2), why should we think there is a price placed on a person in (4)?

Importantly, in MPR, when morphine will shortly kill the person and we foresee this, do we not also exchange a person for his pain relief? If so, the Kantian argument will rule out MPR, though MPR is widely thought to be morally (and legally) permissible. The Exchange Argument would even rule out giving morphine for pain relief when it does not kill, if it has the continuous side effect of knocking out a patient's rational agency and/or capacity for rational agency. (Call this Nonlethal MPR.) Further, consider terminal sedation, which is currently employed when painkillers do not work and which is legally permissible. By "terminal sedation," I mean putting a patient to sleep as long as he is in pain until the underlying disease kills him. (I am not conceiving of it as involving the removal of food and water with the intention of causing death. If one did the latter, the cause of death need not be the preexisting disease but rather starvation and dehydration. Nor am I imagining that the sleep-inducing drug itself causes death.) In terminal sedation, the exercise of rational agency distinctive of persons is also exchanged for pain relief. Hence, terminal sedation may be ruled out by the Kantian objections to physician-assisted suicide or suicide that we are considering, even if it does not hasten death or destroy the capacity for rational agency (it only interferes with its exercise). But is terminal sedation really wrong? I do not think so. If it is not wrong, then this would be reason to think that the Exchange Argument objection to physician-assisted suicide and suicide is not correct.

My tentative conclusion is that neither the Reductio nor the Exchange Arguments show that it is impermissible to eliminate a still-rational person in order to stop his pain because it would involve treating the person as something that has a price rather than dignity.

III

So far, I have mentioned the view that we treat a person as a mere means to his own interests if we attribute no intrinsic value to rational humanity or if we do not attribute to it unconditional and incomparable value relative to what is good for the person. I have said that neither of these senses of "mere means" need be present merely because we do not attribute unconditional and incomparable value to the continued *existence* of the person or we exchange her existence for pain relief. However, there is a third sense of treating the person and the rational humanity in him as a mere means that comes closer to dealing with the objection raised not by Velleman but by supporters of the Doctrine of Double Effect (DDE), who emphasize the moral significance of the intention/foresight distinction: Suppose our balancing pain versus life does not reveal that we see rational humanity in our lives as having no intrinsic weight or no great intrinsic weight. Still, on the occasion when we sacrifice a still-rational person to stop his pain, at least by committing suicide or sometimes assisting suicide, we are (a) acting against rational humanity, (b) with no eventual good for rational humanity per se to be achieved by that act, and (c) because the person's death is an intended causal means to pain relief.[20] This is to treat the *death of the person* as a means and this is the complaint of the DDE. So perhaps, on that occasion, rational humanity in the person is also treated as a mere means. Clause (b) distinguishes between death and doing relaxation techniques to go to sleep, even though sleep will stop the exercise of rational agency. This is because going to sleep at night will help promote further and better functioning of the rational agent qua rational agent in the future. Dying will not.

But when we give morphine in MPR, we also act against rational humanity on an occasion when this will not further it in the future. This is true when death will follow on MPR (as that case has been imagined). It is also true in Nonlethal MPR. If these things (included in conditions [a] and [b]) make what we do objectionable,

MPR and Nonlethal MPR will also be ruled out if physician-assisted suicide is. Nevertheless, only in physician-assisted suicide and not in MPR do we intend the destruction of the person as a causal means. (We can assume that in physician-assisted suicide, this intention is present, at least in the patient, when the act that kills him has no other properties that could justify it, aside from the fact that death is necessary to end pain.) However, even in physician-assisted suicide, we do not specifically intend, though we foresee, the destruction of rational agency per se. That is, the death of the person is treated as a causal means, but that may not mean that rational humanity (or its destruction) in the person is treated as a mere means. In this sense, physician-assisted suicide is not so far from either form of MPR.[21] Suppose it is destruction of rationality that is morally most important, not physical death of a remaining nonrational body. Then, in not aiming at the first, physician-assisted suicide may be morally similar to MPR, from the point of view of those concerned with the intention/foresight distinction as it bears on treating rational humanity as a mere means.

By contrast to death, we could understand a certain imagined sort of terminal sedation to be a form of intentional, not merely foreseen, cessation of rational agency when this is not conducive to future rational agency. In this case, we intend to prevent future rational agency by continuing to give sleep-inducing drugs because (suppose) ending exercise of rational agency is itself the causal means to pain relief. (Call this c′, a variant of c on page 92.) In (c′), the end of the exercise of rational agency is intended as a causal means to pain relief. Hence, if aiming against the continued existence of rational agency, in the sense of its exercise, for the sake of pain relief were what constituted an impermissible use of persons as a mere means, this form of terminal sedation would be ruled out as well as physician-assisted suicide even if it does not hasten death. Indeed, because it more specifically targets eliminating exercise of rational agency for pain relief, it may be worse than suicide and MPR on a Kantian view. But is it really wrong? If it is not wrong, then this would be reason to think that satisfying conditions (a), (b), and (c) is not a sufficient condition for mistreating people.

Suppose now that instead of terminal sedation, we could induce nonterminal brain wasting (dementia) disease as the only causal means to pain relief. We are imagining that, contrary to fact, elimination of the capacity for rational humanity (not just its exercise) will cause pain relief. Could it be morally impermissible to use this route to pain relief even if terminal sedation for pain relief were permitted? Wherein lies the difference? One hypothesis is that dementia is a perversion of consciousness and agency, whereas unending sleep is the simultaneous end of exercising rational agency and of the human being's attempt to act or consciously think at all. Hence no acts or thoughts exhibit a perversion. To induce dementia when the person is not asleep may be disrespectful of the person, while inducing the sleep would not be even if it interferes with exercise of rational agency (as a side effect or means). Death is the simultaneous end of rational agency and of the person, so it too is not a perversion of agency and thought. Hence the moral value of causing it may be closer to terminal sedation than to causing dementia that involves perversion of agency.

However, there are other differences between terminal sedation and death which are worth considering. First, in terminal sedation, we will give sedation whenever pain is present, and we foresee that pain will be continuously present until death. Hence we foresee continuous, deliberate sedation until death. But this is still different from putting someone now into a sleep which cannot be ended once begun because we foresee that pain will continue until the end. Death, by contrast, is permanent. Yet we could imagine a hypothetical case in which putting someone into a sleep that cannot be ended is necessary in order to stop pain, for we cannot keep giving the sedation at times in the future. Here we would intentionally exchange all possibility of someone's exercising consciousness and rational agency for his relief from pain. Call this *superterminal sedation (1)*. A second difference between terminal sedation and death is that only death involves the destruction of the physical ground of the capacity for rational agency. But we could imagine a case in which sedation also has this destructive effect without causing death. Call this *superterminal sedation (2)*. These super states are close to death-for-pain-relief. If it is permissible to use superterminal sedation (1) or (2) for pain relief, with patient consent, then the argument for physician-assisted suicide is strengthened and the argument against it based on the DDE is further weakened.

Notice that Velleman's Kantian position seems not to distinguish between ordinary terminal sedation for pain relief and the two superterminal sedations for pain relief. It rules them all out. Those who would permit terminal sedation but not the superterminal sedations are not concerned with the exchange of rational agency for pain relief per se or even with intending to interfere with rational agency. They are concerned with doing what induces the end of the possibility of any exercise of, or capacity for, rational agency.

IV

These points bear on another argument that Velleman presents against suicide and physician-assisted suicide for purposes of ending pain. I shall refer to it as the *slavery analogy*. He says that entering into slavery is morally wrong if done to acquire goods or avoid harms *for* the person because it attacks the worth *of* the person. Likewise, suicide of a rational being to avoid harms is wrong. But, I suggest, seeking death to avoid harm would be like entering into slavery to avoid harm only if death is like slavery. Its being like slavery should mean that we could substitute it for slavery in other contexts. In order to see if this is so, I shall take a somewhat circuitous route. I shall first consider how Velleman tries to justify some suicides.

Velleman says that suicide is permissible if one's personhood is already being undermined in life. He believes that this may be so even when one is not demented.

Indeed, he thinks that the case I described in which pain is so unbearable that all one can do is focus on it is such a case. Strikingly, he says that in this case, it is the unbearableness of the pain, not its painfulness, that makes suicide justifiable (p. 618). This is because not being able to bear the pain means that it is undermining one as a rational being. One is reduced to simply fleeing pain like an animal. To be like this is to be in a position unworthy of a rational agent. From the moral point of view, someone may permissibly kill himself (and we may permissibly assist him) rather than have him "come undone" as a person or live on as a nonrational being.

Notice that Velleman is here describing someone for whom pain is *not* a reason to end his life. This is not only because it is the inability to bear the pain, not the pain per se, that is the reason to end his life. When someone cannot bear the pain, the pain seems to become a mere cause of, rather than a reason for, his ending his life; it impels him. This implies (as Velleman concedes) that in many cases suicide is permissible only when it *cannot* be the choice of a rational, responsible person at the time it is to be done. This would create problems for the legal requirement of responsible, competent choice for physician-assisted suicide close to the time at which it is to occur. But the fact that the pain is not a reason on which the person acts to kill himself, because it *impels* him, need not mean that the pain could not be a reason why the suicide is justified, apart from its unbearableness. (This would also be true if dementia were a good reason for the suicide of a demented person who cannot himself understand or take it as a reason on which to act.)

I have questions about Velleman's justification of suicide in the case where pain is so unbearable that all one can do is focus on it. He seems to think that if we should help someone in great pain to kill himself, it is to remove him from an undignified state, not out of concern for his being in pain or out of respect for his choice. I think this is the wrong account of why we should act. For example, I think there is more urgency in helping a person in unbearable pain to die than in helping a demented person not in pain to die, yet indignity and the coming undone of the person might be equally present in the two cases (if not greater in the latter case). Does this not show that we act, in good part, to relieve the pain?[22] It is possible, however, that an intermediate position is correct: when someone's rational agency is greatly reduced, the way is open for us to simply focus on the pain. We then sympathize with him as we would with an animal and take the pain as a reason to help him commit suicide. We do not assist him in killing himself to end indignity per se; but it is only because he is in an undignified state that it may be permissible to seek to end pain.[23]

In addition, when we think of someone in great pain, we may think of him as *holding himself together* by focusing on the pain itself. In this case, the pain is not unbearable, though if he does not focus on it, he will fall apart by being subject to it. Some might say that in this situation, though one's rational nature is still being exercised, it has a very restricted scope. I do not think that on Velleman's view this would be a sufficient compromise of rationality to justify suicide. If we nevertheless endorse a chosen suicide in such a case, would it be because such a restriction of the scope of rational agency is unworthy of a person, or rather because the person is in pain? I think it is the latter. For consider a case in which the scope of rational agency is also restricted, but not by pain. For example, a person can only focus on the dots on a wall. Is there urgency in eliminating his life? I do not think so.

Possibly, an intermediate position is available here, too: it is only when the scope of rational agency is so severely limited that we are permitted to focus on the pain and act in order to stop it. If this intermediate position were correct, then it would not be necessary to say that the value of the continuing existence of (wider-ranging) rational agency was overridden by pain in order to justify suicide for the sake of getting rid of pain. On this intermediate view, the claim that avoiding pain cannot be a reason for suicide would be wrong—for it would be the pain, not its unbearableness, that was our reason for action—but the conditions in which avoiding pain could be such a reason would not rule out that enduring pain does not override the continuing *existence* of *unrestricted* rational agency.

This still leaves it open that there may be cases in which the continuing existence of unrestricted rational agency *is* overridden. For example, suppose someone alternates between days on which he totally focuses on pain and others on which he is able to work without pain.[24] Is it not possible that the pain should be so bad when it is present that it could outweigh the possibility of continued unrestricted rational agency on alternate days? Or is it instead the fact that on some days the use of rationality is very restricted which would justify suicide? But sleep also regularly alternates with waking, and sleep radically restricts rational agency when it is present. Yet that is not justification for suicide. So it seems the presence of pain on alternate days is crucial. In this Alternating Days Case, it also seems hard to adopt the intermediate position discussed above and say that because rationality is compromised, it is permissible to focus on the pain as a reason for suicide. This is because there is a lot of unrestricted rationality on alternate days, and alternation itself is not necessarily undignified (as shown by sleep/wake cycles). In the Alternating Days Case, the patient could either take morphine that knocked out the pain but made rational agency impossible on alternate days or commit suicide. If the importance of not exchanging rational agency for relief from pain is paramount, MPR (lethal or not) will be ruled out as well as suicide. If MPR is permitted, suicide cannot be ruled out on grounds of its being wrong to exchange rational agency for pain relief.

Now let us return to the slavery analogy. Suppose, as Velleman argues, it is permissible to end life in order to avoid one's rationality being undermined, and committing suicide and entering into slavery are morally analogous. Then it should be no worse to become a permanent slave if this (somehow) eliminated the pain that was undermining one's rationality than it would be to commit suicide (or go into terminal sedation or take MPR) for this purpose. But I doubt this is so.

Becoming a slave seems more like jumping from the frying pan into the fire, at least with respect to insults to oneself as a rational being. Slavery involves alienating one's rights—giving them over to someone else who then has power of life and death over one. Suicide and taking pain relief that causes death involve waiving one's right to go on living, not turning the right over to someone else.[25] Above, we contrasted death that ended pain with dementia that ended pain. Dementia was characterized as a perversion of ongoing agency and consciousness. Slavery is different: the rationality of the agent is intact, but he is not treated properly by others. Death, I think, contrasts with both dementia and slavery: it simply stops rational agency simultaneously with stopping the person. (No doubt this is a reason why killing oneself is often considered the noble alternative to being made a slave.)

Notes

1. This chapter presents revised parts of my "Physician-Assisted Suicide, the Doctrine of Double Effect, and the Ground of Value," *Ethics* 109 (April 1999): 586–605.

2. J. David Velleman, "A Right of Self-Termination?" *Ethics* 109 (April 1999): 606–28. Velleman criticizes the position I took in "A Right to Choose Death?" *Boston Review* 22 (Summer 1997): 20–23, and in my "Physician-Assisted Suicide." The latter article (and so this one) contained discussion of all but the last part of "A Right of Self-Termination?" The last part was written by Velleman only after he read my comments on the earlier parts of his article. His criticism can be seen as directed at step 3 in the Four-Step Argument (presented in chapter 4 this volume): that if we can destroy a part of the person for his good, we can destroy him for his good. Subsequently, in his "Beyond Price," *Ethics* 118 (January 2008), Velleman says, "I am now dissatisfied with the responses I made to Kamm in my appendix to 'A Right of Self-Termination?'" Hence, he may now accept some of the criticisms of his views that I present in this chapter.

3. These are the same issues I focused on in considering objections to the Four-Step Arguments in chapter 4 this volume, and so I repeat what I said there about these issues and why they are important.

4. See their separate concurring opinions.

5. Velleman agrees that death might be in a person's best interest on occasion, even if seeking what is in a person's best interest is disrespectful of him as a person.

6. See Joel Feinberg, "Voluntary Euthanasia and the Inalienable Right to Life," *Philosophy & Public Affairs* 7 (1978): 93–123.

7. If protecting a person's options were based on the importance of protecting the person's life, it would seem that one could not have an option to do anything that would endanger one's life (e.g., skiing).

8. Though Kant might disagree, as he attributes no intrinsic importance to animals.

9. Perhaps, it might be said, we should kill it because more pain in the world is an intrinsic evil, even if it happens to what does not matter. But could a Kantian argue that this additional pain is a moral evil? In any case, Velleman seems to reject this view.

10. Velleman provides an argument for the permissibility of euthanizing cats when their condition is "unworthy of them," not because it is good for them, in the last section of his article.

11. At the end of his article, Velleman says that he thinks that someone's interests may permissibly serve as a reason for seeking his death when his dignity is already threatened, though the fact that his dignity is already deteriorating does not mean that he does not matter. This implies that Velleman thinks that sometimes acting for someone's interests to eliminate him while he still matters is permissible.

12. I owe this example to Franklin Bruno.

13. Carlos Soto has pointed out that Kant did not think a person's continuing to exist had overriding value; one need not, and sometimes should not, do everything to save one's life, in his view.

14. I owe this point to Franklin Bruno. As noted above (note 7), protecting the person's life might also rule out protecting options that involved risks to his life.

15. Kamm, "A Right to Choose Death," p. 21.

16. It seems that Velleman now accepts this criticism. See his "Beyond Price," p. 192.

17. As David Sanson emphasized to me.

18. See chapter 4 this volume for another discussion of the senses of treating as a mere means.

19. Velleman correctly points out in his response to my argument (in the last part of his paper) that the exchange I describe does not involve destruction of the work of art for money or food. Yet sometimes the latter would also be permissible, I think.

20. As the person who assists someone else's suicide need not always intend the suicide, (c) need not always be true of her. See chapter 2 this volume on this.

21. I owe this point to Janos Kis. He suggests that, in most cases, in aiming at destroying the person, we really aim only at destroying her body which is in pain. If dualism were true, we would be quite happy to have the disembodied mind continue on. (However, could we not also permissibly, specifically eliminate the mind to get rid of severe mental pain if that were necessary?)

22. Note that even if it is suffering and not pain per se that is important, suffering is still distinct from being in an undignified state.

23. I thank Barbara Herman for raising this possibility.

24. I owe this case to David Kaplan.

25. Feinberg draws this distinction in "Voluntary Euthanasia."

6

Brody on Active and Passive Euthanasia

In this chapter, I shall consider Baruch Brody's views on active and passive euthanasia.[1, 2] Some of Brody's important claims are that there is a moral difference between killing and letting die, but we cannot conclude on this basis that killing a patient is not permissible even if letting him die is permissible. Hence, if we conclude that killing a patient is sometimes permissible, it need not be because we assume that there is no moral difference between killing and letting die. I agree with these claims but wish to examine the details of his arguments for them. In section I, I shall summarize and critically reflect on his views about the moral distinction between killing and letting die and its possible clinical significance. In section II, I shall summarize and critically examine his views about how to draw the killing/letting die distinction.[3]

I

A

Brody thinks it is a mistake to conclude on the basis of one set of cases, where all factors are held constant other than that one case is a killing and the other a letting die, that there is no moral difference between killing and letting die. (He criticizes James Rachels for doing this.[4] Rachels compares cases in which someone who lets a child who has slipped in the bathtub drown in order to inherit his money—letting die—with someone who pushes a child into the water to drown him in order to inherit his money—killing). Even if we believe that in one set of cases we should equally morally condemn the killing and the letting die, this need not mean that we should condemn killing and letting die equally in other cases where all factors are held constant. Furthermore, Brody argues, there are different ways in which killing and letting die could make a moral difference: (1) to degree of condemnation; (2) to whether there is a duty not to kill and not to let die; (3) to the strength of the two duties relative to each other and to other duties; and (4) to the efforts required to meet the duty.

I think Brody is correct to consider these various dimensions on which the killing/letting die distinction could make a difference.[5] For it might be that the efforts required to fulfill the duty to aid and the duty not to kill are equally high when considered one at time, and yet the duty not to kill would take precedence over the duty to aid if one had to choose which to perform.

However, Brody is also aware that if, in general, we were morally required to make a greater effort to fulfill one duty than another, it still might be true that, when they conflict, we should choose to carry out the duty judged less strenuous by the efforts test rather than the duty judged more strenuous by the efforts test.[6] For example, I may have to make a great effort to keep a business obligation, but it would be supererogatory of me to make as great an effort to save someone from death. Yet if the choice arose as to whether to keep the business obligation (at minor effort) or to save someone's life (at minor effort), I should do the latter. This phenomenon raises the problem that the four dimensions he describes on which killing and letting die might differ could point in different directions as to which form of conduct is morally more significant. If so, then without further explanation, merely testing on the dimensions would not settle the question of which form of conduct was morally more significant. (In fact, I do not believe that testing killing and letting die on these various dimensions yields conflicting results as to which conduct is more significant. However, I shall not prove that here.)

By the measure of how great an effort we morally must make to avoid killing versus to save life, Brody thinks that not killing is shown to be the weightier duty. He says that if someone will kill you unless you kill a third person, you may not kill the third person.[7] However, if someone will kill you unless you let a third person die, you may leave that person to die. My concern with Brody's argument here is that in the killing case, if you kill someone else, his death would be intended by you (as a mere means to saving your life). By contrast, in the letting die case, it seems that the death of the person you leave to die would be foreseen but not intended by you. Hence, Brody has not equalized all factors besides killing and letting die in these two cases and, therefore, we cannot tell if it is only the killing/letting die distinction that makes the moral difference. We might modify his cases to hold all other factors constant, even including intending death as a means, and then ask if we may let someone die when we aim at his death as a mere means to saving our life because only if the person is dead will a villain not kill us. Alternatively, we could hold *not* intending death constant in both cases. For example, may we let someone die merely foreseeing his death rather than save him in order to avoid our being killed by someone else, and may we do an act (such as releasing a gas) that we only foresee will directly kill someone in order to avoid being killed by someone else? I think we may let die but not kill, and this agrees with Brody's conclusion.

B

What are the clinical implications of this moral distinction between killing and letting die? Brody argues that one implication is that while we need not fund all sorts of lifesaving treatments, we should not kill people in order to avoid paying for their support.[8] Given that Brody thinks that withdrawing lifesaving treatment is letting die, this seems to commit him to the controversial view that it is permissible to terminate lifesaving treatment of patients because we do not want to pay for its continuation. Arguably, some may resist the permissibility of this bedside decision, even if they agree that we need not invest at a social level so that lifesaving treatments are available.

But is Brody entitled to reach his general conclusion even if not this specific one? Recall that in order to be sure that it is the killing/letting die distinction that is accounting for our different judgments, we must hold all other factors constant. When we refuse to fund lifesaving treatment, we foresee additional deaths; we do not intend them. By contrast, if we were to kill people in order to avoid paying for their treatment, we would be intending their deaths. Some might, therefore, conclude that it is not the killing/letting die distinction on its own that accounts for his general conclusion. To test the merits of this objection, Brody might compare a letting die case that involved intending death with a killing case that involved intending death. For example, would it be permissible to let someone die from an easily treatable infection in order not to have to continue expensive lifesaving treatment for another condition he has? If doing this is not permissible, then the general clinical implication that Brody thinks derives from the difference between killing and letting die does not depend on this distinction. Now consider a case where the killing involves foreseen death rather than intended death, to match the merely foreseen death in a letting die case. Would it be permissible not to spend money on improving a medical procedure that we foresee will otherwise cause unintended deaths? If spending this money to prevent doctors unintentionally killing people were more important than spending money on lifesaving equipment, this would be a clinical implication that supports Brody's general claim. But if spending the money on avoiding unintentional killing were no more important than spending money on lifesaving aid, we would still not have derived a clinical implication from the fact that we should make greater efforts to avoid killing than to save life. Indeed, it would show that the effort (or cost, more generally) test does not always work to distinguish killing and letting die.

My point in considering these cases is to raise a methodological concern. Namely, in his argumentation, Brody does not pay enough attention to holding all factors aside from killing and letting die constant. It is only by doing this that one can conclude that it is this distinction and not some other that is making a moral difference.[9]

C

If there is a moral distinction between killing and letting die on some dimensions, what significance does this have for the issue of voluntary euthanasia? (Euthanasia involves killing or letting die intending death, on the grounds that death is in the interest of the patient.) I am here concerned with Brody's discussion of euthanasia and so will not discuss any views he might have on physician-assisted suicide, as the latter is different from active euthanasia (killing) and may also differ from passive euthanasia (letting die). Brody first argues that any duty had by others to give lifesaving aid disappears when a competent adult makes clear that she does not want the aid and waives her right to it.[10] Importantly, Brody wants to argue that this will be true even if a patient and her doctor who would omit the aid both intend the patient's death because they believe it is in her interest. That is, he agrees the patient need not be rejecting the aid merely on the grounds that the aid itself is too unpleasant or intrusive. (Rejecting aid on these grounds would then imply that she is not *seeking* death, as is required for euthanasia.) The patient may permissibly reject aid even when the aid is not intrusive and she is seeking passive euthanasia because life itself is too burdensome for her.[11]

Then Brody makes the important point that even if killing is morally distinct from letting die in some ways, this does not show that the right not to be killed may not be permissibly waived, just as the right to be aided may be waived. This might leave the way open for the permissibility of voluntary active euthanasia because the waiving may imply that the duty not to kill is no longer in force, if the duty is merely the correlative of a waivable right not to be killed. Similarly, the duty to aid would no longer be in force if someone waived his right to be aided, thereby allowing for passive euthanasia. Hence, he claims, we do not have to argue for voluntary active euthanasia on the grounds that passive euthanasia is permissible *and* there is no moral difference between killing and letting die. Nor do we have to conclude that voluntary active euthanasia is impermissible merely on the grounds that there is a moral difference between killing and letting die.

I agree with this argument, but I would like to point out two ways in which it does not go far enough. First, Brody's argument claims that it is *permissible not to provide aid* (there is no duty to aid) when a patient waives his right to it. The stronger additional conclusion is that it is *impermissible to provide the aid* when the competent adult patient waives his right and also makes clear he does not want the aid. Waiving a right to aid need not always imply absence of a desire for it. For example, John may waive his right in order that you be free to decide whether to aid him or another person, but John would be very happy if you chose to aid him. By contrast, a person's rejecting aid because he intends to die can make it impermissible for a doctor to aid, because aiding would involve interfering with the person against his will. Aiding would also involve acting against the interests of the person, if death is indeed in his interest. Hence there is often a duty to let die, rather than just a permission to do so.

Now, suppose that a patient waived his right not to be killed and the only ground for a duty not to kill were such a right. Suppose also that the patient desired to be killed, and it was in his interest to die. There still might not be a duty to kill comparable to the duty to let die, at least on the part of ordinary people and even such hospital personnel as nurses. This is, in part, because if we do not kill someone, we are not interfering with him as an autonomous being, though we may not be promoting his autonomy in the sense of helping to carry out his wishes. The question arises, however, of whether a patient's doctor may have a duty to kill him, either because she has a duty to promote a patient's best medically relevant interests when the patient wants this done or because she has a duty to be the agent of a patient's medically relevant wishes when this is not obviously against a patient's medically relevant interests.[12]

There is a second way in which Brody's argument does not go far enough. When a competent adult waives a right to aid and also desires to die, it still may not be in his interests to die. Nevertheless, I think we still have a duty not to interfere by providing lifesaving aid. (In this case, omitting aid will not be passive euthanasia because the death is not in the patient's interest and is not intended by the person omitting aid.) However, if he waives a right not to be killed and desires to be killed, it may not even be permissible to kill him if this would be against his interests. As Philippa Foot noted,[13] we have a duty not to violate someone's rights, but we can also have a duty not to act against her interests even when this would not violate her rights (and, I would add, not be contrary to her desires).[14] This, however, will not be an argument against voluntary active euthanasia, as euthanasia involves killing only when this is in the interest of the person killed.

Despite arguing that the great strenuousness of the duty not to kill does not show that the right correlative to it cannot be waived, Brody is not sure that voluntary active euthanasia is permissible. He suggests that we investigate whether there are grounds for the wrongness of killing that go beyond any right of the person not to be killed. (So though we would not be wronging the person, we would still be acting wrongly if we killed. Presumably, the grounds would also have to be something other than the interests of the person in not dying because it is being assumed that death would be in his interest.) It may also be, he suggests, that the right not to be killed is not waivable, even if the mere difference in strenuousness of the duty not to kill and the duty not to let die does not show this. I think there is reason to doubt the last claim: the denial of waivability at least suggests that it could not be even a necessary condition for killing a competent patient that he agreed to be killed. In other words, it suggests that whenever other factors weigh in favor of killing a competent patient, the fact that he has *not* agreed to be killed could not stand in the way of killing him. For if his agreeing does not affect the role that his right not to be killed plays, it is not clear why it is so important to seek his agreement. Yet it is important.

II

I have discussed Brody's views on the question of whether there is a moral difference between killing and letting die and the possible clinical significance of this. Now let us consider his views on how to draw the killing/letting die distinction. Brody believes that withholding and withdrawing life support involve letting die, regardless of the intention with which one does it, and giving a lethal drug involves killing. He thinks this is our intuitive judgment and the role of ethical theory is to provide a more precise characterization of the killing/letting die distinction that does not undermine these initial judgments. He considers two possible characterizations of the distinction: (1) an act or omission that involves intending someone's death earlier than it would otherwise have occurred is a killing or, alternatively, (2) killing but not letting die involves causing someone's death earlier than it would have occurred. (His focus on bringing about an earlier death seems to incorrectly exclude the possibility that one kills someone at exactly the time that he would have died anyway. I shall ignore this issue.)

Consider (1). Brody argues, correctly I believe, against the view that intention makes for a killing. His grounds for doing so, however, are merely conservative. That is, he assumes that we need an account that makes a do-not-resuscitate (DNR) order, not giving antibiotics, and withdrawals of treatment be lettings die, even when there is an intention to have the patient die.[15] (Possibly, he will also want it to come out true that these are permissible lettings die rather than impermissible ones.) A nonconservative reason to reject the intending account of killing is that there are clear cases of killing that do not involve intending death; for example, when one runs over someone only because one is determined to get somewhere fast, despite foreseeing that one will kill someone. In the clinical context, giving morphine for pain relief when one foresees with certainty that it will also stop the heart is a killing even when one does not intend the death. It is also often considered permissible. Consider also a case where the omission to aid A is justified by the duty to save B, C, and D instead. Nevertheless, the agent who omits to aid A fulfills his duty to save the greater number instead of helping A only because he recognizes that A is his enemy and he intends A's death. Shall we say in this case that the agent kills A in virtue of his intention, even though another agent who would save B, C, and D instead of A, not intending A's death, would let die but not kill A? I think not.

Now consider (2). Brody considers the view that killing involves *causing* earlier death, whereas letting die is only a necessary condition of an earlier death whose cause is the underlying disease condition of the patient. Some of his concerns with this account are that: (a) It is not clear how to draw the distinction between causes and necessary conditions. (b) Withdrawals of food result in death from starvation, not from the underlying disease condition. Is this then a killing? (c) Most withdrawals of aid are now considered lettings die but it is not clear that they will come out as such on the cause versus necessary condition account. (d) How is one to deal with the fact that when a doctor deliberately withdraws lifesaving treatment intending death we are said to have a letting die, but when a greedy nephew does the same, we are said to have a killing?[16] In regard to (d), Brody provides the following (nonconservative) answer: The greedy nephew does not kill. "He brought about conditions in which the patient's underlying medical problem caused the death and from a reprehensible motive."[17] This, Brody thinks, is as morally bad as the nephew killing.

I think that Brody's analysis of the second characterization of killing (as causing earlier death) is not correct. Let us start with his last point. Suppose the doctor who deliberately withdraws the treatment she was providing, intending death, does so from as reprehensible a motive as the greedy nephew. Is what she does as morally bad as what the nephew does? I do not think so, even if what she does is impermissible because she has a duty to provide life support. Furthermore, I think that the nephew does kill someone, while the doctor lets die (perhaps impermissibly). I believe that what accounts for the difference between the nephew and the doctor is that the doctor stops assistance that she herself (or some entity whose agent she is) is providing. By contrast, the nephew is interfering with assistance that someone else is providing. Proprietary rights over the device that aids (i.e., whether someone is stopping my device or the device of someone else [for whom I am not an agent]) can also be crucial to determining if someone is killing or letting die, even if the letting die is impermissible.[18] (Note that on this account when a person himself pulls out the plug of *doctor's* machine and dies of an underlying disease, he is not killing himself but letting himself die, at least in part, because he is removing *himself*—something over which he has rights that is required in order that assistance be given—from the process of aiding.)

Consider the cases where withdrawal of treatment is a killing even when the patient dies from the underlying disease condition (such as, I have suggested, the nephew's interference with aid.) Does the agent cause the patient's death? If not, the idea that killing necessarily involves causing death will be wrong. I suggest that a distinction might be drawn between *causing death* and *introducing the cause of death*. Hence, Brody's distinction between causing death and providing a necessary condition for death may be too simple; a further breakdown may be called for. When the nephew or the doctor withdraws treatment, I think each causes death by removing protection against it, but that need not mean that they introduce the cause of death. To introduce the cause of death is to induce death. If they removed food, I think they would also remove protection against a cause of death (the cause being starvation), even though the patient does not die of an underlying disease. Does drawing this further distinction helps us answer the question Brody raises in (b): If a patient does not die of an underlying disease when he is starved, is he killed? Food which had always been provided was always warding off another possible underlying cause of death (starvation) that causes death when food is removed. When the doctor removes the things he is providing, though he helps cause death, he does not kill because he neither introduces the cause of death nor interferes with life-sustaining mechanisms that someone else, who is not his agent and for whom he is not an agent, is either providing or has authority over. When the nephew causes death by removing what interferes with it, he kills (as argued for above), though he too does not introduce the cause of death.

Sometimes withdrawing treatment can also introduce the cause of death, thus inducing death. For example, suppose that in a hospital, there is faulty wiring and when the doctor unplugs life support, a painless electric shock is produced that causes the patient's death before anything else can (Faulty Wiring Case).[19] In this case, the doctor kills the patient because he introduces the cause of death. I believe that it may sometimes be no less permissible for him to do this than to withdraw the treatment when there is no faulty wiring, even if voluntary active euthanasia were not, in general, permissible. This can be so when the patient has requested to be disconnected, for the patient should not be required to remain connected to treatment he does not want merely because the painless shock that results from disconnection will cause his death before anything else will.

But suppose the patient did not consent to be disconnected. In the Faulty Wiring Case, as in the case where the doctor withdraws the treatment and the wiring is not faulty, the patient will lose out only on life he would have had by way of the doctor's life-support system. This is a crucial part of what makes the killing in the Faulty Wiring Case have the same moral status as a letting die. Though, of course, both letting die and killing may be impermissible without patient consent.[20]

In sum, I think that Brody may be wrong not to distinguish between causing death and introducing the cause of death (i.e., inducing death), I also think he is wrong not to distinguish between some killings and lettings die on the basis of who is providing aid or proprietary relation to life support, and he is wrong to focus on the motives of an agent (e.g., the bad motives of the nephew versus the good ones of many doctors) as the basis for determining that the nephew's supposed letting die is as wrong as his killing would be.

Notes

1. This chapter is a revised version of my "Brody on Active and Passive Euthanasia," *Pluralistic Casuistry: Balancing Moral Arguments, Economic Realities, and Political Theory*, eds. M. Cherry and A. Ittis. Dordrecht, Netherlands: Springer, 2007.

2. My discussion is an examination of the arguments in his "Withdrawal of Treatment versus Killing of Patients," in *Intending Death: the Ethics of Assisted Suicide and Euthanasia*, ed. Tom L. Beauchamp (Upper Saddle River, NJ: Prentice Hall, 1996). All references to Brody, unless otherwise noted, are to that article.

3. This follows the order in which he himself discusses these issues in the article I am examining.

4. In Rachels's "Passive and Active Euthanasia," *The New England Journal of Medicine* 292 (1975): 78–80.

5. I discuss similar dimensions on which to test the killing/letting die distinction in my "Killing and Letting Die: Methodological and Substantive Issues," *Pacific Philosophical Quarterly* 64 (1983): 297–312, and *Morality, Mortality*, Vol. 2 (New York: Oxford University Press, 1996).

6. He cites my discussion in "Supererogation and Obligation," *The Journal of Philosophy* 82 (March 1985): 118–38, where I tried to show this.

7. Brody, "Withdrawal of Treatment," p. 161.

8. Brody, "Withdrawal of Treatment," p. 162.

9. I emphasize this in my work cited in note 4. In drawing attention to the intention/foresight distinction, I do not mean to suggest that I think that an agent's intention determines the permissibility of an act. It may be the role of death as a required causal means or as the only possible effect of an act, whether it is intended or not, that has a role in determining permissibility. I am only concerned with suggesting that Brody has not answered questions that need to be answered.

10. It is worth asking whether there are not exceptions to this. For example (as John Stuart Mill noted), if someone has obligations to others, he may have a duty not to die until such obligations are fulfilled. In such cases, may not his waiver of the right to lifesaving aid be invalid? I shall ignore this issue henceforth.

11. Brody, "Withdrawal of Treatment," p. 165.

12. I discuss these two grounds for a doctor's role and the relation to a duty to kill in chapter 4 this volume.

13. In her "Euthanasia," *Philosophy & Public Affairs* 6 (1977).

14. This addition is needed because someone might waive his right not to be killed in order to permit you to decide whether to kill him or someone else, and still not want you to kill him.

15. Brody, "Withdrawal of Treatment," p. 169.

16. Brody cites Shelly Kagan in regard to this question.

17. Brody, "Withdrawal of Treatment," p. 169.

18. I have discussed the role of stopping aid one is providing in, for example, "Killing and Letting Die: Methodological and Substantive Issues," and *Morality, Mortality*, Vol. 2. In chapter 2 this volume, I elaborate on the distinction between providing aid and having rights over the device providing aid, a distinction emphasized by Timothy Hall.

19. I first presented this case in "Ronald Dworkin on Abortion and Assisted Suicide," *The Journal of Ethics* 5 (2001), reprinted with emendations in *Dworkin and His Critics*, ed. J. Burley (Malden, MA: Blackwell, 2004) and in chapter 3 this volume.

20. Above I noted that Brody accepts that a duty which is more strenuous by the measure of how much effort we must make to perform it can be weaker by the measure of which duty we ought to perform when we must choose between them. He says this may make trouble for his argument against the permissibility of abortion, which is based on the idea that the duty not to kill is stronger than the duty to aid (as measured by the efforts test). But I think that what really makes trouble for his argument against the permissibility of abortion (based on the idea that the duty not to kill is stronger than the duty to aid) is the fact that in being killed the fetus loses only life it would have received by way of the woman's life-support system. This will make killing it in some ways analogous to what happens when the doctor kills the patient who does not want to die in the Faulty Wiring Case. However, what the doctor does may be impermissible, as impermissible as his not beginning to aid a patient who does not want to die, given that the doctor has a duty to aid a patient who wants to be treated and there are no competing duties he has at the time. By contrast, the pregnant woman, who might be said to kill in having an abortion, may have no duty to provide the aid whose termination may involve killing. For more on my analysis of abortion, inspired by J. J. Thomson's analysis in "A Defense of Abortion," *Philosophy & Public Affairs* 1, no. 1 (Fall 1971), see my *Creation and Abortion* (New York: Oxford University Press, 1992).

7

A Note on Dementia and Advance Directives

A person might make a decision for or against terminating (life-sustaining) treat-ment, suicide, assisted suicide, or euthanasia while he is judged legally competent to make such decisions.[1] He could also carry out the decision (or have it carried out) while judged competent. Additionally, while competent, he may have to de-cide what should be done in the future if he will no longer be competent to give consent to these acts (particularly with respect to terminating treatment and eu-thanasia). One mechanism to allow a person to make decisions for himself about the future is known as a living will. In such a document, a person enumerates what he would like done should various circumstances arise. For example, would he want a lifesaving antibiotic given to him if he is in a persistent vegetative state? One problem with a living will is that circumstances might arise that the per-son did not cover in his will. A second problem is that he might not have enough knowledge about a possible condition to know what he would want done. For example, he might predict that he would not want to go on living with a disability, but once actually disabled, he might prefer to live after all (or vice versa).

An answer to the first problem is known as an advance directive. One part of this document is a living will. But this is supplemented with the designation of another person as a substitute decision-maker (SD), who will have the legal power to make decisions about events not contemplated ex ante if one cannot make them oneself. There are at least two types of reasoning an SD can employ. In "substituted judgment," the SD tries to decide as the person himself would have in the circum-stances. This requires knowing the values and commitments of the person. It does not necessarily result in doing what is in the best interests of the person, if she herself would not have decided in her best interests. It is a way of respecting the person's autonomy. The second type of reasoning in which the SD might engage, if he lacks enough information about the person's values or commitments, is simply deciding what would be in the person's best interest.

Ronald Dworkin has argued that a person has two types of interests.[2] There are "experiential interests" in having good experiences and avoiding bad experi-ences (such as pain and frustration) in one's life. But there are also "critical inter-ests" in having one's life be an objectively good life, a meaningful, worthwhile life. It is possible that a life that is not high in experiential goods is a better life in the second sense. (For example, the life of a creative artist who is often in torment might satisfy his critical interests better than the life in which he is always having pleasant experiences.) One's values will lead one to have a certain view about what really is a good life, but one's view could be mistaken. One's critical interest in really having a good life could then come into conflict with one's autonomous choices, even when they reflect one's values about a meaningful life. Therefore, an SD might not only have to think about respecting someone's autonomy and values, but also sometimes pursue someone's true experiential and critical interests.

Particular problems arise for the use of living wills or advance directives when a person's values and interests change (or seem to change) from the time when these devices were put in force. One type of case involves temporary derangement. Consider a Jehovah's Witness whose values require that he not have blood transfusions even to save his life and who wills this when sane. Suppose that when he is ill, he becomes temporarily deranged and in this state, he requests a transfusion. The problem is whether to heed his most recent, but deranged, request or the directions he gave when sane. (Notice that he might make the request while deranged and then become unconscious at the very time we have to give the transfusion.)

If he is deranged, it is thought that he is not competent to make decisions relating to this matter and that his choice may not reflect his real values. It may also be said that if he were to live on as a result of the transfusion and regain sanity, he would regret having had the transfusion. He is unlike a sane person who undergoes a real change in his values. Hence, if respect for an autonomous choice resulting from one's underlying values takes precedence, an SD should decide as the Jehovah's Witness would have decided when sane. This case shows the importance of a person's history in how we act toward him. Had the deranged person never been sane, it might very well be right to heed his request while deranged for the transfusion, given that having the transfusion is also in his interests as a living being.

It might be argued, however, that attending to values someone last held when sane is correct only in cases where this person will again become sane and be committed to the same values, as was imagined in the Jehovah's Witness case. This could be because it is important whether the person will have to "live with" the results of his decisions made when deranged, in the sense that he will be aware of whether the results are consistent with the values he will again espouse[3] (or perhaps with values he will come to hold for the first time) when he returns to sanity. Therefore, a second case that is important for considering whether to follow a living will or, rather, a contemporary choice involves permanent derangement, as in late-stage dementia.[4] Suppose a person when competent agrees in a living will that when he is in permanent, late-stage dementia, he should be left to die. As he understands it, his life will be a better one if it ends without a period of dementia, even if it is thereby shortened and he is deprived of some simple pleasures. However, when he is demented he resists and expresses a wish to go on living because he gets experiential goods from simple activities in his life. What should be done?

Some have analyzed this case as involving two different persons diachronically occupying the same body.[5] The first person, it is said, has no right to control the fate of the second person. This second person is demented and, let us suppose, incapable of considered judgments and the formulation of values. He has no autonomous will. Nevertheless, he has a desire to remain alive and is having positive experiences in his life. Hence, remaining alive is in his experiential interest and at least not inconsistent with any deep will or values he has, in the view of some. Others might counter that it is worse to be an adult human being in a demented state than to be dead, even if experientially his life is no different from that of a happy rabbit for whom life is not a worse option than death. If the objectively correct critical interests of an adult human are defeated by his staying alive when severely demented, this might trump actual desires and experiences, even on the two-person view that tells us to ignore the "first person's" living will.

An alternative analysis of this case[6] insists that there is only one person who has lived through a competent stage and is now in a demented stage. (Those who believe dementia involves a withering away of the self and the person [understood as a self-conscious being] may speak of the same *individual* rather than the same *person* in two stages.) Only the person in his competent stage has a will that should be taken seriously and that is owed respect. Because he is only deciding for himself in his later stage when he provides a living will, he is not improperly attempting to decide for someone else. If there is only one person throughout, what are the interests of that person? The opinion of the person when he was capable of reasoned thought was, we are assuming, that a demented end would be less consistent with his critical interests than an earlier death would be. Furthermore, the time-relative interests he has when sane (i.e., his interests as the person he is at the time he decides about his future[7]) in having future pleasant experiences while demented are weak. Those interests, therefore, get trumped by his critical interests, which are said to be the same when he is demented and sane, for he is the same person. On this view, though the person could be wrong about what is in his critical interests, if he makes a choice when competent, respect for his autonomy should govern our treatment of him.

The question we are asking is whether this analysis is affected by the fact that the person will not return to sanity, and so will not have to live as a sane person with the results of his being kept alive when demented. If someone answers yes, she might deal differently with the case of permanent derangement and with the following two hypothetical cases: (1) The demented person regains his sanity for one day every year. While he does not have any awareness of having been demented, he always repeats the request he made before becoming demented: not to be kept alive when severely demented. (2) We know that at the very end of his life, the dementia will disappear and the person will regain his sanity. Though he will not remember having been demented, he will express the view that it would have been wrong to have kept him alive after he became demented. In these cases, the person-as-sane does not disappear forever. Some may think that it is this that implies that the person would be wronged by our decision to keep him alive when demented, given his earlier living will.

However, it is important to see that even when the person will remain demented and so could never again form the view that he should not be kept alive when demented, we can wrong the person and harm him in keeping him alive. A ground for thinking this is that we can wrong and harm someone after his death by not carrying out his written will or by destroying his unpublished life's work, though he will not know we do these things nor have to "live with it." (In the dementia case, of course, the person or individual still exists.) This strengthens the case for heeding the advance directive rather than satisfying the desire to live of the demented individual. More generally, it seems problematic to focus too much on whether the sane person will have to live with what the demented person wants. Suppose it were in the interests, and consistent with the desires, of the person *qua* deranged person not to have lifesaving treatment. It would obviously be incorrect not to save the person if, when he was sane, he requested that he be saved and he would return to sanity if he were saved. This is so, even though the person would never have had to live with the decision he made when deranged, had we heeded it, because he would be dead.

The case for respecting the directive of the person when sane is also strengthened, I think, by considering the following hypothetical case. An elderly parent, competent to decide, wants to give an organ to save his child's life. A medicine must be given to the parent a few days prior to surgery to make possible the removal of his organ. Unfortunately, this medicine will cause permanent dementia. The parent knows this and consents nevertheless. When demented, however, the parent refuses to allow the removal of his organ for transplantation (Dementia Transplant Case). Suppose it is morally permissible for the parent to make the dual sacrifice for his child of his organ and his reason. Further, suppose that if he did not object to the transplant when demented, we would follow the instructions he gave when competent. Then, I believe, one should follow these instructions even when he resists them while demented. It would certainly be a cruel waste of his sacrifice of reason not to follow those instructions, and I think it is wrong not to allow the competent parent to sacrifice his reason solely on the ground that we will have to heed what we know will be his wishes while demented not to donate the organ. In this case, of course, the child will benefit if we do *not* heed the wishes of the person when demented. But we would not ordinarily take organs from a demented person when he resists in order to save his child's life. So, it is because the instructions of the person when he was competent are overriding his objections while demented that the transplant is permissible. If they can override in this case, this strengthens the view that they can override in general.

Consider another case in which the life's work that the person produced when sane is at stake. Suppose someone has devoted his life to painting. His works reflect well on his life, though they are not irreplaceable contributions to the general culture. The person is now demented and he has no interest in, or understanding of, his past work. What interests him now is cutting up pieces of paper and canvas that have paint on them. We might even say that this activity gives value and meaning to the person's current life, to the extent to which he still can have the attitudes underlying these concepts.[8] He very much wants to cut up what is, in fact, his life's work of paintings, as they are the only pieces of paper and canvas available. Hence, there may be a conflict between his current values and his past values. Presumably, we should not allow his life's work to be destroyed in order to satisfy the desire (or value) he has when demented, even if there are no other canvases and papers that he could use. Indeed, suppose that the demented person comes to need life-support machinery and the only thing that makes the machine run is the cuttings of his paintings. It seems wrong to destroy his life's work merely so that he can live on in a demented state, even if he requests this when demented, especially if he expressed the view when sane that it would be wrong to destroy his work for such a purpose.[9]

These examples suggest that at least when (1) heeding the wishes (or even interests) of the person when demented would interfere with a life project that was of importance to the critical interests of the person when sane, and (2) the person when sane would have given precedence to his critical interests over the wishes, interests, and values of himself when demented, then it is the critical interests of the sane person that should take precedence.

Nevertheless, we might be reluctant not to medically treat (or to kill) the person in the demented stage simply because the person, when nondemented, wished it. This may be because it is not clear to us that continuing demented life really threatens any interests, values, or products of someone's sane life. After all, ending in a demented state does not, in itself, negate what good one has done in one's past life. A simple concern for the narrative structure of the life seems precious.

As a practical matter, it may be wise for a person who strongly wishes not to live through predictable end-stage dementia to forgo some period of still-worthwhile life in order to end his life while he is still competent to direct this. Then there will be no question of decision-makers having to weigh his present desires and experiences as a demented individual. If such a competent person's concern in seeking death is based only on his belief that his experiences when demented will be bad, he should become well informed about whether this is likely to be true, perhaps on the basis of other people's experiences. However, suppose that a competent person's concerns are rather that, in the light of his values, the demented state itself is demeaning whether or not it is pleasant. Then becoming well informed about his likely experiences when demented is irrelevant. If only particular characteristics associated with dementia, such as becoming violent, are considered demeaning, then a person should become informed about whether he is likely to have such characteristics.

Notes

1. This chapter is drawn from a part of my "Ending Life," in *Blackwell Guide to Medical Ethics*, eds. R. Rhodes, L. Frances, and A. Silvers (Oxford: Wiley-Blackwell, 2007), pp. 142–61.

2. R. M. Dworkin, *Life's Dominion* (New York: Knopf, 1993).

3. Seana Shiffrin, in "Autonomy, Beneficence, and the Permanently Demented," *Dworkin and his Critics*, ed. J. Burley (Malden, MA: Blackwell, 2004), seems to emphasize such a factor.

4. We might also consider a case in which having the transfusion will cause a permanent change in the Jehovah's Witness's values but not through any autonomous reflection or choice. He will then experience no regret at having had the transfusion. Should this affect our judgment of what to do? I think not, as I shall argue.

5. For a view like this, see Rebecca Dresser, "Dworkin on Dementia: Elegant Theory, Questionable Policy," *Hastings Center Report* 25 (November–December 1995): 32–38.

6. For example, provided by Dworkin, *Life's Dominion*.

7. The role of "time relative interests" is emphasized by Jeff McMahan in his *The Morality of Killing: Problems at the Margins of Life* (New York: Oxford University Press, 2004).

8. Carlos Soto has argued that, contrary to what Ronald Dworkin claims, demented persons may still have valuing attitudes. He argues that Dworkin is mistaken to think that one has to be able to take a view of one's whole life in order to have values. That the demented person cannot take such a view does not mean that he cannot value the things of which he is aware. See Soto's *Extending and Ending Life in Health Care and Beyond*, doctoral dissertation, 2010. See also Agnieszka Jaworska's "Respecting the Margins of Agency: Alzheimer's Patients and the Capacity to Value," *Philosophy & Public Affairs* 28(2): 105–38.

9. What if destroying his life's work to run the life-support machines would result in the person's returning to sanity? Then we should consider whether, as a sane person, he would prefer an additional period of sane life or the continued existence of his work.

8

Brain Death and Spontaneous Breathing

When is a person dead?[1, 2] Or more precisely: what criterion should be used to determine when someone is declared dead? The answer may have great practical importance, for perhaps it should determine when medical efforts whose aim is to sustain a patient's life may be discontinued or when a patient's organs may be removed for transplant to others. If the wrong criterion is used—if someone is not already dead when these things are done—then in doing some of them we may kill him (or let him die), and this, many will say, is wrong.

The contemporary debate about this issue focuses on at least four different positions. One is the traditional cardiopulmonary criterion (CPC): a person is dead when his heart permanently stops beating and he permanently does not inhale and exhale air. The possibility of attaching people to respirators that artificially induce respiration has, in the minds of some, created problems for the CPC because, they argue, someone can be dead even though a machine is mechanically producing respiration. Among those who raise this problem for the CPC are the proponents of a second criterion for death, the death of the whole brain (WBC). More accurately, they claim that a person is dead when no part of the brain survives that supports integrated functioning of the organism. It is the latter, they say, that characterizes life, and in the case of humans, it cannot be present when significant parts of the brain die. Cardiopulmonary activity is a sign of life only if it is a sign of such brain activity, and it is not such a sign when produced by machines.

The WBC has come under attack from two different directions. Some have claimed that integrated functioning of the organism can be present when tests for whole brain death are satisfied. For example, growth, healing, neurohormonal regulation, and other organism-wide functioning have been said to occur in those who satisfy these tests.[3] The problem here seems to be that the tests are not adequate to accurately determine death of the whole brain, which would satisfy the WBC. However, at least hypothetically it could be true that the WBC was satisfied and yet integrated functioning of the organism continued. (Indeed, it has been argued that cases presented by Dr. Alan Shewmon do involve integrated functioning in the definite presence of whole brain death.[4]) If integrated functioning of the organism is what characterizes life, then whenever it is still present, death is not. Hence, absence of integrated functioning per se could be peeled apart from the WBC and be used as a third criterion which I shall call the integrated functioning criterion, IFC.

It is my understanding that in cases in which there is said to be integrated functioning when the whole brain is dead and/or the tests for WBC are met there is held to be some spontaneous integrated functioning of the organism although there is also partial artificial life support (e.g., a ventilator). What if the integrated functioning of the organism as a whole was entirely artificially produced? Would it still be a characteristic of life? The WBC was introduced at a time when artificial production of integrated functioning of the organism as a whole was not possible. Robert Truog claims that is now possible.[5] Arguably, a system whose integration is maintained artificially would be alive just in virtue of integrated functions of the whole even if they are mechanically generated. If artificial integration were not sufficient for life, the theory that life is integrated functioning of the organism would face a problem. In addition, higher consciousness is sufficient for life but is not integrated functioning of the organism as a whole. This presents another problem for the idea that integrated functioning characterizes life. Higher consciousness could also be present if there were artificial integration of the organism. If the latter was not sufficient for life but the former was sufficient, then life would not have to be characterized by integration of the organism as a whole. This would be a criticism of the IFC. (It would be a criticism of the WBC only if higher consciousness could be completely artificially continued by an artificial brain when the whole brain has died and this was consistent with the continued identity of the same person.)

The WBC has come under attack from another direction. Some say that death of the person is present when the parts of the brain responsible for higher functioning (e.g., consciousness, perception) are dead, even if the brain stem still supports other functions (e.g., respiration, swallowing, temperature). Call this the higher brain criterion (HBC). Many may believe that if someone is alive according to another criterion but lacks functioning supported by the higher brain, his life has no value to him though he still exists. On this view, the HBC tries to make the loss of value of the life to the person whose life it is coincide with death, but some think that trying to do this is wrong. They think that the HBC should rather be used to tell us *when it does not matter morally if we kill or let die someone who is still alive* (when his life has no value to him). Thus removing the person's organs or stopping life support, even if doing so kills him, would not always be morally wrong according to this position.

In this article, I wish to examine only the WBC, which is currently the accepted criterion for declaring death in many countries. It is important to understand what such a widely used criterion is really trying to capture, as this does not seem to be clear even to its supporters. (For example, one such supporter, James Bernat, has said, "Brain death was accepted before it was conceptually sound."[6]) My discussion has several parts. I shall first try to show that, contrary to what supporters of the WBC say in attacking the CPC, respiration is not important to them merely as such a sign of brain activity. I shall argue that if respiration is not important to them merely as such a sign, this may show that neither brain activity nor integrated functioning of the organism is crucial to them as a characteristic of life. Rather, certain major spontaneous activity (or attempts at it) may be what they see as characteristic of life. Brain activity is a mere sign of these. Finally, I shall suggest that the WBC's supporters would allow that concerted functioning that is supported in part artificially can constitute life and so spontaneity is less important than they seem to think.

I

The cardiopulmonary criterion was the most familiar criterion of death. Those who have made the WBC replace it have argued that when deciding whether someone has died or is still alive, breathing is important only as a sign of brain activity.[7] Hence, when the brain is dead, breathing continued by artificial means does not interfere with a declaration of death, because artificially induced breathing is not a sign of brain activity.[8] Presumably, this means that if someone has lived his life since infancy with an internal mechanical device (e.g., a silicon chip) regulating his breathing, he too will be dead when his brain is dead although he keeps on breathing as he always has.[9]

Why is death of the whole brain important as a criterion of death? Defenders of the WBC claim it is important because the brain is the master organ. Why? Because it makes possible the integrated functioning of the organism and that, they say, is the characteristic (rather than just a sign) of life. It will help in understanding all this to get clearer about such terms as criterion, sign, and also the definitions of life and death. The "new *definition* of death" that lies behind the WBC is irreversible loss of integrated functioning of the organism as a whole. We could also describe this as a theory of when life ends that takes integrated functioning of the organism to constitute or be the characteristic of life. (Recently, some supporters of the WBC have argued that it is only "critical" integrated functioning of the organism that constitutes its life.[10]) Death of all parts of the brain responsible for integrated functioning of the organism is said to be the *criterion* of death. Supporters of the WBC reject the views of those who argue that when functions associated with personhood (such as consciousness) are no longer possible—perhaps because of death of the "higher brain"—the person has died.[11] They point to spontaneous respiration, swallowing, temperature control caused by lower brain activity, and heartbeat, and ask how we could say life is not still present when these phenomena are, as they involve integrated functioning of the organism.[12] Given that they also think a *person* is still alive, they must be identifying a person with an organism even when it lacks a capacity for consciousness, which HBC supporters deny is correct.

A criterion of something is usually thought to be conceptually, not merely causally, connected with that for which it is a criterion. For example, being able to form sentences in English or understand English could be a criterion of knowing English, because we think it makes no sense to say one knows English but not how to do these things. If life is thought of as integrated functioning of the organism, and this conceptually implies an integrator or master organ, death of an integrator can be a criterion of death. However, it is an empirical fact—if it is a fact—that the brain is the integrator, so speaking of brain death as a criterion is speaking loosely, it seems. Defenders of the WBC also call the functioning of any part of the brain that causes integrated functioning of the organism as a whole a "mirror image" of life.[13] This suggests they also think of such brain functioning as a characteristic of life of the organism.

Defenders of the WBC allow that the whole brain *may have died even when some brain cells are still alive* and even when there is some supercellular functioning of brain cells, because there is not enough brain activity to count as, or to support, integrated functioning of the organism as a whole. Similarly, some cells in various parts of the body may continue to live after whole brain death without this disturbing whole brain death as the criterion of death, according to the WBC's supporters, presumably because this is not integrated functioning of the organism. So "whole brain death" should be understood as consistent with life in these cells.

Any property or event empirically correlated with a characteristic or criterion of life can be a sign of it. The distinction between a characteristic of something and a sign of something may be hard to draw precisely, but I think it is intuitively clear. It may be a sign of illness that someone is absent from work, but that is not what constitutes being ill nor is it conceptually connected to it. For supporters of the WBC, breathing is said to be important as a sign of brain activity and is described neither as a characteristic of life (sufficient if not necessary for life) nor as a criterion of it. Signs can be used to test for the presence of the criterion of life and/or characteristic of life, if we have no direct access to the criterion or the characteristic.[14]

There are at least two ways in which we might think of breathing as a sign of brain activity in the absence of artificial support for respiration. First, when it is conceived as the effect of brain activity. Second, when it is conceived as a necessary cause of brain activity via the following loop: respiration provides oxygen so that the heart can survive and circulate oxygen air to the brain, so that the brain can survive (and cause respiration).

II

All of this is background. Now consider the following hypothetical case: Ordinarily during people's lives, the brain prompts respiration. When it does so, respiration is referred to as "spontaneous respiration." That is, "spontaneous" does not mean "not caused by another bodily organ"; it means not caused by an artificial device. Suppose that when the whole brain dies, a toe cell that survives long after the brain is dead begins to prompt respiration instead (Toe Cell Case). That is, another part of the person's body, on its own, without any artificial support, prompts respiration, which continues spontaneously. (This cannot, in fact, happen. This is a purely hypothetical case.) We can also assume that the heart, which in fact (not merely hypothetically) does not need to be controlled by the brain, continues to beat and circulate blood, although this may not be necessary to the hypothetical case. Would those who now support the WBC follow their stated criterion and declare that death has come even in the presence of such *spontaneous* respiration? I doubt it in part because Dr. James Bernat, a defender of the WBC, said he would not declare death.[15] Would this refusal to declare death not show (despite what they say explicitly) that the presence of spontaneous breathing is of significance in itself for them *as a characteristic of life* or as a component of a characteristic (i.e., spontaneous cardiopulmonary activity) rather than just as a sign of brain activity? Indeed, I believe so. (This is true even if spontaneous respiration is not necessary for them to declare life to be present, as in fully conscious people who are on respirators.)

The Toe Cell Case seems to show that there was a crucial mistake in reasoning when WBC supporters jumped from the claim that *artificially* sustained respiration was not important as a sign or characteristic of life to the conclusion that breathing is important only as a sign of brain activity. The mistake was to fail to consider whether *spontaneous* breathing in itself (or with heartbeat)—independent of its being a sign of brain activity—had significance as a characteristic of life. To do so, we must construct a hypothetical case, like the Toe Cell Case, and imagine that spontaneous breathing occurs in the absence of the brain.

Some may ask of what use is the hypothetical case when we know that, *in fact*, there will be no spontaneous breathing when the brain dies. The point of the counterfactual hypothetical is to defeat the view that because spontaneous breathing in fact only occurs when the whole brain is not dead, brain activity but not spontaneous breathing in itself is important to those who support WBC. In general, when two properties, A and B, are as a matter of natural fact conjoined, it is a mistake to conclude that A has significance only as a sign of B, without considering whether A (spontaneous breathing) separate from B (brain activity) (as in the Toe Cell Case) would have significance as a characteristic (or component of a characteristic) of life.

In arguing for the WBC, its supporters have tried to emphasize the connection between the CPC and WBC in the following way:[16] In the absence of artificial support for respiration, the CPC overlaps perfectly with (or as philosophers would say, is extensionally equivalent to) the WBC. This is because with no artificial support for breathing, the absence of breathing means the part of the brain responsible for respiration is dead, and without this respiration, there will be no oxygen to support the rest of the brain (or heart activity) and the whole brain will die.

Hence, WBC supporters say, in the absence of artificial support for respiration, we can take the CPC's concern with breathing to be just concern with a sign of whole brain death.[17] (This argument uses breathing as a sign of brain activity in the second way described above—that is, as a necessary cause of brain activity.) But the Toe Cell Case (where the CPC and WBC can be peeled apart) and the predicted response by WBC supporters reveal something different. They reveal that underlying the attempt to show a union between CPC and WBC is the WBC supporters' belief that spontaneous respiration or cardiopulmonary activity is sufficient (though not necessary) for life, and that the death of *whatever* cell or organ is causing spontaneous respiration is necessary (though not sufficient) for death. I believe they are concerned to show that the spontaneous CPC and WBC really overlap because each is independently important for them.

Notice also that at least in the case of minor cells (like the toe cell), the death of that cell in the Toe Cell Case could be important only as a sign of the termination of spontaneous respiration, not as the absence of what is in itself a characteristic of life. Should this also imply that death of the part of the brain that is responsible only for spontaneous respiration should have significance for those who say they support the WBC only as a *sign* of the termination of spontaneous respiration, rather than as the end of what is in itself a characteristic or criterion of life? It would seem so.

This last conclusion helps us see that there is another way besides using the Toe Cell Case in which to argue for the conclusion that spontaneous respiration (independent of spontaneous heartbeat) is taken as a characteristic of life. Consider the first way in which breathing might be a sign of brain activity—that is, as an effect caused by brain activity. Recall that it is not enough for life according to WBC for just any random brain cells to function.[18] Suppose certain brain cells only cause breathing. If breathing were not a characteristic of life (but just a sign of it), why would the functioning of just those brain cells that cause breathing be important enough to satisfy the criterion for the presence of life and stand in the way of declaring whole brain death? One of the battery of tests that is *actually* used to determine if someone is dead according to the WBC is the apnea test. This test checks to see if there is a spontaneous *attempt* to respire. That is, it is not even successful respiration but only the attempt to respire that is sufficient to prevent a declaration of death by those who use WBC.[19] (Of course, the attempt to respire is not a necessary condition for the presence of life.) If respiration is not important as a characteristic of life, why is the survival of cells that are related only to it considered important? It seems that these brain cells are important only as the sign of respiration (or even of an attempt to respire) rather than respiration being important only as a sign of brain activity.

Consider a reason why some may think the brain cells successfully causing respiration is a characteristic of life but toe cells causing the same functioning would not be a characteristic of life. The brain is the master organ. But "master organ" is defined functionally as the organ that is responsible for much integrated functioning. If "master" is defined functionally, once a part of the organ supports only a few functions of the organism (or even one, such as spontaneous breathing), it is no longer a master organ but merely a part of an organ that once was master. The last "gasp" of a previously master organ could be more important than activity in a toe cell, even though its effects are the same, only to those who think that the *history* of an organ is relevant to deciding if a characteristic of life is present. They would say that if what was once a master organ is still functioning in some way as it used to—still being minimally effective as a cause of a major function—a characteristic of life is present. If some other cell or organ does the same thing but it does not have the same history, this characteristic of life is not present. On this historical view, in order to know whether something is a characteristic of life, we sometimes would have to know the history of the body parts that cause the functioning. But the idea that such history is relevant to the determination of a characteristic of life or the presence or absence of life is implausible.

III

What are some possible responses to my argument so far based on the Toe Cell and Apnea Test Cases? It might be said that all the hypothetical Toe Cell Case shows is that if the brain were not necessary for respiration, it would not be a master organ whose whole death was crucial as a criterion of death. But, in our world, the brain is such a master organ.

There are several problems with this response. First, it seems to imply that being the sole cause of spontaneous breathing is crucial to being the master organ. This implication alone suggests that spontaneous breathing is important in its own right. This would support the view suggested by the Toe Cell Case that defenders of WBC really do think that the presence of spontaneous breathing is in its own right a characteristic of life and not merely a sign of brain activity.

In addition, given how I have constructed the Toe Cell Case, it is difficult to believe that the brain in that imaginary world would not still appropriately be seen as the master organ. After all, in that world, as long as the brain is not totally dead, it *is* in control of what the brain in this world actually controls, including spontaneous respiration. So when the brain in the Toe Cell Case dies, the master organ is dead.

A second possible response is that the toe cell in the hypothetical case, in virtue of its control of respiration after the whole brain dies, is a new master organ. But how can it be, if it does nothing but control respiration? It does not support all the integrated functions that the brain in the actual world supports. So we cannot be concerned with spontaneous breathing merely as a sign of the toe cell qua master organ's survival. It would rather be the reverse: the toe cell's death would be important only as a sign of cessation of spontaneous breathing.

A third possible response is that the toe cell in the hypothetical case is really a *part* of the whole brain, which is to be thought of as distributed throughout the body.[20] Hence, the whole brain will not have died as long as the toe cell is still alive. Once again, it seems that the importance of spontaneous breathing would be leading supporters of the WBC to identify something as part of the brain, rather than their having a criterion for "brain" independent of what causes spontaneous breathing. Identifying the brain in this way suggests that they think spontaneous breathing is a crucial characteristic of life.[21]

A stronger response to the Toe Cell argument is that we should declare life still present when a toe cell or brain cell causes respiration because this *causal relation* is itself an instance of integrated functioning. That is, when one cell is causing some other function, we have integrated functioning of the organism and that is a characteristic of life, not spontaneous breathing per se. (Call this the Integration Objection.) This response might be refined by requiring that the cell cause some "critical" integrated functioning.[22] (Call this the Refined Integration Objection.) If not refined, the objection would imply that if a brain cell caused only toe cells to function, we should not declare death, and this conclusion seems inconsistent with the views of supporters of the WBC.

The first thing to note about these objections is that they fail to account for the Apnea Test Case, which involves no causal relation, only an attempted one. Second, they seem to grant that spontaneous breathing caused by another body part is itself an instance of integrated functioning of the organism, rather than merely a sign of life. Without denying that integrated functioning of the organism is the characteristic of life, spontaneously caused breathing becomes an instance of it. The third thing to notice is that the Refined Integration Objection implies that if in a hypothetical case, a brain or toe cell spontaneously caused the liver to function (or even attempted unsuccessfully to prompt liver function?), there would also be integrated activity and life should be declared present, for if a failed liver is not artificially replaced, the organism will fail. But would spontaneous liver function have the same significance as spontaneous respiration as a characteristic of life? If not, then would this not be because spontaneous breathing per se is considered a characteristic of life?

Fourth, what if breathing was not caused by some other body part? That is, if it were "spontaneous" in a very strict sense, as the heartbeat can be. Would we really think that it had less significance as a characteristic of life because there was no causal relation from another body part to it that counted as integrated functioning?

Most importantly, what is intended by "integrated functioning of the organism" in the theory of life held by supporters of WBC is not present just because one major function is caused spontaneously by another body part. They are concerned with integrated functioning of the organism as a whole. Hence, if supporters of WBC would refuse to declare death in both the Toe Cell Case and in a (hypothetical) case where a toe cell causes liver function, these cases might reveal something else: that the supporters of WBC do not really believe that integrated functioning of the organism as a whole is a necessary characteristic for human life to be present. For this reason, the Toe Cell Case might also be used to criticize the

Integrated Functioning Criterion (IFC). This suggests that at least one possible component of a definition of life of an organism is "spontaneous functioning of some major sort." (I use "major" instead of "critical" to take account of the fact that for supporters of the WBC life can continue without consciousness, but consciousness is sufficient for the presence of life.) However, if a toe or brain cell causing respiration were sufficient for a declaration of life, but a toe or brain cell causing liver function were not, then "spontaneous functioning of some major sort" would *not* be an accurate description of a minimal sufficient condition of life.

Another way to put the Refined Integration Objection to the Toe Cell Case may be more successful in raising an objection to the Toe Cell Argument. It relies on the second way of conceiving of respiration as a sign of integration; that is, it is a sign not because it is caused by some other cell but because it is a cause of other elements in a loop. The objection claims that if respiration is present, then oxygen will be available to maintain the heart, and the heart (stimulated independently) will circulate oxygen to the cell (toe or brain) that is imagined to cause respiration. This loop—not merely the causal relation of toe or brain cell to respiration—is an integrated function and it (not respiration per se) is a characteristic of life. (Call this Refined Integration Objection [2].)

One concern raised by this description of integration is that there could (theoretically) be spontaneous integration of a major (and even critical) subsystem without this involving integration of the organism as a whole. But it is the latter that supporters of WBC emphasize as constituting life. On the other hand, when they point to the relation between brain, lungs, and heart, they seem to allow that at least spontaneous activity of that subsystem counts as life, for they say that functioning heart and lungs are signs that the brain is not dead. But theoretically this could be true when the only cells of the brain that are not dead are those causing respiration, which sustains the heart, which in turn circulates oxygen that sustains the few brain cells causing respiration. Perhaps it is circulation of the oxygen throughout the body that makes the spontaneous functioning of this subsystem also be integration of the organism *as a whole.*

Now consider two possible responses to the Refined Integration Objection (2). The first response asks us to consider a hypothetical but similarly complex spontaneous loop from toe cell to liver function to kidney function and back to the toe cell (in the presence of whole brain death and artificially supported respiration). Would those who say life is still present in the Toe Cell Case say it is present here? If not, then the Toe Cell Case would show that respiration is especially significant as a characteristic of life. But perhaps they would say life *is* present, either because no more than the spontaneous integration of a subsystem is required for life, or because cleansing of all the blood by the kidneys is as much integration of the organism as a whole as is oxygen circulation.

The second response to the Refined Integration Objection (2) involves supposing that there is *no* spontaneous loop from respiration to maintenance of the heart to circulation of oxygen to maintenance of the cell causing respiration. In the Apnea Test Case, this must be so, because there need be no successful respiration but only a spontaneous attempt, and yet death is not declared. This shows that the Refined Integration Objection (2) is wrong. It also seems to be further evidence that spontaneous integration of the organism as a whole is not a required characteristic of life for supporters of WBC.

In the Toe Cell Case, we could imagine that the toe cell that causes respiration functions on a supply of conserved oxygen (or it has an anaerobic source of energy). So there is at least no loop from spontaneous respiration to its cause in this hypothetical case. Conjointly, imagine four further logically possible variations on the Toe Cell Case (called Toe Cell Variant Cases). Either (1) the respiration maintains the life of the heart (whose beat is maintained independently of brain or toe cell) and so oxygen is circulated; or (2) the respiration does not maintain the heart, but the heart has a conserved oxygen supply that keeps it alive and it circulates oxygen; or (3) the respiration does not maintain the heart but the heart is stimulated (or oxygen is circulated) artificially; or (4) the respiration serves no useful function because the oxygen is not circulated. (No doubt someone will soon die in [4], but the question is whether he is already dead.)

If those who agree that life continues in the Toe Cell Case would declare life present when they conceive the case as involving (2) or (3) or (4), then no spontaneous complex integration of a subsystem is required for life in (2) and (3), and no integrated functioning of the organism as a whole is required for life in (4). If they would not declare life present in (2), (3), and (4) but declare it present when they conceive the case as involving (1), then it might be said that while no loop-form of integration is necessary for life, integrated spontaneous cardiopulmonary activity would be sufficient for life. (Possibly this is true although equally integrated spontaneous functioning of other major organs [such as kidney, liver, etc.] that also involve integrated functioning of the organism as a whole would not be sufficient for life.) If life is also present in both (1) and (2), but not in (3) and (4), then it might be said that spontaneous cardiopulmonary activity would be a sufficient characteristic of life even if there is no integrated subsystem. Possibly, equally non-integrated spontaneous functioning of other major systems would be sufficient for life as well. If not, then this would show that spontaneous respiration or respiration with circulation are distinctively important characteristics of life, not mere signs of, or even instances of, integration of subsystems, integration of the organism as a whole, or of brain activity.

Notice, however, that in all these hypothetical variations on cases involving what I have been referring to as integration—for example, when one body part causes other body parts to function, and when the organism as a whole functions—there is no directing, chief integrator locatable at *an apex*. To the extent that it is a mistake to speak of "integration" without an integrator, we should instead speak of "concerted functioning" when one part helps cause another part to function, and of "concerted functioning of the organism as a whole." Perhaps this is the real point of Dr. Shewmon's cases, described as support for IFC, where a patient is said to have "[somatic] integrated unity—the internal harmony, and the over-arching coordination of his body's function . . . in the presence of whole brain death."[23] The quote suggests that something besides the brain is the integrator, but concerted functioning without an integrator is at least a possible alternative. If so, then many supporters of the IFC should really support what I will call the CFC (Concerted Functioning Criterion) of life. (The Toe Cell Case and Apnea Test Case could still be raised as objections to CFC, however.)

However, in Toe Cell Variant Case (2) (page 123), there is not even concerted functioning of subsystems, where one causes another to function; there is mul-tiple, independent functioning (somehow complementary). If we should say life is present if there were either concerted *or* multiple independent functioning of organs (or cells), this is another reason to say that integrated activity is not necessary (although it may be sufficient) in order for life to be present.

In the real (nonhypothetical) world, of course, the death of the whole brain is also a sign of the end of spontaneous respiration, and it may be a *sign* of the end of spontaneous concerted or multiple functioning of organs (or cells) sustaining the organism as a whole. If so, whole brain death may suffice as a *sign* of death. But if the definition of life of the organism (its characteristics and what consti-tutes it) does not *conceptually* imply an integrator because some nonintegrated activity is sufficient for life of the organism, it is not clear why death of an inte-grator is a *criterion* of death rather than just a sign (by being a cause) of death. If, empirically, characteristics sufficient for life could not occur without integration, and an integrator is conceptually required for integration, then the death of the integrator would be a criterion of the end of an empirical, not conceptual, requirement for life.[24]

IV

Let us now examine the idea of a "mirror image." It seems to imply that if A is a characteristic of life, then its mirror image is, too.[25] As noted, the idea of a mirror image is used by WBC supporters to describe the relation between the brain and integrated functioning of the organism. But suppose that in a hypothetical case, a few toe cells were responsible after whole brain death for maintaining the sort of integrated functioning that the brain stem maintains in the real world when the higher brain dies (Toe Cell Integrator Case). WBC supporters would again, I sus-pect, say that life is still present. Perhaps now they would say a second master organ, the toe cells, exists. They would have as much reason to call the functioning of toe cells a mirror image of integrated functioning as they had to say that of the brain stem's functioning.

But if the toe cells are an integrative organ in this hypothetical case, will this organ's functioning be of significance as a *characteristic* of life, which is what the term "mirror image" suggests and which is how WBC supporters seem to think of brain function, or will it be merely a cause and *sign* of multiple major organs functioning successfully? To see, we might consider a case where the toe cells are still alive and sending directions to many body organs but the organs are so damaged that they cannot respond and therefore there is no integrated activity. The same scenario could be imagined using the brain stem as the entity sending directions with no organs capable of responding to it. In these cases, the brain stem or toe cells are imagined to live on quite long on small, conserved amounts of oxygen in their cells. (Call these the Ineffectual Directives Cases.)

Those who say they support WBC might declare life present in these cases, but declaring it not present would be consistent with their refusal to declare life present when there is small supercellular activity unrelated to integrating organ functioning.[26] The unwillingness to declare life present would be some evidence that even when lower brain or toe cell functioning *does regulate effectively*, the regulator's functioning is merely a *sign* (or, at most, a criterion) of characteristics of life (such as integrated functioning of the organism as a whole), not a characteristic of life itself. If so, then even when the entity regulates effectively, it is less than a mirror image of integrated functioning of the organism, for mirror image implies more than a mere sign or criterion of some other characteristic of human life. The Ineffectual Directives Cases are also a way to show that master organ activity and integrated functioning of the organism need not be mirror images of each other because the master organ can function well in sending directives in the absence of integrated activity. (This situation contrasts with the earlier cases we considered in which concerted organic functioning existed with no integrator.)

However, the unwillingness to declare life present in Ineffectual Directive Cases is also consistent with declaring the *effective* functioning of the master organ a characteristic of life, because one organic event in a hierarchical system causing other organic events might itself be a characteristic of life.[27] This is a form of the view discussed above under the rubric of the Integration and Refined Integration Objections. Such a view, however, does not imply that the functioning lower brain, in itself outside of the integrated system, is special in any way as a characteristic of life by comparison with toe cells in the hypothetical case. This brain activity, not spontaneous respiration, is appropriately seen merely as a sign of other characteristics of life. From focusing on integrated functioning of the organism as the characteristic of life, supporters of the WBC who declare brain activity to be its mirror image have come to focus on something quite different as the characteristic of life, namely (some) functioning of (what was once) the integrator. This is another way to understand their declaring the organism still alive when even a small part of the former integrator attempts, even unsuccessfully, to prompt a single major function (as in the Apnea Test Case). This shift in focus seems to have been a mistake.

V

Let me try to summarize some of these results by laying out more saliently the method I have used in getting them. We have been considering whether spontaneous breathing is a characteristic or only a sign of life. In order to see if x is merely a sign (for example, effect or cause) of what is itself a characteristic of life, we should consider it on its own in a hypothetical case. If we consider it as caused by something (as in the Toe Cell Case), we must remember to consider whether a body part spontaneously causing a function is a characteristic of life, even if the function itself or the part's activity itself, considered independently, is not a sufficient characteristic of life. Suppose x is not a mere sign but is a characteristic on its own, though in the real world it cannot exist on its own. Then we should consider whether y, with which x must be conjoined if x occurs spontaneously, is merely a sign of life or is itself also a characteristic of life. We do this by considering spontaneous (e.g., not mechanically produced) y on its own in a hypothetical case. Then we proceed in the same way with any factor z without which y cannot exist in the real world, and so on.

Now I shall briefly repeat how I applied the method in my earlier discussion: (1) The Toe Cell Case suggested that spontaneous breathing would be important in itself (or conjoined with heartbeat) as a characteristic of life for supporters of WBC (despite their explicit rejection of these as any more than a sign of a criterion of life). (2) But suppose that, in the real world, there will be no spontaneous breathing without concerted functioning of the organism. Is concerted functioning of the organism just a sign of life or is it a characteristic on its own? To decide, imagine a case where swallowing, temperature regulation, and other organ activities occur spontaneously without spontaneous respiration (but with mechanical ventilation) and after brain death. Would those who say they support WBC declare life to be present? I believe they would. If so, these activities are not mere signs but characteristics of life. (3) But suppose that in the real world there will be no spontaneous concerted functioning of the organism unless there is an integrator. Is the spontaneously operating integrator a sign or criterion of life, or is it itself a characteristic of life? To answer this question, consider spontaneous directives from a brain stem (or toe cells) without any effect because organs are so damaged they cannot respond. I have suggested that life is *not* present here. (Still, the relation between a part of the body and a function it causes when organs are not so damaged could itself be a characteristic of life.) So the brain (or toe cell) activity imagined here in itself is more a sign of other characteristics of life than a characteristic of life in itself.

The conclusion is that even if in the real world death of the whole brain were a criterion of death, it would not be because brain stem activity is itself a characteristic of human life or even because integrated activity is necessary (rather than sufficient) as a characteristic of life. For example, spontaneous, concerted, major functioning of the organism or spontaneous respiration, at least with circulation of air, should each be sufficient as a characteristic of life of the organism.

VI

So far I have focused on various *spontaneous* activities as characteristics of life. But now we come to a crucial question: is spontaneity necessary? What if the brain stem activity that integrates many bodily functions in vegetative states were not itself spontaneous, but supported by an artificial device? This could be a brain support device external to the body or a silicon chip implanted into the brain.[28] (Neither in the case of artificially assisted brain function nor artificially assisted respiration need we conceive of functioning being totally artificial. That is, some parts of the brain or lungs could be functioning with artificial replacements for missing component functions.)

When supporters of WBC point to cases where the lower brain is supporting all sorts of integrated activities (swallowing, breathing, and so forth) as evidence that human life is still present, they emphasize how the being functions *on its own*.[29] But they also say, "Sometimes, of course, an artificial substitute can forge the link that restores the organism as a whole to unified functioning. Heart or kidney transplants, kidney dialysis, or an iron lung used to replace physically impaired breathing ability in a polio victim, for example, restore the integrated functioning of the organism as they replace the failed function of a part."[30] Would a chip in the brain stem not also do that?

Suppose that when such artificially assisted brain activity produces integrated functioning of the organism life is present. Then it would be possible for respiration that is produced indirectly by such artificially assisted brain activity to still be a characteristic (or a component of a characteristic) of life. This would not necessarily imply that respiration that resulted from direct artificial support had this status. Further, suppose that direct artificial support of respiration is combined with some artificial support of the lower brain that helps cause "lower" integrated functioning of the organism. In this case, supporters of WBC could still say life is present, even if here the breathing itself were not a characteristic (or component of a characteristic) of life. Certainly, if normal mental activity were maintained in someone by the use of artificial support for "higher" brain function and this person were also already on an iron lung, he would be considered alive. Some argument would be needed for why artificiality of cause mattered when "lower" integrated functioning of the organism results but not when "higher" (e.g., normal conscious) functioning results. It turns out then that "spontaneity" in the sense of activity not artificially assisted should not be so important for supporters of WBC when brain activity—even artificially sustained—is present and causing sufficiently great integrated functioning.

Suppose all this is true. Then, barring the patient's consent to removal of life support, those who say they support WBC seem committed to not stopping and *also to starting* an artificial component (brain chip, ventilator) if it would maintain integrated *vegetative* functioning, so long as they also think it is wrong not to save a human life because its quality is not good enough.[31]

Suppose that a set of integrated activities is not such that we should maintain or start the artificial component of the otherwise spontaneous activity. This may indicate that we think it permissible to decide what life to save on the basis of its quality. This is consistent with saying that when these activities are totally spontaneous and do not require assistance, we may not kill such low-quality life by, for example, removing organs. However, suppose we would refuse to provide or continue the artificial component not on the basis of a quality-of-life judgment (or due to patient request), but simply because we think that even with the artificial support, there would not be a human person alive in any case. Then it is hard to see why the completely spontaneous version of the same activities would result in a human person being alive either.

In the Toe Cell Case, spontaneous respiration caused by the artificially unassisted toe cell was sufficient for life as much (or as little) as spontaneous respiration caused by brain activity artificially unassisted. Now imagine that in a hypothetical case, toe cell activity is maintained by artificial assistance in the form of a chip replacing some synapses (Assisted Toe Cell Case). Would the respiration it causes be a characteristic (or component of a characteristic) of life? Some who agree that there is life in the Toe Cell Case might deny there is life in this case because there is no spontaneous concerted or multiple organ functioning *and* respiration is supported artificially, even though there is not complete mechanical support of every aspect of respiration. However, if artificially assisted toe cells supported not only respiration but also other functions common in vegetative patients, advocates of WBC should consider human life as much present as when the similarly assisted brain stem maintains respiration and other functions in vegetative patients.

Suppose all this is true. Then those who say they support WBC should believe that *theoretically*, in the absence of any brain activity and any spontaneous respiration, human life could still be present. This would be the case where artificially assisted toe cells directly produce respiration and/or there is spontaneous concerted or multiple functioning of some major organ systems.

So far we see that (1) multiple functioning of major organs that is *sufficiently (but not entirely) spontaneous* or (2) spontaneous respiration (possibly accompanied by circulation) could be sufficient for life. In the real world, this would be compatible with the WBC only if these characteristics of life could not be present if there were whole brain death. But what we have said in this section implies that whole brain death will not have occurred merely because some artificial assistance to the brain itself is necessary if the rest of the brain is to function.

We have been considering partial spontaneity of brain stem functioning by imagining a chip installed in the brain. However, if *the entire brain stem* were replaceable with an artificial brain stem, the integrated activities it produces could still be in part spontaneous, given that many other organs function without being replaced by artificial parts. Analogously, when we provide support for patients' failing kidneys, we might provide partial support or replace the kidneys entirely with mechanical assistance. If we do the latter, life understood as integrated functioning of the organism would still be present according to supporters of the WBC. It is not clear why completely replacing the component at the apex—the brain stem—should be different from completely replacing a component somewhere else in the system.

One possible source of difference is that total replacement of the brain stem replaces the particular human life that had previously existed with *another* human life. If this is so, then replacing the brain stem would not so much *save* a life as create a new one. The idea behind this objection is that the identity conditions for a particular human life reference that particular brain stem. It is a prominent view that identity conditions of a particular person involve the higher brain (neocortex). If the higher brain were replaced (all at once) with another higher brain (grafted onto the rest of the brain), many philosophers would say that the original person was replaced with another person. But it is not clear why the identity conditions for continuation of a particular human life have to be tied to a particular brain stem in the way that personal identity is said to be tied to the survival of a particular higher brain. If the identity conditions are not so tied, then if the whole brain is dead but an artificial brain stem is put in place, enough partial spontaneity could be present for the *same life* to be present. This would defeat the WBC of death. According to Robert Truog, such artificial replacement for the brain stem is now a realistic option, though it is not practiced.[32] If life is integrated functioning of the organism and replacing the brain stem would not alter the identity of the life, then patients are being left to die when the artificial brain stem is not used. Suppose there is no moral imperative to use the artificial replacement. Then the same questions about what this implies for the connection between quality of life and saving life could be raised as were raised above, about not introducing a partial artificial component into the brain stem.

VII

So far, in considering whether spontaneity is necessary, I have considered partial nonspontaneity where merely a component of a whole system is artificial. However, there is at least one case in which a *completely* artificial system seems compatible with the presence of a person. Imagine a hypothetical case in which we *gradually*, over time, replace all the organic parts of a human being with artificial parts, including an artificial brain. (That is, instead of the gradual replacement of old with new cells that ordinarily occurs in the brain, artificial cells are introduced gradually.) These artificial parts are successful in maintaining consciousness, all higher mental functions, and sentience, and these are experienced as completely continuous with these functions in the original human being. Perhaps what remains is not a human being at all, but still it seems to be the *same* person, or at the very least, a person (if not the same one). If the same person is present through a human and nonhuman stage, we would not declare that person dead and, in that sense, "life" is present, although it makes "life" a nonbiological idea.

Why then is completely artificially supported respiration, with no other major spontaneous functioning, not enough to constrain us from declaring death of a person? So that, for example, the person whose breathing had been directly supported throughout his life by a chip (mentioned at the start of this chapter) remains alive when he continues to respire as he always did, although everything else spontaneous stops, and also the person who is put on a respirator when ill remains alive so long as the respirator keeps him breathing. The theory behind this view is that if a function is important enough to stand in the way of a declaration of death, it does not matter if it is present spontaneously or artificially. If it is not important enough to stand in the way of declaring death when artificially produced, it is not important enough when spontaneously produced. By steps we find ourselves back where we started before the WBC, with CPC, in terms of when life is still present.

Possibly, there are several objections to this conclusion. It may be a mistake to take both consciousness/sentience and intake/output of air as characteristics of life. If so, production of the former by completely artificial means and production of the latter by completely artificial means might not have the same significance for continuation of a life. This may be because consciousness and sentience constitute a subjectivity—what it is like to be something—that the presence of oxygen in an organic system does not. This might be connected to why the latter's being a characteristic of life is tied to its spontaneity. Furthermore, it might be said that consciousnesses and even sentience are conceived as spontaneous activity in themselves, whereas the mere presence and circulation of oxygen are not. Hence, a requirement that there be some major spontaneous functioning for life to be present is satisfied by consciousness/sentience per se, but not by respiration per se.

We should be aware, however, that this view leaves open the skeptical possibility that no merely physical, rather than mental, phenomena are enough to ensure that a life is or has ever been present. This is because it seems coherent to entertain the skeptical thought that behind all the seemingly spontaneous physical functions of the body are "strings" controlled by machines of which we know nothing. If assuring ourselves of spontaneous functioning were crucial to declaring life present, we might be more certain that there are and have been persons than that there is or has been biological life.

I have tried to uncover the theory that supporters of WBC should accept. I have also tried to show that this theory could imply different criteria of death than the WBC; for example, the Concerted Functioning Criterion (CFC) or spontaneous respiration. This is because processes that supporters of WBC have taken to be merely signs of life are really characteristics of it and some things they think of as characteristics of life are really merely signs of it. It turns out then that I have been doing something akin to what supporters of the WBC did when they argued that the point behind the CPC should lead its supporters to accept the WBC. They argued that agreement at a deeper level lay behind apparent disagreement over criteria. That is what my discussion suggests as well. Insofar as there is less conflict than there seemed to be, this is an optimistic result. However, insofar as the CFC or mere respiration (spontaneous and possibly artificial) are insufficient for continuation of a person by contrast to a human life, or for a life that persons should treat as valuable, the question of whether it is morally permissible to end some human lives (even by killing, for example, in order to acquire organs) will arise more frequently.

Notes

1. This chapter is a revised version of an article that appeared in *Philosophy & Public Affairs* 30(3) (2001): 297–320.

2. For comments on earlier versions of the article that constitutes this chapter, I am grateful to Baruch Brody, Elizabeth Harman, Jeff McMahan, Derek Parfit, the editors of *Philosophy & Public Affairs*, Robert Truog, and students in my graduate bioethics class at Harvard University. I thank Baruch Brody and Tristram Engelhardt for encouraging me to write the article. For editorial suggestions, I am indebted to Kathleen Much of the Center for Advanced Studies in the Behavioral Sciences at Stanford, where I wrote part of this article as a Mellon Fellow, supported under grant #2986639, and as an AHRQ/NEH Fellow, grant #FA-36625-01.

3. For an accessible description, see Gary Greenberg, "As Good As Dead," *The New Yorker*, August 13, 2001. Halevy and Brody have emphasized that neurohormonal activity, which is an example of integrated functioning of the organism, can continue after current tests for whole brain death. See Amir Halevy and Baruch Brody, "Brain Death: Reconciling Definitions, Criteria and Tests," *Annals of Internal Medicine* 119 (1993): 519–25.

4. D. A. Shewmon, "Chronic 'Brain Death': Meta-Analysis and Conceptual Consequences," *Neurology* 51(6) (1998): 1538–45.

5. Robert Truog, "Is It Time to Abandon Brain Death?" *Hastings Center Report* 27(1) (1997): 29–37. Truog means that artificial replacement of the brain stem that makes possible integrated functioning of the organism is now possible.

6. As quoted in Greenberg, "As Good As Dead," p. 40.

7. Among the reasons why x could be a sign of y is that y causes x or x causes y. In the latter case, if y is life, x is instrumental to life, even if not a characteristic of life itself.

8. See President's Commission for the Study of Ethical Problems in Medicine and Biomedical and Behavioral Research, *Defining Death: A Report on the Medical, Legal, and Ethical Issues in the Determination of Death* (Washington, DC: U.S. Government Printing Office, 1981), pp. 12–20 and pp. 31–43. Reprinted in *Ethical Issues in Modern Medicine*, 4th ed., eds. J. Arras and B. Steinbock (Mountain View, CA: Mayfield Publishing, 1995), pp. 144–57 (henceforth, *Defining Death*). For example, "But breathing and heartbeat are not life itself. They are simply used as signs—as one window for viewing a deeper and more complex reality: a triangle of interrelated systems with the brain at its apex" (p. 147). "On this view, the heart and lungs are not important as basic prerequisites to continued life but rather because the irreversible cessation of their functions shows that the brain had ceased functioning" (p. 148). According to *Defining Death*: (1) Without air from respiration, the brain cannot live. The brain usually prompts respiration, but if it fails in this respect, respiration can be continued artificially. This is commonly done in people whose brains are

otherwise still functioning well—e.g., polio victims in iron lungs. (2) If the heart does not beat, then even if the brain or respirator causes respiration, the air will not be circulated by the blood and the brain will die. The heart can beat without direction from the brain or artificial stimulation. At the time of *Defining Death*, however, when the heart failed, it could not be sustained artificially for long periods, as respiration could be. My discussion in this article is, in large part, a revisiting of *Defining Death*.

9. Thanks to Baruch Brody for raising the example of the silicon chip implanted early in life.

10. See James Bernat, "Refinements in the Definition and Criterion of Death," in *Definition of Death: Contemporary Controversies*, eds. Stuart Youngner, Robert Arnold, and Renie Schapiro (Baltimore: Johns Hopkins Press, 1999). Bernat seems to think that if life could go on without artificial replacement of a certain sort of integrated functioning of the organism (e.g., neurohormonal integration), it is not a critical function of the organism as a whole. From this he concludes that its presence by itself cannot mean that life is present (pp. 85–86). This conclusion seems problematic. First, life could go on without artificial replacement of consciousness, according to the WBC, and yet Bernat considers its presence a critical characteristic of life (p. 86). Presumably, consciousness is not an example of integrated functioning of the organism as a whole, however. A further problem is that the term "critical" implies *necessary* for life to be present unless artificially replaced, but "noncritical" spontaneous functioning could be *sufficient* for life (even if not necessary) when the so-called critical function ceases to operate spontaneously but is artificially replaced. Apparently, Bernat now thinks that only those integrated functionings of the organism as a whole that would have to be replaced artificially if life is to continue are the sort of integrated functioning of the organism that constitutes its life.

11. Like Robert Veatch. See his "The Impending Collapse of the Whole-Brain Definition of Death," in Arras and Steinbock, *Ethical Issues in Modern Medicine*, pp. 163–72 (henceforth, "The Impending Collapse").

12. See *Defining Death*: "The startling contrast between bodies lacking *all* brain functions and patients with intact brainstems (despite severe neocortical damage) manifests this. The former lie with fixed pupils, motionless except for the chest movements produced by their respirators. The latter can not only breathe, metabolize, maintain temperature and blood pressure, and so forth, *on their own* but also sigh, yawn, track light with their eyes, and react to pain or reflex stimulation. It is not easy to discern precisely what it is about patients in this latter group that makes them alive while those in the other category are not. It is in part that in the case of the first category (i.e., absence of all brain functions) when the mask created by the artificial medical support is stripped away what remains is not an integrated organism but 'merely a group of artificially maintained subsystems'" (p. 149). It is unclear from the last line whether the emphasis is on spontaneous rather than artificial production or on integration of the whole (rather than mere subsystems) which might suffice for life even if artificially maintained.

13. See *Defining Death*: "This process and its denouement are understood in two major ways. Although they are sometimes stated as alternative formulations of a 'whole brain definition' of death, they are actually mirror images of each other. The Commission has found them to be complementary; together they enrich one's understanding of the 'definition.' The first focuses on the integrated functioning of the body's major organ systems, while recognizing the centrality of the whole brain, since it is neither revivable nor replaceable.

The other identifies the functioning of the whole brain as the hallmark of life because the brain is the regulator of the body's integration. The two conceptions are subject to similar criticism and have similar implications for policy" (p. 147). Note that the passage is in error when it speaks of "the whole brain as the hallmark of life" since the WBC allows that brain stem functioning is sufficient for life. It is the death of the whole brain, not the life of the whole brain, that is crucial to the WBC, contrary to what this passage implies.

14. On the related tripartite distinction between definition, criterion, and tests, see Halevy and Brody, "Brain Death: Reconciling Definitions."

15. When I presented this hypothetical case to James Bernat, M.D., he said that he would not declare death in such a hypothetical case. (Response to my question asked from the audience at Bioethics Conference, Bowling Green Center for Social Philosophy and Policy, April 21, 2001.) I first discussed a case of this sort in my *Morality, Mortality*, Vol. 1 (New York: Oxford University Press, 1993), pp. 202–3.

16. See *Defining Death*.

17. As absence of air will also lead to death of the heart, one might take it as a sign of the importance of heart activity (or the activity of any other organ). Nevertheless, supporters of WBC have other reasons for focusing on respiration as a sign of brain activity, because they say the brain (not the heart) is the master organ of integrated functioning of the organism and that is why its death is crucial.

18. Veatch quotes James Bernat in "The Impending Collapse": "Because these isolated nests of neurons no longer contribute to the functioning of the organism as a whole their continued functioning is now irrelevant to the dead organism" (p. 164).

19. I thank Baruch Brody for drawing the apnea test to my attention as support for my argument employing the Toe Cell Case.

20. Suggested by Derek Parfit.

21. A possible counter to this response is to imagine that the toe cell causes what are agreed to be unimportant effects, not characteristics of life, that the "brain during ordinary times" causes. If we identify the toe cell as part of the brain on the basis of these effects, we would not be committed to their being characteristics of life.

22. "Critical" could be understood as described in note 10 (i.e., threat to life would result if there were not artificial replacement for the function).

23. See Greenberg, "As Good As Dead," p. 39.

24. Truog claims that one reason the brain death criterion was introduced was that brain death was always shortly followed by cardiac arrest. (See "Is It Time to Abandon Brain Death?") If so, an argument can also be made that supporters of the WBC really think spontaneous cardiac function by itself is a characteristic of life, rather than just a sign of integrated functioning of the organism. After all, why should the importance of x (brain death) be determined on the basis of its relation to y (cardiac activity) when y is not taken as a sign of anything else, if y is not thought to be a characteristic of life?

25. The term "mirror image" as used by supporters of WBC does not imply that the reflection is less real or substantial than that which it reflects. See note 13. Perhaps "two sides of the same coin" would have been a better phrase to use.

26. See note 18. These cases also bear on the apnea test and why the unsuccessful attempt to respire is a sign of life.

27. An analogue in the theory of value would be that when a process (m) has value only because it is instrumentally useful in causing intrinsically valuable n, it is still *better*

that the valuable characteristic (n) come into existence via m than for n to exist without such a cause. That is, it is to attach additional *intrinsic value to the existence of the instrumental relation*. I do not know of any theory of value that has such an element, but it is logically possible.

28. Veatch raises the issue of artificial support for "higher brain" functioning rather than for brain stem functioning (although not in the presence of such direct artificial support for respiration as an iron lung) in "The Impending Collapse."

29. See note 12.

30. From *Defining Death*, p. 149.

31. I assume that supporters of the WBC think that the *same* human life that once existed continues when only the brain stem functions. Then, I think, they should think the *same* human life continues when the chip is added as support for brain stem function.

32. See "Is It Time to Abandon Brain Death?" Truog also believes that total replacement of the brain stem defeats the WBC of death. But I do not believe he discusses whether the life that would exist with an artificial brain stem replacing the original brain stem is the *same* life as existed previously. This seems to be a crucial issue.

PART TWO

Early Life

9

Using Human Embryos for Biomedical Research

Should scientists seeking to cure human diseases be permitted to use stem cells from human embryos in their research?[1] Proponents of human embryonic stem cell (ESC) research emphasize that it may help in finding cures for diabetes, Parkinson's, heart disease, Lou Gehrig's disease, and other devastating disabilities and illnesses. Critics acknowledge the possible medical benefits, but point out that ESC research destroys embryos. Such destruction, they say, shows insufficient respect for the embryo and, more broadly, insufficient regard for the value of human life. Human embryos, the critics argue, are morally important, and that importance imposes substantial limits on permissible research.

U.S. President George W. Bush came down close to the critics. He announced that taxpayer dollars could be used to finance ESC research only on stem cell lines that had already been extracted from human embryos; federal money could not be used, he said, to "sanction or encourage further destruction of human embryos."[2] Interpretation of this policy softened, making it easier for scientists who accept federal funds to use ESCs in their research, and the policy was rejected by President Obama. But the debate continues, in part because of connections between the use of ESCs and the controversial issue of human cloning. Cloning is one possible source of embryos and many seek to prohibit human cloning for all purposes, including biomedical research. (A majority of President Bush's Council on Bioethics recommended a four-year moratorium on all cloning of human embryos.[3])

The moral problems with ESC research have been exaggerated, I believe. But to answer the critics, it is not enough to show that many lives may well be saved and much suffering avoided by new breakthroughs from ESC-based research. Critics acknowledge those possible benefits but rightly deny that the magnitude of the benefits suffices to justify the research. After all, lethal experimentation on infants is impermissible even if it would generate socially valuable results. To respond, then, we need to address the moral criticism head-on, either by showing that human embryos are devoid of moral importance—like a human fingernail or an appendix or a small clump of human cells—or that the kind of moral importance they have is consistent with using them in biomedical research.

I. The Sources of ESCs

When a human sperm fertilizes a human ovum, a single cell is created with the potential to grow into a human person. A few days after fertilization, a blastocyst develops, comprising an outer layer of cells that forms the placenta and other tissues needed for the fetus to develop and a hollow sphere that contains an inner cell mass. Cells in the inner mass are called "stem cells," and they can go on to form nearly all tissues and specialized cells in the human body (e.g., organs and blood cells). Because of this unusual potential, stem cells—sometimes called *pluripotential cells*—may be useful in treating many illnesses. From this early stage in development until it is nine to ten weeks old, the organism is called an embryo. The embryo passes through a pre-implanted zygote stage, which lasts about seven to fourteen days, and the first eight weeks of gestation. Only after significant cell differentiation has occurred does the organism become known as the fetus. Stem cells can be gathered from the embryo's inner cell mass; thus originates the term *embryonic stem cells.*

ESCs can be obtained from three sources: aborted embryos and early fetuses that still have some such cells; embryos generated for in vitro fertilization (IVF) but not implanted; and embryos created by cloning. However the embryos are obtained, they die when the stem cells are removed. A 1999 government report on guidelines for federally funded research involving ESCs acquired through abortion or IVF (that is, not through cloning)[4] took the view that while human embryos do not have the moral status of human persons, they should be treated with respect. Treating human embryos with respect was said to involve not using them simply as means for achieving some further goal. I shall call this the Mere Means Thesis. (Notice that this thesis does not exclude that one could be using the embryo as a mere means even without intending its death; the death can be merely foreseen as a certain effect of intentionally removing its stem cells for some goal. Supporters of the Doctrine of Double Effect [DDE], which prohibits intending an evil, may not have grounds to condemn using the embryo if its death is a foreseen side effect. However, revisionists about the DDE [such as Warren Quinn] can treat intentionally involving an entity in a way that one foresees will cause its death on par morally with intending its death.[5])

According to the government report, Mere Means has two important corollaries, one concerning the creation of embryos, the other concerning their destruction.

1. *Noncreation.* Embryos should not be created for the purpose of conducting research that will destroy them. In particular, then, embryos should not be created for stem cell research because removing stem cells destroys the embryo. An embryo should only be used in stem cell research if it was created for some other purpose. Otherwise, it is treated as a mere means.

2. *Alternate Destruction.* Even embryos not created for the purpose of conducting research that will destroy them should not be used in research that will
destroy them *unless they would have been destroyed in any case.* Consider,
for example, an embryo left over from an IVF project that will be stored in
a freezer, not destroyed. Alternate Destruction says that a researcher should
not acquire that embryo and use it to acquire stem cells. That, too, would be
to treat it merely as a means and would not show respect.

Together, Noncreation and Alternate Destruction very substantially restrict
morally permissible ways to acquire ESCs; they should only be obtained from embryos that were not created for the purpose of being destroyed but that will in any
case be destroyed.

To appreciate the force of these restrictions, consider how they apply to the
case of cloning as a source of ESCs. Many people have assumed that *reproductive
cloning*—that is, cloning that results in a new human person—should be banned.[6]
But suppose we clone embryos. If reproductive cloning is wrong, then we have a
duty to prevent the cloned embryos from developing into full human persons. So
if a scientist clones ten embryos for the purpose of acquiring ESCs but draws ESCs
from only five, then the other five must not be allowed to survive and grow into
cloned human persons. Unless we can be absolutely certain that if we freeze these
embryos they will never be used, it might seem that we will have a duty to destroy
any that can develop further.[7] But, destroying those that might develop into persons would violate Alternate Destruction, as they would not have died otherwise.
Hence, creation of cloned embryos for research violates Noncreation and destroying those not used violates Alternate Destruction. The result closes off the cloning
option to acquire ESCs altogether.

In a *New York Times* interview several years after the 1999 report,[8] Harold
T. Shapiro, the chair of the federal panel that produced that original report on the
use of ESCs in federally funded research, said that cloning embryos for the purpose of reproduction poses no unique moral problems. Mere Means and Noncreation, however, appear in his panel's report—theses that conflict with cloning for
the purpose of obtaining ESCs for research if, as seems to be the case, destruction
of cloned embryos will occur and indeed would be required were it not that it violates Alternate Destruction.[9]

Perhaps, however, Mere Means need not apply to certain embryos, cloned or
otherwise. How might one arrive at that exemption? One reason for thinking that
embryos ought not to be treated as mere means is that the embryo has the potential to develop into (or give rise to)[10] a person. Embryos, however, could be created
that lack the genetic potential to develop beyond a few days. Some scientists think
that using such embryos for research would obviate many moral problems in using
ESCs from cloned embryos. Let us call this the No-Potential Solution. The proposal is that Mere Means, Noncreation, and Alternate Destruction do not apply to
embryos with such limited genetic potential, even if they apply to embryos with

the genetic potential to develop into human persons. After all, by destroying an embryo lacking the potential to develop into a human person, we would not be interfering with its future development into a person because it could not develop in this way.

An alternative way to reopen the option of cloning as a source of ESCs is to say that an embryo's potential to develop into a human person depends on its environment. Thus U.S. Senator Orrin Hatch, an opponent of abortion, came out in favor of ESC research because "life begins in a woman's womb, not in a petri dish."[11] Hatch's view seems to be that when an embryo is already in a sustaining environment such as the womb, it has the potential to develop into a person. In a petri dish or a freezer, however, it does not have the potential to develop until someone puts it in a sustaining environment. Hence, even cloned embryos that could develop if put in a sustaining environment do not have the potential to develop when they are not and will not be placed in such an environment. Creating and using embryos in laboratories (as is done in IVF) would create no problem according to this view because they would not have the potential for further development. Interestingly, bioethicist Arthur Caplan—who is no opponent of abortion—also holds this view.[12]

Notice that on the view proposed by Hatch and Caplan, we achieve the No-Potential Solution without creating embryos that are genetically unable to develop. If ESCs are to be taken from embryos deliberately created outside a sustaining environment such as the womb, then Mere Means, Noncreation, and Alternate Destruction may not apply. The fact that an embryo will not develop because we will not put it in a sustaining environment is crucial. Achieving the No-Potential Solution in this way would, it might be thought,[13] allow us to obtain ESCs from cloned embryos, from embryos deliberately created for use, and from leftover embryos generated for IVF that would otherwise go into a freezer.

Because he is pro-choice, Caplan may also believe that when an embryo is aborted, it may be destroyed for its ESCs. Senator Hatch, however, may not share this view, for he thinks that abortion, which fatally interferes with an embryo that is in a sustaining environment, is morally wrong. He may believe it is impermissible to take advantage of an immorally aborted embryo. Therefore, depending on one's other beliefs, the No-Potential Solution may or may not allow us to obtain ESCs from aborted fetuses.

II. Problems with Current Policies and Positions

Mere Means and its corollaries impose large restrictions on using ESCs. And, unless we endorse some form of the No-Potential view, they appear to close off completely the option of obtaining ESCs from cloning. I want now to offer some reasons for rejecting Mere Means, Noncreation, and Alternate Destruction, and for thinking that the No-Potential Solution is misguided, incomplete, and even unnecessary. In this part, I shall offer some hypothetical cases that suggest that the three ideas constituting Mere Means are implausible. (It is only later in this chapter that I shall attempt to explain and justify my judgments in these cases.) In part 3, I shall challenge a view that makes the moral importance of embryos depend on their potential to develop into persons, and I shall propose an alternative view of their importance. This alternative should help to justify certain responses to the hypothetical cases. The upshot is that ESC research is morally much less troubling than much current discussion suggests.

A. MERE MEANS

The government report that presents Mere Means seems to be founded on an idea that traces to Immanuel Kant's moral philosophy. The second formulation of Kant's categorical imperative says that we should treat rational humanity "whether in [our] own person or in that of another, always as an end and never as a means only."[14] The embryo is not rational humanity, however, but pre-rational humanity. A pre-rational embryo may have *some* moral significance, but why suppose that the strong Kantian principle applies to it?

To see the force of the question, consider a couple in an IVF clinic. The couple have produced three embryos for implantation and cannot produce any more. The couple hope for at least two children. Two of the embryos run into trouble, but both could be saved by sustaining them with parts of the third embryo. The third embryo is not in any trouble, was about to be implanted in the womb, and would have developed without problems. Arguably, it is permissible to use that one embryo to save the other two, even if it is impermissible to kill one person in order to save two people.[15] Thus, the couple may use one embryo to save two, but they may not, for example, take organs from one infant child to save two others. If this is so, it is not true that human embryos should never be used as mere means. Embryos have a different moral status than human persons.

B. NONCREATION

According to Noncreation, we must not create embryos which we intend to use in research that leads to their destruction.[16] But suppose that a woman dying of heart disease learns that if she becomes pregnant and has a very early abortion that kills the embryo, her body's reaction to the embryo's death will prompt a cure for her disease. Would it be morally permissible for her to become pregnant with the aim of aborting the embryo immediately? The ethos underlying Noncreation implies that she should not do it, even though this destruction does not occur for research purposes. Yet arguably, it is permissible for her to do this.[17] To be sure, the example is very odd, but ask yourself what you think. Now suppose instead that the woman could cure her heart disease by carrying her pregnancy to term and having the infant's heart valves transplanted into her body. In this case, the woman's conduct seems wrong. Once more, moral thought seems to distinguish embryos from other living human beings—a difference obscured by Noncreation.

Suppose it is permissible for the woman to create an embryo for the purpose of destroying it in order to cure her heart disease. Why may she not create it in order to give it to a scientist who will destroy it in an attempt to find a cure for her by doing research with it? Why may she not help create the embryo outside her body in a laboratory, as is done in IVF, for the same research purpose? If a doctor may permissibly help her have the planned abortion in the original case, there is good reason to think a scientist may help her through ESC research using the embryo in a laboratory. Perhaps the likelihood of finding a cure is important for assessing the permissibility of these acts, but this should hold whether or not a scientist is involved. Furthermore, why should it matter that a cure is sought for the very woman whose embryo is donated? Why should she be permitted to create the embryo and have it destroyed in research to help herself but barred from doing this to try to help someone else in the same way?

Another problem for Noncreation is raised by the theoretical possibility that one might need to *create* a spare embryo for IVF in order to use it to keep other embryos alive. (This is an extension of the three-embryo case discussed above.[18]) This case reminds us that creating an embryo in order to have a baby does not necessarily mean creating an embryo that will itself become—or even have a possibility of becoming—a baby. Though Noncreation rules out creating an extra embryo in order to use it to keep other embryos alive, doing this strikes me as morally permissible.

C. ALTERNATE DESTRUCTION

According to Alternate Destruction, we may not destroy an embryo in research unless it would have been destroyed anyway for nonresearch reasons. Suppose, however, a woman undergoing IVF discovers that she has fatal breast cancer just as she is about to implant an embryo. She has every intention of going through with the pregnancy, as this is her chance to leave a child behind for her family. She is then told that if she instead gives the embryo to a scientist, a drug can be developed that will cure her cancer. According to Alternate Destruction, destroying this embryo should be impermissible because the embryo would not otherwise have been destroyed, but implanted. Yet it seems permissible for the woman to save her life in this way. It seems permissible, too, for her to give the embryo to a scientist to save someone else's life.

III. An Alternative View of the Moral Importance of Embryos

The basic principles underlying the 1999 U.S. government report on stem cell research—Mere Means, Noncreation, and Alternate Destruction—all seem misguided. These principles are founded on the perhaps plausible idea that human embryos have some moral importance, but they misrepresent that moral importance.

How, then, *should* we understand the moral importance of embryos? I shall come at this question a bit indirectly through a problem raised by cloning.

My judgments about the hypothetical cases that test Mere Means, Noncreation, and Alternate Destruction imply that it is *permissible* to destroy embryos in more circumstances than if these theses were true. But cloning raises a special problem for these theses. As noted, many believe that allowing a cloned embryo to develop into a human person would be wrong.[19] To avoid that wrong, we might have to destroy any cloned embryo that could develop into a human person. But this itself could be wrong. Even if it is permissible to destroy an embryo for research purposes, it might be thought wholly objectionable to produce embryos that it is not only permissible to kill but that we subsequently could have a *duty* to kill. If an embryo has the potential to develop into a human person, it might be said that we cannot have a duty to kill an entity with such potential. Hatch and Caplan deny that an embryo in a laboratory has any such potential. Imagine, however, that the cloned embryo in question has been mistakenly implanted in a womb (or some external gestation device)[20]—as might happen—and is otherwise fine. Most would agree that this cloned and implanted embryo has the potential to develop into (or give rise to) a person. Could we nevertheless have a duty to kill it? And is it permissible to start projects that might lead to such mistakes and result in such a duty?

The answer to both questions may be "yes" because of the kind of moral importance the embryo has. An embryo is not the sort of entity for which it can be bad to lose its future. An embryo may have some moral value in the sense that its continued existence, *in its own right* (even if it is frozen and will never develop into a person), may give us a reason not to destroy it. This value could only be overridden by some good that we can achieve in destroying it, thus ruling out the useless or gratuitous killing of embryos. But having some reason not to destroy it is not the same as saying that we should not destroy the embryo because that is bad *for the embryo*. (Notice that the latter could be true either because it cannot be bad for the embryo to lose its future or because it does not matter very much morally that something bad happens to the embryo.)

Consider, by way of analogy, a valuable work of art: say, a painting. A painting is valuable in its own right and therefore should not be wantonly destroyed. We could even say that certain things, such as sunlight, are good (or bad) for a painting, meaning that without it (or with it), it will not survive. But this does not mean that we should prevent sunlight from hitting it because it is a benefit for the painting to survive in the sense that it gets something out of this. We do not preserve paintings for the sake of the paintings themselves in the sense that their continued existence can be good *for them*. After all, a painting is not capable of being a conscious or experiencing subject, and this seems to be necessary in order to be able to get anything out of one's existence. Likewise, an embryo is not capable of being a conscious or experiencing subject.[21] In contrast, when we refrain from destroying a bird—even if it is less valuable in its own right than a painting is in its own right—we may be acting for its sake, for it may be good *for the bird* to continue to exist.[22]

Can we be acting for the embryo's sake in not destroying it because it has the *potential* to become a human person able to think, perceive, and experience? I do not think so. Suppose it is good to be a person and there is some sense in which the embryo loses out on becoming a person (by contrast to its being the raw material that gives rise to a very different thing, namely a person). I do not think that it is bad for the embryo to lose its potential because I do not think that an embryo is the sort of entity that can either benefit from the transformation into a person or be harmed by not so transforming.[23] This has something to do with its not being (and never having been) a subject capable of consciousness or sentience, and so (as argued above) its not being capable of being benefited at all, even by turning into the kind of being that can be benefited. Analogously, suppose that a table could, by magic, be made capable of turning into a person. It is not bad for the table if it is destroyed instead of being allowed to transform.[24] (Harming or interfering with a benefit to an entity is not the only way to treat it disrespectfully, of course. For example, overriding a person's will for his or her own good can be disrespectful. But embryos do not have wills and so cannot be treated disrespectfully in this way either.)

Notice that the reasons I have given for the permissibility of destroying embryos for research do not yield a principled distinction between embryos in the first two weeks of life and older embryos. Researchers working with stem cells intend to use embryos in the first two weeks, before the "primitive streak" appears and marks the first point at which the clump of cells begins to be an individual, coordinated embryo. It is possible that some researchers might find it useful to use older embryos. Some have argued for the two-week limit because an embryo can split before the primitive streak appears and form the bases of identical twins. They think this implies that the less mature embryo does not merit the same protection as an embryo that is the basis for a definite individual person.

I am not convinced this is a morally crucial distinction. For suppose it were possible for children to split into identical twins before age four. A child who is "splittable" still merits protection against destruction. What justifies such protection are the characteristics of the entity at the time. A person at, for example, age three has the necessary characteristics that give rise to a right not to be killed, but embryos before and after the primitive streak may not have these characteristics. Nor would it be correct, I believe, to conclude that a child who (it is known) will definitely split into twins can permissibly be killed on the grounds that the child will soon be replaced by two other people and thus cease to exist.

On account of the reasons I have given for it not being bad for the embryo if it is killed, I do not think that it would be wrong to involve ourselves in a project that would result in a duty to destroy a cloned embryo with the potential to become a human person. The grave evil that we associate with the destruction of human life—and more broadly with using people as means to an end—reflects the fact that such destruction—and such use—is either bad *for the persons whose lives are destroyed or who are used* or contrary to their will. Embryos, however, have no will, and their destruction is not bad *for them*. (The same conclusion would follow if it were bad for the embryo to be destroyed but it did not matter morally if this were true.) I also think that many of my judgments about the permissibility of killing the embryo in the hypothetical cases I explored earlier can be justified by this understanding of the moral importance of a human embryo.

Let us now consider in more detail the question of what has the potential to be a person and whether the proposal mentioned earlier of creating an embryo without the potential to develop into a person is an alternative plausible solution to the many moral issues that some think surround ESC research. First, is it correct to say (as Hatch and Caplan have said) that an embryo that is not and will not be in a sustaining environment has no more potential for development than an embryo that is created with a genetic makeup that prohibits development? I do not think so. Consider an embryo that could develop if placed in a sustaining environment but that will be frozen instead. Even if it never develops, its genetic capacity for development arguably makes it more valuable in its own right than an embryo without such a capacity. The potential for developing (or giving rise to) a human person seems to count for *something*.

Imagine a magic wand, capable of producing a great effect, that is locked in a museum case and will never be used. Compare it with a nonmagic wand in the same case. Though neither will ever produce any great effects, the former wand has greater value in its own right in virtue of its potential even though both wands have the same actual instrumental value, namely zero. (I am here accepting the view that a relational property—in this case, having properties that could give rise to an effect—can contribute to the value an entity has in its own right.[25]) The human embryo that could develop into a human person if it were placed in a sustaining environment is like an unused magic wand.

The difference between embryos with no genetic potential and embryos lacking potential because of their environment can also explain why some antiabortionists object to Hatch's position. If one believes that the embryo with genetic potential is very important and its development is important, a possible response is to call for it to be placed in a sustaining environment. This is analogous to how one would treat a child who was in a nonsustaining environment: one would not say that it was permissible to *kill* the child because the child was in a nonsustaining environment and hence lacked potential to go on living anyway. One would instead try to move the child into a better, life-sustaining environment. However, such a position concerning the embryo also implies that leftover embryos from IVF that are frozen should be adopted and transferred to a sustaining environment, at least at reasonable cost. If this is, in fact, not morally necessary, it is because the value of an embryo with genetic potential does not imply that its potential must be developed or even that it cannot be killed for the sake of an important good. What is most important for the permissibility of using human embryos for biomedical research is not that genetically normal embryos in a nonsustaining environment will not have a chance to develop, and in that sense, lack potential, but that such embryos *need not* be placed in a sustaining environment because of what they are.

Finally, is the creation of human embryos without the genetic potential to develop into a person a solution to the current controversies? I believe not. The problem here is that we would first need to show much of what we need to show in order to argue that current embryos may permissibly be used in research projects before we could permissibly create entities that are otherwise like human embryos but lack the genetic potential to develop into persons or to live beyond a few days.

To see why, first notice that there are at least three possible ways in which No-Potential to develop into a person could come about: (1) create a human embryo that has the intrinsic capacity to become (or give rise to) a person but that is made without a gene for longevity beyond a few days; (2) create a human embryo that lacks the intrinsic capacity to become (or give rise to) a person but can go on living indefinitely as a human embryo; (3) create a human embryo that both lacks the intrinsic capacity to become (or give rise to) a person and lacks a gene for longevity beyond a few days.

Now suppose that an embryo already exists with genetic potential to develop into (or give rise to) a person and we seek to take away that genetic potential (without destroying the embryo) in order that we may then destroy it because it lacks genetic potential to become (or give rise to) a person. Doing this would clearly be problematic if we could not first justify our action by showing that embryos are *not* the sort of entities that have a right to retain such genetic potential or for which the loss of this potential is bad. But if we showed these claims to be true, we will have gone a long way in proving that the embryo is the sort of entity that can be destroyed even while it retains this potential.[26]

Suppose we could create an embryo without genetic potential to become (or give rise to) a person rather than removing such potential from an already existing embryo. (This is option [2] from the list above.) To show that this is permissible, we must also first show that an embryo is not the sort of entity for which it is bad not to have the capacity to develop into (or give rise to) a person, assuming continuous identity as the same embryo with and without the capacity.[27] The following analogy may help to understand this. Suppose someone wanted to experiment on human children, but it was objected that this is impermissible because it would lead them to never become adults. Creating a human person with a genetic modification that will make him always remain a child just so that we could experiment on him without thereby causing him any loss of adulthood is not a solution to the research problem. This is because the sort of entity he would be—a person—would thereby not have the potential for adulthood and thus be denied something that is a basic good (adulthood) it could otherwise have had, assuming constant identity as the same person with or without the potential for adulthood.[28] Hence, it is only permissible to make a genetic modification that leads to the inability to become a person to an entity for which it would not be bad to a great degree not to become (or give rise to) a person. If, as I argued earlier, the human embryo is such an entity, then we have already gone a long way in showing that it is the sort of entity that we may destroy even if it has potential for developing into a person. Hence, to defend the permissibility of creating an embryo without potential to develop into a person, we have to defend the very same theses that are crucial to the permissibility of killing an embryo *with such potential.*

Consider again the person who would be created to always remain a child. Even if it was wrong to create him without the capacity to become an adult, it would also be wrong to kill him if he could continue living indefinitely as a child. Would it be comparably wrong to kill an embryo that had been modified to lack the capacity to develop into a person but could continue living on for a long time as an embryo? If not, this too indicates that the embryo, unlike a child, is not the sort of entity that has a claim not to have its distinctive type of life (embryohood) taken from it.[29] This suggests that unlike the child, the embryo's value is completely tied up with its having the potential to develop into (or give rise to) a higher form of being (e.g., a person). This, in turn, helps explain why it is not entitled to retain the potential to become the higher form of being. While we might think the *process* of developing into a person is valuable, this does not mean that the embryo is an entity entitled to undergo that process or that it benefits by undergoing that process. This is supported by the fact that it is not even an entity entitled to life if it lacks its developmental capacity (unlike the child).

Now consider creating an embryo that has the intrinsic capacity to become (or give rise to) a person but is "made" (constructed so as) to die shortly after conception even if we do not kill it (option [1] from the list above). To show that creating such an embryo is permissible, we must first show much of what we would have to show if we were to argue that it would be permissible to *kill* the embryo even if it has potential to develop into a person. Consider the following analogy as an aid to understanding this point. Suppose someone wanted to experiment on human adults but we object that this is impermissible as it would lead them to lose the rest of their lives. The experimenter suggests creating a human person with a genetic modification that will produce an early death (e.g., at age twenty) so that we could experiment on that person just before he dies naturally without the experiment causing him any loss of life he would otherwise have had. This is not a solution to the problem raised by the experiment. This is because the person would be created for a short life span and thus be denied additional life that is a basic good for him as the person he will be. Hence, it is permissible to make a genetic modification that leads to an early natural death for an *embryo* that has the intrinsic capacity to become a person only if such a human embryo is an entity for which it would not be bad to a great degree to not have more life in which it developed into (or gave rise to) a person. This means that to defend the permissibility of option (1), we have to defend the same theses that are crucial to the permissibility of killing an embryo that could go on living and develop into (or give rise to) a person.

What about creating a human embryo that is made both to lack the intrinsic capacity to develop into a person and to die soon after conception even if it is not destroyed (option [3] from the list above)? Would it be permissible to create a human person who cannot develop into an adult and who is given a gene that will make it die early in childhood, just so that we can experiment on it without robbing it of its development into an adult or of its continuing time alive as a child? Presumably not. Hence it is only permissible to make the genetic modifications in option (3) if a human embryo is an entity for which it would not be bad to a great degree to lose out on becoming (or giving rise to) a person and losing out on continuing life as an embryo. Hence, to defend the permissibility of option (3), we have to defend many of the same theses that are crucial to the permissibility of killing an embryo that has intrinsic capacity to develop into a person and to go on living a long time.

In conclusion, I want to recall the context of my argument. The discussion of biomedical research using ESCs begins from two basic considerations: first, that such research may have very large benefits; and second, that the research requires the destruction of embryos. Critics argue that we must forgo the benefits of ESC research because destroying embryos fails to show respect for their moral importance. I have argued that their conclusion is founded on an implausible view of the moral importance of embryos. The correct conclusion is not that we can use human embryos however we want, but that we have no reason to forgo the large benefits that doctors and scientists expect will follow from research on human ESCs.[30]

Notes

1. This chapter is a revised version of my "Embryonic Stem Cell Research: A Moral Defense," *Boston Review* 27 (October/November 2002).

2. Address by U.S. President George W. Bush on stem cell research, August 9, 2001.

3. President's Council on Bioethics, "Human Cloning and Human Dignity: An Ethical Inquiry," available online under "Reports" at: http://www.bioethics.gov.

4. National Bioethics Advisory Commission, "Ethical Issues in Human Stem Cell Research, Executive Summary," September, 1999; http://www.ntis.gov.

5. See Quinn's "Actions, Intentions, and Consequences: The Doctrine of Double Effect," reprinted in his *Morality and Action* (New York: Cambridge University Press, 1994). I discuss Quinn's views in chapter 3 of my *Intricate Ethics* (New York: Oxford University Press, 2007).

6. For discussion of some aspects of that controversy, see chapter 16 this volume.

7. Charles Krauthammer—a columnist, M.D., and member of the President's Commission on Bioethics—points to this as a decisive reason not to allow cloning for research purposes, even though he agrees that the embryo does not have the same moral status as a person. See his "Crossing Lines: A Secular Argument against Research Cloning," *The New Republic*, April 29, 2002. He also supports Noncreation, though the way he puts it is that we must not create human life while *intending* to destroy it.

8. Howard Markel, "A Conversation with Harold Shapiro: Weighing Medical Ethics for Many Years to Come," *New York Times*, July 2, 2002.

9. Of course, Shapiro may not have agreed personally with the panel's report, though no dissent was published. Reports by government panels that aim to provide reasons for their conclusions may well be compromises in their conclusions as well as their reasoning. Such reports appear to propose philosophical rationales, but no one on the panel may fully endorse the rationale. If this is so, it may not be wise to treat the reasoning in these reports as intended to be correct and so rightly subject to critical examination in the search for truth. On the other hand, such a critical examination is important even if only to show that these reports do not embody correct, but only compromise or window-dressing, reasoning. I have examined the reasoning provided in other government reports on organ transplantation and brain death, and also found them wanting. See my "Reflections on the Report of the U.S. Task Force on Organ Transplantation," *The Mount Sinai Journal of Medicine* (May 1989): 207–20 (which was expanded as chapters 11–15 in my *Morality, Mortality*, Vol.1 (New York: Oxford University Press, 1993); and my "Brain Death and Spontaneous Breathing," *Philosophy & Public Affairs* 30(3) (Summer 2001), which is revised as chapter 8 this volume. For a philosopher's discussion of the compromises that are made in serving as advisors to government deliberative panels, see Dan Brock, "Truth or Consequences: The Role of Philosophers in Policymaking," *Ethics* 97(4) (July 1987): 786–91; and the last part of D. Green and D. Wikler, "Brain Death and Personal Identity," *Philosophy & Public Affairs* 9(2) (Winter 1980). On some of the issues they raise, see my "The Philosopher as Insider and Outsider," *Journal of Medicine and Philosophy* 15 (August 1990), which is revised as chapter 23 this volume.

10. Which of these descriptions one accepts depends on which philosophical theory of the person one accepts. For simplicity, I shall use the former expression in a noncommittal way, unless otherwise noted.

11. Sheryl Gay Stolberg, "Key Republican Backs Cloning Research," *New York Times*, May 1, 2002.

12. See his discussion of these issues in "Attack of the Anti-Cloners," *The Nation*, June 17, 2002.

13. The reasons for the qualification will be clear later: I do not think that the No-Potential Solution is really a solution at all.

14. Immanuel Kant, *Foundations of the Metaphysics of Morals*, trans. Lewis White Beck (Chicago: University of Chicago Press, 1950), p. 47.

15. On why we should not kill one person in order to save two, see my *Morality, Mortality*, Vol. 2 (New York: Oxford University Press, 1996). For more on harming or killing embryos to save other entities, see chapter 16 this volume.

16. I shall assume in what follows that creating embryos with the intention to use them for research with foresight of the fact that they will certainly die from such use is as contrary to Noncreation, as is creating embryos while intending their destruction or creating embryos foreseeing that we will intend their destruction.

17. Notice that those who endorse Noncreation and would support its implication for this case could also think that it is, in general, morally permissible to have abortions. For in most abortions, a woman does not get pregnant *in order to* have an abortion. Furthermore, one of the reasons given to support the moral permissibility of most abortions is that the embryo (or fetus) is imposing on the woman's body and its presence is an undue imposition on her. In extreme cases, the embryo may pose a threat to her life, just as heart disease does in the case above. So a person may believe, with no inconsistency, that it is permissible to

destroy an embryo that presents a (morally innocent) threat to a woman but that it is impermissible to create and use an embryo (that is not itself presenting a threat to her) simply because destroying it will help the woman avoid *another* threat that the embryo has not caused, like heart disease.

18. Krauthammer also presents such a case. He thinks that it is analogous to what is involved in cloning—creating when one (supposedly) knows one will destroy—and that it is morally impermissible.

19. I shall not here try to contest this assumption that reproductive cloning is wrong, though it can possibly be contested. See some discussion of this issue in chapter 16 this volume.

20. For discussion of the moral relevance of such external gestation devices for the permissibility of abortion, see F. M. Kamm, *Creation and Abortion* (New York: Oxford University Press, 1992).

21. A being that is capable of sentience or consciousness is not one that merely has the capacity (or potential) to develop into a being that is capable of sentience or consciousness. Also, it is not necessarily a being that has already had sentient experience or consciousness. For example, a being that has never experienced pleasure can still be capable of it, and so it is the sort of being for whose sake I can act in giving it pleasure for the first time and in not depriving it of future life from which it will get pleasure. Here I differ with the view in Bonnie Steinbock, *Life before Birth: The Moral and Legal Status of Embryos and Fetuses* (New York: Oxford University Press, 1992), and Mary Ann Warren in *Moral Status: Obligations to Persons and Other Living Things* (Oxford: Clarendon Press, 1998). They both require that a being having already had experiences in order for it to be possible to harm it (or do something bad for it) by killing it.

22. Notice that even creatures, such as birds, for whose sake we can act in keeping them alive do not necessarily have a right not to be killed. For more discussion of these issues that may be helpful to read in conjunction with this chapter, see chapter 16 this volume.

23. I first made this point in *Creation and Abortion*, pp. 17–18.

24. Even if it is not bad for the embryo to lose its potential, it could be an indication of the value of an embryo if we would try to correct a defect in it that interfered with its achieving its potential rather than dispose of it and create a new embryo without a defect. Similarly, it can be an indication of the value of a painting if we try to rescue it from damage rather than have an equally good painting created in its stead.

25. On this, see chapter 16 this volume.

26. Michael Tooley, in "Abortion and Infanticide" (*Philosophy & Public Affairs* 2[1] [1972]), similarly suggested that if we could permissibly take away the potential to be a person of a kitten that had been modified to have the potential, and then drown it, we should be permitted to drown the kitten while it still has the potential. The two steps can be folded into one.

27. Or that something bad for it does not matter morally. I shall assume this alternative to be understood henceforth.

28. Notice that both in the case of the embryo and the case of the child, I am assuming for the sake of argument that the *same* embryo or *same* child could have been given greater potential; that is, there need be no change in the identity of embryo or person with and without the potential for personhood or adulthood. This is necessary in order to think of the embryo or child being made worse off than *it* would otherwise have been in an entity-affecting

sense, or having something bad for it occur that need not have occurred to it. The alternative is to think that we are dealing with identity-changing properties. Then if creating an embryo that is incapable of becoming a person, or a person who is incapable of becoming an adult, is wrong, this would be not so much for entity-affecting, but for non-entity-affecting reasons. That is, we could instead have created an embryo that could develop into a person, or a person who could develop into an adult. This would be an impersonally better outcome and one it could be wrong not to create instead of the other outcome, but not necessarily an outcome that is better *for* any particular embryo or person. I owe this point to Johann Frick.

29. I first used this example in *Creation and Abortion*, pp. 16–17.

30. I am grateful to Derek Parfit and Jeff McMahan for comments on earlier drafts of *The Boston Review* article and to Joshua Cohen for his work on the article as Editor of *The Boston Review*.

10

Ethical Issues in Using and Not Using Human Embryonic Stem Cells

It is an aim of some to find ways to acquire human stem cells that will raise no ethical objections from any quarter.[1] This is probably an impossible task, as there might be people whose ethical views forbid any scientific research at all. The aim might be rephrased as finding ways to acquire stem cells that will raise no *reasonable* ethical complaint. One problem then is to consider what constitutes reasonable complaints (or what complaints are not unreasonable). But not all reasonable complaints are correct. For example, it might be reasonable given your information at a certain time to think you are being cheated. Nevertheless you could be wrong. So another problem is to consider the correctness of even views that are not unreasonable. Of course, if a view that is initially not unreasonable is conclusively shown to be wrong and one should know this, it might become unreasonable to hold the view.

In the first part of this chapter, I consider a set of objections to acquiring human embryonic stem cells (ESCs) often considered reasonable. I shall argue that although these objections might not be unreasonable, they are nevertheless not correct. In the second part of this chapter, I shall consider alternatives to current methods for acquiring stem cells that are being pursued because they are thought to obviate the objections I considered in the first part of the chapter. I shall consider whether these alternatives could themselves raise ethical objections, and whether and when it is important to seek such alternatives.

I

A

The following objection has been raised to using live human embryos to acquire stem cells: To acquire stem cells, we must do what leads to the destruction of the embryo. But the embryo is an (innocent) human organism and, therefore, it is wrong to destroy it.

By "human organism" is meant at least something with human DNA that is an integrated system organized around an axis. Some say that a one-cell human conceptus has these properties because it has parts that form an integrated single cell system.[2] Further, a defective human organism is still a human organism, at least so long as some underlying integration typical of the species remains. Some add to these conditions on being a human organism the requirement that the system intrinsically be headed in the direction of development typical of human beings. The reference to "intrinsic" means that even though a conceptus will not, in fact, develop in virtue of some extrinsic property (e.g., it will not be in an environment conducive to development), this does not affect its status as a human organism on an account which emphasizes intrinsic trajectory. Further, trajectory to be a defective human being also meets the trajectory requirement.[3] This analysis of the nature of an organism is said to be based on systems biology.

It has been argued that it is wrong to destroy an organism that meets these minimal conditions (e.g., a one-cell human conceptus with a trajectory) because this is the only organism that will develop into an entity that is fit to receive a soul.[4] This is a religious view, but it can be put in secular terms if we think of having a soul as equivalent to being a person. When is a person (soul) present in the organism? The point about the argument I am now discussing is that it takes no position on this. That is, it is not an argument that depends on the view that a person (soul) is present at conception; it is consistent with the argument I am discussing to claim that the person (soul) only comes to be present when complex neural structures develop that support brain activity. This argument merely claims that because the organism is intrinsically able to develop so that it becomes a person (even a defective one), it is wrong to destroy it at any time, even before a soul/person is present. Call this the Organism Argument.[5]

One question to ask about this argument is why something that is not yet a person (ensouled) should be treated in significant ways (e.g., not be killed) as we treat a person? The general principle that is being appealed to by the Organism Argument seems to be: If an organism, in virtue of its intrinsic properties, is intrinsically headed on a trajectory to have property X, it should be treated with as much respect as we treat an entity that has property X. (Call this the Principle.) But this does not seem to be true. Consider an analogy involving a cat conceptus. Cats are entitled to some degree of consideration and are not to be destroyed for any unimportant reason (though they need not be treated as we should treat persons). Does this mean that a cat conceptus that has an intrinsic trajectory to develop into a cat should be treated with as much consideration as a cat? For example, is there no moral difference between destroying a cat and destroying a cat embryo in an experiment? I suggest there is a moral difference, because the properties that develop over time as the cat comes into being (e.g., sentience and consciousness) are relevant to how we should treat it and whether and when we may destroy it. If this is so, the Principle is incorrect.

It is often said that an acorn is not an oak tree. We can add that even if an acorn is an organism of the oak species that has an internal program leading it to become an oak, and even if oaks are not to be treated in certain ways, this does not imply that acorns may not be treated in those ways. We should conclude, I believe, that proving scientifically that something is an organism of a certain species type with an inner program, leading it to develop in a certain way, does nothing to show that it is entitled to be treated with the concern owed to the entity it can become. Evidence from systems biology does nothing to strengthen the argument from potential that was available independent of new scientific evidence.

A second point raised by the Organism Argument concerns the reasons for not destroying things.[6] Some things have value in their own right, independent of their use or relation to other things, and should not be destroyed because of this. But not all entities of this sort are entities "for whose sake" we should not destroy them. One reason we should not destroy a person is that he would get something good out of the life that he could lead, so he benefits, when we do not kill him. By contrast, a great painting is something we should not destroy because of what it is in its own right, but we do not refrain from destroying it for its own sake, for it gets nothing out of its continuing existence. An organism like a human conceptus might have value in its own right, even if not the same degree or type of value as a person, but I believe that it, unlike a person, is not the sort of entity for whose sake we should prevent its destruction. I think that this is because it is not and has never been capable of being sentient or conscious, and because of this it is not a subject who can be benefited by continuing to exist and lose out on a benefit (or be harmed) by not turning into a person.

The point is, whether we do something bad to something in destroying it or whether something bad happening to it is morally important is not only a function of what future life is lost. It is also a function of whether the entity is one for which that loss can be bad or whether it is the sort of entity to which bad things happening matters morally. An analogy may help to make this clearer. Suppose a table is magically given the capacity to develop into a person, but we then destroy the table before it develops. No matter how good it is to be a person, is a table the sort of thing that could suffer something bad happening to it by not being allowed to develop into a person? I do not think so. Knowing that this particular table is a remarkable entity with a unique capacity, and that it could develop into a person for whose sake we could act, still does not make it the sort of entity for whose sake we must protect its continuing development. The potential an entity has to be a person tells us what will not come about if the entity does not transform, but it does not alter the moral status of the entity in the sense that it makes the entity something for whose sake we should act so that it transforms. That sort of moral status depends not on the potential but on other properties the entity has now or has had in the past. The same is true of the embryo, I believe, even if it is a human organism.[7]

B

Let us now put to one side my arguments against the correctness of the Organism Argument and the Principle. Suppose, for the sake of argument, that an embryo that intrinsically has the capacity to develop into a person ought not to be destroyed if it *would* develop into a person. Does this not leave open the possibility that we might destroy embryos as a result of acquiring stem cells if the embryos, as a result of extrinsic factors, will not develop into persons? For example, suppose that embryos will not be placed in a womb, and then will either shortly die or be frozen. And may we not also acquire stem cells and thus destroy embryos that are "nonviable" because something is wrong with them intrinsically that interferes with their developing into (even defective) persons? (To eliminate other possible sources of objection to using such embryos, we might further suppose that they were not created just in order to acquire stem cells and that no one is morally required to put them into her womb. With these assumptions, we would not be the beneficiaries of what some might consider improper creation and abandonment.[8])

The Organism Argument focuses on the nature of the embryo to determine how we should treat it. But the current point is that we should also consider what will happen to the embryo if it is not killed in order to determine how we should treat it. When embryos will shortly die in any case, destroying them deliberately will not put them in any worse situation than they would otherwise be. This, it might be suggested, makes it permissible to destroy such embryos in acquiring stem cells from them. Furthermore, we can ask whether, when embryos would be frozen but not die soon, they lose anything worth having if they are not frozen but killed instead.

Roman Catholic theorists believe there is a reasonable complaint against killing embryos that will soon die anyway. (This also applies to ones that will be frozen.) To see why, recall that the Catholic Church opposes abortion even in the following case: A pregnant woman will die because of the position of the fetus in her womb unless she has an abortion. Suppose that if she dies, the fetus will also die. If an abortion is performed, the woman will live and the fetus will be killed. The Roman Catholic Church's position on this case is that it is morally preferable to not interfere, because we will then let both woman and fetus die merely *foreseeing* their deaths, rather than *intentionally* killing a fetus if we perform an abortion to save the woman.

The rationale for this conclusion comes from the Doctrine of Double Effect (DDE), which says that we may not intend lesser evils to achieve greater goods and either an omission or an action done with this intention is wrong. However, the DDE also holds that it may be permissible to do or omit to do something that leads to lesser evils as unintended side effects if this is necessary to achieve greater goods. (Apparently, the Catholic theorists think that the death of the fetus in an abortion is an evil, even if the fetus would die shortly in the absence of an abortion, because that abortion involves intending its death.)

Hence, the fact that it is foreseen that an embryo in an IVF clinic will die soon in any case as a result of not being put in someone's womb should not—if the

previous case of the pregnant woman and embryo is any indication—license deliberately killing the embryo, according to Roman Catholic doctrine. By contrast, a
policy on stem cells such as recommended by one-time Senate majority leader Bill
Frist allows Federal funding for killing some embryos that will soon die anyway.[9]

However, it might be argued that a fine point is being ignored in the Catholic
position if the position rests on the DDE. For while intentionally removing stem
cells kills the embryo as a foreseen effect, the death of the embryo need not be
intended, and according to the DDE, the distinction between intending and merely
foreseeing death could be sufficient to remove objections to doing what destroys an
embryo if a greater good, such as curing a disease, can thereby be achieved.

If this were true, should not Catholic theologians also permit removing stem
cells even from an embryo that would *not* soon die anyway (e.g., a viable embryo
that was about to be implanted in someone's womb) if a greater good was at stake?
Correctly or incorrectly, Catholic theologians *would* object to removal of stem
cells in such a case. Hence, they must think that the DDE also does not license
taking advantage of the "fine point" when the embryo would otherwise die.

Suppose that some are opposed on these grounds to killing soon-to-be-dead
embryos. Why should we as a community seek a way to acquire stem cells that
could not raise this complaint that we are killing soon-to-die embryos? After all,
we as a community do not endorse a policy (such as the Catholic one described
earlier) that rules out aborting a fetus that will soon die no matter what we do,
when doing this is necessary in order to save the life of the pregnant woman.
While I do not think there is a complete answer to this question, it is worth noting
that, in the abortion case, the fetus may itself be a contributing threat to the
woman. By contrast, the soon-to-be-dead embryo we would kill to acquire stem
cells is not itself a threat to anyone. That is, we would not kill it to stop a threat that
it presents, but rather only to allow us to help people who are threatened by other
diseases. And we do not kill grown persons who are not threats to others and who
will die shortly anyway in order to acquire their organs to save other people from
diseases (though the question may arise whether this should be permissible if we
have their consent to do so). If we take seriously the view that the embryo is morally equivalent to a person, then one can see that there are at least judgments in
related cases that underpin a wish to find ways to acquire stem cells that do not
destroy even soon-to-be-dead embryos. Those who do not think these other judgments are relevant probably do not really think the embryo is the moral equivalent of a person.

II

A

Several alternative ways to acquire human stem cells have been suggested in the
belief that they will obviate objections even to acquiring stem cells from embryos
soon to die. A crucial general factor in morally evaluating alternatives is whether

ESCs *acquired by a process that destroys human embryos* must be used *in order to develop* and test the alternative methods. There are two subdivisions of this question: (1) Will new embryos have to be destroyed? (2) Will only embryos that have already been destroyed be used?

Let us begin by considering the subquestion (1). Suppose that the development of an alternative method will result in killing new embryos. Suppose one takes seriously the claim that the embryo has the moral status of a person. Then one should only use ESCs to develop these alternatives (a) if one would be willing to kill a few people who would not otherwise die shortly in order to develop a new method for fighting diseases that does not require killing people; or (b) if one would be willing to kill a few people who would not otherwise be killed in order to stop scientists from killing many other people in order to find cures for diseases. Would it be permissible to do (a) or (b)? Ordinarily, one should not kill some people even in order to save many others from being killed or dying of natural causes. Furthermore, given that some object to using embryos that will die soon anyway, developing an alternative to use of ESCs that itself uses some of the very same embryos that would otherwise have been killed by current methods of acquiring ESCs should not quiet objections.

However, there are cases (much discussed in moral philosophy) in which we would kill some people who would not otherwise die as a consequence of redirecting a mechanical lethal threat away from a greater number of other people.[10] Many people think such redirection is permissible. This may seem to suggest a possible approach to justifying (b). Suppose scientists were conceived of as already being threats to many embryos and, despite being human agents, they were analogized to mechanical threats. Suppose also that the only way to stop their threat was to redirect the scientists toward carrying out investigations that kill fewer embryos (as a means to finding methods that will kill no embryos). If the analogy to permissible redirection of a mechanical threat were correct, the scientists' killing might be permissible, even if embryos were morally equivalent to persons and those killed would not otherwise have been killed. (This model would require that scientists give up (i.e., be redirected away from) killing many embryos as an ordinary method of acquiring stem cells and only focus on finding new alternatives.) However, it is not clear that it is appropriate to redirect human agents as we would mechanical threats.[11]

Now consider subquestion (2). Suppose that only embryos already killed would be used to develop alternatives. Some groups (e.g., the Roman Catholic Church) did not approve of President Bush's decision post-2001 to allow Federal funding for use of cell lines established before 2001. What problems arise for those who opposed the destruction of embryos that has already occurred, in the use of such embryos' cells to develop alternative methods that will eliminate the future need to kill embryos for stem cells? The most prominent issue for such opponents is whether it is morally permissible to make use of and, more generally, to benefit from the immoral conduct of others, even when one will not thereby encourage further wrongdoing. This issue arises, for example, in deciding whether one should be allowed to make good use of the results of Nazis' experimentation on concentration camp inmates, and in deciding whether there is anything morally wrong with using for transplantation the organs of someone who was murdered. Should labels be put on any pharmaceuticals developed by use of ESCs from already killed embroyos, or by the use of alternatives whose development employed already killed embryos, so that some members of the public can exercise their right not to use such drugs?

This brief discussion of subquestions (1) and (2) suggests that those who are opposed to destroying embryos because they think embryos should be treated as persons might have to complain about some ways of developing alternatives to, as well as about, current methods of getting ESCs. And if they could possibly change the context so that scientists are simply unable to kill or to use already improperly killed embryos, they should prefer this to both killing some embryos to develop alternative procedures or to redirecting scientists to perform fewer killings. Suppose opponents were successful in stopping the use of current methods of acquiring ESCs involving destroyed embryos. Then the mere fact that alternative methods could lead to disease cures should not justify deliberately destroying a few embryos to develop these alternatives, given the premises of the opponents. Those who do not complain about the destruction of some embryos to develop the alternative procedures as much as they would complain about killing people in the same circumstance, and those who do not complain as much about benefiting from the use of already killed embryos as they would complain about benefiting from the use of immorally killed people, thereby indicate that they do not really think the embryo is morally equivalent to a person. This, in turn, would reduce the need to find alternative methods of acquiring ESCs.

B

Now let us consider some proposed alternatives in more detail and see whether they raise other moral problems:

1. Instead of destroying an embryo in getting stem cells, we could remove one cell from an early blastocyst. This would not destroy the embryo and from the cell that is removed we can acquire stem cells. Some might think that several moral problems arise for this procedure. First, perhaps removing one cell could harm the embryo. Many might be concerned about this only if it produced lasting damage that would reduce the chance of a normal child developing from the embryo. But *if* the embryo is thought of as morally equivalent to a person, then perhaps damage to *it*, even if this damage had no effect on the future child, should be a problem. (This would be analogous to the problem of harming a child in research even though the damage would eventually reverse itself and not affect the adult that develops from the child.[12]) Second, if the cell that is removed was totipotent, it could develop into a complete embryo and so it would be equivalent to a one-cell conceptus. Removing stem cells from the one cell would destroy the

equivalent of a one-cell conceptus, thus raising the same problem with which we began. This problem could be obviated if the cell were taken from an embryo far enough along in development so that the cell removed from it would be *pluripotent but not totipotent*. Pluripotent cells can form any type of tissue but they cannot form an entire embryonic organism with capacity to develop further into a person.[13]

2. Another suggestion is that ESCs could be acquired from embryos that have died natural deaths.[14] The model here is said to be the acquisition of organs for organ transplantation after a person dies. For even when an embryo dies, some cells remain alive—just as when an adult dies some cells remain alive—and ESCs could be acquired from these live cells. This procedure should meet the objections of those opposed to using mere dying but not dead embryos. However, complaints might be raised if the cells removed from the dead embryo were totipotent, for (as argued above) if we removed stem cells from those cells, we would be killing what was morally equivalent to a one-cell conceptus. To avoid destroying such a new conceptus in acquiring stem cells, one would have to remove cells only from later-stage dead embryos, when the cell would be pluripotent but not totipotent. Then the cell's dying as a result of removing its stem cells would not interfere with the development of a person.

However, waiting for the cells in the dying embryo to move beyond totipotency raises another ethical issue for those who think the embryo should be treated as a person. For if a totipotent cell were removed from the dead embryo and it developed, it would seem to ensure the survival of the individual who would otherwise have died with the original embryo, at least on some views of individual identity. (Here we see a disanalogy with the organ transplant model. For live cells or whole organs from individual A put into individual B do not literally make A survive.) Hence, refusing to take a totipotent cell and waiting until cells are only pluripotent implies that we will not try to rescue an individual by salvaging a totipotent cell from the dead embryo. Ordinarily, we would not refuse to save a human person's life with equivalent minor effort.

A final concern with using dead embryos is being sure they are dead by the appropriate standard for death. For example, it might be suggested that an embryo that seems to be dead in an extrauterine environment is only dying, and could revive if placed in a uterine environment.[15] To make sure that such problems do not infect the tests used to determine embryo death, we would have to actually place many embryos in someone's womb to check for revival. As it is unlikely that these experiments could deliberately be done, the concern is that we may remain uncertain that an extrauterine embryo really is dead.[16] A more acute problem for the determination of embryo death, I think, is raised by another possible disanalogy with organ transplantation. It is true that people are declared dead even when individual cells and organs are still alive, because there is no integrated functioning of the whole organism, supposedly evinced by brain death.[17] But should we declare an entity dead if, for example, 20 percent of its body cells are still alive and none of its cells ever played a superior regulative role over any other cell (unlike the brain in relation to other body parts)? This would be the case if one cell out of a total of five in an embryo is removed alive. Even if the live cell is pluripotent rather than totipotent, it may be a mistake in determining death to think of there being only one living cell out of very few as an indication of organismic death, even if we think of there being only one living cell in an adult body the rest of whose many cells are dead as an indication of organismic death.

3. Another way to acquire stem cells is to grow human matter that is not an organism at all but that has only pluripotent, nonembryonic stem cells. Examples that occur in nature are teratoma—disorganized tumor-like masses of cells that are often characterized as monstrosities because they have teeth and eyes as parts. If some nonorganisms can be grown that have pluripotent stem cells, it is claimed, there can be no objection to acquiring the stem cells, even if it destroys the nonorganism.[18] One objection that might be raised to this procedure is that it is wrong to deliberately create nonorganisms that are monstrous aberrations. But while doing so is aesthetically unappealing, it does not seem to be morally wrong, if there will be no harm to any entity that could benefit from life.

The bigger problem is that the fact that an entity is a disorganized mass of cells does not, at least logically, ensure that it also lacks properties that might make it wrong to destroy it. For example, imagine that instead of eyes or teeth, a teratoma gave rise to brain tissue that supported consciousness. Consciousness could be sufficient to count against destruction of an entity. Having bodily axes rather than being disorganized may be a necessary condition for being an organism but, at least as a conceptual matter, having axes is not a necessary condition for an entity to be worthy of moral consideration. For if some nonorganism had consciousness, it would be no argument against moral consideration for it that it had no bodily axes! It is only if we could ensure that, as a matter of physical possibility (rather than conceptual possibility), something's being a disorganized nonorganism ensured that it had no other properties that made it worthy of moral consideration, that no complaint could be raised to the destruction of the nonorganism. After all, those who support the Organism Argument (examined in part I) claim that being a human organism is *sufficient* for meriting respect and concern. But this is different from claiming that being a human organism is necessary for meriting respect and concern. (The absence of one sufficient condition does not imply that no other sufficient condition is present.) Those who support the development of nonorganismal entities as sources of stem cells must not only show that what some consider a sufficient condition for respect and concern— being an organism—is absent. They must also show that this condition is, as a matter of physical fact, a necessary condition for the presence of any other sufficient conditions for respect and concern. That is, if it is absent, all other sufficient conditions are also absent.

Finally, it is important to distinguish the deliberate development of nonorganisms from the deliberate development of embryonic organisms programmed to self-destruct or to otherwise lack potential to become a person. If we took seriously the moral equivalence of an embryo and a person, developing an embryo that will self-destruct or not develop properly is comparable to creating a person who will grow to adulthood but to whom a gene for self-destruction or degeneration in youth has been deliberately added. It is obviously a significant bad for a person to be created with such limits in him rather than to be created so that he continues on to a normal life. The fact that nothing would be done to an embryonic organism after its origins to kill or stunt it, the characteristics for delayed destruction being built into it, seems morally irrelevant if the embryonic organism has the same moral status as a person.[19]

Would it be an advance to create nonhuman organisms whose stem cells are compatible with use in humans rather than to create human nonorganisms? Aside from concerns about chimeras resulting from human and nonhuman mixtures, this alternative organism might be a conceptus that has an intrinsic trajectory to be a (nonhuman) person. If destroying a human conceptus raises moral problems, why should not the same moral problem arise in destroying this conceptus?

4. A fourth proposal is that we use adult cells and reverse their development back to pluripotent stem cells. If developing this process requires ESC cytoplasm to be mixed with adult cells, it will raise the problem (discussed in part II, section A) of destroying some embryos to acquire cytoplasm in order to save more embryos from being destroyed. However, if reversal only required using the cytoplasm of an egg cell, it would not raise the same problem.[20]

III

In part I, I presented objections to some arguments against destroying embryos to acquire ESCs. In part II, I put to one side those objections and considered alternatives to current methods of acquiring stem cells and the possible objections to these methods that might be raised by those who believe embryos should be treated as persons. Now let us briefly consider some factors that bear on whether and when it would be morally incumbent on us to pursue the alternatives I have described.

1. The more that moral objections like those raised to destroying soon-to-be-dead embryos can be raised to the alternatives as well, the less we would gain by switching to the alternatives. The less people raise moral objections to the alternatives, though they involve destruction of embryos, that they would raise if analogous methods involved destruction of adult persons, the less reason there is to seek alternatives to current methods that also destroy embryos. This is because we would have evidence that people do not equate the embryo with a person.

2. Suppose that opponents of current methods should reasonably consider some alternatives to be improvements. Suppose those opponents are successfully interfering with funding for research using current methods of acquiring ESCs because embryos are destroyed. This would provide a (i.e., some) reason for our community as a whole to pursue development of alternatives, given the need for cures for diseases that might come from stem cells and the need for funds for research.

3. But a reason to pursue alternatives does not necessarily mean sufficient reason. To decide if there is sufficient reason one would have to consider the costs of pursuing the alternatives by contrast to the cost of overcoming or obviating interference with using current methods. This includes the opportunity cost if there is a redirection of money and research away from current methods using ESCs that could otherwise be used to cure disease. One should also consider the likelihood of success in developing the alternatives to a degree that satisfies the need for stem cells, and how long it will take to develop these alternatives. (The belief that the alternatives would very soon be available could be given as a reason to shut down current efforts, since not much would be lost if the alternatives were truly around the corner. So it is important to be clear about how soon alternatives will be available.)

4. Finally, it is important to distinguish (a) the claim that successful curtailment of funding by opponents of the destruction of embryos gives a reason to consider developing alternatives from (b) the claim that mere respect for the views of these opponents gives such a reason. The latter claim would require much more discussion of the principles of compromise that apply to citizens in a liberal democracy, principles that have nothing to do with the actual power of opponents to impede funding. It would also require more detailed discussion of the relevance to any requirement to compromise of the nature, reasonableness, and correctness of the opponents' views. This is a complex topic in political philosophy that goes beyond anything discussed in this article. (It is not enough to point to the benefit of unanimity. For example, suppose it would be easy to accommodate a hypothetical religious request related to scientific experimentation (e.g., a request that all experiments be blessed). It would still be improper to concede the principle that government funded research does not cater to religious views merely to achieve unanimous support for the research.)

Notes

1. This chapter revises my article "Ethical Issues in Using and Not Using Human Embryonic Stem Cells," *Stem Cell Reviews and Reports* 1 (December 2005). That article arose from my participation in discussions of these issues at the conference sponsored by the Center for Ethics and Technology on June 6–7, 2005, at the University of San Diego (henceforth, referred to as "the conference"). The aim of the chapter is only to report my

thoughts that arose in connection with that meeting. For an earlier discussion of mine, see "Embryonic Stem Cell Research: A Moral Defense," *Boston Review* 27 (October/November 2002), which is revised as chapter 9 this volume.

2. Others deny that a one-cell conceptus is an organism. See Jeff McMahan, *The Ethics of Killing: Problems at the Margins of Life* (New York: Oxford University Press, 2002).

3. These views are drawn from Maureen L. Condic and Samuel B. Condic, "Defining Organisms by Organization," *National Catholic Bioethics Quarterly* 5 (Summer 2005): 331–353.

4. This view was expressed by Father Pacholczyk at the conference. Father Pacholczyk emphasized that this was the position of the Catholic Church and that the Church remained open as to when ensoulment takes place.

5. Does the Organism Argument imply that any skin cell that could, with scientific manipulation, be made intrinsically capable of turning into a person, should also not be destroyed? This would surely be an unreasonable conclusion. The Organism Argument need not yield this conclusion for it can distinguish between entities that already, intrinsically, have properties that lead them onto a trajectory of developing into a person and other entities, like the skin cell, that require scientific manipulation to have this trajectory. Before having been manipulated, the skin cell might not deserve to be protected simply because it could be manipulated so as to have a person-trajectory. As stated, however, the Organism Argument does claim that the human conceptus is the only organism that can become a person (or can come to have a soul). However, suppose there were rational beings of other species. These too would be persons, though nonhuman ones. Why would not their conceptuses also then be organisms that can become persons? To say that they would be *human* organisms alters the meaning of "human" from "having DNA of a certain human sort," as beings of another species would not have that sort of DNA. It also makes it impossible by definition for there to be any nonhuman persons. Now, as a matter of fact, there may not be any nonhuman persons. But if so, this is a matter of empirical fact, not a definitional truth.

6. The remainder of the discussion in section A repeats what appears in chapter 9 this volume.

7. However, I believe there is a broader sense of moral status, according to which an entity's potential could alter the significance of destroying that entity because the potential makes the entity more valuable. For more on this, see chapter 16 this volume. At the conference, after being presented with the Organism Argument, we were asked whether we had gained new respect for the embryo. Respect is an attitude ordinarily thought to be an appropriate response toward a being that is self-governing and to whom we personally can owe things. Not even all entities for whose sake we can act, such as a cat, are thought to be self-governing or to be creatures to whom we can personally owe things. So the embryo can be valuable in virtue of its complex organization and the trajectory it is programmed to follow but this does not make it be an entity that is either owed respect or for whose sake we can act in preserving it.

8. The fact that someone is not morally required to put in her womb even an embryo that she deliberately created for IVF, but may let it die or freeze it, may strike some as reasonable only if the embryo is not already a person. But some have argued (e.g., F. M. Kamm in *Creation and Abortion* [New York: Oxford University Press, 1992]) that it is consistent with assuming that the embryo is a person not to require someone to refrain from deliberately creating it unless she will definitely carry it in her body when it needs this to survive. This is, in part, because the fact that something is a person need not imply that it is wrong to refuse it very costly assistance even if one has created it. If this argument is correct, the

permissibility of letting the embryo die or freezing it when the alternative is very costly assistance does not indicate that it is *not* a person.

9. It is consistent with Frist's policy to be concerned with not doing what might encourage behavior that will lead to there being more embryos that will soon die anyway and to be concerned with encouraging the adoption of embryos so that they would not soon die anyway.

10. A famous example is known as the Trolley Problem.

11. I discuss another case where an analogy between redirecting human agents and mechanical threats might be suggested and discuss possible problems with it in "Harming Some to Save Others from the Nazis," which is chapter 5 in my *The Moral Target: Aiming at Right Conduct in War and Other Conflicts* (New York: Oxford University Press, 2012). That chapter revises an earlier article of the same title published in *Moral Philosophy and the Holocaust*, eds. Gerrard and Scarre (London: Ashgate Press, 2003).

12. In chapter 16 this volume, I discuss this problem in connection with Elizabeth Harman's views about the moral status of embryos that will develop into persons.

13. However, it has been argued that if the only part of the embryo that could not be formed by the removed cell is the trophectoderm (the part forming the placenta), this would not be sufficient to obviate the problem of creating a new embryo. For, arguably, this element is extrinsic to the embryo as an individual organism intrinsically capable of developing into (or giving rise to) a person and only serves to connect it to a source of life support. (See Condic and Condic, "Defining Organisms by Organization.")

14. This was suggested by Howard Zucker.

15. This was suggested by Maureen Condic.

16. However, it has been pointed out (by M. Condic) that in Germany all IVF embryos must be placed in the womb. Perhaps data might be collected on seemingly dead embryos in this context.

17. For possible problems with this criterion of death, see my "Brain Death and Spontaneous Breathing," *Philosophy & Public Affairs* 30 (2002), revised as chapter 8 this volume.

18. William Hurlbut has proposed this alternative.

19. I also discuss problems with this option in chapter 9 this volume. Surprisingly, some theorists' views on what is a human organism suggest otherwise. For example, as I understand them, Condic and Condic believe that an organism with human DNA whose intrinsic nature is heading it toward early destruction would not be a human organism. This would imply that deliberately killing such an organism in order to acquire stem cells should not be objectionable to those who oppose destroying human organisms. I do not think this view is correct.

20. The idea that the makeup of our specialized adult cells is so unstable as to be readily reversible to pluripotency is rather shocking. It suggests the premise of a Hollywood horror (comedy?) film in which human egg cytoplasm is poured over New York, causing its population to decompose into pluripotent cells.

11

Ronald Dworkin's Views on Abortion

In his book *Life's Dominion*, Ronald Dworkin makes certain claims about the nature of the intrinsic value of life, the nature of inviolability, the badness of death, and how these relate to the permissibility of abortion.[1, 2] I shall summarize and then examine several of these claims.

I. Summary

Dworkin begins his discussion by considering how to make sense of survey data on abortion. His interpretive strategy is to find the underlying beliefs that make expressed views consistent (this is known as a "principle of charity"), even if doing this appeals to a view that no one surveyed actually recognizes as her view. Dworkin claims that opposition to abortion is not based on a belief in a fetal (including embryonic) right to life or on a belief that the fetus is a person, because these beliefs cannot explain (make consistent sense of) people's positions on abortion (in survey data). For example: (A) Many say that abortion is wrong but should not be outlawed. However, Dworkin says, "No one can consistently believe that a fetus has a right not to be killed and at the same time hold it wrong for the government to protect that right by the criminal law" (p. 14); or (B): He notes that most people polled believe in exceptions to save a woman's life or even just in the case of rape. However, he says, "this . . . exception would be unacceptable . . . if they really thought that the fetus is a person with protected rights and interests. It is morally and legally impermissible for any third party, such as a doctor, to murder one innocent person even to save the life of another one" (p. 94).

Dworkin thinks that we—both conservatives and liberals with respect to abortion—believe in the sacredness of individual human life (including early fetal life). Though he uses the same term, Dworkin's doctrine of the sacredness of life is very different from what has come to be known as the sanctity-of-life doctrine. (The latter implies that all human life has equal value—regardless of stage of development—and that intentionally killing innocent human life is prohibited.)

Dworkin says that sacredness is a form of intrinsic value, which is, in part, value that something has independently of whether it serves anyone's interests instrumentally. The disconnection from serving interests is complete, since the sacredness of the individual life is independent even of its serving the interests of the entity whose life it is. Dworkin explains that such sacredness holds in the case of the early fetus even though the fetus[3] has no interests that life can serve, as it has never had a mental life (which he thinks is a prerequisite for having interests) (p. 16). Hence Dworkin thinks that the value of the sacred is detached, rather than derivative, from interests (and rights which he conceives of as protecting interests). Further, Dworkin says that the intrinsic value he is describing is also objective value, which is value that exists independently of whether anyone knows or cares about it, and value that can give one a reason to care. The sacred, he says additionally, is nonincremental value: that something sacred is valuable is not a reason to produce more of it, but it is a reason to treat properly what exists of it. Thus one need not maximize sacredness. "Sacred" suggests a religious interpretation of intrinsic, nonincremental, objective value (my acronym for this is INOV), so Dworkin identifies a secular term that he believes conveys what he means by sacred: "inviolable." Furthermore, he says, entities besides human life can be sacred—for example, other species or works of art.

What makes something have intrinsic, nonincremental, objective value? Dworkin considers the sacred primarily in terms of the history of the entity. God, nature, and human action as creative forces give INOV to many of their products; the more investment of these creative forces in the entities, the more INOV they have. (If the sacred is the inviolable, then these causes would also account for something being inviolable, on Dworkin's account.) Also, a bad cause can deprive an entity of INOV; Dworkin believes that this is why some may think that a fetus that results from rape has less INOV than one that does not (p. 95).

The destruction of an entity that has INOV always has some negative weight. (Note that sometimes Dworkin speaks merely of deliberate destruction and sometimes of death from any cause.[4]) He presents a special thesis, which I call the Investment Waste Thesis, as a framework for determining weights. Roughly, a death becomes worse as the ratio between the outcome of a creative investment (numerator) and the creative investment itself (denominator) decreases. Badness seems to track the frustration of investment, given that a payoff would be possible otherwise. However, if one has invested creatively in an entity but it has already returned completely on the investment in it, or it will never return on the investment in it, or it will not return much on the investment in it, then its death is not very bad. He writes: "We regret the waste of a creative investment not just for what we do not have, but because of the special badness of great effort frustrated" (p. 79). This is compatible with the nonincremental nature of INOV, as it is only once life starts that some investment is present. So the death of a 60-year-old person is less bad than that of a 20-year-old person; though more has been invested in the 60-year-old, more return on the investment has also been reaped by that person. But a lot has been invested in the 20-year-old without the person reaping much of a return yet. In the case of an early fetus, much life is lost if it dies, but little has been invested in it, so there is not much waste. The older the fetus becomes, other things being equal, the more investment is lost without return when it dies.

A crucial problem for abortion, in Dworkin's view, is that at least three different types of creative investment are thought to exist—biological/natural, God-driven, and human—and a woman and a fetus will embody all types to greater and lesser degrees (p. 91). For some people, God's or nature's investment is of paramount importance, and the continued existence of that natural or God-given component offers a significant payoff. For other people, the human creative investment and the payoff in terms of human achievement are more important. Most people, Dworkin believes, agree about the three sources of value, but the problem of abortion arises because they weigh and balance the factors differently. Dworkin thinks that how we should balance these sources of intrinsic, nonincremental, objective value—their frustrations and payoffs—in the fetus, in the woman, and in anyone else affected positively or negatively by an abortion is not a matter of philosophical argumentation. It comes closer to being a matter of religious belief (where this does not necessarily imply belief in a deity) about how best to respect the sacredness of life. The state should not interfere with decisions that depend on religious belief.

The fetus and the woman represent different instances of INOV, and the two can conflict, since there is more human investment in the woman, and primarily God's or nature's investment in the fetus. The Investment Waste Thesis also has implications for deciding whether a woman's death, or other losses suffered in the absence of an abortion, is worse than the death of her fetus if it is aborted. Dworkin argues that at least in the view of some, *more* has been invested in the woman than in the fetus, and so it is worse if she, rather than the fetus, is not given the opportunity to return on an investment. But the woman also has interests and rights, since she is a person in a philosophical, a moral, and a constitutional sense. As already noted above, in Dworkin's view it is obvious that the fetus has no interests or rights and is not a person in a philosophical or constitutional sense. Dworkin argues that no one could believe that the early fetus has either interests or rights that protect those interests, since it has never had mental states. When preserving rather than destroying an entity that has INOV would conflict with the rights and interests of a full-fledged person who also has INOV, then the INOV of the less-than-full-fledged person can be overridden, at least legally.

II. Questions

Dworkin attempts to understand the fetus as an entity that has no interests in retaining its future life and in the development of its potential to become a human person. This means that if we were to save its life or allow it to transform into (or give rise to) a person, we could not be doing it *for its sake* in order to benefit it.

Dworkin also attempts to show that even if this is true, a fetus need not therefore lack value. (While Dworkin emphasizes investment in it as the source of its value, an entity's having the potential to develop into a better entity may also contribute to its value.)

I agree with both parts of this analysis. Its plausibility can perhaps be better seen when applied to a nonliving object. For example, Dworkin says that a work of art can have great value—and it could be wrong to destroy it without good reason—but it is not for its sake (on account of its interests in surviving) that we should save it. I would add that a table that magically had been given the potential to turn into a person would also have greater value than an ordinary table but it would not be for its sake that we would allow it to transform.[5] However, I have questions about some of the specifics of Dworkin's views.

DOES DWORKIN SHOW THAT THE VIEW THAT A FETUS IS A PERSON OR HAS A RIGHT TO LIFE CANNOT MAKE SENSE OF CONSERVATIVES' VIEWS?

Consider how we could make sense of claim (A) above, whose expression in surveys Dworkin cites, that abortion is wrong but should not be outlawed. Many may think that their ground for believing that the fetus has a right to life or is a person is a further belief that is not obviously true, so that others could reasonably differ regarding it (e.g., their ground may be the religious claim that the fetus has a soul). Suppose those who hold a purely religious ground for their belief that the fetus is a person also accept the idea that one should not legally enforce views that depend on (are derived from) controversial religious views. For example, they might accept the Rawlsian idea that public reason (i.e., reasons derived from widely shared foundational values of the society) should rule when legal enforcement is in question. Then they could consistently claim that the fetus has a right to life and yet not think abortion should be criminally outlawed. It is surprising that Dworkin does not consider this, as it is the same type of argument that Dworkin himself goes on to offer: people's views of abortion are based on different conceptions of the value of life, and these conceptions should be treated as different religious views and not be legally enforced.

Now consider (B), namely his claim that people cannot really believe the fetus has a right to life if they believe abortion is sometimes permissible. Some claim that it is not inconsistent with the beliefs that some entity has a right to life and is a person to think that we may sometimes kill it to save another person. (Judith Thomson and I hold this view because we think that a person who threatens or imposes on another, even without intending to do so, may sometimes be killed.[6]) Those who hold this view may agree that one cannot "murder" someone if the use of the term "murder" assumes that the killing is wrong, but then the killing that they think is permissible is not a "murder."

Furthermore, as noted, Dworkin expresses as his own the view that "it is morally and legally impermissible for a doctor to murder one innocent person to save the life of another one" (p. 94). Call this view (i). Suppose view (i) is correct. Suppose also that the view that the fetus is a person (view ii) and the view that it is sometimes permissible to kill the fetus in order to save the life of the woman who carries it (view iii) are jointly inconsistent with view (i). (I have just argued above that they are not inconsistent with (i).) Then those who express views (ii) and (iii) will be involved in an inconsistency if they do, in fact, hold view (i). Nevertheless, if, unlike Dworkin, they do not hold view (i)—even if they are wrong not to hold it—they will not necessarily be holding inconsistent views. Dworkin never shows that they do hold (i).

DOES DWORKIN REALLY HAVE A THEORY OF THE INTRINSIC VALUE OF LIFE?

Although a sacred entity is supposed to be valuable intrinsically, Dworkin says that it is sacred because of its history. He says that "the nerve of the sacred lies in the value we attach to a process or enterprise or project rather than to its results considered independently from how they were produced" (p. 78). One might argue that the value of life is not intrinsic if history is at the core of its value, for such a source of value seems to situate the entity (life) in relation to something else (a process leading to life), the combination of which has value. This means that life would have extrinsic rather than intrinsic value—that is, value conditional on its being part of a certain whole. This is consistent, though, with its being valuable as an end, rather than as a mere instrument. (Similarly, happiness might be morally valuable only conditional on desert, but the happiness of those who deserve happiness can be sought for its own sake, not merely as an instrument to something else.) Dworkin makes the mistake of thinking that intrinsic value is to be contrasted with instrumental value, and he is eager to argue that life is valuable not merely instrumentally. But, as Christine Korsgaard has argued[7], intrinsic is to be contrasted with extrinsic, not with instrumental. What is instrumental is to be contrasted with what is an end. Hence Dworkin seems to have a theory about the extrinsic but noninstrumental value of life.

DOES THE VALUE OF LIFE RESPOND TO CHANGES IN ITS CAUSE IN THE WAY THAT DWORKIN DESCRIBES?

In the case of many things (e.g., persons), it may be possible to tell whether they have value by examining their properties independently of their history. Suppose that one's value as a person depended on one's history. Suppose also that one were deceived about one's past, and had come into existence as a rational and self-conscious being only a moment ago by some rape of nature or by mechanical duplication (as in cloning), rather than through a positive creative force. Would one then have less value than one believes? Concluding so seems incorrect, for the properties of rationality and self-consciousness may give equal value regardless of their history.[8] Likewise, in some people's views, instances of life itself (e.g., fetuses, caterpillars) have intrinsic value independently of their histories because of their complexity, animation, or other occurrent characteristics. For this reason, we should doubt Dworkin's argument on behalf of some conservatives that the fetus that results from rape has less intrinsic value because it began in an act contrary to God's will or the frustration of the woman's life (pp. 95–6).

This does not mean that history is irrelevant to the value of all things. Arthur Danto has argued that two physically identical objects can have different value because one was made to express a certain point of view and the other is just the result of a random series of events. The first entity can be a work of art and have properties the other lacks (such as being a statement) in virtue of its history.[9] Still, if Rembrandt had created "The Nightwatch" under coercion and so it had a tainted history (analogous to a fetus from a rape), would the painting have been any less valuable? I do not think so.[10]

CAN AN INTRINSIC VALUE (OR VALUE THAT IS AN END, EVEN DUE TO EXTRINSIC PROPERTIES) BE NONINCREMENTAL?

Dworkin claims that once a human life has begun, it is important that it go well, but this does not entail that the more lives that go well the better. That is, we do not have a reason to create more lives even though each is undoubtedly valuable, in the sense of "sacred," once it exists. The following hypothetical case raises a crucial question about this claim: Suppose that we believe that throughout its history, the world has so far contained 40 billion happy people. Then we discover that in fact we miscalculated, and there have really been 80 billion people in the same time period, each of whom lived a life no better or worse than the 40 billion.[11] Should we think that the history of the world is better in at least one way than we previously thought just because of the increment? If we should think this, then the value of persons' lives would be incremental. But perhaps we should not think that the more populous world is better merely by virtue of the additional people. This would support Dworkin's view about the nonincremental value of human life. (Suppose that we think that the more populous world in the hypothetical scenario is better and the value of human life gives us *a* reason to create more of it, when there is no danger of the species or other valuable things disappearing if we do not so create. This still would not mean that we have an obligation to create more of it, or that there are not countervailing reasons not to create more of it.)

IS DWORKIN'S USE OF "INVIOLABILITY" CORRECT?

Although he says that the secular term that expresses his idea of sacredness is "inviolability," Dworkin's notion of the sacred does not really involve inviolability as commonly understood. This is because the common understanding of inviolability implies the stringent impermissibility of destructive attacks on an inviolable entity, but this is not how Dworkin uses the term. Dworkin says that almost everyone thinks that the fetus is sacred or inviolable (pp. 13, 25). His evidence that even liberals on abortion believe this is that few people view a very early abortion as a morally neutral event, like cutting one's hair; it has negative moral significance, even if it is on the whole justified (pp. 33, 34). He says: "I shall assume that conservatives and liberals all accept that in principle human life is inviolable in the sense that I have defined, that any abortion involves a waste of human life and is therefore . . . a bad thing to happen, a shame" (p. 84). But this is hardly evidence for inviolability as ordinarily understood, since this sort of badness can easily be overridden for many worthy purposes. After all, it is a waste, a bad thing to happen, and a shame if a kitten must be destroyed for scientific research, but a kitten is not inviolable as ordinarily understood. Dworkin's notion of inviolability is merely that something bad happens when something dies or is destroyed, not that it is extremely hard (if not absolutely impossible) to morally override a prohibition on causing its death. But it is the latter that is the mark of inviolability as ordinarily understood.

Most importantly, Dworkin's notion of inviolability is part of the theory of value (which is about good and bad things or states of affairs) rather than part of the theory of the right (which deals with what acts are permissible and impermissible). But when we say some entity is inviolable because there is a strong prohibition on causing its death (or destroying it), we do not mean only that something bad (even *very* bad) will happen if it is destroyed. For if it were just the badness of the destruction that accounted for the prohibition on destroying it, it should be permissible to minimize such badness by destroying one entity in order to *prevent* destruction of more such entities (assuming that more destruction is worse than less). Yet, the inviolability of each entity (such as a person or holy object) ordinarily suggests that such minimization is not permissible.

It seems that Dworkin's idea of sacredness of life could imply that one should create and destroy a fetus if its organs or stem cells would help save the lives of several children in whom much has already been invested. Even if the investment by God were the only value of importance to people, on Dworkin's view they should favor destroying one embryo to save several God-invested lives. Yet those who support exceptional abortions to avoid the death of the pregnant woman would not necessarily support killing a fetus to save the lives of other people in whom God has invested. This suggests that Dworkin's attempt to explain people's allowing some exceptions to a prohibition on abortion (pp. 94–95) on the ground that the exceptions sacrifice something with less value for the sake of something of greater value is not the proper explanation of their views, as it would justify more abortions than they allow.

It would be better if Dworkin had used another term besides "inviolable." For if all Dworkin thinks is entailed by something being "inviolable" is that a bad thing happens when it is destroyed, it is seriously misleading to use this term. (In public debate, just redefining a term that is commonly used in another way can mislead one's audience.) It is also misleading to call an entity "sacred" if one thinks that its destruction involves nothing more than that something bad happens, as this does not capture the idea that the sacredness of an entity presents a greater barrier to its destruction.

IS THE INVESTMENT WASTE THESIS CORRECT?

Let us test the implications of the Investment Waste Thesis. First, are late abortions worse than earlier ones for the reasons that the Investment Waste Thesis provides, namely that there is frustration of more investment? Suppose that one fetus began from conception much more fully developed than fetuses do now, though it still had no sentience or consciousness and it would realize its potential to be a normal human being. This at least seems like a very significant product from little investment. On the other hand, imagine another fetus that has gestated for two years employing many natural processes and at great cost to those who help it grow, yet it is still only at the stage of a normal embryo. If it continues to gestate in its lengthy fashion, it too will realize its potential to be a normal human being. It seems that according to the Investment Waste Thesis, the death of the second fetus is worse than that of the first, because there is more wasted investment. But this seems incorrect.[12] The properties of the first fetus now combined with its future potential seem to make its death worse than that of the second, highly undeveloped fetus, independently of differential investment.

This example involves changes in two variables—product and investment—simultaneously. That is, product A is *better* than product B, and investment x (to produce product A) is *less* than investment y (to produce product B). A simpler set of cases would involve the same product—let us say the better one, A—as a result of differential investment, x in one case and y in the other. I believe that as the product improves, it becomes the dominant factor in deciding how important destruction would be, so that destruction of the entity into which more was invested would not be worse. (The extra investment, we might say, becomes a morally irrelevant factor.) So, contrary to what Dworkin suggests (p. 88), if a first-trimester fetus were to have the properties of a second-trimester fetus, I believe that we would not care less about it than an ordinary second-trimester fetus just because less had been invested in it.

However, in another example of this simpler model, investment might matter more. That is, hold the product constant in the two entities but make it the less good product B—a minimally developed fetus—and imagine that investment x produced B in one case and investment y produced B in the other case. Here it may indeed be worse if the entity due to the greater investment (y) is destroyed. Finally, we could imagine a case in which the products varied but the investments were the same. In this case, it is worse if the better product is destroyed. The intuitive results in these cases suggest that the quality of the product is a more important factor than is the investment in deciding which death is worse. They also suggest that the good that would be lost if an entity dies should make reference to the sort of entity that it already is, rather than just the future we can expect from it relative to investment in it. If a younger, less complex fetus dies, we lose out on more life than if an older, more complex fetus dies. But we also lose a more developed entity if the older fetus dies, and this seems like a bigger loss independent of how much was invested in one fetus or another. (For example, a great deal of natural processes or human efforts might have gone into sustaining the younger one.)

Dworkin has responded to the first case (which I described as involving less investment to produce a more complexly developed fetus and more investment to produce a less complexly developed fetus). He claims that "nature's investment in a fetus is not just a matter of gestation times, but of complexity of development as well."[13] In other words, he denies that the more complex fetus can be the one with less investment in it. (Presumably, he would also describe the death of a more complex fetus as involving a bigger loss of investment, even if it deprives us of less future good than the death of a younger fetus.) But this answer, I think, implies that the boundaries between investment and product are unclear in his theory. Given any property the entity has (for example, consciousness) that one can describe without any knowledge of the entity's history, Dworkin's response seems to imply that we can automatically say that there was investment in it of that property and hence greater investment. We would need no knowledge independent of the entities' current properties to describe an investment history for it. But this idea of investment seems at odds with his view that a crippled child doomed to a short life can make enormous investments in his life (p. 90). For, in this case, not only can there be no future payoff expected but *the current properties of the entity are meager*. This suggests a strong distinction between investment and occurrent properties. Hence, even if we take properties that one entity has that another lacks to be investments in it, there could be a case in which investment in the form of natural and human efforts are greater in one fetus than the occurrent properties "invested" in another fetus. Yet, it would be preferable to preserve the latter because of its occurrent properties, even given similar future payoffs for each.[14]

A second test of Dworkin's Investment Waste Thesis suggests that, independent of any concern about rights, the relative importance of abortion in the lives of two different women could turn on the degree to which the investment in *them* is paid off or interfered with. Suppose that one is a poor, mistreated young woman, who has not invested in herself and who has not been invested in by anyone else apart from her parents in creating her. She becomes pregnant and wants an abortion because she has decided to try to make what little she can of her life and pregnancy would interfere with this. Suppose that the other woman is well cared for and highly educated, someone who has invested time and energy in herself and who has been invested in by parents who creatively raised her. She wants an abortion because pregnancy would interfere with these investments' bearing great fruit. The Investment Waste Thesis alone seems to imply that, because of the differential frustration of investment, it is worse if the second woman does not get an abortion than if the first woman does not. This would be true even if the first woman would, in virtue of efforts she will now start to make, have as good a payoff in the future as the second woman. But this seems wrong simply as a matter of valuing the "sacredness" of life in each of these women.

A third concern about the Investment Waste Thesis is this: In considering investment in a young woman, why assume that a payoff has not already occurred? Many investments, such as education, that should yield future payoffs also give contemporary payoffs, as people enjoy their educational experience. Childhood and youth are simultaneously investments and periods of life worth living in their own right. Hence, it is not clear that more investment would be frustrated if a woman died than if her fetus did. The fact that investment and payoff are often simultaneous, and that achievement of the future goal of an investment is not the only possible payoff, suggests that there is some other ground besides waste of investment for the commitment to keep a life already further along going on.

IS DWORKIN'S ACCOUNT OF CONFLICTS BETWEEN VALUES (WITH AND WITHOUT CONSIDERATION OF RIGHTS) SUFFICIENT TO ACCOUNT FOR THE REASONABLENESS OF SOME PEOPLE'S VIEWS ABOUT ABORTION?

First, consider the outcome of conflicts between a woman and a fetus, taking into account only the creative forces—natural, God-given, and human—that the woman and the fetus represent, and postponing the role of interests and rights. I wish to suggest that, on its own, the discussion of value will not explain as much as Dworkin suggests.

Recall that Dworkin thinks that there is something *prima facie* wrong with a human act that destroys the sacred once it exists (pp. 74, 75, 78, 84); it is an intentional frustration of creative investment. Does Dworkin likewise emphasize active preservation of the sacred? At certain points, he seems to. He says, for example, that it is important that the human race survive and prosper (p. 76) and that sacred things flourish (p. 74), and that premature deaths are a shame (without emphasizing deliberate destruction) (pp. 68–69). But if one were as deeply concerned with preserving the sacred as with not destroying it (or with preventing deliberate destruction), one would have to support efforts to prevent naturally occurring miscarriages as much as to prevent destruction of fetuses. This, of course, might involve harmful interference in women's lives. By contrast, suppose we considered not harming entities that have INOV as more important than aiding them. This would account for allowing miscarriages rather than interfering with women. However, if a woman wants an abortion because she would die without it, and we do not permit the abortion, she (an entity that has INOV) will die because we *do not aid* her. But if we perform the abortion, we actively *destroy* something that has INOV (although perhaps less INOV than the woman). If the harming versus not-aiding distinction were sufficiently morally important, it could outweigh the fact that the woman has greater INOV than the fetus (in the opinion of some). Hence, factors about INOV and investment waste could be held constant in different cases, and in one case (of miscarriage) the woman could take precedence over the fetus, while in the other case (of abortion), the fetus could take precedence over the woman. This suggests that views about differential INOV and investment waste in woman and fetus would not settle matters on their own, or they would settle matters only if the harming/not aiding distinction was either irrelevant or itself tied to views about how to treat sacred entities.

Further, if the abortion issue were only a matter of conflicts between the intrinsic, nonincremental, objective value and investment waste of different entities, independently of the fact that one of the entities that has INOV imposes on the body of the other, one would also probably reach different conclusions. For even if one ought to aid entities that have INOV as well as not destroy them, it is not *generally* true that one is permitted to destroy an entity that has INOV, even one of relatively little value, in order to aid an entity that has a greater amount of INOV and whose loss threatens a greater amount of investment waste. For example, if a woman's fetus were on its own in an external gestation device, not imposing on the woman, it is not clear that it would be appropriate to destroy it in order to help her survive just because it would have been permissible to destroy it to remove it from her body. It seems, therefore, that in order to justify abortion, one might have to take seriously the fact that the fetus that has INOV is imposing on the woman.

Now, let us consider the role of rights. Dworkin seems to assume that rights necessarily protect interests, and so an entity with no interests could have no rights. But some rights, at least, may not protect interests (understood as some aspect of well-being), but rather express the dignity of the subject who has them. For example, subjects that have no interests to be protected could still have rights to freedom of expression or worship because these behaviors are important for reasons other than that they serve the interests of those who have the rights (or even others' interests).[15] However, even if we deny that rights protect only interests, we could grant that an entity that is not a subject at all, like a fetus that has never had mental states (or capacity for them), cannot have rights.

Dworkin does consider that women do not merely have INOV and investment waste potential, but are also persons with interests and rights.[16] When not destroying an entity that has only INOV would interfere in a *serious way* with rights and interests, especially when the value to be attributed to the entity that has only INOV is a matter of religious dispute, Dworkin favors the dominance of rights and interests, at least as a legal matter. But, I would claim, when the *destruction* of an entity that has INOV is at issue, the question arises of *how* not destroying that entity would result in interference with the rights and interests of a person. Consider an art analogy: It is one thing to say that a person with rights and interests may not be severely imposed upon in order to preserve a work of art, and also that we may destroy a work of art in order to stop it from being imposed on a person. It is another thing to say that one may destroy just any work of art because if we do not, something else (such as a disease) will interfere with a person's rights and interests. Again, it seems to me that the details of how the fetus imposes on the woman, and also whether, if we do not destroy it, the woman will wind up aiding it when she is not obligated to, are important to justifying the fetus's destruction. Dworkin does not mention or investigate these points. So it turns out that if one wishes to show that a fetus may permissibly be destroyed in order to help a woman, distinctions other than comparative rights/interests status, INOV, and investment waste will have to be attended to in order to justify abortion. (These are the same distinctions that some think could help justify abortion even if the fetus were a person with interests and rights.[17])

IS DWORKIN CORRECT TO DESCRIBE OPINIONS ON ABORTION INSOFAR AS THEY DEAL WITH THE VALUE OF LIFE AS A MATTER OF CONSTITUTIONALLY PROTECTED RELIGIOUS BELIEF?

Introducing *any* secular equivalent of the sacred, such as inviolability, seems to introduce a different problem. For Dworkin wants to argue that views about the intrinsic value of life and debates about the weighing and balancing of intrinsic value are fundamentally religious rather than philosophical (pp. 93, 156). Dworkin defines a religious view as one that answers questions that religion has dealt with in the past—for example, "What is the ultimate value and meaning of human life?" (p. 163). However, many of these issues have traditionally also been discussed by secular philosophy, which is typically contrasted with religion. For example, secular philosophers have asked: "What is the meaning and point of human life?" and "Does a person's life matter independently of its use to him or her?" Dworkin places these questions under the topic of the sanctity of life, but clearly moral philosophers as well as theologians have discussed them. A clear example is Kant, who said that rational humanity is an end-in-itself and a categorical end; whether people care about their lives or not, they have a duty to make something of their lives.[18] While Dworkin seems to think that moral philosophy deals with the realm of interests and rights rather than the realm of the sacred, as he defines it, this does not seem to be true of such moral philosophers as Kant. Hence, questions he thinks of as religious have been dealt with by philosophy as well as religion.

When Dworkin discusses euthanasia in *Life's Dominion*, he seems to allow more overlap between the realm of interests (dealt with by moral philosophy, in his view) and the realm of the sacred (dealt with by religion in the past, in his view), for he speaks of concern for the dignity of human life in discussing both realms. He says that critical interests represent the concern that one's life has amounted to something, independently of how it merely felt as one was living it (the latter being about one's experiential interests). Indeed, Dworkin says that believing in critical interests is a species of believing in the sacredness of life (p. 215). But if one's critical interests are a matter of moral philosophical reflection, why cannot the worth of life also be a matter of philosophical reflection?

In what sense is such philosophical reflection classifiable as religious? One suggestion, made by Thomas Scanlon,[19] is that Dworkin thinks that certain types of secular philosophical thought (about the meaning and point of life) are religious in the *constitutional sense*; they are to be treated for *constitutional purposes* the way religions are treated. But why are secular philosophical views about the meaning and point of human life *constitutionally religious* while other secular philosophical views are not? After all, philosophical and scientific views that deal with other questions historically dealt with by religion, such as the origins of the universe and of animal life, do not seem to be considered constitutionally religious.

My sense is that Dworkin ultimately wants to use "religious" (or "constitutionally religious") to connote an area of discourse that is not subject to rational proof. This keeps it outside the area of political debate. This could be Dworkin's strategy because unlike John Rawls, he believes that comprehensive philosophical doctrines (e.g., Kantianism, utilitarianism, and in general, the best philosophical arguments available) *do* have a place in legally relevant public discussion of issues.[20] Rawls brackets many philosophical arguments on the grounds that they are part of particular comprehensive doctrines and so no more part of "public reason"[21] than religious views. As Dworkin rejects this position, he must *find some other way* to bracket discussion of certain issues. Dworkin could do this by classifying views that are not subject to rational argument as part of religion, or at least religious for constitutional purposes.

A significant problem for this approach arises, though, if it turns out that these questions, including the relative weight of natural and human creative inputs, are capable of being answered with more rigor and conclusiveness than Dworkin suggests. In that case, such discussion could enter the category of secular philosophy that cannot be classified as religious in a constitutional (or any other) sense. Thus one objection to Dworkin's position derives from the view that a discussion of the meaning of life can be philosophical rather than religious, and so a particular view on this issue can be philosophical rather than religious. Accordingly, the legal enforcement of some views of intrinsic value could not be disallowed on the grounds that they are religious views that the state should not impose.

There is a different problem, internal to Dworkin's own position, concerning the state's involvement with the "religious." That is, Dworkin ultimately does not think that the State must, or should, be totally uninvolved in regulating abortion merely because questions about life's value are at stake. He thinks, for example, that the state should encourage women to make abortion decisions in a responsible way because intrinsic value is at stake.[22] Dworkin, of course, has argued that both conservatives and liberals agree that all human life has some sort of intrinsic value to some degree. But this may not be so, for when philosophers have discussed the meaning and point of human life, some have argued that mere life (the "pulse in the mud," so to speak) is worthwhile only as a *means* to such functions as sentience, rationality, or self-consciousness.[23] This, of course, implies that they have concluded that *life itself* does not have intrinsic value (or value as an end). Dworkin might think that this is either only one possible "religious" position on this question or else a nonreligious view.

Suppose that only some *positive* answer to the question of whether life has intrinsic value is religious. Then Dworkin's view that the state has a "legitimate interest in maintaining a moral environment in which decisions about life and death are taken seriously and treated as matters of moral gravity" (p. 168) involves the state taking sides *with* a religious view and against a nonreligious view (that life per se has no intrinsic value). But separation of church and state should mean that the government cannot side with religion against nonreligion. On the other hand, if making even a negative judgment about whether life has intrinsic value is in itself religious, the state, in intervening to see that women consider abortion to be a matter of moral gravity, would be siding with one religious view over another. This too is ruled out by the separation of church and state. Even if the state intervened just to have people think about what might *possibly* be a matter of gravity from a religious point of view, it would still be in a position analogous to one in which the state encouraged people to think about whether there is a God. This also is something the state may not do if there is separation of church and state.

Finally, recall that Dworkin's notion of the sacred is about value that is not derived from interest and that it does not necessarily take a great deal to override. He himself says that there is something sacred about even a not very good work of art (i.e., one lacking in aesthetic value) (pp. 78–79, 80–81). This suggests that even if all people agree that the fetus is sacred, Dworkin has provided no more reason for state-mandated waiting periods before destroying a fetus than for state-mandated waiting periods before destroying a not very good painting (if the painting were imposing on someone's body).

Despite these criticisms of Dworkin's views, I think there is a valuable insight that lies at the base of his approach. There does seem to be a sense in which people have different conceptions of what makes life valuable and of how to respect the value of life. (Some even seem to accept the view that human life has incremental value, trying to have many children as a way to show that they value human life.) The view that valuing human life is not about preserving it biologically so much as promoting distinctive goods possible in a human life makes sense. Nevertheless, it is hard to make this the basis of a theory of when killing is right and wrong. This is because it seems to lead to permission to kill many living things in order to promote distinctive human goods or prevent waste of investment in such goods.

IS DWORKIN'S HARD-LINE VIEW CORRECT?

Dworkin also holds that abortion would be morally impermissible if the fetus were a person. (I call this his hard-line view.) He takes this position because he thinks, first, that parents have a special duty to support their children (p. 111 nn. 4–5, p. 249),[24] and second, that it is never permissible to kill one innocent person to save even the life of another (pp. 32, 94). I disagree with the hard-line view. With regard to his first claim, I do not think that parents' having a special duty to support their children implies that they must support their child in their body, especially before any parent-child interaction outside the womb has taken place. For example, I do not think that if someone, without your consent, has acquired your genetic material and created a person who is your genetic offspring, you are required to support the person in your body to save his life.

With regard to his second claim, I believe it is permissible sometimes to kill an innocent person who is imposing on someone else, especially when the person killed will lose only life that is being provided by that imposition.[25] Dworkin, I think, believes that such situations represent a conflict of rights, and the stronger right (not to be killed) takes precedence over the weaker right (not to have one's body imposed upon or to have one's life saved). He certainly thinks the right not to be killed takes precedence over an interest in having a fulfilling life (p. 84). We can agree with this in the sense that we would first rescue person A from being killed rather than person B from merely having his body imposed on by person C. But if person A is imposing on person B, and even derives his life from that imposition, the logic of the situation changes; it is no longer clear that the right of the one person not to be killed takes precedence over his supporter's right not to be imposed on or to pursue her own life, let alone to have her life saved from A's deadly imposition. Showing that killing A is permissible even only in this latter case would be enough to defeat Dworkin's argument (p. 94) that it is never permissible to kill one innocent person to save another person.

However, notice that even if it is true that it would sometimes be permissible to abort a fetus even if it were a person from conception on, this alone does not show that we may abort a fetus that has *developed into* (or given rise to) a person after having started as a nonperson.[26] This is because if the fetus were a person from conception, there would be no time when it would be possible to abort a nonperson. Therefore, it matters less whether one has an early or late abortion, for one will be aborting a person whenever one aborts. But if the fetus *develops into* (or gives rise to) a person, then abortion would be possible at a time when we would not then be killing a person. If killing a nonperson is a far less serious matter than killing a person, in failing to abort early we will have lost the opportunity to perform a morally less serious act. Suppose that we want to have an abortion and the fetus has already developed into a person. We cannot simply argue for the permissibility of killing a person in the manner that we would if the fetus were a person from conception on. Rather, we must argue for the permissibility of killing a person given that we failed to take advantage of the opportunity to end the pregnancy without killing a person. This may be harder to do than simply arguing for the permissibility of killing what was always a person. For it may be correct to penalize someone for failing to perform the morally less serious act by restricting permission to perform the more serious act. Likewise, suppose that the fetus develops in morally significant stages and that it is morally worse to kill it at a later stage rather than at an earlier one, even if it is never a person. Then arguments for the permissibility of killing a creature that had always had the properties of a later-stage creature, in order to stop its imposing on a person, need not necessarily justify killing a creature when it has late-stage properties if we could have killed it at an earlier stage when it had different properties.

Hence it is a mistake to argue as follows: (1) either the fetus is a person or it is not a person; (2) it would be permissible to abort it if it is a person; (3) it would be permissible to abort it if it is not a person; (4) hence, it is permissible to abort it. For even if premise (2) were true of a fetus that was always a person, it may not be true of a fetus that develops into (or gives rise to) a person.[27]

III. Conclusion

Dworkin believes that newborn infants should be treated as persons from a moral and legal point of view, even though they are not self-conscious and the latter characteristic may be a requirement for being a person from the philosophical point of view. If we add this and his hard-line view to our previous discussion, we can describe an alternative to Dworkin's views that captures some of what his position commits him to, but revises other components in light of the previous discussion. The alternative involves both *philosophical* (vs. religious) disagreement on the value of the early fetus and agreement that it is not a person.

The alternative position that might be attributed to Dworkin is as follows: The state should not interfere with a person's own decision on abortion when (1) there is still philosophical disagreement (that might eventually be resolved) on the value of a fetus that has never been conscious, and (2) the state's taking one side would impose significantly on the rights and interests of a recognized person. One may enforce a philosophically contested position (for example, redistributive taxation is permissible) on some people only: (i) when there is no large physical impact (by contrast to pregnancy) on any identifiable person; and (ii) when other people's rights and interests are at stake (e.g., those who would benefit from taxation), as they are not known to be in killing an early fetus. If the fetus reaches a point when, like an infant, we should declare it a person for moral and legal purposes, no abortion would be permitted. Just as one cannot kill an infant in order to help its parent, nor kill any person merely in order to help another person, so one may not kill a late fetus that should be treated as a person from a moral and legal point of view in order to help a pregnant woman.

Dworkin may not find this alternative position appealing. First, it does not focus on religion or make use of the constitutional principle of separation of church and state to limit governmental interference with abortion. However, it does emphasize that overriding the recognized liberty interests of women at least requires the Court to be firmly convinced of a position on the status of the fetus that no reasonable person could reject. Second, Dworkin believes in allowing some exceptions for abortion late in pregnancy despite his hard-line view. But given his views on infants and the fact that late fetuses have the same characteristics as many slightly premature infants, he may not be entitled to defend these exceptions unless be rejects the hard-line view.

Notes

1. This chapter is a revised version of part of my "Ronald Dworkin on Abortion and Assisted Suicide," in *Dworkin and His Critics*, ed. J. Burley (Wiley-Blackwell, 2004). I thank Ronald Dworkin for his response to an earlier version of that article in his "Replies to Endicott, Kamm, and Altman," *Journal of Ethics* 5 (2001): 265–66. My first discussion of Dworkin's views on abortion and assisted suicide appeared in "Abortion and the Value of Life: A Discussion of *Life's Dominion*," *Columbia Law Review* 95 (1995): 160–221, on which the later papers rely.

2. Ronald Dworkin, *Life's Dominion: An Argument about Abortion, Euthanasia, and Individual Freedom* (New York: Knopf, 1993). Page references in the text and notes are to this book unless otherwise specified.

3. Like Dworkin, for simplicity, I shall use "fetus" to describe all stages of a conceptus, including the embryo stage.

4. For example, 68–69, 74.

5. I discuss this point in connection with stem cell cloning in "Embryonic Stem Cell Research: A Moral Defense," *Boston Review* 27(5) (October 2002): 20–32 (which is chapter 9 this volume).

6. See J. J. Thomson, "A Defense of Abortion," *Philosophy & Public Affairs* 1 (1971): 47–66; and F. M. Kamm, *Creation and Abortion* (New York: Oxford University Press, 1992).

7. Christine Korsgaard, "Two Distinctions in Goodness," *Philosophical Review* 92 (1983): 169–95.

8. I have argued for the relevance of this point when one considers the moral significance of cloning. If cloning a person is morally wrong, it is not because the person's origins would lower his value. For discussion of this, see my "Cloning and Harm to Offspring," *N.Y.U. Journal of Legislation and Public Policy* 4 (2000–1): 65–76, and chapter 16 this volume.

9. Arthur C. Danto, *The Transfiguration of the Commonplace* (Cambridge, MA: Harvard University Press, 1981), pp. 1–5.

10. In his response to my "Ronald Dworkin on Abortion and Assisted Suicide," *Journal of Ethics* 5 (2001): 218–37. Dworkin agrees with this, but argues that a mechanical copy of "The Nightwatch" (not the result of creative investment at all) would not have the value of the original painted by Rembrandt. I agree. (Indeed, I think that it is another example of Danto's point cited in note 8 above.) But notice that a mechanical copy of an embryo or a human person, which is how we might characterize a clone that is not the result of sexual reproduction, does *not* have less value than the original of which it is a clone. For more on this, see chapter 16 this volume.

11. I owe this case to Leo Katz.

12. The use of a hypothetical case that alters biology as we know it is not meant to deny that, in biology as we know it, the death of a late fetus is worse than the death of an early fetus. The hypothetical case just helps us zero in on why exactly we think that the late fetus's death is worse.

13. Dworkin, "Replies to Endicott, Kamm, and Altman," p. 266.

14. Perhaps we might retain the idea that investment is separable from product, which in turn could be distinguished from future goods that would pay back investment, in the following way: Suppose there are many properties that the entity has. From this, Dworkin might say, one sees that there was investment of these properties and hence much investment has taken place. However, suppose that the properties are all bad ones. So, considered on their own, they would give one no reason not to destroy the entity. However, on Dworkin's view, there has been much investment in the entity with these properties that would be wasted if it died. Does that give us a reason not to destroy it? I think not. Does this conclusion imply that most of the work in determining the degree of badness of the death of a fetus is done by the quality of its properties rather than the investment in it (or a ratio of the two)? Not necessarily, if we imagine that bad qualities will lead to no good future payoff. For Dworkin thinks investment only gives a reason not to destroy something if some good could eventuate from its existence.

15. The fact that people have an interest in worshiping does not mean that worshiping serves their interests.

16. It is worth noting that in allowing that women do have a high degree of INOV or have significant futures in which investment in them might be repaid, as well as rights and interests, Dworkin is taking a position on an issue that, some argue, is at the heart of the abortion debate. This issue is the proper role for women. That is, many think that antiabortion forces really take the view that women have little value relative to fetuses, or at least that investments and payoffs in their nonmaternal futures have little value relative to the lives of fetuses. In allowing that human investment in a woman's capacities counts as a form of valuing life, Dworkin disagrees.

17. On the latter sort of arguments, see Thomson, "A Defense of Abortion," and Kamm, *Creation and Abortion*.

18. See Immanuel Kant, *Fundamental Principles of the Metaphysics of Morals*, trans. Thomas K. Abbot (New York: Macmillan, 1985).

19. Letter from Thomas Scanlon, Professor of Philosophy, Harvard University, to Frances M. Kamm, April 1994.

20. See John Rawls, *Political Liberalism* (New York: Columbia University Press, 1996), which discusses limits on the use of comprehensive doctrines. Dworkin defends judges' use of moral arguments to determine what the general constitutional principles, such as liberty and equality, amount to (pp. 118–27). And, it seems to me, he allows arguments that go beyond what Rawls would think of as part of "public reason."

21. See Elizabeth Wolgast, "The Demands of Public Reason," *Michigan Law Review* 94 (1994): 1936–50.

22. See pp. 168, 170. If someone does not have an abortion, a person will result (a locus of rights and interests as well as INOV). Given this, should Dworkin not also favor the state encouraging pregnant women to think responsibly about *having an abortion* if the child will not be properly cared for?

23. See, for example, Aristotle, *The Nicomachean Ethics*, ed. David Ross (Oxford and New York: Oxford University Press, 1980); Jonathan Glover, *Causing Death and Saving Lives: The Moral Problems of Abortion, Infanticide, Suicide, Euthanasia, Capital Punishment and Other Life-or-Death Choices* (Harmondsworth, UK, and New York: Penguin, 1977).

24. This may be one reason he emphasizes a family connection to the fetus when he notes that while some politicians say they would support their daughter in having an abortion, they could not do so if they believed it meant killing their grandchild (p. 20).

25. Judith Jarvis Thomson first defended the permissibility of some abortions, even if the fetus is a person, in "A Defense of Abortion." My argument against the hard-line view can be found in my "Abortion and the Value of Life: A Discussion of *Life's Dominion*," pp. 160–221, especially pp. 185–221. That section of the article is chapter 12 this volume. A longer version is in my *Creation and Abortion*.

26. I first made this point in *Creation and Abortion*, pp. 174–75. I do not think Thomson considered this gap in her defense of abortion.

27. For more on this issue, see my *Creation and Abortion*, pp. 174–75, and chapter 12 this volume.

12

Creation and Abortion Short

I. The Violinist Case and Some Variations

A. THOMSON'S ARGUMENT

In 1971, Judith Thomson suggested that it would be helpful when discussing abortion to consider the following analogy.[1, 2] Imagine, she said, that you have been kidnapped by a group of people who want to save a dying violinist. The only way to save him is to plug him into your kidneys for nine months. (No one else is available for this use.) You have nothing to do with the fact that he is dying or that he needs your kidneys; nevertheless, the group plugs him into you. In order for you to be freed from the violinist before the nine months are over, a third party must detach the violinist (comparable to a doctor in abortion). In Thomson's case, the violinist will die because he will die without support from you, even if he is safely detached. However, in modified cases he will die because he must be actively killed in the process of, or even as a means of, detaching him from you. Thomson concluded that it would be morally permissible to detach the innocent violinist in any of these ways.[3]

Thomson's argument to support her conclusion is that the violinist's right to life does not imply a right to use someone else's body even in order to save his life. Though he is innocent of aggressing, since it is others who attach him while he is unconscious, still the person to whom he is attached is the victim of an injustice and the violinist is where he ought not to be. (He is a morally innocent threat.) If he is not removed, he will get a right to use your body for nine months, which is something to which, it has been agreed, he has no right. Hence, while his right to life implies a right not to be killed, this must only be a right not to be killed unjustly.

Thomson's argument does not seem complete, for someone may respond with the reverse argument: The violinist's right to life gives him a negative right not to be killed. While it is usually unjust to use your body (even to save someone's life) without your consent, it will not be unjust if this use is a side effect of its not being permissible to kill the violinist in order to remove him. More needs to be said to show why this counterargument is not correct. Furthermore, consider that if someone has no right to use someone's body even to save his life, he certainly has no right to use it if only being attached to someone's body will save his leg (when his life is not in danger). If the Society of Marathon Runners attached an unconscious runner to you in order to save his leg, this would also be unjust. Thomson's argument seems to imply that it would be permissible to kill the innocent runner in this Runner Case to remove him from your body. It also seems to imply that if someone attaches an unconscious person who is in no need of being attached to your body at all, it would be permissible for you to kill him to detach him. While Thomson's Violinist Case focuses on beneficial lifesaving aid that you need not give to someone, her argument seems to imply that even when someone is not getting any benefit or getting less than lifesaving benefit from being attached to your body, it is permissible to kill him to remove him. In the case where no aid at all is forthcoming, the justification for killing would have to be more like an argument from self- (or other-) defense than an argument to discontinue aid.[4]

B. AN ALTERNATIVE ARGUMENT

While it may be true that it is permissible to kill the attached person in all these cases, it seems to me to be easier to justify doing this in the original Violinist Case because of features it does not share with these two other cases. In what follows, I shall try to construct an argument for the permissibility of killing the violinist that shows this.

In addition, *expanding* on Thomson's analogy in other ways is instructive for thinking about the permissibility of abortion because these other ways mimic ways of becoming pregnant. For example, suppose that you attach yourself to the violinist voluntarily with the intention of helping him, or you are attached as a foreseen result of a different voluntary act of yours. Is it permissible to kill him or to have him killed in order to free yourself? Specifically, consider the following variations: (1) Someone attaches the violinist to the supporter's body against the supporter's will. (The costs involved in keeping him attached are similar to those of pregnancy, labor, and delivery.) (2) One performs some action in the normal course of life that has the consequence that, without anyone's deliberate arrangement, the person is attached to one's body; although one knew that this might happen, it was not planned. Subdivide Case (2) and imagine that either (a) one took precautions to prevent this attachment but they failed, or (b) precautions were not taken. (3) One voluntarily attaches the violinist to one's body in order to help him, but without actually promising anyone to keep him there until he is saved.

If one decides that one no longer wants to support this person because one objects to having him attached, is it morally permissible in all these cases to have a third party acting on one's behalf remove the violinist before the nine months are over?

We can combine these variations with variations on the removal procedure mentioned earlier. Considering four procedures will aid our thinking about abortion: (1) The violinist is removed from the person by severing the link between the two and not by directly attacking the violinist. Although the violinist emerges whole, he dies without the support of his host. This is comparable to one type of induced labor. (2) A solution is injected into the supporter that causes the detachment of the dependent violinist. This solution is caustic; it interferes with the dependent's respiration and damages his organs, thereby killing him in the removal process. Thus there is some sort of direct attack on him, even though it is not intentional. This is comparable to a saline abortion. (3) The dependent is detached by directly attacking him—for example, by crushing his skull. The attack on him is intended even though his death is not, strictly speaking. This is comparable to a craniotomy to remove a fetus. (4) The violinist is attacked with the intention of causing his death because (suppose for the sake of argument) unless he dies, it will not be possible to detach him.

Any of these procedures is made painless by giving an anesthetic. If we can justify procedure (4), which seems the most difficult to justify because the attack is intended to cause death, then we can also justify the other three, assuming there is no more pain involved in those procedures than in procedure (4).

Ending a Life in Order to Stop Supporting It

What follows is a possible *general* argument for the moral permissibility of a third party's killing the violinist in manner (4) in order to detach him from the supporting person. It is different from the argument Thomson presents, and it consists of the following five steps, which are commented on in the paragraphs following each.

STEP 1A. NEED ALONE CONFERS NO RIGHT TO HAVE SUPPORT OR DUTY TO SUPPORT: LETTING THE PERSON DIE IS PERMISSIBLE

It is assumed that one has no obligation to attach the violinist to one's body for the sole reason of saving his life, even though it may be commendable to do so. If the violinist has a "right to life," it does not include the right to use another's body solely in order to save his life. Therefore, it would have been permissible to let him die in the first place rather than attach him to the supporting person. Thomson emphasizes this point.

STEP 1B. NEED ALONE CONFERS NO RIGHT TO HAVE CONTINUED AID OR A DUTY TO GIVE IT

Just as the violinist has no right to use another's body initially based on need, he has no right to the continued use of one's body *merely* because this will save his life, even if there are no negative effects on the supporter other than the use of her body. For example, suppose the violinist starts to come detached on his own. The host need not prevent this just because of the need of the violinist.

STEP 2. THERE IS NO OTHER SPECIAL OBLIGATION TO GIVE AID

There is no special obligation to give aid if the attachment was forced on the supporting person. If the supporting person had made a commitment to keep the violinist attached to her body, this could give him a right to stay. However, even voluntarily attaching with the intent of helping him does not *by itself* commit her to allowing him the continued use of her body. Analogously, if a person voluntarily brings a guest into her home, the guest does not have a right to stay longer than the host wants him to, simply because the host brought him in. If the guest's safety were not jeopardized by removal, the host would be justified in removing him even against the guest's wishes.

It may be relevant to Step 2 that the violinist is unconscious and so he does not form any expectations that are then disappointed. But even a declared intention to carry through a project that does raise expectations is not the same as a promise to continue the project (since a promise is an invitation to rely on one's intention).

Suppose that a person does not volunteer to support the violinist but that his attachment is the unintended consequence of some voluntary action by the person that foreseeably had some possibility of having this consequence. In this case, there is still no reason to think that what the person has done, by itself, gives the violinist the right to the continued use of the person's body or gives the person a duty to continue support.

Assume that the continuing attachment of the dependent violinist to one's body against one's wishes is not required merely because he needs help or merely because of one's voluntary actions. The two (his need and one's voluntary acceptance of him) do not create a special obligation, either singly or together.

STEP 3. *IF REMOVED, THE VIOLINIST LOSES ONLY WHAT HE HAS GAINED BY IMPOSING ON HIS SUPPORTER; HE IS NOT HARMED RELATIVE TO HIS PRE-ATTACHMENT OPPORTUNITIES, AND HE LOSES NOTHING THAT THE SUPPORTING PERSON IS MORALLY RESPONSIBLE FOR HIS HAVING THAT HE COULD RETAIN INDEPENDENTLY OF THE SUPPORTER*

Although killing the violinist instead of supporting him is harmful to the violinist, causing such harm may not be wrong; one is only obligated not to harm him relative to the condition he would have been in had he not been attached. If not attached he would have been dead, as there was no one else who could have saved him (by hypothesis). That is, if one has no duty to aid the violinist because of his need or other grounds of special obligation and he had no other opportunities to be saved, then any condition he is in as a result of one's aid is not something he has a claim to keep, at least as long as he needs one's support to maintain it. Therefore, the violinist's improved condition once attached cannot be the baseline relative to which one must not harm him. The baseline is, rather, the condition he would have been in if he had never been attached to his supporter.

The analysis might be different if the violinist could retain what he had received from the supporting person without her, even if not without the aid of others. (This is the point of the last clause of Step 3.) For example, suppose someone finds a person who is dying. She gives him medicine at great cost to herself and he is much improved and no longer needs help. One would not then be justified in killing him simply because he would not be worse off than he would have been (dead) if he had never received aid to which he had no right.

Notice that Step 3 will not be true in the Runner Case, for if the runner is killed, he will lose more than he gets from support and will be worse off than he would have been if never attached. The same is true of someone who is attached but would get no benefit from it at all.

There can be, I believe, a significant moral distinction between killing someone and letting him die. If we let someone die, that person loses only what he would have had as a result of our help at that time; by contrast, when we actively kill someone, he often loses what he would have had independently of us at that time.[5] In certain cases of killing, however, the person loses only what he would have had as a result of our help. This is so for the violinist, for when he is killed he loses only what he would have had with the support of the person to whom he is attached. It is this similarity between killing someone and letting someone die in this particular case that, I am claiming, makes killing him permissible if letting him die is permissible. What may interfere with this conclusion is that, even when killing results in the victim's losing only what he would have had as a result of his supporter's help, killing by method (4) involves actively inducing death, as letting the victim die does not.[6]

This difference, however, may not make the killing impermissible. Rather, it may only increase the costs of support whose avoidance is sufficient to justify killing. For example, we might be justified in fatally attacking the violinist in order to preserve his supporter's physical integrity but not her financial integrity. By contrast, one might be justified in letting someone die rather than impose financial ruin on someone else who could thereby save him.

The difference between killing and letting die suggests the two final steps needed for the argument.

STEP 4. *THE EFFORTS TO SUPPORT THE VIOLINIST ARE SIGNIFICANT ENOUGH THAT, IN CONJUNCTION WITH THE TRUTH OF THE OTHER PREMISES OF THE ARGUMENT, THEY CAN JUSTIFY (SPECIFICALLY) KILLING SOMEONE IN ORDER TO STOP THOSE EFFORTS*

The description of the Violinist Cases above validates this claim. (To justify it in relation to abortion, the costs of life support in pregnancy need to be evaluated.)

STEP 5. *KILLING THE VIOLINIST IS THE ONLY WAY TO END HIS IMPOSITION THAT IS NOT EXCESSIVELY COSTLY TO HIS SUPPORTER, EVEN GIVEN THE AIM OF NOT KILLING A PERSON*

Given the other premises discussed above, killing the attached person is the only means of terminating support that does not require the imposition of additional supererogatory costs on the supporter. Again, the description of the Violinist Cases above supports this claim.

The conclusion of this five-step argument is that killing the violinist in order to detach him from the person on whom he imposes is morally permissible.

C. THE OUTPUT-CUTOFF ARGUMENT

My discussion so far suggests that killing a person is permissible when doing so eliminates the life sustained by that person's imposing on another's body—an imposition not justified by the person's need or by another's special obligation—in order to end that imposition. This is true at least as long as the person killed is no worse off as a result than he would have been had he not been attached to someone's body, and if, in addition, he does not thereby lose anything that the supporter is morally responsible for his having that he could now retain independently of further support. I shall call this the Output-Cutoff Argument because it justifies cutting off the output of imposition—the benefit of life. It also explains why the need to use removal procedures that would kill or harm the attached person does not imply that the supporter has an obligation to continue support when no other factors have that implication.

However, it is not only by way of another's bodily support that the violinist retains his life; his own bodily processes play some role. Does this imply that the benefit of his continued life is a joint product of two people and that one party cannot have it destroyed without the other's permission? (Detaching in way [1] does not raise this issue.) I would argue no, because even the violinist's contribution to the enterprise only occurs because he imposes on the host. That is, his bodily processes continue to work at all only because of the support. Hence, if none of the factors discussed above justifies a requirement of continued support, the host is under no obligation to continue support merely to avoid killing the violinist. This is true despite any contribution the violinist's body may make.

This five-step argument is nonconsequentialist. In other words, whether the violinist should be saved or killed is not decided by determining who will suffer the greater loss—the violinist if he is killed or the supporter if the attachment continues. Rather, my analysis is rights-based: The supporter has a right not to maximize overall good consequences (by bearing a loss that is less than the loss she can prevent). Furthermore, the rights-based nature of this theory does not imply that the more important right in the abstract will always take precedence. Suppose we are asked whom to save—a person merely being imposed upon (by the violinist) or a bystander who is threatened with being killed. We should probably save the second person rather than the first, in order to protect the right not to be killed rather than the right not to be imposed on physically when this is not life threatening. Nevertheless, this is consistent with the view that when the person to be killed is staying alive by imposing on someone's body, he may be killed in order to protect the supporter's bodily integrity, and no one ought to stop this. The Output-Cutoff Argument explains why.

This argument proceeds without arguing that an innocent person has forfeited his right to life. Forfeiture would imply that the person had done something wrong and so had lost his right. One need not say this about the violinist. Rather, the view I am discussing states that the violinist need not be allowed to continue to benefit from his imposition on others.

Finally, I emphasize that in the cases I have used to argue for the permissibility of killing someone who is imposing on someone else, the supporter does not stand to lose her life. The argument would be even stronger if the supporter were going to lose her life if the violinist were not killed.

II. Abortion Cases

Does a variant on the Output-Cutoff Argument imply that killing in an abortion case is permissible? Assuming for the sake of argument that the fetus is a person (or infant) and accepting the Output-Cutoff Argument with the five conditions listed for the Violinist Cases, I shall now present an analogous argument for the permissibility of abortion, with comments following each step. Objections to this argument will be considered later.

A. BASIC ABORTION ARGUMENT (ON THE ASSUMPTION THAT THE FETUS IS A PERSON)

STEP 1A. *NEED ALONE DOES NOT CONFER A RIGHT TO HAVE AID BEGIN, NOR A DUTY TO GIVE IT*

The efforts required in even a normal pregnancy, labor, and delivery are strenuous and risky, not merely inconvenient, and so they extend beyond what a woman is obligated to provide merely because it will save a fetus's life. To give meaning to this observation, imagine a case in which a fetus is growing in a lab but will die unless it is transferred to a woman's body. Is she morally obligated to have it transferred solely because of its need, even if it is a stranger to her?

STEP 1B. *NEED ALONE DOES NOT CONFER A RIGHT TO HAVE CONTINUING SUPPORT, NOR A DUTY TO GIVE IT*

If it is morally permissible to let the fetus die, then its need for survival alone cannot morally require continuing support that has already begun as a result of a pregnancy. Suppose it will fall out of her body after a certain point (this will be a miscarriage). Its need, by itself, does not imply that she must prevent this.

STEP 2. *THERE IS NO SPECIAL OBLIGATION TO AID*

This step is more difficult to argue in the case of pregnancy than in the Violinist Case, for the woman may have created the fetus and thus had a part in *producing its need* for her body. (In the Violinist Case, even voluntarily starting to aid the violinist does not involve giving him his initial need for aid.) The following conditions should be fulfilled for the argument to succeed (though they will not always be fulfilled):

STEP 2A. *THERE IS NO SPECIAL OBLIGATION TO BEGIN SUPPORT*

This condition includes: (a) no obligation to create a fetus; (b) no responsibility in virtue of a woman's actions to begin support if the fetus were growing in a lab; and (c) no responsibility in virtue of the fetus's genetic connection to the woman to begin support if the fetus were growing in a lab.

Consider a case analogous to rape, where someone deliberately intrudes on a woman's body and as a side effect acquires her genetic material. The material happens to fall into a test tube and develops into a fetus growing in a laboratory. The intruder then tells the woman that the fetus will die unless she puts it in her body for nine months (all the while enduring the burdens, changes, and risks of pregnancy and labor). In this case, she has no obligation to support this fetus that someone else created. She is not causally or morally responsible for creating this fetus or for its needing her aid. In addition, I believe, its genetic connection to her would not make it impermissible for her to let the fetus die. Even a genetically related fetus does not have an inherent right to one's bodily support simply because it needs this, nor does one have a duty to provide this.

To be genetically related to our offspring is not the same as being a parent—that is, someone who is in a long-term committed relationship to (what may be) his or her genetically related offspring. Even if we were to assume that a parent is obligated to let a child use her or his body, a genetically related individual may have no such duty. But does even a father have a moral duty to help his sick four-year-old child by allowing him to use his body in the manner of pregnancy? Even when it was foreseen before the child was created that he might need this use? I doubt it.

STEP 2B. *THERE IS NO SPECIAL OBLIGATION TO CONTINUE SUPPORT WHEN A PREGNANCY (ASSUMED TO BEGIN IN THE WOMAN'S BODY) HAS BEGUN*

This condition means that there is no obligation to create the fetus, nor to continue support in virtue of the woman's actions, or because of the genetic connection. It might be claimed that even intentionally and voluntarily creating a fetus—let alone unintentionally becoming pregnant as a result of a voluntary act or of being raped—does not by itself commit a woman to begin or to continue her support of the fetus. This is because people sometimes begin projects, intending to complete them, but stop if the projects become too strenuous; a pregnancy may be such a project, and stopping it might be permissible, at least if the fetus is not harmed because of its supporter's actions relative to an appropriate baseline. Imagine, for example, that a fetus becomes detached quite naturally. If there is no special obligation to continue support, the woman would not be obligated to stop the miscarriage (or reattach the fetus), even though it needs her body to survive. Its support requires her continued efforts, so she might refuse to give further installments. It may be relevant here that the fetus is not conscious and that beginning existence and support arouses in it no expectations. The genetic connection also does not give rise to an obligation to continue support.

Suppose that neither the fetus's need, the types of actions the woman has performed in getting pregnant, nor a genetic connection, alone or together, confers on a fetus a right to be in a woman's body. One possible ground for a woman's being obligated nevertheless to keep the fetus in her body is that its removal would harm it relative to the baseline of opportunities it had before it was attached. But Step 3 will dispute this ground in the case where pregnancy begins in the body.

STEP 3. *THE FETUS THAT IS KILLED IN ORDER TO END A PREGNANCY LOSES ONLY THE LIFE THAT IS PROVIDED BY ITS IMPOSITION ON THE WOMAN AND THE IMPOSITION IS NOT JUSTIFIED (ACCORDING TO 2[B]) BY THE FETUS'S NEED OR ANY SPECIAL OBLIGATION. THE FETUS IS NOT HARMED RELATIVE TO ITS PRE-ATTACHMENT PROSPECTS (AND IT IS NOT WORSE OFF THAN IT WOULD HAVE BEEN IF IT HAD NEVER BEEN IN THE WOMAN'S BODY). KILLING THE FETUS DOES NOT CAUSE IT TO LOSE ANYTHING THAT THE WOMAN IS MORALLY RESPONSIBLE FOR ITS HAVING AND THAT IT COULD RETAIN INDEPENDENTLY OF HER*

The fetus had no opportunities before it was attached to the woman's body (that is, before its conception) of which it would be deprived; and it had no opportunities other than being attached to the woman's body, in that before it was attached to her there was (by hypothesis) no one else to whose body it could have been attached. Thus, although killing the fetus makes it worse off than it would be if the woman continued to support it, harming it in this way may not be wrong. One may only be obliged not to harm it relative to the condition it would have been in if it had not been attached. If the woman has no duty to aid it because of its need or other grounds of special obligation, any condition it is in as a result of imposing on her is not something it has a claim to keep, at least as long as it continues to need her support to maintain its condition. Therefore, the condition it is in when attached cannot be the baseline relative to which it must not be harmed.

If a fetus begun in a lab is left to die (versus being killed), it similarly is not harmed relative to its precreation opportunities (of which there were none) or relative to other opportunities it had (e.g., one does not interfere with someone else attaching it to her body who would have carried it to term). This observation, together with Steps 1A, 2A, and 2B, suggests that one may let the lab fetus die, even if it is not the result of an intruder's actions.

STEP 4. *EFFORTS INVOLVED IN SUPPORTING AND/OR DELIVERING THE FETUS ARE SUFFICIENT, IN CONJUNCTION WITH THE TRUTH OF THE OTHER CONDITIONS, TO JUSTIFY KILLING THE FETUS IN ORDER TO STOP THESE EFFORTS*

STEP 5. *KILLING THE FETUS IS THE ONLY WAY TO END ITS IMPOSITION THAT IS NOT EXCESSIVELY COSTLY TO THE WOMAN, EVEN GIVEN THE AIM OF NOT KILLING A PERSON*

The basic strategy of this argument, which I shall call the Cutoff Abortion Argument, is similar to that of the Output-Cutoff Argument in the Violinist Cases. It aims to justify abortion in cases in which a woman does not want to continue a normal pregnancy because of the effort it requires (including labor), not because she will die. It is nonconsequentialist in that it does not consider whether her life is more valuable than that of the person she would bear, or whether she stands to lose more if she continues the pregnancy than the fetus will lose if she does not.

Consider Step 3 further. Unlike the violinist who existed prior to being in someone's body and who needed to be attached to another person, the fetus did not exist before it was attached to the woman's body. Is the fetus therefore worse off if it is killed than if it had never been in the woman's body (i.e., nonexistent), or is it harmed relative to its pre-attachment opportunities (none)? One possible claim is that it need be no worse for a person to live a short time and then be permissibly and painlessly killed than never to live at all.[7] One reason for this is that the principal misfortune of death is not receiving any more of the goods of life;[8] and it might be argued that not receiving more goods is not worse for a person than not receiving any originally due to nonexistence. Furthermore, if the killing were permissible, no injustice would enter into the life.

To say that the fetus if killed is harmed (or not harmed) as compared to its precreation prospects seems odd, since it had no such prospects as it did not exist. Nonetheless, I believe that if the fetus were living a life of uninterrupted pain, there would be a sense in which it would be harmed by being created, relative to the prospect of never being created.[9] But such pain is not involved in abortion.

To strengthen the claim that the fetus which is aborted is not harmed (in this sense) relative to the prospect of never being created, and is no worse for living a short time and dying rather than never having lived at all, consider the case of a woman who deliberately becomes pregnant even though she knows that she has a very high risk of miscarriage. If some life and an early death were worse for the fetus than never living at all—if creating that short life were comparable to making an existing innocent bystander worse off by exposing him to a cause of death that he otherwise would not have faced—then this woman should be required to do a great deal to avoid becoming pregnant. However, women who know that they bear a substantial risk of losing their fetuses are still encouraged to become pregnant if they want a child, or at least are not discouraged for the fetus's sake, even by people who currently believe that a fetus is a person.[10]

Assume that it is no worse for the fetus to live for only a short time than never to live at all, and that it is not harmed relative to its pre-attachment prospects (nonexistence and no one else to whom to be attached) if it is aborted. It may still be true that a *world* in which a creature that had the chance to live a long life but never fulfills its potential is worse than a world in which such a creature never lived. The first world contains a waste; the second does not.[11] If this is so, the next question is: how much effort should someone expend in order not to produce such a worse state of the world (even if it is still not worse relative to the appropriate baseline for judging its effect *for* the fetus, namely the fetus's pre-attachment prospects)? The answer may be that one is not obligated to make a large sacrifice to prevent waste that is not worse for anyone than his relevant baseline. Perhaps one should also balance the waste of destruction of the fetus against the possible waste of opportunities in the life of the person who would have to carry it.[12]

B. VIABILITY

Suppose that at a certain point the fetus were, what I shall call, *superviable*. This is the (unrealistic) state of not needing and also not deriving sustenance from the woman's body on which it imposes, but not being removable from the woman. In this case, the fetus would have lived outside her body if its attachment had safely ended. If the fetus is still inside the woman because it cannot be removed, then the fetus's residence is still part of the process necessary to give it life, even though the woman's body no longer provides it sustenance. Therefore, if one removes it in a way that kills it, one is taking away the fetus's benefit (life) resulting from its residence as a whole—from the point it is attached to the point of detachment—in order to end its continued residence. If this continued residence and labor needed for exit, which is necessary for the fetus's life, has not been donated and is more than the fetus has a right to, abortion will be permissible.

The superviability case bears on the relevance of normal viability to the permissibility of abortion. At viability, the fetus can live outside the womb (albeit with mechanical support), though it is still in the womb and in fact derives sustenance from the woman. Suppose that its safe removal before a nine-month attachment is not physically possible. Then killing the fetus to remove it ends a process that, as a whole, is necessary for giving life to it, and the fetus loses what, in fact, it cannot have without using the woman. Suppose, alternatively, that its safe removal is possible, but at a cost which is beyond what the woman would be obligated to endure in order to avoid killing the fetus. Then the fetus is no worse off for being killed than it has any right to be, since it has no right to the means necessary to be safely removed from her and no right to all the body support it needs otherwise.

How does the fate of a fetus that does not receive the costly things it needs from the woman in order that it be alive compare with the fate of that fetus if it is killed? Suppose safe exit from the woman's body is possible only at an excessive cost to the woman and the fetus would remain alive if it stayed in her body. In this case, the fetus would need the period in her body that she has not donated and need not donate and that extends beyond the point of viability to birth. Therefore, the baseline for considering whether one may kill the fetus is how the fetus would be without either of the things it needs from the woman: the cost to her of its safe exit or the remaining period of residence and labor. Without these things, it would not continue to exist, so the relevant baseline for judging the permissibility of abortion is its nonexistence.

This leaves the case in which it is not too costly to the woman to transfer the fetus to an external womb. In this case, a woman who prevented a fetus from being safely removed and then had it killed to effect its removal would be making the fetus worse off than it had a right to be. She would have harmed it relative to prospects to which it had a right. Abortion should not then be permissible. Therefore, one reason that viability may be morally significant is that viability is the point at which it is possible for a woman to make the fetus worse off than it would be in an alternative state to which it had a right, namely being easily removed. Notice that in this last case, the fetus still could not retain its life independently of her efforts if it remains in the womb, but either it has a right to those efforts or she has a duty to give them given that she does not permit easy removal.

C. PROBLEMS WITH THE CUTOFF ABORTION ARGUMENT AND THE SIGNIFICANCE OF CREATION

The Cutoff Abortion Argument is analogous to the Output-Cutoff Argument, but it has problems that the latter does not have. One problem is that when creating a new person, merely making sure that the new person will be both no worse off than if she had never existed and not harmed relative to prospects she had before being attached (if these differ and assuming these comparisons can be made sense of) are not sufficient conditions for morally correct reproduction. In discussing this objection to the Cutoff Abortion Argument, I shall examine the role of creating the fetus in an argument for or against abortion.

a. The Fetus Versus the Violinist

It has been argued that although killing the violinist deprives him of the life he could have had, this might be permissible because it does not necessarily harm him relative to his prospects before his attachment. But the satisfaction of the same factors (in some sense) in the case of the fetus may not make killing it permissible. When a person kills the violinist, he brings about a bad state of affairs that would have existed anyway—the violinist's death—in order to stop the aid that would prevent his death. In contrast, the bad state of affairs for the fetus—its being dead—would never have existed if the fetus had never been created. There is no one in existence before his or her creation who needs to be created or who is worse off if not created, so why bring about for the first time the possibility of someone's losing further life after only a short time alive? (By contrast, in the Violinist Case someone needs to be attached to a body and it will be worse for him if he is not attached than if he is attached.)

b. Why Death Is Bad

My earlier discussion suggested that death is bad primarily because it deprives a person of more of life's goods.[13] But perhaps other things may make death bad, and these may also make living a short while and then dying worse (in some sense) for a person than not living at all. I shall refer to the goods and bads that are important to us when we consider our lives from the outside as the *formal* (or structural) goods and bads, and those which are important to us only as we live our lives as the *experienced* (or experiential) goods and bads. The latter may lead us, for example, to prefer avoiding as much pain as possible *in the future* even if this meant that there will have been more pain in our lives overall because there will have been more pain in the past.[14]

Among the formal bads of death, but not of total nonexistence, may be its taking from someone what he already has (life) and what he already is; it happens *to* someone and demonstrates his vulnerability. By contrast, nonexistence does not happen to someone who already exists; it does not take what one already has, and no one is shown to be vulnerable because he did not exist. Death is a decline (from the good of life, if life is good), whereas not going from nonexistence to life (if life is good) can be considered a failure to incline in a formal sense. These factors make death a sort of insult to a person that total nonexistence is not, whether or not a person is aware of the insult.[15]

Death, of course, also represents the *impossibility* of any future experienced goods for the dead person. This can be distinguished from simply not obtaining more such goods of life. For example, someone might enter a limbo state containing no goods of life and then return to complete his conscious time alive, thus extending his time alive without increasing the total goods in his life (call him the Limbo Man). He would do this merely to delay his end and the end of the possibility of obtaining more goods, since as long as he stays in limbo there is the possibility of return. Suppose this person is not unreasonable in preferring to go into limbo rather than having the same amount of goods and length of consciously experienced life continuously. Then one will have found yet another reason for death being bad besides the reduction of total goods of life: it involves the end of the possibility of good life.[16]

c. Is Mere Fetal Life a Harm?

If the fetus is a person (as we are assuming for the sake of argument), it will lose many goods of life it might have had and suffer an (unfelt) insult if its life is taken from it. Also, it is worse for the world when waste results because a creature dies young, never having had compensatory goods. Is it still possible, however, that someone is not harmed overall by having a bit of life and then losing so much, even if it is possible for someone to be harmed (in some sense) in being created to a very bad life? If so, it would not be for this person's sake that we should not create him. If the formal characteristics of his life are not good (because he lost out on practically everything and was insulted), should this influence us more than the fact that his experiences are not bad and perhaps even good? I am sympathetic to the view that respect for persons should lead us to emphasize the poor formal characteristics of the life of a short-lived person. If this were so, we would have a reason to avoid creating out of respect for the fetus-person. Nevertheless, a love for life itself (a pro-life view, in a sense) might lead us to see no harm in creating such a short life if it had sufficient positive experiences.

In sum, I will assume that in the experiential sense, the fetus is no worse for living and dying than if it had never lived (assuming there is a sense in which we can make such comparisons), nor is it harmed relative to prospects it (nonliterally) had prior to conception. That is, it does not have overall bad experiences and it is not deprived of any goods of experience and activity which it might have had if it had not been conceived. I leave open that there may be some other *formal* sense in which the fetus is harmed in being created and living only a short life. To indicate this, I shall say that the fetus is not *experientially* worse off and not *experientially* harmed. I shall not assume that if it is harmed in the formal sense, much sacrifice is morally required to avoid the formal harm per se. Nevertheless, I believe that a new person is owed more from its creators than just not to be overall harmed experientially by its life. This leads me to want to present an alternative to the Cutoff Abortion Argument, for that argument relies on the satisfaction of the "not experientially worse off" condition. The alternative argument tries (in broad outline) to develop a different ethic of creating new people.

D. THE BENEFIT-BURDEN APPROACH AND THE MINIMA

I shall now present such an alternative, which I call the Benefit-Burden Approach to abortion.[17] It builds on the Cutoff Abortion Argument. It may be best to understand this argument as an attempt to explain the reasons that someone who holds certain views about abortion could give for these views and to show how these reasons are consistent with common views about the limits of parental obligations in creating new people. It is not presented as a knockdown argument for holding such views. Some distinctive elements of the argument are: (1) the view that it is legitimate to impose some risks on the fetus for the sake of its getting what is comparable to a benefit of life; (2) the emphasis on the possible burdens of abstaining from sex, refraining from having a child, and carrying and delivering a fetus; and (3) the emphasis on the benefits to the creator of creating a person. It is because of the emphasis on these factors that I call this approach to abortion the Benefit-Burden Approach. Now consider the argument in detail.[18]

Suppose that persons ought not be created at will unless it is believed that they can have some number of years of life with some degree of health and welfare. I shall call these things which they ought to have the *minima*.[19] It may be true that one should not begin creating a person without aiming for the minima. But this does not mean that once people actually have been conceived, they should not be kept alive even if they will not obtain the minima. Hence, a woman may refuse to take advantage of the moral permissibility of abortion on the grounds that it is in the interest of a person once conceived to remain alive as long as its life is better for it than nonexistence, even if this standard is below having the minima.

A crucial question in relation to abortion is how much and what kind of effort persons are entitled to, and from whom, if they are either to have the minima or not be created at all. In particular, do they have a right to the minima at such costs and sacrifices as: (1) being carried in someone's body (this includes labor, delivery, and the risks and changes of pregnancy); (2) someone's forgoing a heterosexual sex life for their entire reproductive years; or (3) surgery on someone's body (in caesarean section or fetal therapy)? I shall refer to these costs and sacrifices as *carriage, abstinence,* and *surgery,* respectively. There may be additional personal costs of an unwanted pregnancy (for instance, the woman may be thought of as a mere part of nature; she may lose her sense of separateness as a person; economic, career, or familial troubles may ensue) as well as social costs if abortion is not available (for example, more social inequality between the sexes). Even if one rejects the Cutoff Abortion Argument, one should keep these other costs in mind in constructing the Benefit-Burden Approach and ask whether a fetus has a right to bodily aid to get the minima when these costs ensue as well. Though I shall not refer to these other costs repeatedly, they can be considered costs of status.

a. Veil of Ignorance

One way of determining acceptable costs for achieving the minima or avoiding lives without the minima might be to reason from behind a veil of ignorance.[20] The veil deprives people of knowledge about the particulars of their circumstances in society, so they are unable to allow a bias in their favor to influence decisions as to what social policies should be established. It might seem that this exercise would result in a decision that abortion is impermissible, for the following reason: From behind a veil of ignorance, one would not know whether one was a pregnant woman or a fetus. If the fetus is assumed to be a person, and the woman has lived longer than the fetus has and will not die if the pregnancy continues, would not decision-makers behind the veil choose to ban abortions in order to improve the prospects of the worst-off person?

This way of reasoning behind the veil, however, would have radical implications if applied elsewhere. For example, if one cared only about the length of life and maximum number of lives saved, one would also decide from behind the veil on a policy to kill older persons to save younger ones, or to kill one person to save five people. Yet we do not institute such policies. Perhaps this is because other factors should direct our reasoning even from behind the veil.[21] For example, it may be important to recognize the status that people have of being in certain ways inviolable. This status could imply that one does not have to endure some impositions for the sake of others.

Suppose that from behind a veil of ignorance one would be concerned with equality. Suppose also that a cost of the impermissibility of abortion would be greater inequality between the sexes. If one is concerned about this cost because of concern about inequality in general, ought one not be concerned that a more severe inequality will occur if the fetus is a person and abortions are permitted? That is, if it is assumed that the fetus is a person and it will be killed at a young age, then surely it will be the worst-off person.

Ought one correct for inequality between the sexes at the cost of a more severe inequality?[22] A related point is to note that every woman who may suffer inequality if abortions are not permitted would herself have been in danger of having been killed as a fetus. Arguably this is a worse fate than adult sex inequality.

However, perhaps it is not unreasonable to be concerned about one type of inequality being generated as a result of trying to relieve an even worse form of inequality. Consider that everyone who is now an adult was once a child. Suppose that only adult blacks turned out to have the capacity to save children (both black and white) by giving them certain of their organs. Could one not object, out of concern for racial equality, to a policy that required adult blacks to give up their organs to save the lives of young children, even though dying at ten years old is worse than being required to donate on the basis of race at forty?

b. Factors that Determine Efforts

I suggest that the following factors should be part of one's reasoning about how much a person is obligated to do to provide the minima for a fetus (on the continuing assumption it is a person) or to avoid creating persons without the minima, even if we do not rely on reasoning from behind a veil of ignorance.

1. The new person should be experientially no worse off having lived even without the minima than never having lived at all, and should not be experientially harmed relative to prospects he had prior to conception. (I shall continue to interpret these phrases nonliterally and shall not rely merely on the fact that this person literally had no prior prospects and would not have existed. We can imagine nonexistence as a zero and pluses or minuses being added by life with good and bad experiences.) These conditions should set an upper limit on the sacrifices required in order to prevent the occurrence of a life without minima. This factor helps reduce the sacrifices one is obligated to make for the minima, as it is relatively easy to be made no worse off experientially than zero.

2. When determining the efforts required of a creator to create, one should not necessarily compare the new person's actual condition with his condition had other people cared for him. For example, that a millionaire offers my child a better life does not mean that I must meet that standard in order to avoid losing rights to my child. Therefore, this factor helps reduce the sacrifices one is obligated to make for the minima.

3. There is an "internal logic" associated with creating a new person that may include some idea of human normality. That is, it would be wrong to create a human being who was in a happy psychological state, but who lived a life functionally equivalent to that of a normal rabbit. This internal logic may also include the idea that some efforts are required to make the next generation at least as well off as the present one is, and the idea that persons should not be created solely as tools for others independent of consideration of their own interests. These ideas set

minimum standards and in this sense increase sacrifices for minima. But they also imply that one need not make great efforts to exceed the standards set by the minima.

To clarify the idea of an internal logic of creating, I shall compare it with the ideals and requirements for entertaining a guest. These also apply independently of whether abiding by them makes one's guest better or worse off than he would have been had he spent the weekend somewhere else. However, if the host is morally responsible for bringing the guest to his house, then in addition to any obligations inherent in the role of host, he should ensure that his guest is no worse off than he would have been elsewhere, in particular as someone else's guest. This is one difference between the logic of being a host and that of being a creator, as emphasized by factor (2) above.

4. A creator's treatment of a new person is constrained, minimally, by the requirements that a stranger would have to meet. For example, one must respect the new person's individual rights. Creators do not own the persons they create and ought not treat them less well than strangers ought to simply because they have given them life. Therefore, this factor helps increase the sacrifices one has to make for the minima.

5. Since one does not exist before conception, one cannot literally be benefited by coming to life, nor is one literally harmed by not being created. Yet I consider creating a good life to be in some ways similar to bestowing a benefit on someone. People in good conscience can think of themselves as creating a good new life for the sake of the created person when the new person will live a good life.[23] I consider this a pro-life assumption.[24]

Factor (5) can help reduce the sacrifices one is obligated to make in order to ensure the presence of the minima. Here is one reason why. Assume that this pro-life view of creation treats the new person to some degree as if he is benefiting from receiving life. Then might it not be fair to require him to bear some risks, including that of a short life, in order to obtain this benefit? After all, even committed parents need not provide a complete insurance policy against all risks that will be faced by the children they create. If a child needed a parent to lay down his life to save him, the parent is not morally obligated to do this merely in virtue of having created the child. (Though many parents would make such a sacrifice from love.) Might not the risks to a new person even include some risk of being worse off than if he had never existed (that is, the risk of living a life of pain)? Is not the (hypothetical) willingness to accept such risks part of a (pro-life) view that life is like a great gift to the person created? This factor helps reduce the sacrifices one is obligated to make for the minima.

6. Intentionally providing a benefit to someone is a good thing to do (assuming that creating a good life is in some ways like giving a benefit). This factor may help reduce the sacrifices one is obligated to make for the minima.

7. Intentionally creating usually means creating with the knowledge that fetal needs will then exist that would not exist otherwise. This factor helps increase the sacrifices one is obligated to make for the minima.

8. As things are now, the newly created person requires significant efforts (i.e., pregnancy) from others to meet its needs, efforts that are not usually required on behalf of just anyone. This factor helps reduce the requirement to make the sacrifices necessary for the minima.

9. Although the need for the efforts involved in pregnancy are usually foreseen as inevitable, the creators (at least given current technology) do not choose to make the new person dependent on these efforts when it could have been independent. This factor helps reduce the sacrifices they are obligated to make for the minima.

10. There may even be weighty sacrifices necessary if one is to avoid creating the new person. These may include not having a heterosexual sex life, using dangerous contraceptive drugs, or not trying to have children when one strongly desires them. At this point, it is relevant to recall the imperatives of humanity as a whole, and of some individuals in particular, to reproduce. There are costs of not reproducing that correspond to these imperatives. Not permitting abortion can interfere with a need to have children that is not all-consuming, because it can dissuade people from attempting a pregnancy for fear it cannot be ended. This factor, therefore, helps reduce the sacrifices one is obliged to make for the minima.

11. Factor (10) implies that voluntary creators themselves can obtain benefits from creating; that is, they do not create for totally altruistic reasons. Rather, they want children and, in some cases, need children. This factor helps increase the sacrifices they are obligated to make for the minima. (On account, for example, that one should bear risks to get a benefit for oneself, as was suggested above in the case of the fetus.)

In sum, I believe that, in some respects, factors (1) to (3) and (5) to (10) help to reduce the sacrifices that a creator is obligated to make either to support the fetus or to prevent its conception. In some respects, factors (3), (4), (8), and (11) help to increase such sacrifices. I shall refer to this set of eleven factors as the Creation Factors.

c. Objections to Creation Factor (5)

Before proceeding further I wish to consider some objections to creation factor (5). One objection to what it proposes is raised by Seana Shiffrin. Shiffrin is willing to accept that being created to a good life is something like a benefit for the person created. However, she argues that acts that bring about risks of harm or actual harms to people who are created cannot be justified by the possibility or, importantly, even the actuality of goods greater than the harms coming to them.[25] This includes risks that are unavoidable if the person is to be created to a good life, not just risks that could be avoided. Her argument concerning procreation stems from a more general argument about harms and benefits in nonprocreative contexts. It is important to emphasize that her argument focuses on harms that are less than the goods achievable, not merely on risks of harms or actual harms that are greater than goods that could be achieved.

Let us first consider her discussion of the nonprocreative contexts. One part of her position is that harms are separable events that may occur even when a person is overall better off as a result of another's action. For example, if we can save an adult from dying only by doing what breaks his leg, his having a broken leg is a harm to him even though it helps him avoid the worse harm of losing his life and so he is overall better off. Another part of her position is that imposing harms on (or allowing harms to befall) someone without his consent can be permissible in order to prevent greater harm coming to him but not in order to produce (or prevent the loss of) what she calls "pure benefits." The case we just considered involves the first option and she holds that though one harms the person without his consent, he is not wronged and no compensation is owed to him. Pure benefits are goods whose absence would not involve someone being in what she calls a harmed state, such as suffering bodily injury or serious frustration of his will. (Note that she believes that one can be put in such a harmed state even if one is not made worse off relative to a previous state one was in or to a state one could otherwise have been in. Her notion of harm is, as she says, noncomparative.)

She presents a case to illustrate the point about not imposing harms for pure benefits: A rich person, Wealthy, wishes to benefit a group of already well-off people by giving each of them an immense fortune. The only way to get the fortune to them is to drop gold cubes on them from above with the risk that someone will be injured even though care is taken; there is no way to communicate with them so as to get their consent to this. One person, Unlucky, does suffer a broken arm in receiving his fortune. (Call this the Gold Cube Case.) The fortune is a pure benefit because, while one will be worse off in life without the fortune, one will not be in a harmed state. Shiffrin claims that it is impermissible to drop the gold cubes even though overall Unlucky is better off with the fortune and the broken arm than with no fortune and no broken arm. She claims that this case is support for her view that without consent, it is impermissible to harm or risk harm to someone in order to provide a pure benefit.

She applies this view to procreation, for even if creating life is conceived as like (though not as literally) giving a benefit, it is a pure benefit since no one will be in a harmed state if we do not create him. Furthermore, there are unavoidable harms associated with being alive. Among these harms, Shiffrin thinks, are the burdens of moral choice, having to deal with eventual death, typical risks of physical and psychological injuries that are run in every human life and the fruition of these risks in some cases, and the absence of an easy exit from these burdens (as suicide is difficult). Since it is impossible to get consent to his creation from the person created, her conclusion is that providing the pure benefit is at least morally problematic on the ground that it wrongs the person created even if the benefit is reasonably expected to be (and in fact will be) greater than the harm. (The Gold

Cube Case seems to suggest a stronger conclusion, namely that procreation is pro tanto morally impermissible.) She further suggests that the explanation for parents' duties to provide extensive care for their offspring, beyond making his life merely on balance good, is that this is compensation owed for wronging him by creation.

I have concerns about Shiffrin's analysis of the Gold Cube Case and the implications she draws from it for what is owed as a result of creating people who will live normal lives. However, here my first concern is to consider the implications of her views for the permissibility of aborting a person before he becomes conscious, forms preferences about living his life, or exercises his will. Imagine a variant of the Gold Cube case in which the gold cube fell into Unlucky's garden but evaporated shortly thereafter (hence his being unlucky in this case) without his knowing that he had ever had the cube or that it had evaporated. Would Shiffrin believe that Unlucky had been harmed in losing this pure benefit even though he would not have been harmed in not receiving it in the first place? If not, it is not clear how the Gold Cube Case would help us conclude that creating a person who will die never having been conscious of his life harms him in depriving him of a pure benefit. (This is not to say that he is not harmed in losing his life—even if he is not worse off overall relative to nonexistence in getting and losing the benefit—only that Shiffrin's analogy and her notions of noncomparative harm and benefit do not seem to have this implication.)

However, if abortion involved pain to the fetus, this would be a harm. Then Shiffrin's position would imply that it is wrong to create with even the risk that an abortion (or unavoidable miscarriage) painful to the fetus will take place even if this were a lesser harm relative to the good of life. However, this problem with abortion could be eliminated if anesthetics for the fetus were used.

Of course, abortion (unlike natural miscarriage) involves someone taking the pure benefit away in order to stop a burdensome process needed to provide the benefit. To capture this in a variant of the Gold Cube Case, we should imagine that after the cube falls in Unlucky's garden, Wealthy evaporates it in order to prevent further cost to himself due to maintaining the cube. One question raised by this variant is whether Wealthy's doing this wrongs Unlucky; another is whether it harms him. Shiffrin holds that wrongs can be harms even if they do not involve harmed states. (Suppose for argument's sake that this is true.) To determine whether Unlucky is harmed when Wealthy does the evaporation if Unlucky is not harmed simply by the evaporation, one would have to *first* decide if Wealthy's action is pro tanto wrong and a wronging of Unlucky. Hence, one could not show that Wealthy's action was wrong *because* it harmed Unlucky. This would be analogous to our first determining that abortion of a person is wrong and then concluding that it therefore harms him. However, at this point in the Benefit-Burden Approach we are trying to decide *whether* abortion is wrong *because* it impermissibly harms or risks harm. We cannot make use of any argument that *assumes* that deliberate removal of a pure benefit is wrong and therefore a harm.

I will not here discuss Shiffrin's views insofar as they bear on the question of parental responsibilities for offspring who are not aborted.[26] However, it is important to realize that the Benefit-Burden Argument for the minima according to which it could be wrong to create a person without the minima does not rely on a view like Shiffrin's that compensation is owed for creating without consent when lesser harms may occur. To see how the two views diverge, suppose it were certain that even without parental intervention offspring would have the minima in their lives. The Benefit-Burden Argument would not imply that parents had further responsibilities in virtue of creating. By contrast, Shiffrin's view implies that no matter how much the goods of life outweigh the harms, further goods of compensation are still owed by parents for what they did in creating.

Having relied on the Gold Cube case and the distinction between causing lesser harms to avoid greater harms and causing lesser harms to produce pure benefits to support her argument about procreation, it is only near the end of her article that Shiffrin notes a difference between procreation and nonprocreation cases. Namely, if someone does not get the pure benefit of the gold cube, he will go on living in a less good condition (even if not a harmed state). By contrast, if someone is not created (and so does not get life that is like the pure benefit), there will not be a person who exists in a less good condition. It is possible that this distinction will make it wrong to provide what is like a pure benefit in creating with the risk of abortion, because if not created, no one would live less well. So a second objection to the view presented in (5) is that because a person is not waiting to be created and no one is literally benefited by being created, an agent for all future fetuses might easily hold out for better terms—that is, no risks at all for them of less than the minima. Suppose such a model involving a bargaining agent were the appropriate basis for determining what is due any given fetus. In this case, an aborted fetus would indeed have been harmed relative to better prospects it had a right to have.

I do not believe that this view of creating—which gives the fetus essentially a veto right—is morally required or is even morally acceptable. Weight must be given to the fact that there is no real moral alternative to procreation, in view of two imperatives. The first is reproduction of the species, or, more appropriately, the continuation of humanity, insofar as this phrase expresses not mere biological continuation but continuation of intelligent beings with capacities for worthwhile lives. The second imperative is the need of many individual human beings to reproduce (as a biological desire) and to pass on their individual humanity (in the nonbiological sense). In the face of such strong reasons to reproduce, demanding complete security and the best possible outcome for the fetus seems unreasonable. Indeed, even in the absence of an overwhelming personal desire to reproduce, many people consider there to be strong reasons to create because of the worth of continuing humanity and the importance of involving oneself personally in creating a new generation.

Given this background, fetuses-to-be sometimes may be treated as if (in a nonliteral sense) they were under an obligation to allow themselves to be created consistent with certain outcomes for them. They must play their part in the human enterprise. It seems true, however, that people take advantage of a given fetus's nonexistence in requiring such participation. For if one needed the involvement of an already existing person in such projects, and the person might be made worse off overall, one probably could not justify involving him without his consent (except in extremes, such as the prospect of humanity's extinction), even if he had a good chance of receiving a large benefit. But if it were necessary to gain the consent of those who are created, no creation would be morally permissible at all.[27]

Suppose that fetuses have been permissibly "called upon" (or drafted) to participate in the human enterprise, and that creators' reasons for creating are (in part at least) as just described. Then there must be some sort of balancing of interests and rights in deciding what freedoms the creators have and what the fetuses are owed in order to get the minima, keeping in mind that the fetuses may eventually themselves be creators.[28]

d. Relation Between the Cutoff Abortion Argument and the Minima

Suppose that the fetus has a right to a certain effort on its creators' part to obtain the minima and a woman has a duty to provide it. If the fetus were then killed to stop that effort, it would lose more than the benefit (life) of efforts to which it had no right and that the woman had no duty to provide. But assume that there are efforts to which the fetus has no right, and that the woman has no duty to provide, in order that the fetus obtain the minima. Then one can assert that there is no special obligation to provide minima at certain costs (following from Steps 2a and 2b in the Cutoff Abortion Argument), and proceed with the rest of the Cutoff Abortion Argument to explain the permissibility of killing. Therefore, despite criticism of it, the Cutoff Abortion Argument still provides the structure for the Benefit-Burden Approach, which tries to demonstrate the moral plausibility of certain positions permitting abortion.

Put formally, I propose that at most there is a duty to provide the minima at no more than cost m if one could not avoid being pregnant at a cost less than c. Alternatively, if it was foreseen that much more than m (an additional cost x) would be required for the minima and the cost to avoid being pregnant was less than c, then there could be a duty to provide the minima at cost $m + x$.[29] The fact that a new person may be treated as though he benefits from creation, and so may appropriately be asked to take risks for that benefit, has a role in setting the values of m, x, and c. If being created would always be experientially worse than never existing or if there were a very small chance of "benefiting" from creation, c, m, and x would represent greater efforts. In what follows, I shall formulate possible proposals for different degrees of responsibility had by creators to provide the minima based on different degrees of responsibility for creating a new person. My aim is to explain the reasoning behind each proposal—what would have to be true if the proposal is to be correct (though it may not be correct).

e. Proposal One for Voluntary Creation without Foreseeing a Need for Carriage

1

People who, voluntarily and not for "reasons of state,"[30] create a new person must attempt to obtain the minima for the new person[31] and provide these minima by undergoing up to cost m, where m is less costly than carriage, abstinence, or surgery. Alternatively, they may find someone else to provide the minima for no more than cost m. They need not provide the minima by means of carriage, abstinence,[32] or surgery if, before creating the person, they could not reasonably predict the need for these in order to provide the minima. (Admittedly, it is highly unlikely for it to be reasonable not to foresee the need for carriage.)

Let me clarify this proposal. First, the relation between a voluntary creator and a fetus is weaker than that between a parent and a child because (I assume) the latter relation but not the former involves acceptance of a long-standing commitment to a dependent person. A point of Proposal One is that one need not be an accepting, committed parent in order to have some obligations to the person that one has voluntarily caused to exist.

Proposal One is consistent with refusing to require even parents to give up their bodily organs or bodily products (such as bone marrow) for their children if in those cases the parents could not have reasonably predicted the need for those things when they created the child. The parents' willingness to undergo carriage, abstinence, and surgery for their children (if contrary to fact, these were useful for older children) could be retained as an ideal without its being a moral requirement. Even if parents were morally required to do these things in order to provide the minima, voluntary creators and bearers of a fetus who are not yet so committed may not have such duties. Although the fetus is assumed to be a person, it is not one with whom someone has been involved in a committed or long-term relationship, especially one where expectations have built up.

Cost m is defined as lower than the cost of carriage, abstinence, or surgery. But suppose that cost m comprised something comparable to the ordinary responsibilities of raising a child for several years. How can one then say that cost m is lower than nine months of bodily support?

The distinction, if there is one, between the use of someone's body and other costs and sacrifices must be drawn qualitatively, in terms of privacy or bodily integrity. It cannot be drawn in terms of strenuousness of effort alone. In this sense, saying that cost m is lower than that of carriage or surgery is misleading.[33] Likewise, working for forty hours a week may be more of a burden to someone than having his body examined. Yet society thinks it has a right to sentence a criminal to hard labor (or service to the community) but not to physical testing or involvement in (even low-risk) research experiments that intrude on his body. Furthermore, bodily intrusions themselves can differ qualitatively. A forced bone marrow transplant may be strenuous, if not very damaging in the long run. But a nonvoluntary rectal exam, which causes less damage and is not strenuous, may be humiliating. Sexualized bodily impositions can be like this, and real pregnancy (if not the ersatz one in the Violinist Case) is a sexualized imposition as well as a strenuous use of a body.

What is the rationale behind not ensuring that a new person always obtains the minima at the cost of carriage, abstinence, or surgery (let alone at a higher cost), given that even in the highly unusual case we are now discussing (in which there is no foresight to the need for carriage) one could foresee that there may be a slight chance that the new person will need aid at these costs? One proposed rationale is based on the fact that being created into a nice life is like a benefit that requires a rather unusual cost for its provision. Therefore, it is appropriate to have the new person accept risks for the sake of a sufficiently high probability (but not a guarantee) of gaining the benefit of life with the minima.

2

Suppose that Proposal One is correct for the unusual case it describes and that such a creator is not obligated to provide carriage, surgery, or lifetime abstinence in order for its fetus to receive the minima. We can apply this result to the Cutoff Abortion Arguments Steps 2a and 2b concerning special obligations to aid in a case where there was voluntary action and it was not unreasonable to lack foreknowledge of the need for carriage. In this case, there is no special responsibility to aid in these ways, in part because it is permissible to impose on the fetus the risk of not receiving a benefit and in part because absence of foreknowledge to the need for more than m was not unreasonable. However, I have noted that the efforts that should be made rather than kill someone (even to stop aiding him) may be somewhat greater than the efforts required to aid someone.[34] Therefore, showing that carriage, abstinence, and surgery are not necessary to aid a fetus does not show that they are not necessary to avoid having it killed.

The next question is whether carriage, surgery, and abstinence are great enough impositions that killing the fetus is permissible in order to avoid them, given the other crucial properties of the abortion case. If they are, then Step 4 in the Cutoff Abortion Argument can be accepted. Assume that the qualitative line between certain bodily invasions and other losses is taken seriously or that the invasive surgery is major. It seems reasonable to regard the losses as significant enough so that if they are not required as aid, then killing the fetus in order to end them is justified, given that other conditions in the Cutoff Abortion Argument are met. What remains is Step 5, that there are no other alternatives that are not excessively costly to the creator.

I shall assume for each subsequent proposal that it fits into the structure of the Cutoff Abortion Argument in a similar way.

f. Proposal Two for Voluntary Creators Foreseeing a Need for Carriage

Now suppose that the voluntary creators know before creating a new person that it will definitely need carriage if it is to have any chance at all of receiving the minima. This is so for most voluntary creators in ordinary pregnancies. It also would be true for a male creator who was told before conceiving his child that when his child was one day old, it would need to be attached to the father's body for nine months in order to survive. Proposal Two states that voluntary creators are morally required to provide carriage for the fetus if they could easily have avoided creating it. For example, they would be required to provide carriage if all that had been required to avoid a pregnancy was that they not deliberately create.

However, one possible problem with Proposal Two is that refraining from deliberately creating has a cost. This is the cost of not having a child that one might otherwise have had because one would, in fact, have completed the carriage. (Strictly speaking, this cost should be the value of the child to oneself multiplied by the probability that one would have completed carriage.) Call this the *refraining cost*.[35] I appeal to this cost of not having a child to explain why a person would want to be given the opportunity to start a pregnancy without giving up the option to end such efforts as carriage. If one could not retain this option, the cost of starting the pregnancy might seem great enough that one would never attempt it and one would, thereby, suffer a lesser but still significant refraining cost.

g. Proposal Three for Voluntary Creators Foreseeing Need for Carriage

The third proposal also applies to situations in which voluntary creators foresee with certainty the need for carriage. However, unlike Proposal Two, it takes into account the refraining cost and requires only some chance of carriage being completed. In this way, it reduces the efforts required of creators, in part because it assumes that if the cost of avoiding a pregnancy is great, the cost required to complete pregnancy should be less.

The refraining cost is defined as the loss of the good to the creator that would have been produced by creating. The emphasis is on the fact that the person who creates instead of refraining stands to gain a benefit from acting. It might be argued that the refraining cost should not reduce the efforts that one is morally required to make after conceiving a child in order to provide the minima for it. The argument would be that when the cost of refraining is only the loss of the benefit that would result from not refraining, the cost does not justify one's not refraining from harming someone nor from becoming pregnant. Here are some reasons to reject this view.

(i) *The Need to Benefit.* I distinguish pregnancy in two ways from those cases in which it is *im*permissible to include the loss of the benefit of a particular behavior as part of the cost of refraining from that behavior. First, not having a child may be a serious loss and having a child can be a need. Second, creating a person, unlike harming someone, does not take away something from someone in order to satisfy one's need. Rather, it creates someone and, in a nonliteral sense, "gives" him life and thereby (nonliterally) benefits him. Indeed, a creator does these things in order to satisfy his own need. So, it might be said, someone needs to (do something like) benefit someone. However, it is still true that the fetus will be killed if the pregnancy is discontinued. In nonpregnancy cases, would the fact that someone truly needs to "benefit" someone else (and suffers a loss in not doing this) play a role in relieving him of some responsibility for continuing to "benefit" that person? The claim is that it could play such a role if other factors hold, such as the condition that the potential beneficiary will not be experientially harmed if aid is discontinued relative to prospects he had beforehand.[36]

If the refraining cost is not large, its role in reducing requirements in pregnancy will likewise be diminished, unless the creation of children has objective value. If it does have objective value, then what may be relevant is that people *should* sorely miss the children they could have, whether or not they actually miss them. If trying to have children is something they should do, then this may also help to reduce the requirements of pregnancy. This is so because if one had something like a duty to have children, then beginning a pregnancy should not be seen as exercising an option for which one should pay in higher costs to achieve the minima. (This assumes that one need not discharge the duty at such a large cost as carriage, abstinence, or surgery anyway.)

(ii) *Proposal Three and the Chance of Being Born.* Proposal Three also considers it sufficient that there be some significant chance of the offspring's receiving the minima at the foreseen cost to the woman of carriage.[37] That is, it would allow the new person to bear the risk of being aborted in exchange for its having a significant chance of gaining (what is like) a benefit of a life with the minima, taking into account the costs to the creator both of refraining from becoming pregnant and of the significant imposition represented by carriage. More specifically, suppose it was foreseen with certainty (by everyone) that the fetus would need carriage in order to receive the minima. At what level would Proposal Three set the acceptable risk of the fetus's not receiving the carriage that it would need? Perhaps at the same level of risk at which the fetus could permissibly be denied carriage by its creators when there was a chance of its developing a special condition for which it would need carriage, when carriage was not routinely necessary. (Call this level of risk *y*.)

Consider an extension of Proposal Three. Suppose that a voluntary creator decides in the middle of her pregnancy that she no longer wants to raise a child. That is, she no longer is willing to do all of *m*, which comes to something like eighteen years of child raising. Furthermore, assume that there is no one available to adopt this new person. A proponent of Proposal Three might concede that the creator knew that *m* was necessary in order for the new person to receive the minima, and that *m* is, in fact, required of voluntary bearers at some point if adoption is impossible. Yet this proponent might also claim that because *m* is significant, voluntary bearers may stop carriage at certain times because they are not willing to do all of *m*. In support of this claim, the proponent might also point to the high refraining cost. (The proponent of this view may still deny that it is permissible for creators to have abortions because they are not willing to do merely some parts of *m*.)

This further-liberalized Proposal Three is, in fact, a revision of Proposal One. Proposal One suggested that all voluntary bearers, rather than just parents, must do all of *m* for a voluntarily created person if no one else can. Proposal Three involves a moral requirement for voluntary bearers to do all of *m* only after a grace period, even if need for *m* was foreseen, Again, the suggested grounds for this grace period—persuasive or not—might be the claim that, given the size of *m*, it is permissible to make a fetus bear risks of not getting *m* in order to receive benefits, especially given the refraining cost.

h. Brief Summary

Let me summarize the overall strategy I have used up to this point in deciding how much aid the voluntarily created fetus has a right to receive and how much aid the creator has a duty to give. Voluntary creation of the fetus and foresight to its need for aid move us in the direction of greater responsibility to aid. On the other side, there are the (supposed) facts that: (1) the fetus is (in a nonliteral sense) benefited by a life with the minima; (2) a creator can create a life that (in a nonliteral sense) benefits the person born; and (3) the costs involved both in refraining from creating and in supporting a new person are great. These factors move us in the direction of less responsibility to aid and the permissibility of imposing risks on the fetus. It may seem paradoxical that deliberate creation has factors that move morally in two different directions—toward and away from greater responsibility to bear costs. Yet, I believe, this is a plausible portrayal of the role of deliberate creation in a theory of the morality of creating people. Finally, the fact that the fetus is (or is reasonably expected to be) experientially no worse off living and dying than it would be if it had never lived helps set an upper limit to efforts that might be demanded for the sake of preserving it. This is so even in the context of an ethic that demands more for it than merely having it be experientially no worse off than if it had never lived.

i. Proposal Four for Unintentional Creation but Voluntary Sex

Consider a fourth type of case: Suppose a woman unintentionally becomes pregnant as a result of a voluntary sex act. She always intended to end any unwanted pregnancy; she has a legal right to end such a pregnancy; and she would have had to give up her sex life during her reproductive years in order to avoid the chance of becoming pregnant. Such a person consciously refused to abstain from heterosexual sex, even though she knew that abstaining was necessary to ensure the nonexistence of a new person who would have no significant chance of receiving the minima (given her commitment to aborting it).

For this situation, consider Proposal Four: Since this woman would have needed to make the sacrifice of abstinence in order to avoid a pregnancy in which carriage was necessary for her fetus to receive the minima, the magnitude of the sacrifice relieves her of any responsibility for providing carriage. (This is on the assumption that she had no good reason to believe that the fetus would be much worse off experientially than if it had never existed at all if it is not carried.)

Hence Proposal Four states that it is morally permissible for this woman to use her legal right to abort. The basis for this proposal is the claim that neither men nor women are morally required to abstain totally from sex to avoid causing pregnancy. Nor need one carry someone in one's body if, hypothetically, this prevented pregnancy. If making these sacrifices were the only way to be certain of avoiding pregnancy, then if a woman becomes pregnant, she will not be morally responsible for providing carriage. The following discussion elaborates on issues related to voluntary sex but unintentional creation.

(i) *The Cost of Not Having Heterosexual Sex.* Some people may believe that for women, heterosexual sex is hardly ever truly voluntary.[38] They may believe that coercion, both blatant and subtle, often makes sexual relations compulsory for women. Suppose, for the sake of argument, that this view is correct. Then the cost of abstaining would not only be losing the good involved in sexual relations per se, but also whatever (supposed) penalty is imposed on women for not having sexual relations (for example, bad economic or social consequences, and physical or mental abuse).

Social encouragement of sexual relations transmits the message that it is right and good to have sexual relations even when no pregnancy is intended. If women follow this advice and then become pregnant, something like "moral coercion" will have put them in the position of being pregnant. Then one of the costs of not having sex will be the sense that one has failed to do something right, perhaps one's duty. But if the cost to them of doing the right act—which social encouragement says sex is— were uninterrupted carriage, then they would not truly have been morally obligated to have sex. If women were convinced by society, nevertheless, that they ought to perform this act and if this made them faultless for being pregnant, then this may be grounds for thinking that they do not have to assume responsibility for continuing carriage. Even if they had a duty to have sex, they would not have such a duty at the cost of carriage. If the cost of carriage does not relieve them of the duty to have sex, they may perform the duty without paying the cost.

Suppose that even if heterosexual relations were not thought to be important, they were important—reflecting the pursuit of real value. Suppose, in other words, that such sexual relations represented a type of activity one should invent if it did not already exist. The real value of such relations and the real cost of abstaining, despite beliefs about their value, might count in a pro-choice argument as well. But if sex that cannot cause pregnancy were an alternative good option, then abstinence from sex that can cause pregnancy would not be as costly.

Hence, the conclusion of an argument concerning the morality of abortion may vary depending on one's view of the value or necessity of heterosexual sexual relations, and on the extent to which women are encouraged or pressured to have such sex (more frequently than for intentional reproduction).

(ii) *What If Sex Should Be Avoided?* Ordinarily, if an activity should be avoided because it is bad, engaging in it could not justify the resulting harm to others. An interesting possibility is that this may not be true when what makes the activity bad is also a characteristic of the consequences of the activity, and one wants to harm someone in order to end these consequences. For example, suppose it were claimed that heterosexual sex encourages passivity and loss of independence in women.[39] Suppose also that pregnancy fostered some of these same dispositions and that these were dispositions worth avoiding. If a woman could not protect herself from becoming passive and dependent by avoiding sex, it might be argued that she should try at least to avoid the passivity and loss of independence caused by pregnancy. Notice that this sort of argument for the permissibility of abortion will succeed only if one has a moral duty to avoid certain types of character traits, or to prevent certain states of the world (for example, the control of women by men). It will not succeed if one merely has a prudent interest in avoiding certain dispositions and burdens, because it may behoove one to endure dispositions and burdens that are the result of not doing what one should have done to avoid them in the first place. (There may be other reasons to avoid sex which have this feature of being reasons to avoid pregnancy as well. For example, a person may be too young to engage in it. If one should avoid sex because one is too young, one presumably should also avoid childbearing for the same reason.)

(iii) *Abstinence to Avoid Miscarriage?* A case worth thinking about in connection with responsibilities due to voluntary sex is one in which abstinence would be physically required to avoid pregnancies that we accurately foresee will unavoidably miscarry. That is, consider a woman who cannot tell in advance on which occasion of intercourse she will conceive, and she always miscarries whenever she does conceive. In her case, total abstinence would be required to avoid pregnancies that will certainly miscarry. Suppose that she has no moral responsibility to abstain in order to prevent conceiving a fetus without the minima coming about in *this* way, on the assumption that the fetus will be experientially no worse off living and dying than it would be if it had never lived. Then should she have to abstain to avoid becoming pregnant or else, if she becomes pregnant, be required to provide carriage if this will help the fetus gain the minima?

The answer to this question is complicated by the fact that it may be morally permissible to require less sacrifice in order to avoid creating a person who will definitely be miscarried than in order to save that person once conceived. There are at least two separate reasons why this might be so. First, the efforts made to avoid a pregnancy, unlike comparable efforts made after conception to save the fetus's life, do not result in a new person living a good life. Second, one cannot be sure that abstinence is in fact necessary on each occasion it is practiced to prevent a fetus without the minima (that is, not all sex acts would result in pregnancy). Therefore, most of the sacrifice of abstinence is probably wasted.

Suppose that the efforts that could be required to avoid creation were lower than those that could be required to save the resulting fetus. Then one could not automatically conclude that one need not provide carriage in order to save a life just because one need not abstain over a reproductive lifetime (or, hypothetically, make prenatal efforts comparable to carriage) to prevent conceiving a fetus that could not possibly be saved once it was conceived.

Perhaps the following is the correct way to show that abstinence is so large a sacrifice that failing to make it will not result in responsibility for carrying a fetus: One should not require a woman to abstain from sex during her childbearing years by total abstinence when *all* sex leads to pregnancies that miscarry, just to prevent a fetus that will not have the minima. One also should not require a woman to perform carriage (or abstinence) if this were necessary to save an existing fetus that she did *not* create. If a woman is pregnant as a result of not completely abstaining, the costs required of her to save her fetus should be no greater than that of a woman who did not create the fetus, as the woman who created it has done nothing to merit raising the costs she must pay relative to those the women who did not create the fetus must pay.

In addition, the fact that abstaining is necessary to avoid becoming pregnant might relieve one of the responsibility to pay the lesser cost m once the fetus has been conceived. This is so even if these efforts are required of voluntary creators. This amounts to the claim that those who voluntarily create new persons have greater responsibilities for them than nonvoluntary creators do.

Would a woman be obligated to pay cost m (or its equivalent) to avoid becoming pregnant with a fetus that will definitely miscarry? (I am supposing that this cost would be useful in this way, as abstinence in fact is.) It might be argued that she would not, because: (1) paying the cost on any given occasion is of uncertain usefulness; (2) no fetus will exist who is helped to live a better life because of such costs; and (3) she is not in a voluntary bearer relationship to a fetus. Suppose it were known on which occasion she would conceive so that (1) did not apply. Would a woman have to pay cost m to avoid conceiving on this occasion? I do not think so. Would just any woman (analogous to an innocent bystander) be morally obligated to pay cost m once she confronts an existing fetus who needs to have cost m expended in order to receive the minima? Presumably not. Has a woman who has conceived because of a blameless voluntary act (i.e., not doing m to avoid the act) thereby increased her responsibility to pay cost m for the sake of the fetus? It seems not. Hence, she too should not be required to do m for her fetus.

The responsibility for paying cost m in order to save a fetus once it exists should be tied (if it is tied to anything) to having performed a voluntary act that could easily have been avoided, if one foresaw that the act would create a fetus. Alternatively, paying cost m should be tied to having intentionally conceived a fetus when the cost of avoiding intentional conception was not too high (as argued previously).

(iv) *Contraception.* The use of contraceptive devices is a way of reducing both the chances of pregnancy and the cost of avoiding pregnancy (by comparison to abstinence). Nevertheless, contraception does not diminish the chances of becoming pregnant as much as abstinence does, and using contraception has its own possible health cost. It is useful to reconsider my discussion of unintentional pregnancy resulting from voluntary acts to evaluate whether refusal to pay the cost of contraception (rather than abstinence, *m*, or carriage, if these were useful [hypothetically] in avoiding pregnancy) should make people responsible for providing carriage in order to ensure that their fetuses obtain the minima.

Suppose that contraception were relatively costless (on all dimensions). Then its use could well be required and a woman who did not use it and became pregnant could have a responsibility to carry the fetus. If a woman did use contraceptives, then it might be argued that this not only reduces the possibility of pregnancy but also how much she owes to an unintended fetus. That is, it may be seen as a way of engaging in sex nonnegligently, in which case it should limit the extent of the effort a woman would have to make if she became pregnant anyway. This assumes, first, that she need not abstain over the course of a reproductive life to avoid becoming pregnant or else provide carriage simply because she did not abstain in this way, and, second, that the chance of pregnancy with contraception is sufficiently small.

The general idea here is that, in itself, avoiding a life that will be without the minima may be worth imposing cost $m - x$ (for some value of x) on those who have not caused such a fetus's conception as well as on those who cause it as a mere side effect of sex. Intentionally causing pregnancy can change the required efforts to cost m. But not taking small precautions to prevent the pregnancy, in the absence of attempting to create a good new life and a significant chance for the new person to gain such a benefit, can raise the required efforts to cost $m + x$ = carriage. Therefore, the wrong of not taking simple precautions could be said to raise the required efforts above even those required in an intentional pregnancy.

j. A Proposal for Fetuses Conceived by Rape

In the case of rape, no act undertaken by the woman gives her any responsibility to undergo carriage, abstinence, or surgery for the sake of her genetically related fetus, even though it ought to have the minima. Furthermore, if it is aborted, the fetus is not experientially harmed relative to prospects it had before conception, and it does not lose anything that the woman is morally responsible for its having that it could retain independently of her.

k. Overall Summary

In sum, the arguments for various types of pregnancies based on the Benefit-Burden Approach assume that if a fetus is a person, it has a right to have its voluntary creators try to provide the minima for it at cost *m* to themselves. The voluntary creators (or their substitutes) have a duty to pay cost m, which is assumed to be less than carriage, abstinence, or surgery. The fetal person then also has a right, at most, to have other parties who may potentially cause its existence pay cost m or less to avoid its being without the minima. These claims will be correct at least if the fetus is not experientially worse off without the minima than never living at all, and also if it had a significant chance to gain the benefits of life from voluntary creators. Alternatively, this significant chance may compensate it for ending up experientially worse off than never living. The responsibility of the potential creator includes efforts that she morally must make to prevent the fetus's conception. Suppose that efforts up to cost m could be required but are useless to prevent conception because (hypothetically) only carriage, abstinence, or surgery alone would be sufficient. Then carriage, abstinence, or surgery cannot be required of a creator if the pregnancy occurs and these would help provide minima. Carriage, abstinence, or surgery can be required to keep a fetus alive only if the creator failed to do what he or she should have done to avoid conception. Note that both sexes can be required to make efforts to avoid conception and to make postnatal sacrifices.

Furthermore, it is actually less than cost m that should be required of someone to prevent conception. Before conception, no voluntary bearer relationship exists. There is no life that will be saved or benefited by paying cost m, only one that can be prevented. Possibly efforts may also be wasted if conception would not have occurred each time the participants had sex. The problem here is to find out how much a potential creator, who is not involved in any voluntary bearer relation with a new person, is morally obligated to do in order to prevent that person from being conceived, when the new person ideally should not exist without the minima, should be provided with the minima at up to cost m from voluntary creators, but can itself be expected to bear some risks.

The proposals for particular cases we have discussed generally acknowledge the responsibility for avoiding the conception of a life that will not have the minima. But because life is seen as a good thing to be born into, the proposals also emphasize that it is acceptable to impose risk on the fetus and even to reduce the responsibilities of those who can produce a good new life. In some respects, those who attempt to create a child have greater responsibilities than do those who try to avoid pregnancy but become pregnant anyway. And in some respects, they have fewer responsibilities than do those who do not make sufficient efforts to avoid pregnancy. This view takes seriously whether there is a real chance for a new life with the goods of life and also how people become pregnant.

The Benefit-Burden Approach builds on the Cutoff Abortion Argument but incorporates a great concern for providing the minima. Step 5 in the Cutoff Abortion Argument permits a woman to refuse to make efforts that, *considered individually*, are greater than she would have to make in order to avoid having the fetus killed, given the other circumstances of the abortion. However, if there is great concern about providing the minima, then a differential standard may be more appropriate. That is, one should compare the cost to the woman of the procedure resulting in death of the fetus (abortion) with the cost to her of the procedure that preserves fetal life, and determine whether *the difference* required for the life-preserving procedure is greater than the cost that someone would be obligated to bear to avoid having the fetus killed. The costs may include the later bad consequences to the woman of that life-preserving procedure, but may not include the later bad consequences to her of the mere success of that procedure (that is, the consequences of the newly created person being alive). This leaves it open that it is permissible not to endure a procedure whose cost, in comparison with the alternatives, is greater than necessary to avoid having the fetus killed, even if the desire not to endure the procedure stems from concern over the mere success of the procedure. That is, the woman need not make the excessive effort to bring about a state of affairs that she wants to avoid (such as the existence of a person genetically related to her).

One significant limitation on requiring a procedure that is only a bit more burdensome than an abortion is that even when an additional burden is small, it may come in addition to so much already endured that it simply cannot be demanded.

I. Steps in the Benefit-Burden Approach Corresponding to Those in the Cutoff Abortion Argument

On the basis of the previous proposals for different types of pregnancies, let me now describe five conditions of the Benefit-Burden Approach corresponding to the conditions in the Cutoff Abortion Argument, for three types of cases. Satisfying these conditions would make abortions permissible.

(1) RAPE

Step 1a. Need for support in a woman's body (carriage) does not by itself give a right to have such aid begin, or a duty to begin it, even for a person who may claim the minima from someone.

Step 1b. Need alone does not give a right to have continuing support, or a duty to provide it.

Step 2a. The woman has no special obligations to begin such support.

Step 2b. The woman has no special obligations to continue such support.

Step 3. By being killed, the fetus loses only the life provided by its imposition on the woman's body that is justified by neither need nor special obligation. The fetus is not experientially harmed relative to prospects it (nonliterally) had before being conceived,[40] and it does not lose anything the woman is morally responsible for its having that it could retain independently of her.

Step 4. One may kill the fetus in order to stop efforts significant enough to justify such killing, given the other conditions.

Step 5. In this context, the increase in cost to the woman in using any other procedure that could save the fetus's life is excessively large relative to abortion, even given the aim of not killing the fetus.

(2) VOLUNTARY PREGNANCY FORESEEING THE NEED FOR CARRIAGE

Step 1a. Same as the preceding Step 1a.

Step 1b. Same as the preceding Step 1b.

Step 2a. The woman has no special obligation to begin carriage for a fetus she voluntarily created but which is gestating in a lab if the refraining cost is sufficiently high, if the fetus is not experientially harmed by living and dying relative to (nonliteral) preconception prospects, or if the chance of its receiving the "benefit" of life is sufficiently high so that it would be permissible to impose a risk of the fetus's not receiving it. (Perhaps the chance is so high that it would be permissible to impose a risk of the fetus's being experientially harmed relative to never existing.)

Step 2b. The woman has no special obligation to continue carriage of a fetus begun in her body (for example, to prevent a miscarriage) for the reasons given in Step 2a.

Step 3. Same as the preceding Step 3.

Step 4. Same as the preceding Step 4.

Step 5. Same as the preceding Step 5.

(3) VOLUNTARY SEX FORESEEING (A POSSIBILITY OF) PREGNANCY AND ITS REQUIREMENTS

Step 1a. Same as the preceding Step 1a.

Step 1b. Same as the preceding Step 1b.

Step 2a. The woman has no special obligation to provide carriage if the abstaining cost is sufficiently high and if the fetus is not experientially harmed by living and dying relative to its preconception prospects.[41]

Step 2b. The woman has no special obligation to continue carriage, for the reasons given in Step 2a.

Step 3. Same as the preceding Step 3.

Step 4. Same as the preceding Step 4.

Step 5. Same as the preceding Step 5.

m. Limits to the Approach

1

I have argued on the assumption that the fetus is a person throughout pregnancy. I emphasize this, for it is not necessarily possible to use either the Cutoff Abortion Argument or the Benefit-Burden Approach to justify aborting a fetus at a stage when it is a person *if* it is not a person throughout pregnancy. In other words, if the fetus were a person from conception, there would be no time when it would be possible to abort a nonperson. Therefore, it matters less whether one has an early or late abortion, for one will be aborting a person whenever one aborts. However, if the fetus develops into (or gives rise to) a person, then abortion would be possible at a time when one would not be killing a person. If killing a nonperson (even one with the potential to become a person) is a far less serious matter than killing a person, one will have lost the opportunity to perform a morally less serious act by failing to abort early.[42]

Suppose that a woman wants to have an abortion, and the fetus has already *developed* into (or given rise to) a person. She cannot simply argue for the permissibility of killing a person in the manner that either Thomson or I have used. Rather, she must argue for the permissibility of killing a person given that she failed to take advantage of the opportunity to end her pregnancy without killing a person. This may be harder to do than simply arguing for the permissibility of killing what was always a person. Indeed, the general structure of one's thinking about this issue is a variant of the general question I have already considered in discussing voluntary sex with unintended pregnancy: How much must one do in order to avoid producing a person whom one will then kill? Having an abortion early then becomes analogous to avoiding the conception of a person. As we did when considering avoiding conception, we would have to consider whether an early abortion was not undertaken because of coercion (comparable to rape), because of the efforts required (comparable to abstinence), or because of a voluntary decision.

It is ironic that those who take the view that a person exists from conception onward provide a premise that could make later abortions more permissible than do those who work with the premise that the fetus develops into a person. (On the other hand, those who accept the development premise make the justification for having conceived less crucial, given that it is a less serious matter to conceive and quickly abort what is not yet a person.)

2

Means of gestation external to the womb that eliminate the need for the creator's carriage present interesting problems for both the Benefit-Burden Approach and the Cutoff Abortion Argument on the assumption that the fetus is a person.[43]

Assume that there are at least two different types of mechanical external gestation (MEG) devices: a partial (PEG) one and a total (TEG) one. A PEG pregnancy must begin in the womb, but it essentially provides early viability for a fetus who can be removed from the womb. Both the Benefit-Burden Approach and the Cutoff Abortion Argument are in certain ways connected to the view that (nonliterally) the fetus would be no worse off if it were killed than if it had never been in the woman's body. Of course, this is far from being a sufficient—and in the Benefit-Burden Approach not even a necessary—condition for the permissibility of abortion. (That is, we allowed that the risk of being worse off than if one had never existed might be worth the chance of a life with minima, or at least be acceptable given the chance for minima along with other factors in creating people that point in the direction of reduced costs for creators.)

However, if it is possible to move a fetus to a PEG, another relevant comparison is introduced: The fetus will be worse off if it is aborted than it would be in a machine, where it does not need to impose on the woman in order to continue living. If there is a better alternative for the fetus than death by abortion, which also removes it from a woman's body with no additional costs to her, why should a woman be permitted to have an abortion? Perhaps she should be morally obligated either to go through with the pregnancy or to transfer the fetus safely.

Suppose also that the fetus would have a safer gestation in a machine than in a woman *who is willing* to carry it. Then the woman's body, which the fetus does not need, would stand in the way of the fetus's better prospects. What right has she then to continue the pregnancy rather than to transfer the fetus to a PEG?

These considerations help explain the significance of viability accompanied by actual removal for the abortion discussion, independently of identifying viability with a crucial stage in fetal development. Consideration of a PEG method also reveals the possibility of a dilemma for those who are both concerned for the fetus's welfare and intent on having women be gestating mothers. The reason is that removing a fetus from a woman's womb might often improve its welfare. That is, the interests of fetuses and women may conflict if it were only in the woman's interest to continue pregnancy.

What can we say about these considerations? First, they may depend on its being true that the procedure to remove the fetus from the woman itself requires no greater sacrifice than the woman would have to make in order to save the fetus's life or to avoid having it killed. If this were not so and removal did require a greater sacrifice, a woman need not make it. There would then be no morally relevant alternative to abortion that promised a better existence for the fetus that could be used for comparative purposes: The fetus may be worse off if killed than if transferred to PEG, but not worse off than it had a right to be.

We have already noted that the Benefit-Burden Approach may have a result different from that of the Cutoff Abortion Argument on the issue of whether we consider burdens differentially or nondifferentially. That is, given the approach's concern for achieving the minima, what is crucial is whether the difference in burden between removal to a machine and abortion is greater than the woman would have to endure in order to ensure that the fetus obtained the minima. If concern for the fetus getting the minima were the sole determining factor, the same should be true when a woman wants to carry through with a pregnancy: We should see whether the difference in physical cost between transferring the fetus to a machine and continuing the pregnancy is greater than the woman would have to pay in order to avoid imposing the risks on the fetus that come from its being in her womb.

What if the abortion procedure or live birth involves equal or greater risk for the woman than the fetus's removal to the machine, but the latter effort is still greater than required in order to help the fetus? Should its removal, which is better for the fetus, then be required?

Consider abortion first. To prefer running a big risk in abortion so as not to produce a person whose mere existence would be a disturbance to oneself seems morally suspect (even though the alternative would be to have surgery, a cost that one need not pay to bring about an end that one does not like). Given how the Benefit-Burden Approach derives a right not to continue with carriage, it would not endorse this abortion. This is also the conclusion of the Benefit-Burden Approach when PEG is not available, and carriage is necessary to avoid an abortion that is even more risky than carriage. Then the woman's not wanting to contribute great efforts to produce an outcome that will be burdensome to her on account of the fetus's mere existence is not an acceptable reason for having an abortion. Furthermore, in the case of voluntary creation, in which one conceives because of the desire to produce a new person, changing one's mind and paying a higher price in abortion than in carriage to avoid the new person's existence would not be permitted. These restrictions on avoiding great efforts (carriage) which are nevertheless comparatively smaller than some others (in this imagined abortion) stem from the concern for what is owed to a new person. It is only if differential effort necessary to save the fetus is greater than what the woman would need to do to help the fetus that she is not required to make the effort. This is true even if she decides not to make the effort because she prefers the new person not exist.

Now consider the arguments for requiring the fetus's removal to a PEG even if a woman wants to continue carrying. These arguments depend on the assumption that if someone or something is available to do more for the fetus than its current bearer would do, the current bearer who chooses to continue must do as much for the fetus as the alternative or else lose the fetus to the other bearer. As noted when discussing the Creation Factors, this is not a standard to which we hold even voluntary parents, although it is a standard to which we often hold other caretakers. That is, we sometimes know even before pregnancy that potential adoptive parents would do much more for the new person than its natural parents would. But we still do not raise the requirements of acceptable parenthood for the natural parents. We do not expect them to do what the adoptive parents would have done, on pain of losing their newborns. Likewise, if a parent refuses to rush into a burning building to save his newborn infant, the fact that someone else is willing to rush in does not mean that the parent will lose custody of the infant, so long as running into burning buildings has not been established as a parental duty.

This noncomparative determination of parental duties might help explain why a person who wanted to be pregnant would not be obligated to give up the fetus to a PEG. The interests of voluntary bearers and parents in keeping their offspring, not only the minima interests of offspring, must be considered when these interests conflict. The psychological cost to the pregnant person who wants to be pregnant of making the fetus better off by not going through with the pregnancy herself is, perhaps, greater than she must endure.

The noncomparative determination of duties is also relevant to the view that someone whose fetus survives an abortion has lost any right to it, as she abandoned it in trying to have an abortion. If having an abortion is a way of refusing residence in one's body and the erstwhile bearer has no obligation to provide such residence, then she will be refusing nothing she was required to give. Legal abandonment means only a refusal to give what one is required to give. Therefore, a woman might still have a claim to her fetus if it survived abortion.

Now suppose that TEG (total external gestation) became available. How would this affect the Benefit-Burden Approach? The effect of PEG was limited in part by the possibility that the removal procedure might itself be an impermissible imposition on the woman for the fetus's sake. But TEG does not include such a procedure. Rather, in a voluntary pregnancy it means choosing between beginning the pregnancy in an external device and beginning it in one's body. Suppose that a woman chooses to have the pregnancy in her body, even if it were predicted that a machine would gestate the fetus safely. It might be argued that she should be prohibited from having an abortion (assuming the fetus is a person) on any ground at all. The reason is that she would then deprive the fetus of a safe environment which it could have had without imposing on her. This may result in her being obligated, on pain of making the fetus worse off than it would have been without her assistance, to provide it with just as good a gestation. (The same problem would arise for someone who started a pregnancy in a machine and then decided to implant it in her body rather than keep it in the machine.)

We already noted that in pregnancy as it is now, we foresee that a fetus will be dependent. However, the creator does not make it dependent when it could have been independent. If TEG were available and a woman did not use it, she would be choosing to make a fetus dependent on her when it could exist without being dependent on her and (unlike PEG) there would be no physical imposition on her required in order to use TEG. (The problems that stem from voluntarily creating dependencies that can be avoided will also increase if we are ever able to decide whether people begin life as fully developed adults or as infants.)

The claim that technology that may help increase the freedom of women should not have bad consequences for them seems an inappropriate response to the conclusion that a woman who does not use TEG may not have an abortion. The argument uses ordinary reasoning that could apply as well to the following case: Suppose that men had special capacities to help dying violinists and sometimes voluntarily let their bodies be so used. Then an artificial device was developed to help the violinists. If a man still insisted on helping, there is good reason to believe he must meet the standard of the machine since he deprived the violinist of that alternative.

Here is a possible counterargument: The loss to at least some women of not carrying a fetus in their own bodies may be so great—even though with TEG this no longer means not having a genetically related child—that they would rather not have children than have them in TEG. But by not having children, they will suffer a large personal cost and also prevent the existence of a new life. The violinist will be plugged into the machine if not into the man, but there will be no fetus to plug into a machine if the woman refuses the options of either using a TEG or being committed to an uninterruptible pregnancy. Given these costs (no fetus, unhappy woman), should we refuse to raise the requirements of pregnancy so as to ensure the same outcome as we could achieve by using a machine?

Unless there is a shortage of children, the threat of not having a child is not very effective, especially because there is no person who is literally deprived by not being created. We therefore are left with the costs to the woman as the dominant consideration.

We need to decide in regard to machine substitutes whether there is a morally crucial difference between pregnancy and the case of the violinist. This difference may be that once again, the standard to which parents and bearers are held when we decide what they are obligated to do for their offspring is not set by the best that would be done for the offspring by others. Why is this? Both the desire of some people to bear children in their bodies and the cost to them of not having children in this way may be so significant that they compete with the interests of the fetus. This may account for the permissibility of not having to sacrifice a womb pregnancy and of our not raising the amount of risk that women must take during that pregnancy in order to match the good outcome of a TEG.

E. THE IMMIGRATION ARGUMENT

The Benefit-Burden Approach emphasizes that creators may owe their creations more than people ordinarily owe to other people. However, there is another approach to abortion that I wish briefly to explore. I shall call this approach the Immigration Argument. It suggests that although creators have greater responsibilities than merely ensuring that their creations will be experientially no worse off than if they had never existed, abortion is permissible because creators owe to new persons still in the womb *less* than they owe to other people.

Thomson's approach to abortion assumes that one is not obligated to share one's body for a long period with a violinist in order to save his life.[44] But suppose that people were entitled by law to share each other's bodies; there might be a social contract to this effect because it would maximize the number of lives saved or maximize the ex-ante probability of each person's survival. Would it follow then that in such a society, a fetus (assumed to be a person) also had a right to use another person's body? It might not follow if one thought of the fetus as analogous to an immigrant who was on his way into the society rather than as someone who is already a member of the society—it could be a person but not yet a citizen. Assume that one understood the right to bodily support in order to save a life not as a universal right of persons—that is, something to which persons have a right (or come to have a right) just because they are persons—but as a special right granted to members of the particular society in which the special contract is enforced. In addition, suppose that the members of the society were those who had already made the "immigration journey"—that is, the passage requiring assistance in someone's body that began with nonexistence. Then it might be that the immigration journey into the society and the need for support during that journey would not be covered by the rights enjoyed by people who had already made the journey.

Would it be morally unreasonable for citizens of such a society to decide whether immigrants should have rights equal to those of established citizens, based on factors such as those presented by the Benefit-Burden Approach? That is, deciding, based on how much the immigrants' having such full-fledged rights would impose on the full-fledged citizens, and on how badly off the immigrants would be without full-fledged rights in comparison to how they otherwise would have been if they had not started the journey (what risks for benefits they might be expected to bear, etc.)?[45]

F. INFANTICIDE AND CHILD ABANDONMENT

Is it true that if it were permissible to kill a fetus that is a person, then infanticide would also be permissible, as Ronald Dworkin suggests?[46] The argument I have given for killing the fetus justifies killing in order to stop residence in a woman's body. It does not justify killing an infant who is not attached to the woman's body, since we do not then need to kill it in order for it not to be imposing on the woman's body. Is it true, as Dworkin suggests (p. 111), that if it were permissible to kill a fetus that is a person, it would also be permissible to abandon one's children? I have argued for a distinction between being voluntary creators and parents. In addition, I have argued that there are duties of parents that do not involve imposition on their bodies in the manner of pregnancy. Perhaps even parents are not morally required to let their bodies be used in this way, but that does not mean that they may refuse to perform other tasks for their children.

G. WAITING PERIODS AND INFORMED CONSENT

Dworkin argues that it may be permissible for the State to require women to wait or to obtain certain information before making an abortion decision, so long as this does not interfere with their right to abort. His reason is that the State has a right to encourage its citizens to think responsibly about matters of life and death (pp. 153–54). However, he thinks that those who believe the fetus is a person should not be satisfied with required waiting periods and information (p. 244 note 8).

I have argued that if the fetus were a person, it may be permissible to abort it. I have not argued that if the fetus were a person, the decision to abort should be left *entirely* to the woman. If one assumes that the fetus is a person, some organ of the State, such as the Supreme Court, would be needed to decide when it is permissible to kill a person residing in a woman. Then, within the officially endorsed range of permissibility, it would be up to the woman to decide whether she will seek assistance in killing the person or not. If abortion were morally and legally permissible in all types of pregnancies, even if the fetus were a person, there would be no chance that the woman would do what is morally or legally prohibited in having an abortion.

Still it is an important decision whether to have a person killed or not, and so waiting periods and requirements of full information might be acceptable.[47] But the information provided should include not only reasons why one might not choose abortion, but also arguments for the permissibility of abortion and reasons why abortion might be the right choice to make. Just because a person desires an abortion, it does not follow that she realizes that her desire does not contravene any moral requirements or that it is supported by good reasons. Furthermore, if having an abortion is morally permissible killing that terminates aid, cases of abortion and other cases in which people will die if not aided should be handled consistently. For example, if the State requires information and waiting periods in abortion, the State might also require information and waiting periods for people who are refusing to give organs to others who will die without a transplant.

Notes

1. This is a revised version of the summary of my book *Creation and Abortion: A Study in Moral and Legal Philosophy* (New York: Oxford University Press, 1992), which appeared as part of "Review: Abortion and the Value of Life: A Discussion of 'Life's Dominion'" (a review of *Life's Dominion: An Argument about Abortion, Euthanasia, and Individual Freedom* by Ronald Dworkin), *Columbia Law Review* 95(1) (January 1995): 160–222. A revised version of the first part of that review is chapter 11, this volume

2. See Judith J. Thomson, "A Defense of Abortion," *Philosophy & Public Affairs* 1(1) (1971): 47, 48–49.

3. She thought that mere detaching was a killing. I think it is not a killing. Given that a third party acts as your agent to end support you are providing, this seems to be a letting die. Nevertheless, Thomson considered active killing in her next article on the topic, "Rights and Deaths," *Philosophy & Public Affairs* 2(2) (1973), and considered that this would be permissible, too. In *Creation and Abortion*, I tried to take account of all the ways the violinist (and fetus) might die due to removal from someone's body.

4. We could also imagine cases where someone does not need to be attached to your body but, once attached, becomes dependent on your body for life support.

5. I note "at that time" (and shall assume it henceforth) in order to avoid cases in which someone we kill loses only what he would have had as a result of our help given years ago.

6. Though mere detaching by method (1) is *active*, it is (arguably) a letting die.

7. I am here assuming that abortion is permissible only in order to determine whether a life that ends with no injustice would still be worse than never living. Some may think that the reason for concern with abortion is the possible pain to the fetus. A life with pain and no goods is worse than nonexistence, but this cannot be the problem with abortion. If it were, the moral problem of abortion would disappear if we gave the fetus an anesthetic, as we are assuming is possible in all our cases.

8. This view is well expressed in Thomas Nagel, "Death," reprinted in his *Mortal Questions* (Cambridge: Cambridge University Press, 1979), pp. 1–10.

9. For more on this issue, see chapter 15 this volume.

10. I first used the case of women who miscarry in F. M. Kamm, "The Problem of Abortion," in *Ethics for Modern Life*, 2nd ed., eds. Raziel Abelson and Marie Friquegnon (Boston: St. Martins, 1982), pp. 103, 111. Dr. Robert Morris, of the New York University Medical Center, confirmed my suspicions that women who know they run a high risk of miscarrying are not blamed for trying to conceive. Of course, actual attitudes of many people may be based on the supposition that the fetus is not a person. Telephone interview with Robert Morris, New York University Medical Center, 1980.

11. Dworkin's view on abortion emphasizes this. See chapter 11 this volume.

12. Notice that I have not relied on an equality-of-the-sexes argument in constructing the Cutoff Abortion Argument. Indeed, I believe that one may want to question an Equality Argument for abortion on three points: (1) It may be wrong if it suggests that abortion would be morally *im*permissible if its permissibility were not necessary to achieve social equality of the sexes. In other words, if women were socially dominant over men, or if both men and women could get pregnant, would abortion be impermissible? (2) It may be wrong if it claims that one may kill someone simply because this is necessary for social equality. It would not be permissible to kill infants, detached from anyone's body, if their existence led to social inequality because women but not men could not resist taking care of them. (3) The Equality Argument would be wrong if it suggested that abortion would not be permissible if a right to decide whether to abort actually reduced women's power relative to men's overall because, hypothetically, women's power stems from having many children.

This does not mean, however, that we should not consider a role for equality in the Cutoff Abortion Argument. For instance, equality might be a reason that justifies exercising one's right to decide whether to have an abortion, a right that is justified on grounds other than a concern for equality. Alternatively, concern for equality might combine with the fact that in pregnancy one's body is being used to provide someone with life. For example, if even a small imposition on the woman's body resulted in large inequality for a particular woman, avoiding this cost to her could play a role in the Cutoff Abortion Argument's Steps 4 and 5 if added to efforts in pregnancy.

13. See note 8 and accompanying text.

14. For a discussion of this distinction, see F. M. Kamm, *Morality, Mortality*, Vol. 1 (New York: Oxford University Press, 1993).

15. These are factors I have pointed to in comparing pre-natal nonexistense of a *living person* with his death. See, for example, *Morality, Mortality*, Vol. 1. Here I discuss them in comparing total nonexistence of a person with death of a person.

16. On what makes death bad, see also chapter 1 this volume and *Morality, Mortality*, Vol. 1.

17. I also discuss the ethics of creating people in chapter 15 and chapter 16 this volume.

18. I first suggested an approach along these lines in 1972. See F. M. Kamm, "Abortion: A Philosophical Analysis," *Feminist Studies* 1 (1972): 49–62. I developed it in detail in *Creation and Abortion*.

19. I deliberately leave open the number and quality of years.

20. See John Rawls, *A Theory of Justice* (Cambridge, MA: Harvard University Press, 1971), pp. 136–42. Rawls himself does not consider whether the fetus should be treated as a person from behind the veil.

21. I discuss these issues in F. M. Kamm, "Harming Some to Save Others," *Philosophical Studies* 57 (1989): 227; in *Morality, Mortality*, Vol. 2 (New York: Oxford University Press, 1996); and in *Intricate Ethics* (New York: Oxford University Press, 2007).

22. Response by Ronald Dworkin to comments by F. M. Kamm, New York University Law School Colloquium on Law, Philosophy, and Social Theory, October 31, 1991.

23. Again, I realize that much needs to be said to defend this claim, and also much might be said to oppose it. But I am concerned here with identifying certain factors that have some plausibility, to see what they would imply if they were true.

24. If human life were not worth living and were for this reason unlike a benefit, then the fetus would not be deprived of much if it was aborted.

25. In her "Wrongful Life, Procreative Responsibility, and the Significance of Harm," *Legal Theory* 5 (1999): 117–48. My discussion on Shiffrin has not been previously published and was added subsequent to publication of the article on which this chapter is based.

26. In chapter 15 this volume, I discuss Shiffrin's argument when the issue is not abortion but the quality of longer lives for the people we create. However, my discussion there bears on the part of Step (5) that points to the ordinary limits of parents' responsibilities to assume burdens for their offspring as grounds for limits on their responsibilities to prevent harm to the fetus. Though I have raised the question of whether, on Shiffrin's account of life as a pure benefit and the Gold Cube Case, she can think that death of a fetus person is a harm to it, I am willing to assume that death would be a harm to a fetal person.

27. For more on whether prospect of benefits can outweigh lesser harms or risk of greater harms in deciding to create, see further discussion in chapters 15 and 16 this volume. Notice that I have helped myself to the idea of a quasi-obligation to participate in the human enterprise. Yet I also believe that having the right to decide whether to procreate saves the procreator from thinking of herself as a mere part of nature. For these two approaches to be consistent, it would have to be claimed that, once in existence, a person may choose whether to participate in the ongoing human enterprise via biological reproduction, but there is no such requirement of choice on being created to be a choosing person.

28. For more on these issues, see chapter 15 this volume.

29. This part of the summary was phrased by Shelly Kagan.

30. Increasingly, there is a call in Western societies for people to reproduce when they do not want to, in order to stop a falling birth rate or to preserve certain so-called desirable genes in the gene pool. Individuals who would not otherwise reproduce but who respond to this call voluntarily are, strictly speaking, voluntary creators. In fact, however, they can be compared with soldiers who respond to their nation's call: They believe that they are obligated to reproduce. The following discussion of voluntary creators does not necessarily apply to them, or to others who reproduce as a matter of duty.

31. An exception to this—the case in which someone can produce only a significantly handicapped child—is discussed at note 36.

32. While abstinence is realistically a way of avoiding an unintended pregnancy, it also may be imagined to be a sacrifice required of a voluntary creator to obtain the minima for his creation. I am imagining, for purposes of argument, a hypothetical case in which a creator's abstinence for the rest of his reproductive years would help him provide the minima to the person he created.

33. It may also be worth distinguishing in other ways among the different efforts encompassed by cost *m*. For example, suppose the activities typically carried out by mothers are not activities they would engage in if they were not necessary for raising a family. Suppose the activities typically carried out by fathers (e.g., their jobs) are activities they would engage in even if they had no family to support. This may suggest that the latter have some intrinsic value missing in the former, and are in that sense less of a burden.

34. See above, part I, discussion of Step 3 (pp. 187–188).

35. This cost of refraining from deliberately creating a child should, obviously, be distinguished from the cost of abstaining from sexual intercourse.

36. The fact that there is a cost in not deliberately attempting to have a child is also relevant to a decision about the morality of creating a child when one cannot aim at the minima because it is impossible to obtain them. That is, consider someone who can give birth only to a handicapped child of limited intelligence who will not suffer over its twenty-year lifetime. Would it be immoral to create such a child in order to fulfill one's desire to have genetically related offspring? It might be argued that if the refraining cost is understandably high—that is, if it is not unreasonable to want such a child very much given the absence of an alternative—it is permissible to conceive the child.

37. How this significant chance comes about may also be relevant. That is, perhaps the chance must be present because there is some intention to have the child, rather than because one foresees that abortions will be difficult to obtain. Those who think intention is not relevant to permissibility would dispute this.

38. Catherine MacKinnon seems to take this view. See her *Feminism Unmodified: Discourses on Life and Law* (Cambridge, MA: Harvard University Press, 1987).

39. Freud's view inverts this causal order: Passivity precedes and causes a desire for heterosexual intercourse. See his "The Psychology of Women" in *Sigmund Freud: New Introductory Lectures on Psychoanalysis*, ed. James Strachey (New York: W.W. Norton, 1964).

40. According to both the Benefit-Burden Approach and the Cutoff Abortion Argument, in cases of rape many abortions may be permissible even if the fetus would be experientially harmed relative to its preconception prospects. Therefore, this condition is sufficient but not necessary.

41. I cannot here add, "and/or the probability of a pregnancy in which the fetus will be experientially harmed is sufficiently low." This is because the Benefit-Burden Approach does not allow one to run such risks to the fetus unless there is expected benefit to the fetus, and I have assumed there is none in this type of pregnancy because an abortion will definitely be sought.

42. I am assuming knowledge of the pregnancy and an opportunity to end it from conception onward. If the fetus never becomes a person during pregnancy, the issue I am discussing does not arise. I first discussed this issue in *Creation and Abortion*.

43. I first discussed this issue in *Creation and Abortion*.

44. See note 2 and accompanying text.

45. In his discussion of my *Creation and Abortion*, Jeff McMahan criticizes some of the arguments I have presented in Part II, sections A-E. See Jeff McMahan, "The Right to Choose an Abortion," *Philosophy & Public Affairs* 22 (1993): 331. McMahan discusses only the case of voluntary sex with unintended pregnancy and argues against the permissibility of abortion in this case, assuming for the sake of argument that the fetus is a person. He does not dispute the permissibility of killing in rape cases. Let me take this opportunity to respond briefly.

McMahan argues by using his Dependent Child Case, in which a biological mother is called upon to aid her child with carriage when the child is three. In this case, (a) the child was the product of voluntary sex with precautions, and abstinence would have been the cost to avoid any risk of pregnancy; (b) it was foreseen before pregnancy that the child would need carriage at age three to live; (c) the child was adopted by someone else, so there is no parental commitment on the part of the biological mother; and (d) it is a case in which what is at stake is letting the child die rather than killing it. McMahan says the biological mother has a duty to provide carriage. From this he concludes she would also have to provide bodily support in a pregnancy that resulted from voluntary sex rather than have an abortion to avoid carriage. (See McMahan, "The Right to Choose an Abortion," pp. 338–41.)

Consider a variant on the Dependent Child Case called "Pre-adoption": It is foreseen that in order for an adoption to be possible, the newborn infant must be placed in the body of one of its creators for nine months. (Also factor in any other negative effects this might have, comparable to social and status effects of no abortion, if there are any.) Would the biological creator have to do it? I believe not. This suggests that the pregnant woman need not provide bodily support in pregnancy. Why is this Pre-adoption Case intuitively different from the Dependent Child Case, and more like pregnancy? Here are some suggestions: (a) The child in the Dependent Child Case is around in our society longer—for three years; (b) it may be imagined that the biological parents played a part in arranging for the adoption, so they are partly responsible for the parenthood of the adoptive parents; and (c) there are committed adoptive parents who will lose a child, and there may be an obligation to help them once they are committed parents. Furthermore, in both the original and Pre-adoption variation, the woman's having already given continuing support during pregnancy may actually lead her, not unreasonably, to feel bound to the child. By contrast, if she wanted an early abortion, this would not be true.

It is also useful to compare the Dependent Child Case to the Car Driving Case I used in *Creation and Abortion*, pp. 95–96. McMahan uses car-driving cases to conclude that drivers who injure bystanders owe aid even though they have driven nonnegligently. I reach a conclusion that distinguishes among the efforts people must make to aid. In these cases, I suppose that there are good reasons for the driver to drive, and there is a sufficiently low probability of an accident that society endorses his driving under these circumstances. In my case, the accident victim needs to be attached to the body of the driver and would have to be supported for nine months in order to live. Does the driver have to do this? Even though the Car Driving Case involves making someone *worse off* than he would have been if he had not been hit and attached, I do not think such bodily support is required. (We could change this case to make it more like the condition of the fetus. For example, imagine that the victim will be failing to get something important if aid is stopped but not getting it does not make him worse off than he would have been if he had not been attached. This is because a tree would have fallen on him and killed him if he had not been hit and attached.)

McMahan says that in the Dependent Child Case, carriage is required because: (1) there will be a big benefit to the child and a lesser loss to the woman; (2) the child exists because the woman did not forgo the benefits of an activity (sex); and (3) the child's life would not have the minima. But comparable reasons exist in the Car Driving Case: (1) there will be a big benefit to the victim and a lesser loss to the driver who aids by carriage; (2) the accident occurred because the driver did not forgo the benefits of driving; and (3) the victim will not have basic goods if he is not helped. Yet, I do not think the driver has to go so far as to provide carriage.

46. In Dworkin, *Life's Dominion* (New York: Alfred A. Knopf, 1993), p. 111. All subsequent references to Dworkin are to this book.

47. For a discussion on requiring the provision of information before an abortion, see my *Creation and Abortion*, pp. 193–97, 220.

13

McMahan on the Ethics of Killing at the Margins of Life

I

Jeff McMahan's book, *The Ethics of Killing: Problems at the Margins of Life*, aims to answer practical questions (such as whether and when abortion and euthanasia are permissible and how we should treat persons with mental retardation and animals) by answering such theoretical questions as what we are, when we begin and cease to exist, when it is worth caring about the continuation of our lives, and who is entitled to respect.[1] McMahan provides detailed, rigorously argued, comprehensive, and often unconventional answers to both the theoretical and the practical questions. The book is an enormous achievement. It should be required reading for anyone concerned with questions of personal identity, issues of life and death, and the morality governing relations with animals.

The detailed nature of the analysis makes for slow reading in many sections, but never because the text is unclear. McMahan's method of argument relies heavily on intuitive judgments in hypothetical cases. However, he believes that not all our intuitive judgments will cohere and some will simply have to be ignored in formulating a correct theory. (Below I raise some questions about why he chooses to ignore some and not others.) Those who would be less willing than he to reject intuitive judgments might argue that the need to ignore some judgments is an indication that we simply have not yet found the correct theory which would accommodate all the judgments.

A striking example of McMahan's willingness to reject some intuitive judgments is his view that a human infant whose genetic makeup determines that she will have only the potential to be severely retarded from conception on is no more unfortunate than a normal animal that has the same potential. McMahan thinks that neither the normal animal nor the infant is unfortunate in virtue of its limited potential. (Although he thinks that the *absence of* a better potential is not a misfortune, he holds that the *loss of* a better potential once had *is* a misfortune.) It is also striking that he accepts the following implication of this view: It is morally permissible for someone who wants a human pet, rather than a nonhuman pet, to deliberately choose to develop a human embryo that only has the potential to be severely retarded.[2] (McMahan does not believe that we have a duty to maximize the good. Hence, he cannot rule out choosing such an embryo on grounds that we could have created a human of greater intelligence, so long as he permits people to breed nonhuman animals as pets.)

II

According to McMahan, we are embodied minds and we begin to exist when fetal development reaches the point where the nervous system has the capacity to support consciousness. We cease to exist when the area of our brain that has supported our capacity for consciousness no longer exists or functions. To say that we are essentially embodied minds is not to say that we are essentially persons. By "person" he means a self-conscious being with some degree of rationality and, apparently, psychological interconnections between temporal stages. We might survive the person-stage of our lives if our mind continues on in a demented form.

McMahan also rejects the view that we are essentially organisms; he thinks that our organism began when cells specialized and functioned in an integrated way. However, this is not sufficient for us to exist on his account of what we are. He also rejects the view that the early embryo becomes us. This is because he thinks that while the changes undergone in the transition from an embryo to a late fetus preserve the identity of the organism, the organism is not identical to the entity that has capacity for consciousness (us).

Here are some possible concerns about McMahan's account of what we are. The early embryo is the beginning of our organism and part of our organism is a brain. (McMahan argues that self-conscious twins who share the same body from the neck down share the same organism, and yet they are different persons. He concludes from this that persons are not organisms. But this argument seems to ignore the fact that the twins do not share the same brain, and so they do not completely share the same organism.) If the part of the organism that is the brain is the source of the mind, and the embryo is the beginning of an organism that will have a brain, it is not clear why the embryo is not the beginning of us—us under construction—even though it is not yet us (i.e., an embodied mind).

A second type of concern is raised by McMahan's insistence that in order for the same mind to be present, the material substrate of consciousness must remain the same. It is for this reason that he rejects the view that we could survive teletransportation; the psychology at the other end of the teletransporter would be embodied in a completely different physical material than the original psychology was. He recognizes, of course, that normally cells die and are replaced in our brains, but he claims that so long as this happens slowly—in the sense that at any given time new cells are a small fraction of the total cells in the part of the brain that supports consciousness—this is consistent with the same part of the brain giving rise to the same mind. However, on his account, if too large a proportion of brain cells is replaced at a given time, the original embodied mind would not survive. (It seems that cells could turn over at a very rapid rate consistent with identity of a mind, so long as they did not turn over in a great mass.) Furthermore, he claims that if at t_1, part A of a brain supports consciousness and at t_2, part A dies but part B of the same brain supports consciousness—"shining its light" on all the same memories and thoughts once supported by part A—there would be different minds at t_1 and t_2, and no identity of a mind over time.

Are these requirements on identity excessively strict? For example, suppose it turned out to have always been true of our brains that the seat of consciousness moves, as cells in a previous area die en masse, with a seamless flow of consciousness throughout. Would we really think that no one had ever survived as long as we had previously thought? Or suppose (counterfactually) that one way by which our brains could naturally prevent dementia would be to grow replacements for 75 percent of our brain cells that had been destroyed by a virus. Would a particular person who could survive as a mildly demented person with 25 percent of his "original" brain cells be extinguished if such a rapid internal dementia cure took place? Would a particular person be extinguished if we cured dementia by rapidly replacing most of the brain cells supporting consciousness and self-consciousness using his own stem cells? If so, this would make current research for such a type of cure self-defeating, at least if personal survival is what one is after.

Suppose, contrary to what McMahan's view suggests, identity of a person and/or mind would be retained in these hypothetical cases. Then what would distinguish the cases from teletransportation? Intuitively, at least, it seems that if the death of cells in the brain leads the brain to provide new cells that support consciousness, there could be survival of the same mind or person, but when an intervening agency (as in teletransportation) supplies matter that is unrelated to either the original brain cells or the person's own stem cells, there would be no such survival.

III

Of course, McMahan thinks that whether we survive and whether it matters if we survive are two different questions. He thinks that the presence of properties that account for survival are not sufficient to account for its mattering much to us that we survive. This will be true even though more and more goods will be present in our life if we survive and, on what he calls the whole life comparative account, we will have a better life if we survive than if we die. The alternative view he supports is that in cases where we do not split into different branching lives, concern for survival should be a function of what our interests are at a particular time in surviving. (He calls these time-relative interests.) These time-relative interests will be a function of (1) the strength of (what he calls) the prudential unity relations between ourselves at that time and at the times we would live through if we survive, and of (2) the quality of life we would have if we survive. (The most important part of prudential unity relations depends on overlapping chains of psychological continuity and connectedness between different times of our lives, though the mere survival of the embodied mind provides some prudential unity relations.) In the absence of any strong prudential unity relations there is little difference from the point of view of the interests of an entity whether it continues or a new entity appears in its place.

To illustrate his point, McMahan describes someone who is an "isolated subject," forever under the impression that he has just come into existence and with no thought of his future. McMahan's views lead him to believe that there is no strong reason to care for the sake of an isolated subject that it continue in existence, not because of the inadequate content of each of its present moments but because there is no psychological connectedness and continuity in the life. This seems to imply that there is little more reason for its sake to rescue an isolated subject from death than to rescue an animal whose natural life span is one minute.

I do not think this conclusion about an isolated subject is correct, and it is a reason to be concerned about the importance of prudential unity relations. For if the isolated subject is a self-conscious being who continually thinks that he has just come into existence, he can be a person even if there is little or no psychological connectedness and continuity in his life. This is a synchronic rather than a diachronic conception of personhood. And what if the content of each of this person's moments was extremely good and different from other moments? Does the fact that this subject is not aware of any accumulation of these good moments in his life make his life not significantly more worth preserving for his sake than that of a very short-lived animal? I find this hard to believe.

A further concern about the importance of prudential unity relations stems from McMahan's views about a person who would survive from t_1 to t_2 (i.e., be the same embodied mind) but go through psychological changes resulting in no psychological continuity at t_2 with his present (t_1) state. He thinks this person would still have reason at t_1 to fear being tortured at t_2. If such significant concern for what condition one will be in *if* one survives makes sense even without psychological continuity and strong prudential unity relations, why cannot it make sense to have significant concern for *whether* one survives—whether one's embodied mind continues—despite the absence of psychological continuity and strong prudential unity relations?

To further consider these issues, McMahan presents the Cure Case, in which an adult will die in a year unless he takes a cure immediately. If he takes the cure, he will survive and have a nice future life, but with no psychological connection to his past life. McMahan thinks that the adult in this case has no time-relative interests in surviving and, therefore, has no reason to choose the cure rather than die in a year. I think this is the wrong conclusion and that the cure is to be preferred. For suppose it is a five-year-old child who will die in a year unless he takes a cure now, and the cure will put him in a coma for twenty years after which he will awaken to a normal life. This life will have few prudential unity relations with his five-year-old self. Presumably, it would be correct for him to have the cure, other things equal. If the cure is to be preferred, this suggests that the whole life comparative account gives a better answer to this case than the time-relative interest account. It may also give a better answer to McMahan's Cure Case.

Suppose there is reason from the point of view of time-relative interests to care whether one dies. This implies that death can be good or bad for one. But if death involves nonexistence, its goodness or badness cannot be due to death's intrinsic properties, McMahan argues. Rather, he holds that death's goodness or badness for one is due to nonexistence being comparatively better or worse than what would have occurred in the future life with which one would have had prudential unity relations. McMahan also agrees with the following views (for which I also have argued): (1) often the fact that one's future life would not have involved relevant goods, and so death could not deprive one of them, is what is really bad even if this makes death itself less bad; (2) we should not hesitate to make death itself worse for people if this happens by making their prospects for further goods (with which death can interfere) better; and (3) the badness of a future loss should be discounted by goods one has already had in the past.[3]

In connection with the latter point, the question should arise for McMahan, given his emphasis on prudential unity relations in evaluating the loss of future goods, whether only those goods in the past with which one has significant prudential unity relations at the time one would die should be used to discount future losses caused by death. This seems incorrect to me. For suppose someone had undergone a radical psychological change accompanied by amnesia. If prudential unity relations with the past were important in discounting future losses, then the fact that he had had in the past a long, wonderful creative life would count for very little against the losses he would incur in dying, making his death quite as tragic as that of someone who had had none of these goods. This is implausible, I believe. This matter could be of significance in deciding to whom to give a scarce lifesaving medical treatment. I believe that how much good life each candidate has already had should be relevant in deciding to whom to give more good life.[4] Suppose one candidate has lived five hundred good years already. He is now bound to have very weak prudential unity relations to hundreds of years of his past life. Does that mean that they should not be counted in deciding whether to save him or someone who has only lived seventy years? This seems wrong to me. Again, the whole life comparative account which would count all the good in someone's life, not just prudential unity related goods, seems to yield a more reasonable conclusion.

Given his view that death is a bad relative to the prudential unity related goods to be had in further life, it is surprising that McMahan does not deal with whether a simple outweighing of prudential unity related goods by prudential unity related bads in further life would make death not be comparatively bad.

Philippa Foot argued against this when she suggested that having certain basic (on McMahan's view, prudential unity related) goods in future life would be sufficient to make death be comparatively bad. [5] Nor does McMahan consider the possibility that someone's life being all over is an intrinsically bad aspect of death, independent of its diminishing the amount of goods of life. If this possibility were true, then the fact that death involves nonexistence need not mean that it is only comparatively bad in virtue of interfering with more goods of life. Rather, on account of this other source of the badness of death, though one might decide to die in order to avoid further life with only bad things in it, one could regret that this entailed the end of oneself as a conscious being. One might even try to put off this end, without increasing total prudential-unity related goods in one's life, by going into a so-called limbo state simply to extend one's life. [6]

IV

Can an account of the badness of death, understood as involving the loss of future goods, provide us with an account of the wrongness of killing, so that wrongness varies with badness? McMahan argues that it does so only for beings who fall below the threshold of ever having been persons. In the case of persons (or individuals who used to be persons), the morality of harm is combined with the morality of respect for what a person wills. Hence, in the case of innocent persons, killing is said to be wrong in virtue of its either harming someone or going contrary to what he wills. [7] I assume that some sort of harming/not aiding distinction is embedded in this view. Then refusing to save someone's life, against his wishes, need not be as wrong as killing someone, other things being equal.

One of McMahan's primary concerns is to see how what he calls the Equal Wrongness Thesis can be defended. This is the view that it is equally wrong to kill a person who will be harmed greatly in dying and a person who will not be harmed greatly in dying. The measure of being harmed greatly is that one will lose out on many goods that one would have had if one had not died. (But, I would note, death could be worse for someone who will die having had very little in his life even if he would not have had many goods had he lived on. The truth of the Equal Wrongness Thesis should also be tested using this measure of harm.) Since the properties on which respect is based (e.g., rationality, autonomous will) can also come in degrees in different people, a threshold level of these properties must be both necessary and sufficient for the equal wrongness of killing any person.

McMahan thinks that a problematic case for this view is the one he calls the Deluded Pessimist. This involves someone who competently (i.e., with full information and understanding) waives his right to life and asks to be killed even though his death would be bad for him, as he is under the mistaken impression that his future life will be worse than nonexistence. [8] (Making such mistakes is consistent with being competent, though the use of the description "deluded" is not ideal to convey this.) McMahan thinks both that we would not be showing disrespect for this person's will if we kill him and that it would be wrong to kill him. But if the Equal Wrongness Thesis depends on giving priority to what someone wills, out of respect, it should not condemn the killing. He concludes that concern for a person's interests (including not harming him) must be part of respect for that person. However, Carlos Soto has pointed out that if concern for interests is a part of respect, [9] this threatens to undermine the Equal Wrongness Thesis, for will it not be less respectful to kill someone who would lose a lot in dying than to kill someone who would lose little? Perhaps the answer to this problem is that there is a threshold account of interests in the theory of respect comparable to thresholds of rationality and autonomy. Alternatively, perhaps respect for persons is neither merely a matter of respecting their choices nor a matter of acting from concern for their interests, after all.

McMahan's account of the wrongness of killing (innocent, nonthreatening) persons may also be incomplete for other reasons. For there seem to be cases in which harm is done to someone and there is interference with his will, and yet the acts are not wrong. For example, McMahan does not attempt to explain why killing someone by redirecting a trolley away from two other people toward him may not be wrong, even though he is harmed and we act against his will. If turning the trolley is permissible, accounting for the wrongness of killing will also require taking account of *how* we harm someone against his will.

Also, consider a case in which someone is attached to my experimental and very expensive life-support system, though he had no right to be attached. I decide not to continue the support, though the beneficiary is opposed to this and could gain many years of life if I did continue. It happens that there is faulty wiring in our facility and I know that when I unplug my machine, the attached person will experience an electric shock that painlessly causes his death. In this Faulty Wiring Case, I actually kill the person against his will. It could also be argued that I harm him, as I interfere with his having many years of good life.[10] What distinguishes this case from many cases of killing, such that it may be permissible? I have argued that it is that the person who dies loses only life he would have had with my support at the time, rather than what he would have had independently of such support. This is a property that is conceptually true of letting die, not of killing, but it may be present in some cases of killing (as in Faulty Wiring).[11] I believe that someone's acting contrary to a person's will and harming him will often not account for the wrongness of killing him if he does not thereby lose what he would have had independently of the support of those who kill him. An account of the wrongness of killing may, therefore, need to make some reference to what distinguishes many cases of killing from all cases of letting die.[12]

McMahan's discussion of the Equal Wrongness Thesis is an instance in which he refuses to ignore an intuitive judgment (that the Equal Wrongness Thesis is correct), even though he raises objections to it and accepts that he cannot yet find a theory that adequately accounts for it. He must find his intuitive judgment favoring the thesis to be stronger than the intuitive judgment that always-retarded humans have a different moral status from animals with the same potential. For he is willing to ignore the latter intuition when he cannot find a theory that adequately accounts for it. But some might argue that, for all McMahan says and in the absence of a justified double standard, there is as much or as little reason to retain the one intuitive judgment as the other.

V

McMahan's views on abortion follow from his views on identity, death, and the wrongness of killing. The conceptus prior to having the capacity for mind is not a subject, and so there is no one to lose anything in dying. The later fetus may be an individual subject who loses its future as a person (a stage in the life of an embodied mind), but the individual has very weak prudential unity relations with that later stage, and so is not harmed much by death. To the extent that one is skeptical about the significance of strong prudential unity relations in determining how bad death is for someone at a given time, this account of why one might think that even late abortion and infanticide are not morally problematic will not be convincing.

McMahan, however, is critical of the view that abortion would often be permissible even if the fetus were a person, as some (such as Judith Thomson[13] and I[14]) have argued. He thinks that it is hard to see how abortion could be permissible if (1) one is responsible for a person's having a need for bodily support, even if the person would not have a fate that compared unfavorably with never existing if his needs were not met; (2) the person is one's biological offspring; and (3) one would have to kill the person to stop providing it bodily support. McMahan admits that he finds the relevance of (1) and (2) to the impermissibility of abortion puzzling; but he joins people who are intuitively drawn to them and their relevance. This is another instance in which McMahan refuses to ignore intuitive responses, despite his inability to find an adequate justification for them, and it contrasts with the way he deals with the intuitive judgment concerning the moral difference between humans and other animals of identical potential. The question is why the standards for accepting (1) and (2) are lower than the standard for accepting this other intuitive judgment.

In my *Creation and Abortion*, which is argued on the hypothetical assumption that the fetus is a person, I was drawn to the view (similar to McMahan's) that one owes a person that one is responsible for creating more than his or her just not having a fate that compares unfavorably with never existing. (I was willing to accept this even if the person one created was not one's biological offspring but a person one manufactured.) However, unlike McMahan, I thought there were greater limits on what a creator could be morally required to sacrifice in order to see to it that his creation had certain goods appropriate to a person (what I call "the minima") when the creator had not yet formed a true parental relation with his creation, as would be true if the fetus were a person.[15]

Furthermore, the emphasis that McMahan places on killing (rather than letting die) in (3) may be wrong. For he allows that it may be permissible to let die one's biological offspring, for whose creation one is responsible, rather than carry it in one's body. But (as I argued in *Creation and Abortion*) killing someone when he will thereby lose no more than what he gets from bodily support to which he would have no right merely to save his life may be no more wrong than letting the person die. (This will be especially true when what the person gets from the bodily support [i.e., his continuing life] causes him to be imposing on the person providing support.[16])

McMahan's views about aborting a person are further complicated by the fact that he thinks that killing a person who is a morally nonresponsible threat in order to help the person he threatens is no more permissible than killing an innocent bystander in order to help someone avoid a threat. I find this an implausible view. McMahan supports his view by presenting the Trapped Miners Case: Due to a shift in rocks, miner A was hurled against supports that had prevented the collapse of a mine, thereby causing the mine to partially collapse. The collapse reduces the oxygen available to miners in one part of the mine. May these miners kill A (who has enough oxygen in his part of the mine) if only this will make available to them enough oxygen to survive? If we think they may not kill A (the morally nonresponsible threat who caused the collapse), why should we think that they could permissibly have killed him when he was in the process of being a threat, in order to stop his impact on the supports? And yet it does seem to me that while A is hurtling toward causing the collapse, it would be permissible to kill him if one knew that this alone would stop his impact. The issue at stake here is, I believe, whether (a) the permissibility of harming someone to stop the process through which he would cause harm implies (b) the permissibility of harming someone so that there is no harm that he will have caused. It is (b) but not (a) that would license our imposing losses on morally nonresponsible threats to undo the damage they have caused (or to prevent such damage as will still result) after their involvement in a harmful process is over. (This is on the assumption that the losses could permissibly have been imposed on them to stop their causing the harm in the first place.) The (admittedly theoretically puzzling) idea is that a process can be bad only because of the harm it will cause, and yet one may permissibly make the harm not exist in a way that deliberately harms a morally nonresponsible person who is a part of the harmful process only to stop the bad process itself.[17]

Notes

1. This chapter is a revised version of a review of Jeff McMahan's *The Ethics of Killing: Problems at the Margins of Life* (New York: Oxford University Press, 2002) that appeared in *The Philosophical Review* 116 (2) (2007).

2. He agreed this was an implication of his view in responding to a question from me verbally.

3. For my discussion of these points, see my *Morality, Mortality*, Vol. 1 (New York: Oxford University Press, 1993). Points (1) and (2) are found in the section on death. Point (3) is connected to my claim that those who have had more goods of life are, in general, less in need of having more of them, at least from a moral point of view. That point is found in the section on allocating scarce lifesaving resources.

4. See my discussion of this issue in *Morality, Mortality*, Vol. 1.

5. In her "Euthanasia," *Philosophy & Public Affairs* 6 (1977): 85–112.

6. For more on this, see my discussion of the Limbo Man in chapters 1 and 12 this volume, and *Morality, Mortality*, Vol. 1.

7. The idea that people are worthy of respect, McMahan says, is different from the idea of the sanctity of life. The latter makes no reference to rationality and willing. However, McMahan (p. 242) also says that to kill a person "is to show contempt for that which demands reverence," and this may blur the difference.

8. Philippa Foot discussed a similar case for a different purpose in her "Euthanasia."

9. In Carlos Soto, *Extending and Ending Life in Health Care and Beyond* (unpublished manuscript).

10. I discuss these sorts of cases in chapter 3 this volume.

11. See my *Morality, Mortality*, Vol. 2 (New York: Oxford University Press, 1996) for discussion of this.

12. A possible alternative is to argue that if the person loses only what he would get from aid, he may be killed but he is not harmed, only not aided.

13. In her "A Defense of Abortion," *Philosophy & Public Affairs* 1 (1971).

14. In my *Creation and Abortion* (New York: Oxford University Press, 1992). See also chapter 12 this volume.

15. McMahan says that I claim in *Creation and Abortion* that giving up sexual relations is too much to demand of a woman in order to avoid a pregnancy ending in abortion of a person. However, I only said that this claim would have to be true in order for an argument for the permissibility of abortion in cases of voluntary sex to be justified. If giving up sexual relations was good or an easily accomplished task, there would be little reason not to avoid pregnancy that will end in abortion of a person and this might affect the permissibility of an abortion.

16. In arguing against abortion if the fetus were a person, McMahan also appeals to intuitive judgments about his Dependent Child Case. For my discussion of this case, see chapter 12 this volume, note 35.

17. I first discussed this problematic issue in my "The Insanity Defense, Innocent Threats, and Limited Alternatives," *Criminal Justice Ethics* 6 (1987): 61–76, and again in my *Morality, Mortality*, Vol. 2, among other places. I discuss it again, coming to a somewhat different conclusion in connection with morally responsible threats, in "Torture: During and After Action," in my *Ethics for Enemies: Terror, Torture, and War* (Oxford: Oxford University Press, 2011). I am grateful to Jeff McMahan and Carlos Soto for comments on a draft of the review on which this chapter is based.

14

Some Conceptual and Ethical Issues in Munchausen Syndrome by Proxy

Introduction

Munchausen Syndrome by Proxy (MSBP) involves a caregiver's lying about and possibly even inducing her charge's symptoms while persistently presenting the charge (most commonly the child of the caregiver) for medical assessment.[1, 2] Doctors are most interested in getting advice on morally permissible means of collecting evidence that MSBP is occurring, as a way to stop harm to the patient. However, there are also other issues of a conceptual nature raised by MSBP, such as its relation to child abuse, the distinction between deceiving and harming, and the distinction between diagnosis and prevention of harm. In this chapter I will first discuss conceptual issues and then move on to the more clearly ethical concerns related to diagnosis, prevention of harm, and collecting evidence.

I. Conceptual Issues

A. THE USE OF THE TERM "SYNDROME"

Suppose a small percentage of doctors deliberately gave their patients laxatives inappropriately and wrote notes in the patients' records, on which other physicians and nurses in a hospital rely, attesting to the patients' being diarrhetic. Would it be most appropriate to refer to the doctors' behavior as a "syndrome" and think that confirming its occurrence was most appropriately referred to as "diagnosing" the doctors' problem? Surely this would be inappropriate language to use, because it medicalizes what is essentially criminal behavior. Similarly, finding out if A was poisoned by B is not best described as diagnosing the cause of A's ill health. Crime may be bad for people's health, but trying to find out which particular person committed the crime as a result of which A's health is jeopardized is not best described, I think, as a diagnosis of A's ill health. Yet, when a parent[3] does essentially what the doctors in my imaginary case have done, it is referred to as a syndrome and finding evidence confirming her action is sometimes described as diagnosing the child's medical problem.[4] Here is a quote (to which I shall return to make several different points) from an article on MSBP:

> In general, once MSBP is a part of the differential diagnosis, hidden camera or other monitoring may be viewed as a diagnostic tool like any other. Monitoring is not performed to collect evidence of criminal activity against the parents, but to make an appropriate diagnostic finding and to protect the child. The evidence may subsequently be used in child protective proceedings.[5]

Perhaps both the doctors in my imaginary case and the parent in MSBP are discovered to have psychiatric problems and so should themselves be thought of as patients. But it is odd to think that this could turn discovery of their problem into a diagnosis of a syndrome from which their victims are suffering (as MSBP is sometimes used).

Why might one medicalize a criminal act so that confirming its occurrence is thought of as diagnosing the cause of its outcome? Perhaps because, as the quote above suggests, we think we could more easily justify ordinarily impermissible means of collecting evidence of criminal acts if we can label these means "diagnostic tests." This is one way the conceptual point about ways of describing an act can bear on the ethical issues to which I shall turn later.

B. COMPONENTS OF MSBP

Commonly, cases of MSBP involve (1) a parent deceiving a doctor about (i) symptoms had by a child, and/or about (ii) the causes of these symptoms. It is worth distinguishing (i) and (ii), because if the parent actually makes the child diarrhetic, she is not lying if she says he is diarrhetic. The cases also involve (2) something harmful happening to the child either because (i) the parent does something potentially harmful to the child (e.g., giving him laxatives), or (ii) because she does something that leads the doctor to do something at least potentially harmful to the child (i.e., excessive tests). When a parent adds blood to an infant's diaper so that doctors will do tests, but does not cause the infant to bleed, we have (2)(ii) and not (2)(i).

Factor (2)(ii) is interesting in highlighting the role that doctors can play in themselves harming patients, since they are made the instruments of the parent's attempt to harm the child. In turn, the parent becomes the powerful, manipulating figure. This also makes MSBP interesting because it has usually been doctors who have deceived patients, especially in the days before informed consent and full disclosure of diagnostic findings. Doctors' shock at the violation of their trust in the parent of the patient is great in MSBP. This may not be because they are shocked at lies per se, having themselves lied to patients, but because they think that health and diagnosis, of all things, are goods that should not be interfered with. It would be useful to know if the desire to switch power roles in the medical scenario plays a part in the parent's motivation, especially since it is reported that a large number of the Munchausen parents have lower-level medical roles in their work-life.

Note also that a child could have real symptoms some of which the parent deliberately omits to report to the doctor. If the parent truthfully reports only some symptoms, this can prompt the doctor to do tests, and yet they may fail to reveal the real illness because of the missing information. In this case, no lies are told and yet the deliberate withholding of information with the intention of misleading should lead us to classify the behavior as MSBP. Hence, factor (1) should include a parent's intentional omission of information in order to mislead as well as a parent's lying.

C. MSBP AND CHILD ABUSE

Often, in ordinary cases of child abuse, the abuser harms the child (so (2)(i) is present) and then lies about it or otherwise deceives only if, contrary to his or her wishes, someone finds out about the harm already done. Sometimes, the abuser takes a child to a doctor so that the harm can be discovered in order to have it treated, and lies about its cause. Both these scenarios differ from MSBP, where one aim that motivates the activity that is harmful to the child is to deceive doctors while continuing to harm the child and to involve doctors in harming the child. It is also (theoretically) possible that the deceiving and harming criteria for MSBP are met, and yet we would be reluctant to call the case one of child abuse because the aim is not to make the child worse off overall, either as a means (to a goal like obtaining power over doctors) or as an end in itself. (This is consistent with there being an aim to cause some harm.) For example, suppose a homeless mother believes correctly that her child will be better off overall in a hospital than living on the streets, even if unnecessary tests risking harm are done. Deception and doing some harm may be the only way to get hospital admission. Of course, a child could be harmed in the ordinary way (e.g., beaten up) for this same reason, as well. Hence certain types of justification for the harm and deception will defeat an ascription of MSBP.

D. DOCTORS' AIMS

We can distinguish three aims doctors may have in relation to their patient: (a) to diagnose why the child is ill, (b) to treat the child, (c) to prevent further harm to the child. These are distinct. For example, we might need to diagnose why the child was ill, even if the parent is no longer in a position to do further harm and there is no need to treat. In MSBP, (b) often collapses into (c), because there may be no need for treatment of past harm done (e.g., bruises induced during tests) and future harm is prevented by a treatment which involves separating parent and child.

II. Ethical Issues

A. GENERAL CONSIDERATIONS

As I have noted, doctors are most concerned with what it is morally permissible to do in order to discover the cause of the child's illness. (I shall use "discover" instead of "diagnose" so as not to over-medicalize.) This question should be distinguished from whether the permissible acts are effectual. For example, what is morally permissible may be ineffectual because it scares the mother into taking the child elsewhere. So we could refuse to do something not because it would be intrinsically unethical but because it would be ineffectual or even counterproductive.

Let us first consider the question of permissibility. Consider again the quote cited above. It says that secret monitoring is like any diagnostic technique. This may be true in the sense that many diagnostic techniques invade privacy, but just because this is so, it would be prima facie unethical to use them without the consent of the person on whom they are to be used (or his or her authorized proxy decision maker). But secret monitoring in the cases under consideration seems to be done without consent of the person monitored. This is the ethical issue. Notice that posting warning signs to the effect that secret monitoring will take place does not ensure that someone has consented to their use simply by entering the premises. And signed contracts that do not make explicit the specific kind of monitoring that may take place also do not satisfy the requirements of informed consent.[6] There is also the conceptual problem of a concealing description. Just as "diagnosis" did not seem the best word to use when speaking of uncovering an act that victimized someone, so "diagnostic technique" conceals the moral impact of what is done in secret monitoring. Analogously, if a doctor's lying to a patient prompts the latter to do something that reveals the cause of his illness, the lie is a diagnostic technique, but this description conceals morally relevant properties of that technique.

The quote also suggests that the monitoring may be permissible merely because doctors are not aiming at collecting evidence for a criminal prosecution of the parent. But ordinary diagnostic techniques are also not used in order to collect criminal evidence and yet using them without appropriate consent can be unethical. In addition, it is noted that "the evidence may subsequently be included in child protective proceedings." Even if this is not intended by doctors, a foreseen consequence of one's acts could be morally relevant in deciding what to do. Possibly, the evidence might also be used in criminal prosecution of the parent, unless the evidence were barred for that purpose because of the way in which it was obtained (for it might be legally permissible to collect evidence in a certain way for some purposes and not for others). An ethical (not legal) question is what we should do if we know that the evidence would not be barred from use in criminal prosecution.

As an aid in considering this situation further, let us hypothesize a situation in which a patient lies to a doctor about her own condition, though she does not fabricate an illness. Suppose having an abortion is a criminal act and a doctor is required to report any person she knows to have had an abortion. The patient has a gynecological problem but conceals its origin in an abortion, though knowledge of the origin of the problem would be helpful in treatment. If the doctor searches out secret records without the patient's permission and finds that the patient had an abortion, this will aid her in diagnosis and treatment. But once she has the knowledge of an abortion, she is required to turn over the patient for trial. The patient can thus be made overall worse off as a result of getting superior medical treatment than if inferior treatment had taken place. Should the doctor not consider the ultimate result and also the illicit means she uses, and refrain from getting a perfect diagnosis?

So far, we have seen that acting without patient consent to uncover truth about the cause of an illness is not necessarily permissible merely because one does not aim at criminal prosecution. But, of course, one important difference between the case in which a patient lies about him- or herself and MSBP is that, in the latter, the deceiver is harming someone else, and if collection of evidence can prevent that harm to another—harm which the liar either induces and/or helps cause—it may possibly be justified, even if it involves non-consensual monitoring and ultimately leads to prosecution. Whether this is so must now be considered.

B. A POSSIBLE ARGUMENT

Let us consider some arguments that aim to justify secret monitoring and secret bag searches when preventing harm to others is at issue. One argument takes note of the fact that doctors are increasingly permitted to detect and report on patients who pose a threat to others. For example: One may draw blood with a patient's consent and, without telling a patient, search for a particular disease and report the results to others who are at risk because of the patient. Suppose a doctor is taught to conceive of the patient's family—for example, his mother—as his patient as well. Why not monitor this patient (the mother) to prevent harm she may do to others?[7] Call this the Parent-As-Patient Argument.

There are problems with this argument. First, taking a blood test is not done without the patient's consent, even if searching for an item in his or her blood and reporting this information to others is done without the patient's consent. Absence of permission also differs from absence of information, because a patient may be told what the doctor will do even if the patient's permission to do it is not requested. But secret monitoring is begun not only without the person's permission but also without his or her knowledge. Second, while a doctor may have to take account of the child's family in treating the child, that alone does not mean the parent is also a patient in the sense of having sought treatment or agreed to some diagnostic procedure. The parent is primarily the child's agent until proven otherwise.

C. TWO OTHER ARGUMENTS

It is interesting to compare MSBP with a case in which the parent harms the child but not deliberately and there is no deception—for example, in a case of folie à deux involving parent and child. In this case, we can think of the parent as what philosophers call a morally innocent threat. Suppose secret monitoring were the only way to uncover the effect of a mother on a child in such a case. Since there is no attempt by the mother to harm or deceive, we could assume that given her current motives and intentions, she would want the discovery technique to be used and would consent to it, were it not that her knowledge of the monitoring would interfere with its effectiveness. The fact that we could presume her hypothetical consent to the investigation in the absence of her actual consent, based on her current motives and intentions, makes it easier to proceed with secret monitoring in this case, I believe. However, since there is an intention to harm and to deceive in MSBP (a morally guilty state of mind), we cannot assume the same hypothetical consent based on current motives and intentions in MSBP in order to help justify secret monitoring.[8]

Nevertheless, it might be suggested, hypothetical consent could play a role in a possible justification of monitoring in MSBP. First point: If we knew for certain that the mother was lying and trying to harm the child, we would know she has forfeited her moral right not to be lied to or even harmed in the process of stopping harm to the child. Second point: If we have only a suspicion of her guilt, it is possible that we should proceed as we would if we were certain. An argument for doing so is that if she is morally innocent, she probably would want the interests of her child to be protected even by secret monitoring of herself. This is a hypothetical-consent justification based on *possibly* current motives and intentions. It is an analogue of the justification given above for monitoring, where the woman is harming her child without intending to do so. For example, if secretly monitoring a morally innocent mother, who also caused no harm, was (somehow) the only way to stop a third person from harming her child, she would probably want it to be done.

Putting the two points together, it might be thought that we can get a four-step argument: (1) If she is morally guilty, she has no right not to be monitored to prevent harm she will cause. (2) If she is morally innocent, she would want to be monitored to prevent harm. (3) She is either morally guilty or innocent. (4) Hence, it is permissible to secretly monitor her. Call this the Hypothetical-Consent Argument (for the permissibility of secret monitoring).[9]

There are several problems with this argument. First, if there is any reason to secretly monitor a morally innocent parent, it must be to gather information to prevent harm. But (by hypothesis) the only way in which the harm is coming about in MSBP is if the parent is *not* morally innocent, because there is no chance that she is a threat without knowing that she is one. Hence, she is either morally guilty or there is no avoidable harm that monitoring a morally innocent person will prevent. This means step (2) is confused.

I think this problem can be remedied as follows. If a mother were morally innocent, she would want us to be so vigilant about the welfare of her child that we would even try to find out if she were guilty. Further, we need not even assume she hypothetically approves of being monitored. We need only assume that she hypothetically approves of our having an attitude (vigilance), one of whose necessary side effects is that we suspect even her. An analogy may help here. Suppose a chief of police wants all his officers to guard a VIP by checking the ID of everyone who comes in the building. When the chief himself tries to enter the building, his officers demand even his ID. He may be angry with this, but he can see that it is a consequence of their fulfilling his orders.

In sum, we should change the Hypothetical-Consent Argument for monitoring in MSBP so that we no longer hypothesize both that the parent is morally innocent and that monitoring is necessary to stop harm. Instead, we hypothesize that the morally innocent mother would wish us to be vigilant and a side effect of this is our suspecting her of being guilty. In particular, we can revise the argument slightly to produce Hypothetical-Consent Argument II: (1) If she is guilty, she has no right not to be monitored to prevent the harm she will cause. (2) If she is morally innocent, she would want us to be vigilant and this permits us to secretly monitor her. (3) She is either morally guilty or innocent. (4) Hence, it is permissible to secretly monitor her.

There is still a problem with the first premise of this argument. If someone is guilty, he has forfeited certain rights. But at the time we collect evidence to prove someone guilty, we do not know that he is guilty and so we do not know that he has forfeited rights. Hence, it was wrong of us to act on the assumption that he had forfeited rights. Put another way, even if someone is found to be guilty, that does not mean that we did not do anything wrong when we collected the evidence of his guilt before his guilt was proven. In the collection of evidence, even those who will turn out to be guilty are to be treated no worse than those who will turn out to be innocent.[10]

But step (2) in the argument claims that it *would* be permissible to secretly monitor someone who is, in fact, innocent. Hence, it seems we can construct a new, shorter Hypothetical-Consent Argument III: (1) We should treat those we do not yet know are guilty no worse than the innocent. (2) If a parent is innocent, she would want us to be vigilant even if this leads us to secretly monitor her. (3) Hence, it is permissible to secretly monitor the parent. Notice that treating those who turn out to be guilty no worse than the innocent may result in more problems for them, if the evidence leads to a criminal prosecution. But this does not invalidate the argument. When the fact of guilt alters the effect of otherwise permissible procedures, the additional bad effects are not a reasonable complaint against those procedures.

I do not think this Hypothetical-Consent Argument III is airtight. First, even a parent who was innocent of MSBP still might not be the sort of parent who cared more about her child's welfare than about not being secretly monitored. She might not want us to be so vigilant that we suspect even her. She might be insulted that we would suspect her and also wish not to be embarrassed if monitoring reveals her doing other things she should not be doing the prevention of which would not justify monitoring. She may also be correct to insist that we had to have strong grounds to think harm was going to be done to her child before we were justified in monitoring her. Furthermore, she might believe that privacy is necessary in order for her to interact with the child in ways beneficial to that child.[11]

In other words, the Hypothetical-Consent Argument seems to depend upon it being reasonable to attribute a certain state of mind to a parent innocent of MSBP, namely that she cares more about her child than about aspects of her own dignity. It also depends upon this not being an unreasonable standard to which to hold a parent.[12] It also seems to depend on the view that a parent's beneficial interaction with a child does not require an assurance of privacy.

There is a further problem with Hypothetical-Consent Argument III, however. It may also justify searching a parent's bag in secret, for would not a morally innocent good parent want us to be so vigilant that we even do this? Yet, intuitively, there seems to be a big moral difference between secret monitoring and secret bag searches. If this is so, then the argument is too strong. Finally, we should consider that the Hypothetical-Consent Argument III is in a way too weak and so may be unnecessary. Many people besides the parent can come into the child's room and so be subject to secret monitoring. It is true that we may not intend this monitoring; observing them is a side effect of targeting the parent. But we could imagine that we had no idea who was making a child sick and truly aimed to observe everyone. These people, if morally innocent, cannot be assumed to be so concerned with the child that they would want us to maintain a degree of vigilance that leads us to monitor them secretly without their explicit prior consent. If we could nevertheless justify intentionally monitoring everyone simply because avoiding harm to the child justifies this intrusion, regardless of what these people would want given their concerns, we do not need step (2) in the Hypothetical-Consent Argument III in order to justify secretly monitoring the parent.

D. TWO OTHER ARGUMENTS

An alternative argument, unlike the Parent-As-Patient and the various Hypothetical-Consent Arguments, would not focus on the parent in particular. One such argument claims that privacy is not expected in a hospital room; it is understood to be part of a public place and no more immune from secret surveillance than hospital corridors. Furthermore, bag checks of which one is aware as a condition for admission to a patient's room are no more impermissible than as a condition for admission to the hospital first. Let us call this the Expected-Public-Zone Argument. I do not think it is correct. First, if visitors did not expect that privacy was achievable in a hospital room, why would they bother to close the door or draw a curtain? Why would they whisper (under the impression that then they would not be heard)? Even in an emergency room or hospital corridor where one least expects privacy, one may not expect explicit violations of privacy. That is, one may expect that people will be able to observe patients and family, but not by secret video or audio machines. Second, undergoing a bag check when one retains the option of simply not entering if one refuses is different from a secret bag check that is, therefore, beyond one's control. Ordinarily, people expect surveillance in a public space only if a sign gives warning of it, as is done in banks.

Still, it might be said, a hospital has a right to monitor its property and hence people have no (or an easily overridden) right to privacy in a hospital, even if people do not expect to be monitored. Residents on a hospital's property (i.e., patients) are like guests, but unlike those in a hotel, they are guests whose welfare is of special concern to the hospital. (They are also guests who would presumably consent to losing much of their own privacy for the sake of their own well-being.) The hospital seeks to protect its residents from "visitors." This account helps explain why, while the hospital may monitor its property without being given permission by visitors, it may not search visitors' bags without their permission. The bag is the visitor's property, not the hospital's.[13]

According to this argument, which I shall call the Public-Zone Argument (by contrast to the Expected-Public-Zone Argument), the primary moral problem in justifying secret monitoring is not showing that people's right to privacy may permissibly be overridden in a hospital. That has just been done. The moral problem is that in order for monitoring to be effective (i.e., for it to stop harm), it must be kept a secret. If we defeat the public's expectation of privacy by announcing the fact that the hospital will exercise its right to monitor without permission, monitoring will not be effective. Acting without someone's consent is different from acting without his or her knowledge. The ability to effectively monitor in order to rule out a diagnosis of MSBP and prevent harm depends upon parents believing they are not being monitored. Hence the moral problem, according to the Public-Zone Argument, turns out to be having to either lie or not be open about acting on a right to monitor.

The next step in the Public-Zone Argument, therefore, would be to show that we have a right to lie or not be open in this way. Such a right may depend on how urgent it is to resolve the diagnosis and what alternative means there are to this end. A possible solution is to post notices or to include in admission agreements paragraphs saying "The hospital reserves the right to monitor in the interests of its patients without giving further notice when there is good reason and alternatives are not available." This makes it rational to still believe one might not be monitored when doing something wrong, and hence it does not completely eliminate the effectiveness of monitoring.

Suppose some argument justifies secret monitoring. This still does not mean that we do not wrong the person we monitor in the course of doing what is permissible; there may be "wrong-making and wronging characteristics" still present in what we do, even though they are overridden by "right-making characteristics" that speak in favor of the act. For example, it may be overall right (not wrong) to do what involves wronging someone, as when I lie to an innocent person to save a life, and while the result is tainted, the victim of the lie should not complain about what I did. Sometimes, I believe, we may even permissibly wrong someone in the course of doing what is justifiable despite the fact that person might legitimately resist our doing to him or her what we are justifiably doing.[14]

What wrong we do to the morally innocent or those we are obliged to treat as morally innocent depends on what makes deception and invasion of privacy wrong. Even if a person is guilty and has forfeited his right not to be lied to or misled, there could be reasons aside from violating his right that make our lying or misleading morally offensive. For example, it may simply be inappropriate to someone's nature as a rational being—even criminals can have this nature—not to be dealt with honestly. These wrong-making considerations can speak in favor of using other means besides deception and invasion of privacy if they are as (or nearly as) effective in stopping harm to the child.

Now let us consider the issue of the effectiveness of various discovery procedures and what sort of balance we can achieve between them and moral considerations. There seem to be essentially two types of procedures for finding out whether the parent is involved in causing the child's illness: (1) those that stop her from doing harmful things, whereupon the child improves; and (2) those that catch her while she is doing harmful things. The second may give a more definitive proof of wrongful acts, since some ways of stopping her acts (e.g., barring her presence) leave it open that it is merely her psychological interaction with the child that causes the problem. Hence, the second type of procedure would also be more useful in yielding evidence (if it were admissible) for a criminal proceeding or child-custody case. However, since the medical establishment's aim is not criminal prosecution or child custody per se, this cannot provide a reason for choosing a type (2) over a type (1) discovery procedure.

Consider four specific procedures that fall under these two types: (A) the parent is barred from the child's room; (B) a nurse is obviously present at all times; (C) secret monitoring; and (D) secret alarming of the child's IV line or other equipment so that tampering will be detected if it occurs. (The last option is not one described in the literature I have read.) Procedures (A) and (B) are type (1); (C) and (D) are type (2). We could evaluate each of these procedures with respect to (i) their effectiveness, and (ii) moral considerations as they bear on (a) innocent people and (b) those people we must treat as innocent until proven guilty. (It is possible that if something is objectionable from the perspective of the innocent, that should count against it more than if it is objectionable from the perspective of those proven to be guilty.)

Procedure (D) seems best from all points of view, since only if one is doing what one should not does any monitoring or interference by others take place. The question is whether it is feasible and effective. Now consider procedures (A) and (C). The innocent would probably find being barred from the child's room more objectionable than being monitored. Secret monitoring is also more effective if barring a guilty parent may lead her to remove the child from the hospital. Hence, it would seem there is more to be said for secret monitoring than for barring. But we should keep in mind that even if the innocent would hypothetically prefer monitoring to barring, monitoring which involves deception seems intrinsically morally more objectionable than simply not allowing someone in a room. That is, secret monitoring is more disrespectful of the person, even if it causes less suffering to an innocent parent and her child. (This helps bring out the difference between wronging someone and harming him.) If it were possible to prevent a parent from removing a child from the hospital, or to alert other hospitals in the vicinity if there is an attempt to transfer, this would increase the effectiveness of barring. Finally, consider procedure (B). Having a nurse in the room seems as effective as barring in catching the guilty and imposes less of a burden on the innocent.

On the basis of all this, a possible ranking of the four procedures in order of overall preference is (D), (B), (A), and (C), but monitoring would move up on the list if (A) and (B) would lead to the child being removed.

Finally, we might consider telling the truth about our suspicions. Suppose we openly suggest (nonsecret) monitoring or alarming. The innocent might be tempted to reject it because they are insulted. But would they risk the health of their child by removing the child from the hospital, especially if all hospitals had the same policy? I doubt it. If someone refuses nonsecret monitoring and removes the child, I think we have at least enough grounds for further investigation by child-abuse authorities, as well as grounds for temporarily restraining the parent from removing the child from the hospital.[15]

Summary

Having first characterized MSBP, I have considered possible approaches to justifying secret monitoring of a parent. One approach relies on what a good parent would hypothetically be willing to agree to undergo. A second approach focuses on the right of a hospital to monitor its premises but faces the moral problem of the need to conceal whether it is acting on its right. Finally, I have evaluated, on effectiveness and moral grounds, several specific means that might be used to deter and stop wrongful behavior.

Notes

1. This chapter is a revised version of a chapter originally published in *Ethical Dilemmas in Pediatrics: Cases and Commentaries*, eds. Lorry R. Frankel, Amnon Goldworth, Mary V. Rorty, and William A. Silverman (New York: Cambridge University Press, 2005). I thank Derek Parfit, Roger Crisp, Rosamond Rhodes, Arthur Applbaum, the editors of *Ethical Dilemmas in Pediatrics*, and the audience at the Oxford–Mt. Sinai Colloquium on

Medical Ethics, New York, April 1999, for helpful comments on previous versions of this chapter.

2. Since this article was originally submitted for publication, there has been increasing skepticism about whether many cases presumably thought to involve MSBP actually did so. There has also been concern that hostility to women may sometimes have prompted the MSBP diagnosis. I shall simply assume for the sake of argument that MSBP actually occurs at least sometimes.

3. For stylistic reasons, this chapter generally uses "mother" and "she" in referring to the parent, although fathers and male caretakers have also been associated with MSBP.

4. According to the DSM-IV the diagnosis is applied to the perpetrator. But according to the OED the diagnosis can be given to the victim. I thank Olivia Bailey for research on this.

5. J. A. Wilde and A. T. Pedron, "Privacy Rights in Munchausen Syndrome," *Contemporary Pediatrics*, November 1993, 86.

6. R. Connelly, "Ethical Issues in the Use of Covert Video Surveillance in the Diagnosis of Munchausen Syndrome by Proxy: The Atlanta Study, An Ethical Challenge for Medicine," *HEC Forum* 15 (2003): 21–41.

7. This argument was made to me by Dr. Kurt Hirschorn, at the time head of the Ethics Committee of Mt. Sinai Hospital, New York City.

8. I do not wish to foreclose the possibility that the reason the parent has the morally guilty state of mind is that she is psychiatrically ill, and this may be an excusing condition that makes it wrong to declare her legally guilty.

9. An alternative strategy is to focus on our expectation that an innocent parent would endorse our behavior after the fact when it is revealed.

10. Derek Parfit emphasized this point to me.

11. Connolly, "Ethical Issues."

12. Much more would have to be said about why we should hold parents to the standard of a good parent.

13. Hospitals may have a right to monitor, but suppose it was generally known that they did not take advantage of that right. Then it would be reasonable for people not to expect to be monitored, although they would not be entitled to expect not to be monitored.

14. Notice that there is a distinction between wronging and harming; a lie can be a wronging of someone even if it does not harm him. Paternalistic action is by definition action that promotes someone's interest, and yet it can be a wronging of a person.

15. Wilde and Pedron, "Privacy Rights in Munchausen Syndrome," seem to think it is a more serious step to keep a parent from a child than to monitor her secretly. This may be true in terms of burden on an innocent mother and child, but barring access lacks some of the moral problems of secret monitoring.

PART THREE

Genetic and Other Enhancements

15

Genes, Justice, and Obligations in Creating People

REFLECTIONS ON *FROM CHANCE TO CHOICE* AND
ON VIEWS OF NAGEL, SHIFFRIN, AND SINGER

I. Introduction

In this chapter, I shall discuss ethical issues that arise with our increasing ability
to affect the genetic makeup of the human population.[1] These effects can be produced directly by altering the genotype (through germline or somatic changes),[2]
or indirectly by aborting, not conceiving, or treating individuals because of their
genetic makeup in ways made possible by genetic pharmacology. I shall refer to
all of these sorts of procedures collectively as the Procedures. Some of the ethical
issues the Procedures raise are old, arising quite generally when we can affect the
well-being of people, even in the absence of the ability to affect them in the ways
just described. My examination of these issues is prompted by the in-depth discussion of them, in *From Chance to Choice* (henceforth *CC*), by Allen Buchanan, Dan
Brock, Norman Daniels, and Daniel Wikler.[3]

I shall begin in part II by offering what is for the most part a summary of some
of the topics and views presented in *CC*, with interspersed critical remarks. In part
III, I address several of the topics examined in *CC* in greater detail. I raise further
questions about *CC*'s analyses and about discussions by Thomas Nagel, Seana
Shiffrin, and Peter Singer of some related issues. I also offer my own somewhat
different views on these various matters.[4]

II. Overview of *From Chance to Choice*

In the immediate future, our ability to alter humankind by way of some of the
Procedures may not be great. (Our most immediate ability may not be to alter a
genetic condition, but rather to diagnose it and avoid having progeny that have
it. Several of the Procedures related to controlling reproduction— for example,

avoiding conception or having an abortion—have been feasible for some time.) However, let us, like the authors of *CC*, take a long view, which is not necessarily science-fictional. Two possibilities for change by way of the Procedures involve (1) eliminating diseases that interfere with normal species functioning (NSF), and (2) enhancement of NSF. It is a merit of *CC* that it recognizes that enhancement itself may take two forms: (a) improving humans so that they fare better than any current human with respect to some characteristic; and (b) bringing people to have good characteristics, whose absence in them would not be a disease, that are now already common to many but not all humans (e.g., high intelligence). Furthermore, since the same condition—for example, a height of 4' 10"—can be caused by low-range NSF in one person and by a disease in another, enhancement in one person could result in nothing more than what eliminating a disease would cause in someone else. For something to be an enhancement, it must be in some way good. Even NSF should not be pursued unless it is good in some way. Does this mean that, in deciding to treat or enhance people, we must adopt a uniform and controversial theory of what traits are good? Not necessarily, as the authors of *CC* believe that we can reach reasoned agreement on certain primary natural goods and evils in order to guide a social program; beyond that, *CC*'s authors suggest, individuals, independent of social agreement, might be free within limits to alter themselves or their children based on different conceptions of the good.

This raises the question in *CC* of who, individual or society, should instigate treatment or enhancement. A primary reason why *CC* claims that eugenics as a social goal and eugenics as an individual undertaking can dovetail is that the legitimate goals of society coincide with at least many of the goals that parents may suitably have for their children. That is, both society and parents want children who have what all can agree are primary natural goods. I shall call this the Coincidence Thesis. However, *CC* claims near its conclusion that society can engage in eugenic alteration beyond changes related to basic, socially agreed-upon defects and excellences without violating liberal neutrality with respect to controversial views about the good life. They claim this is possible because if we vote on which traits to alter, society is acting on aggregated preferences rather than on an enforced scheme of values. I find this claim quite problematic. First, some may think that democracy ideally involves deliberation rather than the mere aggregation of preferences. But even if democracy is merely preference-aggregation, I think it is worrying that a temporary majority should be able, on the basis of its controversial preferences, to introduce widespread eugenic changes that would be difficult to reverse (and that may also vary from nation to nation).

If society does engage in eugenic planning, is the question of whether to treat or enhance a matter of justice or a matter of some social goal beyond justice? In considering this issue, *CC* for the most part understands justice deontologically— that is, as a side constraint on the production of good states of affairs. (Although the authors depart from this understanding on occasion, I shall argue.) Justice so understood is something for the sake of which we may have to sacrifice various goods, such as efficiency and the creation of overall wealth. Modern theories of *social* justice (e.g., Rawls's)[5] deal with how the goods of a cooperating unit such as a nation-state should be distributed justly. Such theories take it as given who the participants in cooperation are and what naturally given individual characteristics they will have. It is assumed that people do not deserve to have the set of natural characteristics with which they find themselves; what one gets is simply a matter of (good or bad) luck in the natural lottery. CC notes that since the Procedures will make possible the donation and alteration of natural characteristics, we may move beyond the natural lottery and face the question of whether justice requires any particular distribution of genetic material. I shall call this question the Just Creation Question. One way to phrase the query is as follows: assuming genes influence abilities, does justice require that we create people either roughly equal in abilities or unequal in a way that is in the interest of those who turn out to be worst off? (This particular formulation is modeled on what is known as the "maximin solution" for just distribution of primary goods in Rawls's theory of justice. Part of Rawls's second principle of justice, known as the Difference Principle, says that inequality is not unjust if it is necessary to serve those who will be worst off.)

Suppose justice does not require us to enforce a systematic social plan as an answer to the Just Creation Question, but some individuals do engage in treatment and enhancement at the individual level. The social effects of this may be that some people who are not treated or enhanced will be at a disadvantage or even unable to participate in what becomes society's dominant cooperative framework. CC asks if it is at least a requirement of justice that society monitor individually instigated changes to ensure that everyone be able to participate minimally in the dominant cooperative framework and not be excluded. (I shall call this the Just Inclusion Question.) This could be done by seeing to it that the dominant cooperative framework does not change so that some people cannot participate in it. Alternatively, society could make provisions, as a requirement of justice, to allow people to be created or altered so that they meet the requirements for participation in a dominant cooperative framework that becomes much revised as a result of optional treatment and enhancement by individuals.

Put very briefly, CC's answer to the Just Creation and Just Inclusion Questions is that correcting for defects so as to provide NSF is required of society by that part of Rawls's theory of social justice concerned with fair equality of opportunity (FEO), as is any enhancement necessary for minimal-level participation in the dominant cooperative framework. In addition, CC argues that if other enhancements are widespread and very valuable, those who lack the enhancements have a claim, based on justice, to receive them.[6] (It is important to realize what these requirements do not include. Suppose that prior to a radical change in the dominant cooperative framework, being a secretary satisfies the requirement for minimal inclusion. Now suppose that enhancements undertaken by individuals cause a radical change in the dominant cooperative framework so that many individuals who were previously high-level executives can now fill only secretarial positions.

According to *CC*, these individuals have no claim on society, as a matter of justice, for enhancements that would allow them to reclaim their prior executive status. This is because they can be secretaries.)

Suppose we are in a situation in which we face a choice between changing the dominant cooperative framework to match people or changing people to match the dominant cooperative framework. *CC* says that the interest in a more excellent dominant cooperative framework could mandate changing people. But suppose we can obtain a much-improved dominant cooperative framework, with the caveat that some people, even after we do whatever enhancements for them that we can, would be incapable of minimal-level participation in the new framework. According to *CC*, whether we keep the dominant cooperative framework from improving for most people should be decided by balancing the legitimate interest in being inclusive against the legitimate interest in there being a more excellent dominant cooperative framework, with inclusion being given some but not absolute priority. Indeed, *CC* says that justice, at this point, is a matter of balancing the interests.[7] This balancing view suggests that the interest in inclusion could be outweighed in certain circumstances. At the very least, balancing implies that inclusion would not be treated as a matter of the FEO component in Rawls's theory of justice. This is because in Rawls's scheme FEO has lexical priority over achieving great goods in general and even over the Difference Principle. I think that by accepting the balancing of inclusion and dominant cooperative framework excellence, *CC* modifies to some degree the deontological conception of justice with which it begins.[8]

For the authors of *CC*, three moral duties that apply to society and to individuals are as basic as the requirements of social justice. Two of these duties are the duty not to harm persons and the duty to prevent harm to persons. In *CC*, the first of these duties is exemplified by the duty of a pregnant person not to expose herself to a toxin that would cause damage to a fetus (which *CC* assumes is not already a person) from which a defective person will arise.

As for the duty to prevent harm to persons (even at moderate cost to oneself), *CC* claims that this duty could justifiably lead to restrictions on reproductive freedom. This is because fetuses will ultimately give rise to persons, and the authors think we can prevent harm to those future persons by acting so as to prevent certain types of naturally occurring conditions in fetuses. The duty to prevent harm entails a subsidiary duty to prevent (even at moderate cost to oneself) lives that are not worth living (or lives worth not living—e.g., lives full of so much pain and suffering that a state of affairs without those lives would be a better one, other things being equal).[9] According to *CC*, we can satisfy this duty by not conceiving such a life, by aborting it before it reaches a developmental stage where it has the right not to be destroyed, or by altering the future person's characteristics in some way. (I might add that if its life is not worth living, it is not clear that prior to having a will of its own, a being ever reaches a developmental stage where it is impermissible to destroy it.)

The duty to prevent harm also entails, *CC* claims, a subsidiary duty to prevent (even at moderate cost to oneself) the existence of a person whose life would be worth living but who would be disabled in some significant respect. This duty applies straightforwardly if we can prevent the disability in a given person. The duty can be modified, *CC* argues, so as to also give us a duty to substitute for an individual who will be disabled another individual who will not be disabled, and who will otherwise have a life as much worth living. When we can prevent the disability in a given person, the duty derives from a "person-affecting" moral principle of preventing harm. Person-affecting principles are those that apply when the person affected if we perform some action is the very same person who is affected if we do not.[10] When we can substitute another individual for the one with the disability, the duty derives from a "nonperson-affecting" moral principle of preventing harm—that is, a principle of preventing harm that applies when our performing some action results in an entirely different individual being formed.[11] In the case of a disability, the relevant action is our substituting the creation of one person without a disability for the creation of another person with it. The "substituted" person who lives without the disability is not better off than she otherwise would have been, since the person with the disability in the alternative state of affairs would not have been her, but someone else entirely. On the other hand, if we do not engage in these sorts of substitutions, no person will be worse off than *he* or *she* otherwise would have been, and the disabled person who is created would have a life worth living (according to the stipulations described at the beginning of the paragraph). However, *CC* claims that we could nevertheless have a duty to make these sorts of substitutions.

Suppose someone cannot prevent the only offspring he could have from being severely disabled or living only a short time, when this offspring would have a life worth living. *CC* claims that so long as one is prepared to take care of such an offspring, it is permissible—and even good—to produce it.

The third duty that *CC* claims pertains to both society and individuals involved in creating people is a duty correlative to the right of a child to an open future. This is the right of a child not to have her set of potential options in life narrowed too much through genetic manipulation or other means. Though *CC* does not raise the issue, a possible problem with such a right to an open future is that it would also imply that we should use genetic manipulation to alter the makeup of individuals who would naturally have an excessively constricted range of options, even if those options are very good ones. For example, if the right to an open future implied that it is wrong to actively predispose someone to exercise one particular great intellectual gift, it could also call for altering someone who is already strongly genetically predisposed to exercise such a gift. Because this latter position seems implausible to me, I worry about the existence of a right to an open future, unless it is construed as a negative right not to have one's options closed rather than a positive right to have one's options expanded.

Construed as a negative right, the right to an open future may be very important, I believe. The authors of *CC*, unlike some who think that the free choices of parents rather than a state program should determine genetic alterations, do not forget that the freedom of any children produced is also an issue. The parents, after all, are not merely making self-concerned choices; they are affecting a third party.[12] For example, suppose parents were free to "hardwire" gender stereotyping. Then in the absence of an antidote, the options of girls and boys would be greatly narrowed given that there is currently some capacity for nonstereotypic behavior. The traits parents choose may make their child more "successful" within a sex-stereotyped system when it might be better to question that system itself.

However, I think there remains a danger that an open future will be thought of in terms of the *number* of options that people retain. Perhaps it would be better to think of having an open future as having the higher-order ability to think rationally, evaluate, and act in accord with the reasons there really are for living and acting in certain ways, whatever those ways are. It may be safe to enhance this higher-order ability.

The combination of duties that *CC* outlines, following from FEO and from our duties not to cause harm, to prevent harm, and not to violate a right to an open future, are important. But it is also important to see that these duties do not completely foreclose what intuitively seem like morally objectionable genetic selections. For example, altering genetic material so that someone develops who is heterosexual or male rather than homosexual or female does not seem to foreclose to that individual a sufficiently open future, nor does it harm that individual. It might nevertheless be morally wrong to genetically select for heterosexuality or maleness if homosexuality and femaleness are equally nonharmful states and offer an adequately open future.[13]

CC discusses the issues involved in controlling genes in a history-sensitive manner. Its authors realize that they are talking about eugenics and that eugenics, especially when state-run, has a bad history. They believe that eugenics pursued as a useful social goal (even if not required by justice) can be appropriate so long as we are conscious of ethical requirements that previous generations ignored. Some of these I have already discussed, such as our duty to socially subsidize people's inclusion in a changing dominant cooperative framework and our duties to not harm and to preserve open futures. The other requirements include our duty to take the inviolability of persons seriously (i.e., so that we do not kill people who are imperfect, even as we try to eliminate imperfections by not creating people who will have them), our duty to take the separateness of persons seriously (i.e., so that we do not produce great aggregate goods by providing only small goods to each of a great number of people while neglecting to prevent great ills that occur to each of a small number of people), and our duty to take the autonomy of persons seriously (i.e., so that we do not coerce use of the Procedures to produce a social good).

I would summarize the advice of *CC* by saying that it provides two overriding principles that should guide any individual or social eugenic project, including projects that rank the objective worth of traits. First, always aim to improve and not make worse the life of every individual person, subject to the person's consent. Persons' lives will not be improved if they are eliminated when they have lives well worth living from their point of view, even if they lack traits it would be better to have. Second, temper individuals' freedom to determine the traits of others by developing social controls that express concern for (a) the welfare and freedom of those others whose traits would be determined, and (b) the effect that genetic control can have on equality of opportunity in society. The authors believe the point of eugenic change is the improvement of an individual's life from his own point of view. But they deny that this goal is to be achieved by an individualistic, unregulated "supermarket" in genetic alteration, or licenses the absence of a social project to improve the citizenry.

Unfortunately, *CC* does not attend sufficiently to the possibility that many societies will not be able to proceed safely with eugenics, since they are not appropriately noncoercive and socially just, and will not be able to enforce the ethical requirements that *CC* emphasizes. *CC* barely discusses this issue, which concerns what to do when there will be imperfect compliance with justice and other moral requirements.

III. Alternative Proposals

In this part, I first focus in more detail on aspects of the Just Creation Question and on what FEO requires in the way of treatment and enhancement. I consider not only *CC*'s positions but also the views of Thomas Nagel. I then move on to consider the issues of duties to prevent and not cause harm when producing future people and the effect of genetic selection on the disabled. Finally, I deal with the Coincidence Thesis.

A. JUST CREATION: DIFFERENT CONCEPTIONS OF EQUAL CONCERN AND RESPECT

Many of the hypothetical cases moral philosophers like to discuss involve the question of whether it is permissible to take some good away from one person who has it in abundance in order to redistribute it more equally among a greater number (either including the original person or not). For example, if one person has two healthy eyes, may we take one to give to someone else who is blind? Nonconsequentialists typically say it is impermissible to do this, even if the state of the world in which the good is more equally distributed is a better one. The inviolability of the person or his right to bodily integrity is appealed to as a side-constraint on the production of the best state of affairs. But if we are about to create people, no one's claim to bodily integrity stands in the way of our distributing traits equally if this is in our power.

Suppose I am going to create from scratch three new people. Further, suppose, by hypothesis, that certain genetic material is known to be correlated with talents and opportunities in life. Am I morally obligated to distribute these materials equally, or unequally if this will thereby (somehow) make the absolute position of the resulting worst-off person better than it would be in an equal distribution? I do not think I am obligated in either of these ways. It would be permissible for me to distribute in other ways, even though (by hypothesis) no one deserves to be better off than anyone else. It may be said that I will owe each person who will result equal concern and respect and so should create them in the same spirit. But I want to suggest that a requirement to treat others with equal concern and respect is satisfied if I simply give each person what he is owed as a person by the person who creates him (his creator). I think creators do owe their creations certain important goods or a significant chance at them.[14] Once I give this to each of the people I create, as a byproduct they will be equals with respect to getting what each is owed as an individual by his creator. Having done this, I might choose to give more to one person than I am required to give to just any person I create, not because he deserves it, but simply because I would like to create a certain type of person—for example, one with great musical talent—and I cannot do this if I am equally generous to all my creations.

This understanding of "equal concern and respect" may be further illustrated by examining how we understand the phrase in other contexts. For example, when we say that a doctor owes each of her patients equal concern and respect, we mean that they are entitled to be treated as equals with respect to their medical needs. We do not mean that it would be wrong of the doctor not to be concerned with her patients' educational needs, or wrong of her to give a present to one patient and not another. We first have in mind certain things to which patients are entitled from their doctor, and a doctor's equal concern and respect pertains to the provision of these things. Similarly, I believe, when we say that one's government owes each citizen equal concern and respect, we mean that with respect to those things that a citizen is entitled to from its government, citizens must be treated with equal concern and respect.

On this view, we cannot derive what a doctor owes her patient, what a government owes its citizens, or what a creator owes her progeny from the idea of equal concern and respect itself. This idea is applied only after we know what the entitlements are. This interpretation of owing equal concern and respect contrasts with one that tries, for example, to derive what a citizen is owed by his or her government from the idea that the government owes each citizen equal concern and respect.[15] This second interpretation can immediately lead to what I would call a "totalist" theory—for example, one in which the state must be concerned with how citizens fare overall on any dimension that could be relevant to judging if people are faring equally. By contrast, on a "nontotalist" view of the state, once the state has fulfilled its responsibilities, whatever they may be, equally to all its citizens, inequalities (even those that are side effects of state policies) are not necessarily violations of equal concern and respect.

The nontotalist interpretation of equal concern and respect on the part of creators of people (or the state) allows for inequality in the distribution of natural
traits, at least so long as the inequality does not result in the disappearance of
important goods such as an atmosphere of mutual understanding or equal political
participation. A nontotalist view is, I think, morally permissible so long as we do
not think of available genes as common property belonging to all past, present, and
potential future members of the human race. The common-property view might
imply that we are obligated to distribute genes equally or in accord with maximin,
as a similar result is often argued for with respect to products of social cooperation.
But why should we think genes or possible talents are common property? Is it
because no one deserves to have the ones they have, and this is thought to imply
that if traits do not already inhere in individuals, everyone who will exist is entitled
to an equal share? This would seem to be a possible presupposition of an egalitarian (or maximin) requirement on the distribution of genes. But it is, at the very
least, a problematic presupposition.

Since *CC*'s authors argue that justice does not require us to distribute genes or
talents equally or in accord with maximin, I take my conclusion to be in line with
theirs. However, the authors also take the view that society, as a matter of justice,
does have an obligation to provide NSF (e.g., eliminate disease) and also to provide
people with enhancements that are either necessary for minimal participation in
the dominant cooperative framework or necessary in order to have valuable enhancements that are already widespread. They argue that the satisfaction of Rawls's
FEO principle requires us to see to it that people with equal talent and motivation
fare roughly similarly, so ill health should not interfere with one person if it does
not interfere with others who are equally talented and motivated. However, note
that, strictly speaking, it is compatible with FEO so understood that equal *ill* health
be present within a talent/motivation set, for then two people with equal talent
and motivation will fare roughly similarly. The real point *CC* is making, I take it, is
that it may be a matter of FEO that people's outcomes not be a function of ill health
or disability, whether these are equally or unequally present, but rather of their
talents and motivations.[16]

Suppose we adopt this (somewhat revised) view of FEO. It implies that if we
can control the distribution of genes, it is a matter of social justice that there be a
social program to genetically treat diseases and disabilities that interfere with
people exercising their talent/motivation packages. Though this program would
involve the control of genes, why should it be seen as radically different from
public health programs that now try to control bacteria that cause paralysis,
blindness, or deafness? (This is not to deny that there would be distinct ethical
problems—which *CC* recognizes—in the state requiring forms of genetic control
that include abortion, destruction of embryos, or participation in projects that
involve public knowledge of private data.) As *CC* notes, this view of FEO does
not call for equal or maximin distribution of genes relating to talents and motivation themselves.

I suggest we might put this point about the treatment of conditions that interfere with talents, by contrast to general enhancement, in the following way: If, because I am ill, I have the opportunities open to me of someone with an IQ of 110 even though I have an IQ of 130, then my ill health stands in the way of my expressing my nature. In contrast, if the reason I have the opportunities of a person with an IQ of 110 rather than those of someone with an IQ of 130 is that I have an IQ of 110 (which is within NSF), the failure to provide me with 20 additional IQ points does not prevent me from expressing my nature. The question is whether this distinction is so morally crucial that it can justify providing treatment of diseases while not providing equally costly enhancements that would have the same results.[17]

B. NAGEL ON FEO

Let us now take note of the fact that not everyone accepts that justice requires us to seek NSF in order to ensure FEO. Thomas Nagel, for example, seems to reject this view.[18] He argues that Rawlsian FEO is intended to address only socially caused— not naturally caused—impediments that lead to different opportunities for people of equal talent and motivation. For example, some social inequalities are just since they result from incentives permitted by the Difference Principle. Yet according to Rawls, if these inequalities impact equal opportunity in the next generation, these effects must be corrected. By contrast, Nagel claims, if someone is born with an illness not due to social causes that would limit his opportunities in any society, correcting it does not have the priority of a deontological claim of justice. (This does not mean it should not be corrected by society. It is just that correcting it must be balanced against all the other good things that one could do with social resources, and it does not have the deontological priority of justice.) Nagel does recognize that there are a class of effects on opportunities that are the result of the interaction of society and nature; that is, if society were not structured as it is, certain physical differences would not make a difference to people's opportunities. He argues that we must first decide what is to be deemed the cause of these differences in opportunity—society, nature, or both—and then decide who has responsibility for dealing with them. Nagel believes that it is appropriate to say that nature, not society, causes the problem if (1) there is no intent to structure society in order to hold back people with the relevant physical or mental differences, (2) there is a good independent reason for society's being structured the way it is, and (3) it would be very socially costly to change society so that these differences did not affect opportunity. In Nagel's view, identifying the cause of the differences in opportunity still does not settle the question of whether society is responsible *as a matter of justice* for correcting what it does not cause, but he doubts that it is responsible as a function of either FEO or the Difference Principle.

I wish to raise several questions about Nagel's analysis. First, I find puzzling his way of determining whether society can be said to cause a lack of equal opportunity.

The three factors he cites as indicating that nature rather than society is the source of the problem—the lack of an intent to differentially affect people's opportunities; the existence of a good independent reason for the social structure; and the large cost of changing the society—do not seem to have anything to do with determining the cause of a problem. To see this, consider the role of three factors like Nagel's in another context. Suppose I am driving a car fast and run over someone. Suppose further that I did not intend to hit him, that I acted for the good independent reason of needing to rush five people to an emergency room, and that I would have suffered the big expense of ruining my car had I instead swerved. These facts do not imply that the primary cause of the accident was my victim's crossing the road rather than my driving fast. I may have a good excuse (or even a justification) for causing the accident, but I am still identified as the cause. Why should the three factors Nagel points to be any more relevant to determining whether it is society or nature that is the primary cause of lack of opportunity?

Now consider a particular social situation. Suppose there is a small difference between people—some have an extra knuckle on their ring finger that has never before had any social importance. Imagine that this difference comes to be very important in operating computers that are crucial to social production and we cannot alter the computers without great cost; hence, people's opportunities are very different, depending on whether they have the knuckle. Nagel's analysis of causation yields the conclusion that these differences in opportunities for people are *caused by* the natural difference rather than by the nature of the society. But this conclusion about causation seems clearly wrong, even if this does not determine whether it is impermissible for society to have this causal effect.

Nagel's analysis of causation may even imply that the inequalities in opportunity that he himself says are socially caused and should be corrected as a matter of justice are *not* socially caused and so need not be corrected as a matter of justice. Suppose the economic inequalities due to incentives are not introduced merely in order to create unequal opportunities for equally talented children of the next generation, that there are good reasons licensed by Rawls's Difference Principle for introducing the incentives, and that the social costs of not having such incentives would be great. Does not Nagel's analysis of causation imply that the differences in opportunity that are the effects of the incentives are not socially caused?[19] If so, on what grounds should society, as a matter of justice, be responsible for correcting the differences in opportunities of the next generation that result from incentives—for example, by providing scholarships for educating poor but talented students—if it is not responsible as a matter of justice for correcting other inequalities that it does not cause according to the same explanation of causation?

Suppose that my discussion shows that there is some problem with Nagel's analysis of causation. Suppose also that society is required by justice to undo certain effects of even just wealth inequality when they affect equally talented and motivated people differently. This means that if rich, talented children get higher education, then society should pay for higher education for poor, talented children as a matter of FEO. Now suppose that the rich use their money for health-care treatment, or even for greater genetic enhancement of their talents, so as to correct naturally caused limitations. The resulting inequalities in health and talents between rich and poor would be as socially caused as the unequal access to education. (In the case of talent enhancement, there would be socially caused unequal opportunity for those of equally low talents to acquire more talents.) Why then should there not be as strong (or weak) a claim based on justice for social help in equalizing health care and enhancement resources as there is for social help in equalizing education resources? On the view I am now describing (unlike *CC*'s), if *no one* were using extra wealth to acquire health care for NSF or enhancement, there might be no claim on the part of anyone for social help in correcting any natural differences in health (even to achieve NSF) or in talents *as a matter of justice*. But suppose some are acquiring these services (even if they are not widespread and do not affect the dominant cooperative framework) because of socially caused economic differences in wealth (even just ones). Then the claim for social help seems justified by the grounds that Nagel himself puts forward to support FEO.[20] (Of course, this conclusion might lead some to reconsider the correctness of these grounds in general.)

Finally, note that when Nagel discusses the nature/society interaction, he does so in the context of imagining an illness that is clearly caused independently of society, even though its impact on opportunity may be a function of society. But recent data indicates that wealth inequality may be a cause of—not merely correlated with—differential health. For example, wealth inequality may not be merely correlated with health by way of differential access to cures for illness; rather, whether illnesses appear in the first place seems to vary inversely with wealth.[21] The claim is that the less talented are sicker than others with more talents in a society where wealth is (roughly) distributed in accord with natural talents, but they would not be sicker than others in a society with a more egalitarian distribution of wealth. (In other words, the claim denies that the less talented become sicker for reasons unrelated to such social determinants as wealth incentives.)

If this claim is correct, social justice might mandate treatment (including genetic treatment) to achieve NSF, if we think that a society chooses its incentive structure and in doing so actually causes unequal health. A possible objection to this conclusion is that social causation of illness is not sufficient for social responsibility for treatment if those who are caused to be less healthy are still better off overall with the incentive structure than they would be in a more equal society.

C. REPRODUCTION

1. Preventing Harm, Causing Harm, and Enabling Harm

CC notes that if someone is born to a life not worth living that could have been avoided only by his nonexistence, he has not, in the strict sense, been harmed. This is because he has not been made worse off than he would otherwise have been, as he would not otherwise have been at all. However, as *CC* notes, if we save someone from death, she will also not strictly have been benefited, since she is not better off than she would have otherwise been (given the assumption that death involves her nonexistence). Yet we reasonably would treat saving a person to a good life as benefiting her and causing her to die when she would have had a good life as harming her. Hence, even if these cases do not strictly involve harming and benefiting, *CC* thinks it is reasonable to treat them as involving what is *identical* in moral respects to harming and benefiting. *CC* also argues that if having three more years of bad life at the end of life is worse than having zero additional years at the end of life, then it is also true that having three bad years of life is worse than having zero years due to noncreation.

Let us consider possible implications of these views. From the premise that creating lives not worth living (really lives worth not living[22]) can be wrong and can be treated morally like straightforward harming, *CC* concludes that we have a duty to prevent such lives stemming from a duty to *prevent harm*. But notice that in creating someone with a life not worth living, we could *do* something like harming, rather than just allow something like harming to occur. This seems clearly so when parents create with genes that will definitely cause spina bifida. Why then does *CC* say that our duty in this situation falls under the duty to *prevent* harm—a duty that is thought to apply when we should rescue someone from harm that we do not cause—rather than the duty *not* to *cause* harm? *CC* says that the duty not to cause harm applies if a pregnant woman were to take a toxin that would cause a defect in her fetus. This suggests that the authors think that if a creator does not deliberately give genes that cause a bad life in someone (as in spina bifida when parents could not have given different genes), a creator does not cause harm. This seems wrong. Consider a case involving someone who is already alive: I want the person to be close to me. The only way to accomplish this is to bring her through a route where naturally occurring x-rays will unavoidably cause her great damage. (Call this the Bring Close Case.) This bad effect is only a foreseen side effect of my bringing her close to me. Indeed, my actions do not even cause the x-rays but only expose her to them. Nevertheless, if I bring the person through the route, knowingly exposing her to harmful rays, I will have harmed her, not merely failed to prevent harm.[23] (Designating this a harming is not inconsistent with thinking that if one arranges for the harmful rays to work when one could have avoided this, or if one uses this route when one could have used another harmless route, one will have committed a more serious wrong.) Furthermore, if there is no possible benefit to the other person in coming close to me, doing what harms her is wrong.

I believe that the costs that one must incur in order not to cause harm are higher than the costs that even a parent-to-be must incur to merely *prevent* harm to his creation that he has not caused. My own view is that at least when it is known for *certain* that a life not worth living (understood as worth not living) will result from the act of creation that provides harmful genes, it is the duty not to cause harm and the costs one should pay to perform that duty that are relevant, rather than the duty to prevent harm that one did not cause and that duty's associated costs.

Now, consider cases in which there is only a small risk that a life not worth living will result but the risk comes about by the *chance* that harmful genes will be given. Since no one would be harmed by not existing, and no one's noncreation represents a strict failure to be benefited, does not exposing one to this risk fall under the duty not to cause a risk of harm rather than the duty to prevent a risk of harm? After all, merely deliberately exposing already existing people to a risk of their lives not being worth living, when this provides them with no possible improvements in their condition, can be considered causing a risk of harm and is prima facie wrong. For example, consider a variation on the Bring Close Case in which there is only a small risk of exposure to x-rays causing the great damage. Even a great need to have the person close might not justify moving her through the route with x-rays when there could be no benefit to her in doing so.

The fact that it is permissible, when we create, to expose someone to the risk of having a terrible life either by possibly giving bad genes or by introducing our creation into a physical environment that may cause very bad states—and to some extent this is what we always do when we reproduce—may suggest that we implicitly think the following: The possibility of creating someone with a good life (i.e., a life that is worth living to a degree high enough to meet the standard that should be a goal in creating a person) is *like* the possibility of giving someone who is *already* in existence a benefit for which it is acceptable for him to run a risk of harm.[24]

Previously, we noted that saving someone from death is *like an ordinary benefit*, even though the already-existing person will not be better off than he would otherwise *be*. Now we are extending the connection to an ordinary benefit so that even those who do not already exist can be treated as though they are benefited in being created to a good life. Perhaps this is really already presupposed by our having said that we can do something like harming someone who does not already exist by creating him to a life worth not living. Nevertheless, I think that saving a life is closer to the ordinary notion of benefit than is creating a good new life because, in the former case, an individual already existed to whom more good life will come. We might, therefore, think of three categories: benefit, benefit(a), and benefit(b). Benefit strictly involves comparative states of a person (e.g., he will be better off than he would otherwise be); benefit(a) involves keeping someone in a good state (rather than his going out of existence) so that one possible trajectory of his life is better than another in that it goes on longer in a good state; benefit(b) involves creating someone to a good state. (It seems impossible to fail to benefit[b] by not creating someone since no one will exist if we do not benefit[b], and yet it is possible for the person one creates to be benefited[b].[25])

This benefit(b) to the potential person would also make sense of the idea that when we create new people, it is appropriate to think that we can do so for the sake of the good life *they* will enjoy (not only for our enjoyment). This is so even though in the strict sense we do not benefit them when we create them, since we do not make them better off than they were or would have been. We may also think that independent of benefits to a person, the moral importance of being a person (and of there being persons) justifies exposing someone to certain risks involved in the process of creation.[26]

CC goes beyond this view, I think. For from the fact that someone is benefited(a) by living three extra good years of life rather than dying, *CC* seems to conclude that three good years are better than nonexistence (represented by zero). From this, *CC*'s authors seem to further conclude that three good years is always better than zero, even when the choice before us is whether or not to create a new person who would exist for three good years and then die (assuming we could not create anything better). This leads to their view that if one cannot have any other child, it is fine to have such a child. This, I think, may be a mistake. The end of life is a morally different context from the beginning of it. When someone already exists, his dying (becoming zero) is harm(a) to him. Although there are no strict comparative states of the person involved, there is a shorter versus longer (better) trajectory of an existing person's life at stake. However, because a person we could create will not exist if we do not create him, there is no one who can be harmed or harmed(a) by not having three good years. Hence, it is possible that when no one would be harmed or harmed(a) if the three good years did not come to pass, creating the three good years may not be morally better than zero. This need not necessarily be because in creating someone who will die after three years of life we create someone who will be greatly harmed(a) (by being deprived of more life by death). That is, we need not be refraining from creating in order to avoid there being someone to whom a deprivation of life occurs. (Although it is true that we could prevent such a deprivation by not creating any life at all, as there would then be no subject who is deprived of life.[27]) Rather, we may refrain from creating because three years of life is not an appropriate goal to have when creating a person rather than a rabbit.

Indeed, I think that when we create a new life, we are obligated to try to provide it with what I call the "minima" appropriate to the life of a person, and these (despite the use of the term "minima") go beyond what makes a life minimally worth living.[28] For example, the sort of life that would consist of pleasure for a few years may be an appropriate goal if we create a rabbit, but may not be if we create a person. This is a reason to refrain from creating a short-lived person.[29]

Of course, one would have to explain in more detail why it is wrong to create if there is no hope of providing the minima. Here I only wish to note a possible connection between two claims: the claim that if human beings and nonhuman beings are functionally alike, they should be treated alike (a view for which Peter Singer and Jeff McMahan have argued),[30] and the claim that the type of being that will be created does not affect whether it is appropriate to create a being with a certain type of life. Some deny the first claim. They think that a human being who has failed to meet the standard of normality for its species-type by being much lower than the norm should be treated differently from a functionally equivalent being who is perfectly normal for its type (e.g., a rabbit). I think this view may be connected to the denial of the second claim and support for the view that we should avoid creating failures of the human type, even if they would be functionally equivalent to happy rabbits that it is permissible to create.[31]

To summarize a bit, I suggest that for the following reasons, we might wrong people even if we create them with lives worth living:

1. No one is harmed or fails to be benefited and no one is harmed(a) or fails to be benefited(a) by not being created because there is no one in existence if we do not create someone. (Also, no one fails to be benefited[b] or is harmed[b] in not being created since there will then be no subject.) Once someone exists, his losing his life can constitute a harm(a) to him, though it is not clear that this sort of harm(a) is a reason why one should not create him.

2. In part due to (1), we can set a high standard for permissibly creating people, demanding that people create lives with the minima for persons, lives that are more than minimally satisfactory.

3. Furthermore, if new people have a right to such lives, then we could violate their rights by creating them without meeting this standard. One way to avoid the violation is by not creating them, which would involve no violation of their rights nor any harm, harm(a), failure to benefit, or failure to benefit(a).

4. We can wrong people by violating their rights.

This view, unlike *CC*'s, implies that even if we are unable to create anything better, there are strong reasons not to create a very short life, even if it will be worth living for the person being created. These reasons might be overridden by the desire of individuals to parent, but there is something negative to be overridden.

Suppose creating a person unavoidably carries with it a small risk of creating a life worth not living and in a particular case a life worth not living is created by unavoidable donation of certain genes. The parents have done what is like causing harm, but it may have been acceptable to impose the risk of this on the new person in the light of the benefit(b) he might have had. If so, then the parents' duties in creating and to the offspring should be determined as though the parents did *not* do what is like causing harm or at least as though it was permissible of them to run the risk of doing this to produce benefits. I believe, for example, that the costs one morally ought to expend to reduce the risk of creating a life not worth living in risk cases are more like the costs that are implied by a duty to prevent harm that one does not cause than like the costs that are implied by a duty not to cause harm simpliciter. Likewise, the personal reasons (such as the strong desire to have bio-logically related offspring to which *CC* refers) might serve as adequate justification for creating only if we conceive of creating as like running a risk of causing harm to someone for the sake of benefiting him or as like not preventing risk of harm one does not cause. Such reasoning can make sense of *CC*'s speaking of the duty to prevent (rather than not cause) harm in many cases.[32]

Now consider creating lives that will be worth living but that will *definitely* have some serious disability due to unavoidable absence of some genetic element. I said above that there may be a reason, stemming from what is owed a person who will be created and the fact that no one will exist who is deprived of life, not to create a seriously disabled life (below the minima) even though it is still worth living. As a result, *not* creating what we know will definitely be such a life should have the moral significance of a duty not to *do* something wrong that would also wrong the person who will come to exist, even if it does not involve anything like *causing* harm. This is by contrast to not creating such a child having the significance of the duty to prevent a wrong (e.g., that someone else would cause).

2. Shiffrin on Harm and Procreating

I have been discussing the risk of creating lives not worth living[33] (really, worth not living) or without the minima owed to persons, when such lives come about by creators doing what seems like causing an outcome in the ordinary sense. I have suggested that one way to justify such risks may be to think of a good enough life for a person as something like a benefit for which it is worth the person-to-be running some such risks. Some opponents of this view hold the radical position that even the risk (and actuality) of relatively small burdens in an otherwise wonderful life can make creating impermissible (or at least morally problematic) even if (i) being created is assumed to be something like a benefit and (ii) the burdens do not come about by creators doing what seems like ordinary causation of an outcome. Let us consider the arguments of one proponent of this position.[34]

Seana Shiffrin is willing to accept that being created to a good life is something like a benefit for the person created. However, she argues that acts that bring about risks of harm or actual harms to people who are created cannot be justified by the possibility or, importantly, even the actuality of goods greater than the harms coming to them.[35] This includes risks and harms that are unavoidable if the person is to be created to a good life, not just risks and harms that could be avoided. Her argument concerning procreation stems from a more general argument about harms and benefits in nonprocreative contexts. It is important to emphasize that her argument focuses on harms that are less than the goods achievable, not merely risks of harms or actual harms that are greater than goods that could be achieved.

Let us first consider her discussion of the nonprocreative contexts. One part of her position is that harms are separable events that occur even when a person is overall better off as a result of someone else's action. For example, if we can save an adult from dying only by doing what breaks his leg, his having a broken leg is a harm to him even though it helps him avoid the worse harm of losing his life and so he is overall better off. Another part of her position is that causing (or allowing) harms to befall someone without his consent can be permissible in order to prevent greater harm coming to him but not in order to produce (or prevent the loss of) what she calls "pure benefits." The case we just considered involves the first option and she holds that though one harms the person without his consent, he is not wronged and no compensation is owed to him. Pure benefits are goods whose absence would not involve someone being in what she calls a harmed state, such as having bodily injury or some other condition that involves serious frustration of his will. (Note that she believes that one can be put in such a harmed state even if one is not made worse off relative to one's previous or alternative future state. Her notion of harm is, as she says, noncomparative.)

She presents a case to illustrate the point about not imposing harms for pure benefits: A rich person, Wealthy, wishes to benefit a group of already well-off people by giving each of them an immense fortune. The only way to get the fortune to them is to drop gold cubes on them from above, with the risk that someone will be injured even though care is taken; there is no way to communicate with them so as to get their consent to this. One person, Unlucky, does suffer a broken arm in receiving his fortune. (Call this the Gold Cube Case.) The fortune is a pure benefit because, while one will be worse off in life without the fortune, one will not be in a harmed state. Shiffrin claims that it is impermissible to drop the gold cubes even though, overall, Unlucky is better off with the fortune and the broken arm than with no fortune and no broken arm. She claims that this case is support for her view that without consent, it is impermissible to harm or risk harm to someone in order to provide a pure benefit.

She applies this view to procreation, for even if creating life is conceived of as like (but not literally the same as) giving a benefit, it is a pure benefit since no one will be in a harmed state if we do not create him. Furthermore, there are unavoidable harms associated with being alive. Among these harms, Shiffrin thinks, are the burdens of moral choice, and having to deal with eventual death. There is also the burden of typical risks of physical and psychological injuries that are run in every human life and the fruition of these risks in some cases, and the absence of an easy exit from these burdens (as suicide is difficult). Since it is impossible to get consent to his creation from the person created, her conclusion is that providing the pure benefit is at least morally problematic on the ground that it wrongs the person created even if the benefit is reasonably expected to be (and in fact will be) greater than the harm. (The Gold Cube Case seems to suggest a stronger conclusion, namely that procreation is pro tanto morally impermissible.) She further suggests that the explanation for parents' duties to provide extensive care for their offspring, beyond making his life merely on balance good, is that this is compensation owed for wronging him by creation.

I have concerns about Shiffrin's analysis of the Gold Cube Case and the implications she draws from it for creating people. Let us first consider Shiffrin's Gold Cube Case itself. It involves the provision of a pure benefit, not the prevention of its loss. The latter would be a better analog, still involving a pure benefit, to preventing a greater harm (as in the case where we break a leg to prevent a greater harm). For example, consider whether one may risk imposing lesser harms in order to prevent someone from losing a gold cube that is his already. It is even more important, I think, to consider *how* lesser harms could come to people in the course of providing (or preventing the loss of) the gold cubes and *what* sort of lesser harms occur. The chart in figure 15.1 presents some possibilities.

Chart: Where H= harm; B = benefit; GH= greater harm; PB= pure benefit

Some Issues in Intrapersonal H/B Case:	To stop GH	To give PB	To prevent loss of PB
1. Cause lesser harm Lesser harm as means			
Lesser harm as side effect of means			
Lesser harm as effect of good (no GH or no loss of PB) a. w/o intervening act/decision			
b. w/ intervening act/decision of i. beneficiary			
ii. of other agent			
2. Don't prevent lesser harm (Repeat subcategories as above)			

FIGURE 15.1

Shiffrin's case involves harm to Unlucky coming about as a side effect of the means to provide the benefit (i.e., dropping the cube). In another version of the case, the harm could itself be a means to his getting the cube (as when breaking his arm or running the risk of doing this is what makes it possible to drop the cube). But it is also possible that some lesser harms arise from his having the cube itself, for given the harms that Shiffrin sees as unavoidable in life, we can identify comparable harms that would come to someone who received the cube by way of harmless means. For example, once someone has golden cube riches, he has to decide what to do with them (e.g., whether to keep them for himself, or to share them with others and with whom). These are like the burdens of moral and prudential choice that Shiffrin sees as burdens of human life that could make creation of a person who will have these burdens morally problematic. Even deciding whether to avoid these burdens by giving up the pure benefit will be a difficult choice, just as Shiffrin says giving up life by suicide would be burdensome.[36] Notice that these burdens are effects of a conscious being with a will having the pure benefit independent of any further acts by himself or other agents. It does not seem reasonable to think that the Wealthy must avoid giving someone the pure benefit of a large fortune simply because the person will face these sorts of burdens.

Shiffrin arrived at her conclusion that without the person's consent we must not provide pure benefits when this also involves harms by considering a case where the means to providing the benefit itself caused a certain sort of harm (broken arm). But this case is inadequate to support her general conclusion, given that it seems permissible to provide a pure benefit to someone by innocent means when his having it causes other sorts of conditions that she also considers to be burdens to him (e.g., moral and prudential choices that she groups together with other harmed states).

Furthermore, we should also consider cases where the means to having the pure benefit caused such other sorts of burdens. So suppose that dropping the gold cube (rather than having it) itself caused people to start wondering what they would do with their wealth when they got it and so burdened them even before they received the wealth. Presumably this would not be a reason not to provide them with the wealth.

Next, the chart in figure 15.1 includes cases in which the harms that result from having the good result from the intervening agency of either the beneficiary or some other agent. So there may be burdens and harmed states of all sorts that result from the beneficiary's use (or misuse) of the benefit. There may be similar harms and burdens due to other agents' responses to his having the wealth (e.g., the threat of being robbed and suffering not only loss of part of the benefit but also a broken arm). It does not seem that the chance of such lesser harms or even foresight to their certain occurrence is a sufficient reason for Wealthy not to provide the pure benefit in the absence of consent. Shiffrin notes that some might dispute that the donor causes rather than exposes the beneficiary to harm, but she argues that exposing someone to a foreseen and certain harm (such as an avalanche) is not morally different from causing the harm. However, suppose we foresee that the cube recipient himself or another agent may by an intervening future act harm the cube recipient. *Enabling* him to face this problem by providing the wealth is not morally equivalent to either causing the harm or exposing the recipient to harmful events such as an avalanche, in part because the latter do not depend on future intervening agency of others, I believe.[37]

The next part of the chart involves cases where we do not cause the lesser harm but fail to prevent it. (This is in keeping with Shiffrin's claim that both of these have greater significance than providing pure benefits.) So imagine that Wealthy must choose whether to (a) prevent Joe from running into and breaking Unlucky's arm or (b) drop the gold cube into Unlucky's garden. (In this case, letting Unlucky's arm be broken is a side effect of doing something that gives him the cube.) It is not clear to me that Wealthy should do the former and that it is impermissible for him to do the latter instead.

Consider a case of this sort involving Unlucky's burden of deciding what to do with his life, a burden he has independently of Wealthy's acts. Should Wealthy do what alleviates the decision problem or instead drop the gold cube (on the assumption that the wealth will not solve the decision problem)? It does not seem impermissible to give the pure benefit rather than alleviate the burden.

I conclude that Shiffrin does not consider a wide enough range of ways in which different types of (what she considers to be) lesser harms can occur. Furthermore, consideration of a wider range does not support her conclusion that in general it wrongs someone to provide a pure benefit when this will be accompanied by a lesser harm in nonprocreation cases. Therefore, her discussion of the Gold Cube Case does not provide support for a comparable general conclusion in procreation cases.

For the sake of completeness, let us now consider procreation cases that fall under figure 15.1's categories. There will be cases in which the means involved in procreation cause lesser harm or risk of harm and such cases will be analogous to the way in which harm comes about in the Shiffrin's original Gold Cube Case. The use of a drug in order to become pregnant whose side effect may be a minor disability in the person created would be an example. A case in which causing or risking a lesser harm is itself the means to providing life might involve deliberately removing cells necessary for the growth of a person's finger from a blastula when doing this is necessary to save a pregnancy. (Only if a blastula were already a person might this be seen as harming a person for the sake of preventing the greater harm of his death. I here assume the blastula is not already a person.) Finally, there will be cases in which being alive as a conscious, intelligent being itself leads to burdens of deciding what to do with one's life. Being alive can also put the person created in the position of making decisions that cause him lesser harms relative to the goods in his life. It can put the person created in the position of being caused lesser harms by other agents.

Suppose the Gold Cube Cases that I discussed were appropriate guides to whether it is impermissible or problematic to procreate in these cases I have just brought up. Then creating in the case where life itself enables there to be decision problems and many types of intervening acts by others should be permissible and not problematic. However, if procreating by using the drug or removing the cells were also permissible, this would indicate that the Gold Cube Cases are not good guides to procreating since the comparable Gold Cube Cases seemed to involve impermissible acts by Wealthy. One possible ground for the difference is that in the Cube Cases we are interfering with a body that belongs to a person. If the fetus is not a person, what the parent does may affect a person ultimately but it is done to a nonperson (e.g., removing cells from a blastula) and may consist in tailoring the endowment she gives to her offspring. (I discuss this further in subsection 3.)

In addition, having relied on the Gold Cube Case and the distinction between avoiding greater harms and producing pure benefits to support her argument about procreation, it is only near the end of her article that Shiffrin notes the following difference between procreation and nonprocreation cases: If someone does not get the pure benefit of the gold cube, he will go on living in a less good condition (even if not a harmed state). By contrast, if someone is not created (and so does not get life that is like the pure benefit), there will not be a person who exists in a less good condition. She suggests that it is possible that this factor will make it a more serious wrong to provide what is like a pure benefit with the risk of harm in creating. However, it actually seems morally *easier* to justify imposing harms as a means to creation than as a means to providing pure benefits within life (as suggested by our earlier discussion). If this is so, then the fact that the alternative is nonexistence would be shown to make our acts have less (not more) significance in some ways. In any case, Shiffrin's arguments do not recognize this possibility.

An additional reason to think that the Gold Cube Cases are not guides to procreation is that a natural way to resolve the dilemma in them would be morally inappropriate when procreating.[38] In the Gold Cube Case, it would be correct to reduce the danger of harm by reducing the size of the benefit given if this were possible. The analogous course in procreation would be to reduce the goods one creates to the point necessary to eliminate the problems that life may bring. Hence, Shiffrin's argument would lead one to conclude that creating creatures incapable of moral choice, never in pain, and unaware of unpleasant truths like the prospect of death—such as extremely happy, long-lived rabbits that had no other problems—would be preferable to creating human persons as they are now. But I think this is the wrong conclusion. It would be wrong and would have been wrong at the beginning of (some hypothetical) creation to substitute such creatures for humanity. This may be not only because of the benefits to people of distinctively human lives but also because of the worth *of* persons' lives independent of any benefit this provides *to* persons.[39]

Of course, Shiffrin emphasizes that in the Gold Cube Case, when it is not possible to bestow a benefit in a nonrisky way, it is still wrong to drop the cube and one must compensate those hit. My point is that this does not show that when it is not possible to create people in a nonrisky way, it is still wrong to procreate and one must compensate offspring. Reducing benefits to avoid problems is what should be done in the Gold Cube Case if it were possible, but reducing distinctive benefits or the value of human life to avoid certain problems is not what should be done in procreation if it were possible. If one should not get rid of the problems at the cost of reducing benefits or value even if one could, this supports the conclusion that one should not be liable to compensate for these problems if they unavoidably arise in the course of procreating.

3. Affecting Persons and Future Persons

I now wish to examine a view that underlies *CC's person-affecting* principles of (a) not causing harm and (b) preventing harm. The view is that we have a duty to a *definite potential person* not to do things (and also to prevent things) at the fetal stage (here assuming the fetus is not already a person) that will result in the person being worse off than he might have been. This duty is thought to be as strong as the one we would have to the person if he were already in existence (i.e., if he were past the fetal stage) to see to it that he does not become worse off than he might be.[40] That is, CC holds that if we have duties while there is only a fetus, it is because of the person it will develop into. CC's authors think it follows from this premise that duties that exist while there is only a fetus should be as strong and of the same type as duties that we have to the person once he has developed, if we are certain that the fetus will develop into a person. I wish to argue that the premise does not have this implication, both with respect to doing what causes a person to be worse off than he might have been (harming) and with respect to helping him to avoid being worse off (preventing harm).[41]

Here is an example in which, I believe, it is permissible to affect a future person by doing something to the fetus from which he develops, though it is not permissible to affect the person in the same way by doing something to him once he exists. Suppose a woman has given (via the natural lottery) a fetus genes that will result in a person with an IQ of 160. She decides this is too smart, not because it is against the interests of the person who has the high IQ but because it is against the interests of the family. As a result, she takes a drug during early pregnancy to reduce the future person's IQ to 140. I shall call this the 160 IQ Case. It is a case of causing a person to be worse off than he would otherwise have been.[42] I believe her action is permissible (for reasons to be given below). But it would not be permissible, I believe, for the woman to give her child, once it is a person outside her body, a pill that reduces its IQ from 160 to 140.

What explains the difference between affecting the person by affecting the fetus and directly affecting the person himself? One possible explanation is that a fetus, not yet being a person, is not the sort of entity that is entitled to keep a characteristic that it has, such as a genetic makeup that will generate a 160 IQ. In addition, the person who will develop from the fetus will not fall below an acceptable level of life for a person if he has only a 140 IQ, so he is not owed a 160 IQ. (A 140 IQ is already far above the minima standard owed to the people we create.) These two facts are crucial to the permissibility of taking back from the fetus IQ points that the parent gave it. But since a child is already a person (I assume), it is entitled to keep a beneficial characteristic it has, even if doing so raises the child far beyond the standard it is owed and negatively impacts the family. Hence, I believe, it is impermissible to give the pill to the child, even if doing so would not cause his IQ to fall below the minima owed to one's child.[43] By contrast, suppose we owe a good chance of an IQ of at least 100 to people we create. In this case, doing something in pregnancy to a fetus that results in a person who develops with an IQ below 100 may well be as impermissible as doing to the later child something that lowers its IQ to below 100.

Because the fetus is not yet a person—and even though it will become (or give rise to) one—taking away characteristics it has (which would have an impact on the person it will be) is no different from not giving it those characteristics to begin with. And presumably, one would have a right not to give a future person that one created genes sufficient for a 160 IQ. (Note that it is not strictly the absence of personhood that is crucial here, but rather the absence of an entitlement to keep what one has been given. For we can imagine the following Million Dollar Case that involves a person all along and has the same general characteristics as the 160 IQ Case: I put a million dollars into a box that a person will be entitled to take out tomorrow. Before tomorrow comes, I change my mind and take the money back. This is all permissible, though my second act makes the person worse off than she would have been had I only performed the first act. It is permissible because she is not entitled to get that amount of money to begin with or to keep the money until she comes into possession of it.)

The analysis of the 160 IQ Case does not strictly require that it is the woman who gave the 160 IQ to the fetus. For suppose it is the father's genetic material that is primarily responsible for the high IQ. The woman's services as the carrier of the fetus are still needed to bring this potential IQ to fruition. Imagine that she reduces the excellence of these services (for instance, by deliberately exposing herself to a toxin or engaging in an activity so as to bring down the future person's IQ to 140). This too can be permissible, for the same reasons as given above. Furthermore, if a pregnant woman may deliberately reduce the fetus's IQ in the way I have described, it would also be permissible for her to do certain things while she is pregnant, such as eat certain foods or take certain drugs that, as a *foreseen though unintended* side effect, would change the fetus and make the person that arises from it worse off in comparable ways. But I do not think it would necessarily be permissible for her to engage in these activities when somehow they cause the loss of the 160 IQ in a child of hers living outside her body who has reached the stage where it is entitled to keep its advantageous properties.

Suppose now that the fetus is not in the woman's body, dependent on her services in carrying it. Instead, it is growing in a mechanical external gestation device (MEG).[44] Imagine that the world is such that if the woman engages in an activity such as exercising (no matter where), this has the effect of altering the fetus so that the person who develops will have an IQ of 140 rather than 160. Call this the MEG Case. Would it be permissible for her to exercise? First, consider the variant in which she has given the fetus its intelligence genes. Here I think it is permissible for her to do what causes the drop in IQ; it is a way for her to give 140 versus 160, which is a permissible donation. However, it would be prima facie impermissible for her to engage in the same activity when it would affect a child of hers also outside her body who is already in possession of the higher IQ, a trait he is entitled not to be deprived of.[45]

Now consider the variant of this case in which it is the father who gave the fetus growing in the MEG device the intelligence genes. It is true that the fetus is not entitled to keep these genes, but that does not mean that just anyone may permissibly do what takes them away from it. Since the woman in this case is not contributing any service necessary for the fruition of the genes, I think that she may not do those things that lead to a drop in IQ to 140. (Nor may any other entity, such as a government, do those things without the father's permission, other things being equal. In this connection, it may help to recall the Million Dollar Case: If the million dollars is in the box because I have put it there for you, not just anyone can come and take it out before you have laid claim to it.)

What about the permissibility of a parent not rendering assistance to a fetus in order to prevent a natural change that will lead the person who develops from the fetus to have a 140 IQ rather than the 160 IQ that would have otherwise come about? If the change would occur in the fetus before it is entitled to keep the traits that will cause the 160 IQ, I believe that one need not make as great an effort to stop the fall in IQ as one should make once one is the parent of the child who has the

160 IQ. A parent's duty to help his child keep a trait (whether thought of as a potential for the 160 IQ or the 160 IQ itself) that the child already is entitled to keep can be stronger than a parent's duty to see to it that his fetus who is developing will acquire or retain that trait.[46]

Finally, what I have said here also bears on cases in which *CC* might appeal to nonperson-affecting principles: Suppose I can have a child with an IQ of 160 if I refrain from an important project, but will have a different child with an IQ of 140 if I do not refrain. It could be morally permissible to pursue the project even if it would be morally impermissible for a parent to pursue it if this would (somehow) cause, or even involve him in failing to prevent, a comparable drop in the 160 IQ of his child. (*CC* itself rejects the "No Difference" View for how to treat person-affecting and nonperson-affecting cases.)

I draw these conclusions even though I believe that the creator of what will become or give rise to a new person has stronger responsibilities—and ones that have a different source—than those that other people who are bystanders have. A creator's responsibility not to create a child whose life is not worth living does not stem from the duty we *all* (including bystanders) have to prevent harm to others. The creator is not merely a bystander; he can be in the position of causing a life that is not worth living. The duties of creators not to cause such harms(b) can be greater, I think, than the duties of bystanders to help prevent or stop those harms(b). Nevertheless, I believe that this is consistent with a creator's changing a fetus so that the person stemming from it is worse off than he would otherwise have been, in the ways I previously described for the reasons I previously gave.[47, 48]

4. The Disabled

CC claims that some characteristics (for example, blindness and paralysis) constitute impairments that in many circumstances result in one's being disabled. (This is because one cannot do certain things and one has no choice as to whether one will or will not do certain things, such as seeing.) It is truly better not to have these impairments (other things being equal). That impairments are bad is commonly thought to be the basis for our attempts to prevent and cure such conditions as blindness and paralysis through common medical practice, on the assumption that no other compensatory goods accompany the impairments.[49] *CC*'s authors conclude that we should prevent these impairments by using the Procedures, even if one can have a life worth living with the impairments and even if, through large-scale social change, we could reduce the degree to which an impairment makes one disabled. I agree with this claim. *CC* argues further that disfavoring disabilities does not imply having less respect and concern for those who actually have them. For example, wanting to prevent someone from having a disability does not imply that we would try to rid ourselves of a person who exists with it. Nor does it necessarily imply that if we have a scarce medical resource and we can extend (to an equal extent) either the life of a disabled person or the life of one who is not disabled, but not both, that we should favor the nondisabled person. (In contrast,

Peter Singer argues that it is rational to save the life of the person without the disability because that person will have a better life.[50] As a consequentialist, Singer is interested in maximizing the good of an outcome, but the authors of *CC* are not committed to doing this.) I agree with *CC*'s authors that differences in outcomes caused by preexisting disabilities can often be irrelevant to the distribution of scarce resources.[51]

CC claims that disfavoring disability implies that we should delay conception to prevent the existence of a disabled person if we can do so easily, even if this means that a different person will exist than would exist if we do not delay. Does this imply that we wish that those actually born with impairments had never been born? (Wishing that someone had never been born is, of course, different from wishing that his or her life would end once it has started.) I do not believe *CC* deals with this question. I wish to deal with it in order to further strengthen *CC*'s conclusion that preventing the existence of disabled people by not creating them (rather than by altering the environment so that impairments do not disable) need not imply negative attitudes toward existing disabled people.

Suppose it would be better for someone if he did not have a serious disability. Then that is some reason to forestall the creation of a seriously impaired person before that person actually comes into existence and create a nonimpaired person instead, as this is a much easier and more complete way to stop disability than making large alterations in environments. Once a disabled person is in existence, the preference that he never have existed may be a preference that a better state of affairs (e.g., one with a different, nondisabled person) exist instead. But we need not prefer that a better state of affairs exist if it would mean the absence of the particular person who exists now (even by his never having existed rather than his dying). Our concern for and commitment to this person can be inconsistent with, and take precedence over, wishing that the world were better and that it would afford someone else a life that is better for him.[52] True, if we did wish that he had never existed, we would be wishing for something that would *not* have harmed him or strictly failed to benefit him, since he would never have existed to be harmed or not to be benefited. But we would still be wishing for a world that is worse from the perspective of the actual person who exists and has a life worth living, since he would not exist in that other world. For this reason, we do not wish it.

If this is so, it means that prior to the existence of a person, we could know that even if we create a disabled person (with a life worth living) rather than waiting and creating a different, nondisabled person, we will reasonably not regret the existence of the disabled person. We will reasonably not wish that someone else without the disability had been created instead. This does not show, however, that if we have a choice, it is not morally correct to create the nonimpaired person rather than the impaired one who will be disabled. It only shows that the criterion for correct action is not merely whether we will reasonably regret the state of affairs that results from what we have done.[53]

CC endorses the permissibility not merely of delaying conception but also of aborting at least an early embryo in order to prevent the existence of an impaired person. This position can raise the following possible objection with which, I think, *CC does not deal.* When we cure someone of an impairment, he remains alive. When we change an embryo so that it will not give rise to an impaired person, the embryo is not destroyed and (arguably) the same person that would otherwise have existed will exist. By contrast, if we end a pregnancy simply because we find out that it would give rise to an impaired person, we decide on the basis of that one characteristic to prevent the existence of the person, even though that embryo will give rise to a person with many other good characteristics and abilities. Is this not like prejudice against the disabled, namely treating actually existing people with impairments only in the light of their disability, ignoring their other good characteristics and abilities? Will treating the embryo in this way not encourage prejudice against existing disabled people?[54]

I think the answer to this objection is as follows: Prejudice as described does not merely involve acting on the view that impairment is bad for the person who has it (otherwise surgery to cure it would involve prejudice as well). Treating existing disabled people only in the light of their disability is wrong because it deprives them of opportunities that would benefit them. But destroying an embryo merely in the light of the fact that it will give rise to an impaired person does not deprive a person of opportunities that would benefit him because the potential person does not yet exist. (If the early embryo is not a subject, then it too is not harmed by being destroyed.) Furthermore, if another child is created without the impairment, all the good properties that would have been present in the person whose existence was prevented can still be present in the new person, minus the impairment.

I suggest that it is only if one takes seriously the destruction of the embryo itself, either because it matters or because interrupting the process of its development matters, that one will be concerned with deciding to replace an embryo because of one of its bad properties. For suppose the destruction of the embryo and the interruption of its development had no moral significance per se. Then destroying it would be no different from what we do in the following Blueprint Case: Suppose we have written down a plan for the creation of a new person that will be put in action unless we intervene. We then notice that one of the gene sequences we have written down will give rise to an impairment, though the other sequences will give rise to many good properties. We can change the gene sequence that gives rise to the impairment, but this will result in a person with all the other good properties only if we change other sequences that determine the personal identity of the individual who will be created. Hence we would have to create a plan for a different person. Suppose those concerned about the rights of actual disabled people would not think it morally wrong to change the plan as described in order to avoid the impairment. They might think it is not wrong because there is no one who will suffer the harm of having her other good characteristics ignored.

This would show that it is not deciding whether a person exists or not on the basis of an impairment that is wrong. If someone still objects to destroying an embryo because it will give rise to an impaired person, this must be because he views the embryo or its process of development as having some independent significance.

Some who object to destroying an embryo solely because it will give rise to an impaired person have said that they do not object to parents destroying such embryos in order to avoid additional hardship to them in raising an impaired child.[55] However, suppose someone thinks that it is permissible to act in the Blueprint Case but not permissible to destroy an embryo to avoid an impairment. Then it is not clear that parents trying to avoid hardship will have an adequate reason to destroy an embryo either. This is because it would be concern over the status of the embryo or its process of development, rather than concern over selecting on account of an impairment, that would underlie the objection to destroying the embryo, and concern to avoid hardship might not override this consideration.

It is possible, however, that even if concern for the parents' hardship was not an adequate reason to abort, concern for the person who will be impaired might be. This is a point that may come out if we consider the following question: May some disabilities be permissibly prevented by altering a particular (nonidentity crucial) genome in a fetus, though avoiding the disabilities is a wrong reason for not reproducing or for destroying a fetus? I think that this question is best answered by considering several factors: (1) The characteristics of different particular disabilities. (2) What means we would use to prevent these disabilities—for example, delaying conception so that we have a different fetus or having no fetus at all, aborting a fetus, or treating a particular fetus. (3) For whose sake or out of respect for whom we would prevent the disabilities. For example, is it for the sake of or out of respect for the person who would come to be, or for the sake of or out of respect for the potential parents?

Consider having a clubfoot, arguably not a major disability. Is there anything morally wrong with not conceiving a child that one knows will have a clubfoot, out of concern for the child who would exist? I do not think so. This is true even though once one is in existence as a person, it would not be worth ending one's life just so as not to live with a clubfoot and one would have a life well above the minimum owed in creating people. Similarly, it could be wrong (for reasons given above) to wish that someone already in existence with a clubfoot had not come into existence. But this does not mean that before there is such a person, we may not decide, out of concern for the person who would come to exist, not to create him because he would have a clubfoot. I think this is because he would have an additional difficulty in his life, and there is no one who would lose anything by not being created. The parents could also decide for *their* sake not to create such a child, because it would be difficult for them and, again, there is no one who would lose anything by not being created. (However, if thus acting for their own sakes involved parents giving up the chance for any child, it exhibits either a weak desire for a child or a misunderstanding of what to care about in a child.)

Now consider the abortion option on the assumption that a fetus is not a person. Out of concern for the person who would have to live with a clubfoot, I believe it would be permissible to abort the fetus that would develop into that person, for the same reasons as we could give for not creating that fetus. Does this conclusion imply that it would also be morally appropriate for parents to abort in order to avoid the difficulty *for themselves* of having such a child, as it was permissible for them to avoid conception for their own sake? Possibly not. This is not because they would be inappropriately putting their interests ahead of those of the person who would develop from the fetus, for we have already seen that it might be appropriate to abort out of concern for that potential person. Hence, there is no conflict of interests. Rather, the fact that a life has begun and is developing toward a life worth living may be an *impersonal value*, respect for which, some might say, overshadows the potential parents' interests. Perhaps this is why some think that it is wrong to abort for the sake of avoiding minor disabilities. If so, this would reveal an interesting asymmetry: The impersonal value of a developing life may override the parents' interests in not having a child with a disability, so that the fact that the abortion would make their lives better would not be a sufficient reason to abort. But the impersonal value might not override effects on the person whose life it would be and who would have to live the disabled life.[56]

Now suppose it were possible to cure the clubfoot by altering genes in the fetus. If only effects on the potential person are at issue, I do not think it matters whether we alter the genes or abort the fetus that would develop into the person. But if there is impersonal value in continuing a life-process, we should cure instead of abort, even if doing so is somewhat more costly to parents.

Suppose there is some disability that, when we just consider effects on the future person, does not provide a sufficient reason for not reproducing or for interrupting reproduction. If the disability provides the potential parents with an interest-based reason to interrupt reproduction, their interest might not be strong enough to outweigh the impersonal value of continuing a life-process once it has started. Here again, however, we might seek a cure in order to serve the parental interests rather than to prevent effects in the potential person.

Suppose that there were disabilities that should be avoided by delaying conception or by altering a gene, but not by destroying a developing embryo or fetus. This class of disabilities could serve as a ground for rejecting the Preventive Principle that Peter Singer proposes. According to this principle, "For any condition X, if it would be a form of child abuse for parents to inflict X on their child soon after birth, then it must, other things being equal, at least be permissible to take steps to prevent one's child [from] having that condition." (Among the steps Singer allows here are genetic alteration, abortion, and embryo destruction.[57]) I assume that Singer's point is that seeking to eliminate condition X is a reason that helps justify taking steps before birth. It is not merely that since taking steps before birth is anyway permissible, it does not matter what reason one gives for doing it. (Although the latter may be true.)

It would be a form of child abuse for parents, soon after their child's birth, to deliberately cut off the top of its middle finger (even painlessly). According to Singer's principle, this implies that it is at least permissible to abort a fetus if one knows it will develop into a person with this part of his finger missing, in the sense that the missing part provides a reason that helps justify the abortion. I believe that this may be incorrect. The Preventive Principle has even more far-reaching results that I also think are suspect. It is an implication of what I have said earlier in section C, subsection 2, that if a parent does something to her child that interferes with its 160 IQ so that the child only has a 140 IQ, this would be child abuse. The Preventive Principle thus implies here that if a fetus quite naturally develops an illness that will reduce its potential IQ from 160 to 140, it is at least permissible to terminate the pregnancy, in the sense that the potential person's only having a 140 IQ justifies abortion. This case shows that Singer's Preventive Principle fails to take account of the fact that inflicting condition X may be abusive merely because such infliction is a rights violation that makes the child worse than it would have been, even when there is nothing intrinsically wrong with condition X. When X is the original condition of the fetus, or the outcome of a natural event, there may be nothing about it worth preventing. I conclude that the fact that it would be wrong of a parent to inflict certain conditions on a child does not show that they provide an adequate reason for terminating reproduction (if some reason were required). In some cases, acting on this nonjustifying reason may be wrong because of the impersonal value of the developing life, a factor that Singer's principle also does not take into account.

The following is a (conservative) alternative to Singer's Preventive Principle that may avoid some of the objections I have raised: For any condition X, if it would be permissible for parents to prevent or eliminate it after birth by physical means, then it must, other things being equal, at least be permissible for them to prevent or eliminate it before birth by altering a particular conceptus or (when there is no need for an additional person) by not conceiving.

I have been discussing the degree to which disabilities give us reason to use the Procedures. I do not necessarily mean to include under this description conditions that become disabilities only because the incorrect values of a society give them too much weight (e.g., not having blonde hair and blue eyes). If we wish to raise children so that they have correct values, it is hard (though not always impossible) to justify giving in to such incorrect values in creating children simply because this will give them easier lives.

D. THE COINCIDENCE THESIS

CC places great emphasis on the need to control *individual* ventures in eugenic improvement for the sake of social justice. It also suggests that society itself might pursue eugenic modification beyond "primary values" on which there is an overlapping consensus. I have already expressed concern about CC's suggestion that a majority vote could legitimate controversial society-sponsored "improvements." Now I want to point out that some conflicts between society and individuals could arise even if society pursues only treatments or enhancements on which there is very widespread agreement.

One argument *CC* gives for the coincidence of social interests and individual interests—*CC*'s Coincidence Thesis—is reminiscent of Mill's argument for the Principle of Utility and has some of the same problems purported to afflict the latter. *CC* points to three statements that I present below (with some modification for clarity and simplicity):

1. I want genetic intervention for my child because I want my child to have the best genes (consistent with it still being my biological child).
2. We each want genetic intervention for each of our children because we each want each of our children to have the best genes (consistent with each child still being the biological child of its parents).
3. I (a state official) favor genetic intervention for each of our state's children because I want our state's children to have the best genes (consistent with each child still being the biological child of its parents), given that each parent wants this.[58]

These statements could be taken to form an argument to show that there is no conflict between what individuals want for their children and what a state official in a eugenics program would want. I shall therefore call it the Coincidence Thesis Argument.

Mill's Argument contains the following statements:

1. My happiness matters to me.
2. The happiness of each matters to each.
3. The happiness of all matters to all.[59]

To which we could add a further conclusion analogous to that in the Coincidence Thesis Argument:

4. The happiness of all matters to me as a state official, given that each citizen favors it.

Step (3) in Mill's Argument equivocates between (a) a simple aggregation of the wants of individuals, each of whom may care only about his own happiness, and (b) the formation of a new object of each person's desire—namely, the happiness of all. It is fallacious to deduce (b) from steps of the argument; we can only deduce interpretation (a) of step (3) in Mill's Argument. But the official in Mill's Argument step (4) has as the object of her concern the happiness of all. This only coincides with what we all individually want if interpretation (b) of step (3) in Mill's Argument holds. But, I have said, we have no right to assume this.

Similar problems can afflict the Coincidence Thesis Argument because step (2) can be understood (a) as a simple aggregation of the wants of each parent for his own child, or (b) as involving the formation of a new object of each person's desire—namely, the welfare of all children. It is fallacious to deduce (b), but the official in the Coincidence Thesis Argument's last step does have this new object of desire—the genetic welfare of all children.

Due to this, the way is open for conflict between the official who wants the good of all children and an individual parent who in the first instance desires the good of his own child. Suppose the official wants the good of each child but cannot have it; it might be argued that she should achieve the good of as many as she can instead. This might require her to sacrifice the good of some. It may be a question of not treating one child in order to treat a greater number of other children. What the state official wants in this case will be in conflict with what the parent of that one child wants, since the parent primarily wants his child's welfare, not the welfare of everyone's children. (He may want the latter only as a means of pursuing his primary interest in his own child's welfare, since if all children are treated his will be among them.)

There is another somewhat problematic relation between the official's interest and the parent's. Suppose a parent wants genetic intervention for his child. In this case, he primarily wants the intervention; he does not primarily want that his desire for the intervention be satisfied. But it is an important issue whether the public official in a democracy should primarily want that the parent's desire be satisfied (so long as it is for good, not evil) rather than that there be genetic intervention per se. Or put alternatively, should the official primarily want genetic intervention but only *on condition* that the parent wants it and not otherwise? (The last clause in step (3) is ambiguous as between these two interpretations).[60]

When the interventions at issue are to eliminate what are widely agreed to be defects, the day may come when parents will not be thought to have a veto that can prevent such interventions, any more than Christian Scientist parents can have a veto on their children's getting blood transfusions. It is not that there will not be conflicts between society and parents; it is just that these conflicts may be settled in the light of the interests (or wishes) of the offspring rather than the preferences of the parents.

IV. Conclusion

We have seen that the ability to influence the genetic makeup of the population in various ways raises important questions about what society owes individuals as a matter of justice and about how much control parents should have over genetic changes in their offspring. It also raises important questions about what parents owe their offspring and about the status of those who, in one way or another, do meet the standard of functioning that will be met by most people. I have suggested that neither social justice nor parental obligations make it morally mandatory to seek great improvements in a future person's genetic makeup. However, certain changes would uncontroversially be improvements whose pursuit is compatible with respect for all persons.

NOTES

1. This chapter is a revised version of "Genes, Justice, and Obligations to Future People," originally published in *Social Philosophy and Policy* 19(2) (July 2002): 360–88. For comments on an earlier version of that article, I am grateful to Allen Buchanan, Dan W. Brock, Norman Daniels, Richard Arneson, and the contributors to that volume, as well as to audiences at the American Philosophical Association (Pacific Division) and Vanderbilt Law School. It incorporates some parts of "Baselines and Compensation," *San Diego Law Review* 40 (2004): 1367–86.

2. Germline changes will be carried into future generations; somatic changes only genetically affect the individual altered.

3. Allen Buchanan, Dan W. Brock, Norman Daniels, and Daniel Wikler, *From Chance to Choice: Genetics and Justice* (Cambridge: Cambridge University Press, 2000) (hereafter, *CC*).

4. Discussion of Shiffrin was added subsequent to publication of the article on which this chapter is based.

5. See John Rawls, *A Theory of Justice* (Cambridge, MA: Harvard University Press, 1970).

6. I base this summary on what *CC* says in chapters 3–7. I interpret the last sentence as applying only to valuable enhancements. I do not believe *CC* claims that if a very valuable trait were widespread without this being the result of an enhancement, the minority is entitled to that trait as a matter of justice. The question is, why the difference? Perhaps what is said in part III, section B, pertains to this question.

7. *CC*, pp. 292–94.

8. Related to this is *CC*'s refusal to speak of *rights* to reproductive freedom. *CC*'s authors consciously choose to speak of interests in reproductive freedom, which suggests that they think the balancing of interests is appropriate in this area. But how, without the idea of a right, can we explain why a less important interest of one person (e.g., a woman's interest in bodily integrity) may trump a more important interest of another person (e.g., if the fetus were a person, its interest in staying alive)? Judith Jarvis Thomson, in her "A Defense of Abortion," *Philosophy & Public Affairs* 1(1) (Autumn 1971): 47–66, and F. M. Kamm, in her *Creation and Abortion* (New York: Oxford University Press, 1992), have argued that the weaker interest can trump the stronger one because it is backed by a right.

9. I think it is better to call the sort of lives described in the parenthetical as "lives worth not living," since they are worse than comatose states that also are lives not worth living. Derek Parfit suggested (in conversation) this new phrase. I assume throughout that *CC*'s "lives not worth living" refers to such worse lives.

10. In discussing prevention of disabilities, *CC*'s authors assume that eliminating a person's serious disability is not enough of a change to make that person go out of existence and be replaced by someone else. Elsewhere in the book, however, they argue that our phenotype (the set of our actual properties, which are the result of genetic and nongenetic factors) is crucial to our identity, to who we are. Preventing a given person from being

severely retarded so that he is nonretarded leads to a big change in his phenotype; does this mean that by preventing such retardation in someone we change something crucial to his identity in the sense that we have a new person? *CC*'s authors must be denying this in the case when we affect the same biological individual. Typically, the philosophically strict sense of identity allows that one can undergo large changes in phenotype yet remain the same individual person.

11. The distinction between person-affecting and nonperson-affecting principles was first offered by Derek Parfit. See his *Reasons and Persons* (Oxford: Oxford University Press, 1984), p. 370.

12. In a public lecture delivered at Stanford University on October 25, 2001, Peter Singer said that a regime of individual parents "shopping at the genetic supermarket" preserves free choice, unlike a regime featuring a state genetic program. See Peter Singer, "Shopping at the Genetic Supermarket," in S.Y. Song, Y.M. Koo, and D.R.J. Macer (eds.), *Asian Bioethics in the 21st Century* (Tsukuba, 2003), pp. 143–156. But this does not seem correct, because free choice for all is not necessarily preserved when some are given the right to determine outcomes for another person—namely, a child. For more on whether genetic enhancement limits freedom of offspring, see chapter 17 this volume.

13. Admittedly, it must be shown why this would be wrong. In the lecture cited in note 12, Peter Singer noted that the policy of eliminating more female fetuses than male fetuses would come back to haunt societies when men looked for brides. But even if women who were selectively aborted would not have become brides, there may, I believe, be a moral problem with their elimination (even if abortion itself is not wrong). Furthermore, suppose that the number of males and females is equal, due to some people eliminating fetuses because they do not want males and others eliminating fetuses because they do not want females. The moral issue could remain of whether action based on such individual preferences for females or males should be permitted.

14. For more on this, see my *Creation and Abortion* and chapter 12 this volume.

15. This latter use of the idea of equal concern and respect seems to lie at the heart of Ronald Dworkin's political philosophy. Hence, my remarks may serve as a criticism of his views.

16. For more about this and other concerns I have regarding the relation of FEO to health, see chapter 19 this volume.

17. Pibbe Jogge has argued that the authors of *CC* fail to distinguish between (a) treating a disease and (b) bringing someone to the state he would have been in without the disease without, however, treating the disease. She argues that (b) is no more implied by the idea of treatment than is enhancement. (Hers is certainly a narrow notion of treatment.) So consider *CC*'s case contrasting someone who is very short because of a disease preventing him from producing his own growth hormone with someone who is very short but within a normal range because his parents are short (see *CC*, p. 115). Jogge's view seems to imply that giving growth hormone to someone with the disease without curing the disease is as little mandated by a theory that would require us to treat the disease as is giving growth hormone to someone who is short through no abnormality. See Pibbe Jogge, *Does Billy Have a Right to Grow Up? The Moral Relevance of the Distinction between Treatment and Enhancement* (unpublished manuscript). Suppose we think that we should give the hormone to someone with the disease (Jogge's case) but agree that this does not constitute treating the disease. Then this supports providing height enhancement as well.

18. See Thomas Nagel, "Justice and Nature," *Oxford Journal of Legal Studies* 17(2) (1997): 303.

19. Of course, in this case, there is no *other* factor such as nature that is assigned the causal role. But why should Nagel's procedure for deciding what factor causes an effect apply only when we are considering *which* one of several factors is the cause?

20. *CC* also draws attention to the analogy between education and other enhancements; see *CC*, pp. 189–90. Note also that while initially only the rich may be able to afford the Procedures, the market itself may eventually lead to lower prices, removing the need for state subsidies. (I would now add: If some acquired the treatments or enhancements using only money acquired *without* incentives—just distributing their equal economic share differently from others—the present argument for support for treatments or enhancements would not apply.)

21. For the data on this point, see Norman Daniels, "Justice, Health, and Healthcare," *American Journal of Bioethics* 1(2) (2001): 2–16.

22. As noted earlier (in note 9), the latter description is owed to Derek Parfit. It applies to lives worse than nonexistence. By contrast, living in a coma seems a life not worth living but it may not be worse than nonexistence.

23. This case shows that drawing a distinction between inducing a cause (as in the spina bifida case) and exposing to a cause will not usually help distinguish between harming and not harming.

24. I suggested this in *Creation and Abortion* and in chapter 12 this volume. (I would now add that it may make moral difference whether [1] a given person will run a risk of a life worth not living when he has a chance of a good life, or [2] there is a risk of creating a person who can only have a life worth not living rather than creating a different person who will have a good life. In [2], what makes the life worth not living is connected to identity-determining properties so there was no chance of a good life for this person.) On whether this makes a moral difference, see unpublished work by Johann Frick.

25. I would now add that while it seems just as wrong to create someone to a life worth not living as to make someone already in existence have a life worth not living, it is not morally important in the same way to create people with good lives as to benefit and benefit(b) those already in existence.

26. Johann Frick notes (in unpublished work) that even if one does not create a person *in order* to benefit him, one may decide to create only *because* he will have goods in his life that outweigh bads. I argued in favor of a distinction between acting "in order that" and "because of" in chapter 4 of my *Intricate Ethics* (New York: Oxford University Press, 2007). I make similar use of this distinction when I discuss a case in which soldiers must not act in order to help civilians, but they may bomb a munitions plant that will cause these civilians property damage only because the bombing will also benefit the same civilians in a greater way. See my *Ethics for Enemies* (Oxford: Oxford University Press, 2011), chapter 3.

27. For this reason, it does not seem entirely correct to say that not creating any life is no solution to the problem of death interfering with more life. This is because the latter but not the former occurs *to* someone, and this problem can be avoided by not creating.

28. I discuss these "minima" in my *Creation and Abortion* and in chapter 12 this volume.

29. This position contrasts with the one Jeff McMahan proposes in *The Ethics of Killing: Problems at the Margins of Life* (New York: Oxford University Press, 2002).

30. See Peter Singer, *Practical Ethics*, 2d ed. (Cambridge: Cambridge University Press, 1993), and McMahan's *The Ethics of Killing*.

31. We should distinguish between creating (i) a short-lived person and (ii) a nonperson human being. Both can involve lives that are experientially good for the creatures that have them. However, CC, Singer, and McMahan all believe it may be wrong to create a short-lived person when one could make that same person be long-lived. By contrast, McMahan thinks that deliberately creating a short-lived human nonperson (e.g., a human pet) is permissible even when one could create something better (e.g., a human person). See my discussion of this point in chapter 13 this volume.

32. Such reasoning would also imply that creating a person is in many respects analogous to the following case (which was put to me by Dan Brock): Suppose I see someone at the point of losing a leg. It would be in his interest for me to drive him to a hospital, and I start to do so. There is a small chance of a car accident happening, and the accident does in fact happen on the way (not due to negligence). It causes him to lose both legs. Though what I do causes the greater harm, the fact that it was in his interest for me to do what exposed him to the possibility of harm alters my responsibilities to him from what they would have been if I had exposed him to such harm when it was not connected with doing something that was in his interest. My duties to my injured passenger are instead closer to the duties I would have as someone who can help but who did not cause the car accident. For more on all this, see my *Creation and Abortion*, chapter 5, and chapter 12 this volume.

33. This section was added subsequent to the publication of the article on which this chapter is based.

34. The first part of the following discussion, which describes Seana Shiffrin's views, repeats some of what was said in chapter 12 this volume. There I was concerned only with the relation of her views to abortion.

35. In her "Wrongful Life, Procreative Responsibility, and the Significance of Harm," *Legal Theory* 5 (1999): 117–48.

36. We could also imagine a case in which Unlucky could (magically) immediately get rid of his broken arm, caused by the means used to get him the cube, merely by returning the cube. Presumably, Shiffrin will hold that the difficulty of giving up the cube still helps make causing the broken arm wrong. If the burdens are less than the good of having the benefit, it also seems foolish to give up the good. In cases where the burden is greater than the good, there may still be some difficulty in giving up the good even if it is worse not to.

37. Determining the moral significance of others' intervening agency for limiting responsibility of an initial agent is a big intellectual problem. Here I can only point to its possible role. I discussed it a bit in my "Substitution, Subordination, and Responsibliity," in *Philosophy and Phenomenological Research* 80(3) (2010): 702–22.

38. I made this point in "Baselines and Compensation," and in the article on which chapter 16 this volume is based.

39. I make this point again in chapter 16 this volume. However, in that chapter's discussion of disability, I also argue that one may not impose avoidable harms on people without their consent merely in order to make their lives have exceptional worth. For example, one should not give a person a mental illness merely because this will lead to her exceptional artistic achievement. It would require further argument to explain why creating some benefits and valuable states but not others licenses risk of unconsented harms.

40. *CC* does, however, distinguish these cases from ones in which we create a fetus that will give rise to a person with a worse life rather than *another* fetus that would have given rise to a different person with a better life.

41. Similarly, Jeff McMahan, in his *Ethics of Killing*, discusses cases where a woman takes a drug during pregnancy. He says (with my substituting X for "sterile" and Y for "have children"): "If an act causes a person to be X, it hardly seems to matter whether the act was done early in the victim's life or later when the victim would be more closely psychologically connected to himself at the time that he might desire to Y" (with which X will interfere) (p. 282). And "The important consideration is whether one's action frustrates a time-relative interest; it does not matter whether the act is done before the time-relative interest exists" (p. 283). (For explanation of "time-relative interest," see chapter 13 this volume.) And "The primary moral reason the agent would have not to inflict the prenatal injury would be just as strong as his reason not to inflict a comparable harm on another person now" (p. 286). So my arguments against the views of *CC* apply as well to McMahan's view.

42. Subsequent to publishing the article on which this chapter is based, I created a variant on this case in which a woman alters her egg (not the fetus) so that the child will have an IQ of 140 instead of 160. This is the Egg 160 IQ Case discussed in chapter 16 this volume. It first appears in my "Affecting Definite Future People," *APA Newsletter* 9(2) (Spring 2010).

43. I first presented this argument in *Creation and Abortion*, p. 207.

44. I discuss these in *Creation and Abortion* and in chapter 12 this volume.

45. I would now add: The point of using a MEG Case is to show that it is not just the fetus being in the woman's body and her affecting it by doing something to her body that makes it permissible for her to reduce the IQ. The MEG Case may not succeed in showing this, however, because the woman's exercising is still something she does to her body. An even purer MEG Case would involve her giving a drug to the fetus to reduce the IQ. I suggest that this too is permissible. One might also construct a case in which the child (not fetus) with the 160 IQ is in the woman's body. If it were not permissible to reduce the child's IQ (when this had no other effects), this too would help show that it is not merely being in the woman's body that explains the permissibility of reducing the IQ.

46. Unlike the duty not to take away from (what is already) a person what she is entitled to keep, the duty to provide aid does not rely so strongly on the existence of the person. For this reason, one may sense less of a difference in the fetus and child variants of cases when aiding is in question. For additional variants on the 160 IQ Case and discussions of related matters, see chapter 16 this volume.

47. Note that nothing I have said implies that it is better for someone acting in the interests of a future person to (1) cause a large loss to the future person by acting at his fetal stage rather than (2) cause a small loss to that person through an action one takes when he exists. Here is an argument for this: If I know that I have to do one or the other, it is ex ante in the future person's interest to waive his right against my doing (2) so that I do not do (1). Hence, I think I should do (2) rather than (1) in this case. A second argument is based on what I call the Principle of Secondary Permissibility. Very roughly, it implies that if I will permissibly cause someone a harm in one way, it may become permissible (and even the only permissible harmful act) to cause him a lesser harm in a way that would otherwise be impermissible, because this will be better for him. (For more on this principle, see my

Intricate Ethics, chapter 5.) On these grounds, I should do (2) in this case. I thank Richard Arneson for the question to which this is a response.

48. The material on future generations that occurred at this point in the original version of the article on which this chapter is based has been omitted here. It may be found in its entirety in chapter 16 this volume, as part of it was also a part of the original version of the article on which chapter 16 is based.

49. On the importance of this assumption, see chapter 21 this volume.

50. See Singer's "Shopping at the Genetic Supermarket."

51. I argue for this in chapter 21 this volume, but there I also argue for ways in which disability can be relevant to the distribution of scarce resources. See also chapter 22 this volume.

52. I believe Robert Adams originally made this point. The example he gives is someone who marries a particular woman. If he loves this woman, he does not wish that he had instead loved someone else with whom his life would have been objectively better. See Robert Adams, "Existence, Self-Interest, and the Problem of Evil," *Noûs* 13 (1979): 53–65.

53. This is a contrast between the ex-ante and ex-post attitude. I note another way in which ex-post and ex-ante attitudes can differ in chapter 17 this volume: Parents can wish for a child with enhanced talents, though they know they will care as much for the actual child they will have whether it has enhancements or not. In chapter 21 this volume, I note that a disabled person could prefer to have a better life without the disability while caring as much about the less good life he has as someone else cares about the better life he has. In the latter case, however, one could actually prefer that one's life be changed for the better because one would continue to exist with the improvement. By contrast, a loving parent would not care to have the better child (even if this child would have a life better for it) if it means the nonexistence of the child who actually exists and whom the parent actually loves.

54. An objection like this is to be found in A. Asch and D. Wasserman, "the Uncertain Rationale for Prenatal Disability Screening," *Virtual Mentor* 8(1) (2006): 53–56.

55. For example, Adrienne Asch in "Can Aborting 'Imperfect' Children Be Immoral?" In *Ethical Issues in Modern Medicine*, 4th ed., eds. J. Arras and B. Steinbrek (Mountain View, CA: Mayfield, 1995), pp. 386–89.

56. This point may also bear on the legitimacy of suicide in cases of illness. Ronald Dworkin emphasizes the impersonal value of a life considered independently from its value for the person who will live it; see *Life's Dominion* (New York: Knopf, 1993). I contrasted the value of a life to a person as seen from the "outside" and as experienced from "inside" in my *Morality, Morality*, vol. 1 (New York: Oxford University Press, 1993).

57. See Singer, "Shopping at the Genetic Supermarket."

58. *CC*, p. 53.

59. See John Stuart Mill, *Utilitarianism*, ed. Oskar Piest (Indianapolis, IN: Bobbs-Merrill, 1957), for Mill's Proof of the Principle of Utility.

60. *CC* itself notes this problem; see *CC*, p. 54. I think that *CC*'s authors mistakenly believe that they deal with the problem by noting that parents' desires are not sufficient for social intervention (if parents want something bad). But the question is whether parents' desires are necessary for social intervention.

16

Moral Status, Personal Identity, and Substitutability

CLONES, EMBRYOS, AND FUTURE GENERATIONS

I. Introduction

The permissibility of our actions can sometimes depend on the identities of those who will be affected by them.[1] Investigating this phenomenon has been a traditional focus of deontological ethics. Deontological ethics claims that what we ought to do is not always a function of what will produce the best outcome. For example, we could be morally constrained from producing the best outcome because it would require harming someone who would not benefit from our action, though others would.[2] John Rawls referred to this as the moral relevance of the separateness of persons.[3] One way of expressing this idea has been that persons are not, in general, substitutable for one another when we do a calculation of harms and benefits for moral purposes. More precisely, from a moral point of view, harm to A may not be compensated for by benefit to B even if it would be compensated for by the same benefit to A himself. In part II of this chapter, I shall briefly canvass some ways in which the differing identities of those affected by our acts can bear on the permissibility of imposing harm on one person without any accompanying benefit for that person. I shall also consider what sorts of properties an entity must have such that harms imposed upon it may not be morally compensated by benefits to another.

In part III, I shall examine the validity of concerns about reproductive cloning that focus on the fear that cloned people will become completely substitutable for each other. In part IV, I shall consider whether compensation of harms by benefits that would be impermissible interpersonally would be permissible when we act on embryos, even when there will be continuity between any such embryo and the person who will arise from it so that there is identity over time of a human being (if not a person). If such cross-embryo compensation is permissible, this will serve as a criticism of those who argue that the moral status of an embryo should be that of a person if the embryo will definitely give rise to a person (as opposed to merely having the potential to give rise to a person). I shall also consider how all this bears on what is called the Non-Identity Problem and the distinction between person-affecting and nonperson-affecting moral principles.

II. Types of Entities and the Importance of Personal Identity

A. WAYS OF MATTERING MORALLY

In one sense, moral status can be defined as what is morally permissible or impermissible to do to some entity.[4] In this sense, rocks may have the moral status of entities to which, just considering them, it is morally permissible to do anything. This is what we can call the "broad sense" of moral status. An important point in talking about status in the broad sense is to distinguish it from what actually happens to an entity. For example, if your moral status makes it impermissible for someone to kill you, you do not lose that moral status merely because you are impermissibly killed. One way to reduce the number of morally bad things that happen in the world is merely to populate it with entities whose status is such that it is permissible to do anything whatsoever to them. Yet most would not think that such a world—for example, one with only rocks in it—would be a morally ideal world, better than one in which there are entities it would be morally impermissible to treat in certain ways, even if it happens that they are sometimes actually treated impermissibly. Presumably, this is because the more important an entity is, the more it matters how one treats it, and it is better to have a world populated by more important entities.[5]

There is a different sense of moral status where the contrast is not between what it is permissible to do to an entity and what is actually done to it. It might be suggested that the contrast is between entities that in some important sense "count" morally in their own right, and so are said to have moral status, and other entities that do not count morally in their own right. "Counting morally in their own right" is a narrower sense of moral status. This implies that in the broad sense of moral status described above, some entities have no narrower moral status. For example, ordinary rocks do not count morally in their own right. But there are also different ways to count morally and, perhaps, different degrees to which one may count in any given way.

When we say that something counts morally in its own right, we are often said to be thinking of its intrinsic worth or value rather than of its instrumental value. If it were morally right to treat animals well only because this would promote kindness between persons, animals would count morally only instrumentally. That is, they should be treated well not because they count in their own right, but only because of the effect on others of treating them well. But Christine Korsgaard has argued that the true contrast to mere instrumental value is having value as an end, not having intrinsic value.[6] For example, if an animal counts morally in its own right, there is no further end that need be served by our treating the animal well in order for us to have a reason to treat it well. If something is an end (in this limited sense), it need not mean that it has value that can never be trumped, nor that it should never be treated as a mere means.[7] At minimum, it means only that its condition can provide a reason (even if an overrideable one) for, for example, attitudes of concern or actions on its behalf independent of other considerations.

Korsgaard argues that some things may be ends in virtue of their intrinsic properties that give them their intrinsic value but others may be ends in virtue of their extrinsic properties. The intrinsic properties are all of an entity's nonrelational properties.[8] Its extrinsic properties are properties that it has in virtue of its standing in relation to other things. For example, Ronald Dworkin claims to have a theory of the intrinsic value of even nonsentient, nonconscious life such as is found in an early embryo. But he also says that this value comes from the history of the embryo, in particular the investment that nature or God has made in it. This is not a theory of the intrinsic value of a life but of its extrinsic value. This is because it derives the value of the embryo from its particular history and its relating to God or nature rather than from properties it has independent of its history and relations.[9] An entity's ability to produce an effect (i.e., be an instrument) is a relational property between it and the effect. It is possible, given what Korsgaard has said, that something could be worth treating as an end because it is capable of causing an effect, even if it never does.[10] Hence, I take it that the narrower sense of moral status involves, at least, something having value as an end rather than as an instrument whether because of its intrinsic or because of its extrinsic properties.

A work of art or a tree may count in its own right in the sense that it gives us reason to constrain our behavior toward it (for example, to not destroy it) just because that would preserve this entity. That is, independent of valuing and seeking the pleasure or enlightenment it can cause in people, a thing of artistic value gives us (I think) reason not to destroy it. In that sense, it counts morally. But this is still to be distinguished from constraining ourselves *for the sake of* the work of art or the tree. I do not act for its sake when I save a work of art, because I do not think of its good and how continuing existence would be good for it when I save it. I cannot do these things because neither the tree nor the work of art is a subject. (Nor do I think of its willing to go on existing. Acting for the sake of what an entity wills might also involve acting for its sake, though it need not involve seeking what is good for it.) Rather, I think of the good *of* the work of art, its worth as an art object, if I save it for no other reason than that it will continue to exist.

We could say that sunlight is good for a tree, meaning that without it the tree will not have life. However, this does not mean that we should avoid blocking the sunlight because it is a benefit for a tree to be alive in the sense that it gets something out of being alive. It is not capable of getting anything out of being alive. Hence, it is not something that in its own right *and* for its own sake merits being kept alive.

By contrast, when I save a bird, I can do it for its sake, because it will get something out of continuing to exist, and it could be bad for it not to continue because it will not get goods it could have had. It seems that something must already have or have had the capacity for sentience or consciousness in order for it to be bad for it not to continue on in existence.[11] This is because an entity having such characteristics—being a subject—seems to be necessary for it to be a beneficiary or victim. It must be able to get something out of its continuing existence, and capacity for sentience or consciousness seems to be necessary for this. (I do not think that the capacity for both is a necessary condition for us to be able to act for the sake of the entity, since each without the other is sufficient.) Having the capacity is not the same as actually being, for example, sentient. It is also not the same as merely having the potential to be sentient, as the latter is consistent with an entity merely having the potential to have the capacity that then gets exercised.[12]

So, we see that within the class of entities that count in their own right, there are those entities that *in their own right and for their own sake* could give us reason to act. I think that it is this that people have in mind when they ordinarily attribute moral status to an entity. So, henceforth, I shall distinguish between an entity's counting morally in its own right (which might be true of a tree) and its having moral status. I shall say that *an entity has moral status when in its own right and for its own sake it can give us reason to do things such as not destroy it or help it.*

On this account, a nonsentient, nonconscious embryo lacks moral status but could count morally in itself (e.g., give us reason in its own right not to destroy it) because of its intrinsic and extrinsic properties, such as its potential. This is different from its merely having instrumental value because it will give rise to a person who has moral status. For even if the embryo is not instrumental to there being a person because it is deprived of an environment in which to develop, its having the potential to develop could still give it greater value than an embryo that lacks the potential. (Similarly, a Chippendale dining table may have value in itself and more value as a work of decorative art if it can also turn into a magnificent writing desk, though it will not.) Notice that an embryo can have greater value in its own right if it has the potential to become an extraordinary person (e.g., Beethoven) rather than an ordinary person, even if these persons would, were they to exist, have the same moral status, and even if the embryo will not, in fact, generate anyone. (The instrumental value of an embryo will also be greater if it will generate Beethoven rather than an ordinary person, even if these two persons' moral status does not differ.)

If an embryo can matter in its own right, this does not mean that its continued existence is good for it, or that it is harmed by not continuing on, or that we can act for its sake in saving its life. Similarly, suppose an ordinary table by magic is turned into a table that has the capacity to develop into a person. It may be good to be a person, but can a table be the sort of thing for which it is bad not to get the fulfillment of this capacity? It does not seem so.[13] The person who would come from the embryo or the table also cannot be harmed or have something bad happen to him by never coming to exist. But we can act for the sake of a person who will arise from the embryo by doing things to the embryo, not for its sake, but for the sake of the person who will exist. (I shall return to this issue below.) The fact that an embryo may have value as an end in virtue of its extrinsic properties could account for why it might be wrong to use it for frivolous purposes. If so, the ground for objecting to such acts would be like the ground for objecting to making lampshades of the flesh of deceased human persons (who had died of natural causes). The flesh has no moral status (as I am now using the term), so we do not act for the sake of what it can gain, but it has an extrinsic relation to once-living human persons who had moral status. Hence, the value it has in its own right in virtue of its extrinsic properties may give us reason not to use it in certain ways. (The embryo's particular intrinsic and extrinsic properties, of course, differ from those of the dead flesh.)[14]

Those things for whose sake we can act when we save their lives may or may not give us as much reason to save them as entities whose existence cannot be extended for their own sake. For example, if we had to choose whether to destroy the Grand Canyon or a bird (holding constant the number of people who would get pleasure or be enlightened by each), it could be morally wrong to choose to destroy the Grand Canyon. This illustrates how something can count morally because it can get something out of life, and so have moral status, without this giving us more reason to act in its favor than in favor of another thing whose continuing existence, in its own right, is more significant even though it gets nothing from its existence. Sometimes, something's remarkableness or uniqueness calls for more protection than does something else's moral status.

We can have duties to behave in certain ways toward entities that count in their own right and, as a subset, toward entities that have moral status.[15] However, having duties to behave in certain ways *toward* entities still does not imply that *we owe it to* these entities to behave in these ways. There is a difference between one's having a duty to do something and having a duty *to a specific entity* to do it. The latter is known as a "directed duty," and typically it has a correlative; that is, a right or claim had by the entity to which the duty is owed against the person who owes it.[16] Correspondingly, there is a difference between doing the wrong thing (for example, in not fulfilling a nondirected duty, such as a duty to promote the good) and *wronging* some entity in failing to perform the duty owed to her.[17] The entity to whom a duty is owed is not necessarily the entity who is benefited or affected by the object of the duty. For example, if you owe it to me to take care of my mother, it is ordinarily thought that I am the right-holder, not my mother, even though the object of the duty is to benefit her. It is ordinarily thought that you wrong me, not my mother, if you fail to help her, though she is the one who fails to be benefited.[18]

Arguably, the ideas of respect for persons and the dignity of the person are connected to the idea that one can *owe it to* a person to behave in certain ways, and also that what we owe to the person can depend on what the person wills (e.g., whether or not she releases us from a claim she has against us), rather than on what is good for her. Hence, she has some authority over what is owed to her and can authorize others to act. This is in contrast to it merely being wrong to treat someone in certain ways because, for example, one owes it to God not to, or because it would not maximize utility to do so and one has a general duty as a rational being—but not owed to anyone—to maximize utility. Hence, just as only some entities that count in their own right are entities that have moral status (as I defined it), so it may be that only some entities that have moral status are owed things and have rights against us at least in part in virtue of what they will and what they can authorize. These are entities for whose sake and in response to whose will we can act on directed duties.

It is tempting to think that these entities have a *higher* moral status than other entities that also have moral status (as I defined it). At the very least, there are reasons to do things with regard to them that do not apply to other entities; that is, we owe it to them and they will it. (The distinction is analogous to the one that applies in cases where A needs assistance but has not been promised it while B is equally needy, has also been promised assistance, and wishes the promise fulfilled.)

The possibility of wronging some entities opens up the further possibility that moral status in the broad sense (with which we began) may not be completely defined by how it is permissible to treat an entity. This would be so if it were sometimes permissible to do something to an entity and yet one still wronged it in the course of acting permissibly. (This might occur if we had to lie to an innocent bystander in order to save someone's life.) Those entities which could be wronged in the course of a permissible act would have a different moral status from those which, while capable of being wronged in other situations, could not be wronged in the course of the same permissible act. It is tempting to think that those we could wrong in the course of a permissible act would also have a higher moral status than those not so wronged. Hence, another indication of moral status could be expressed by whether one could be wronged in the course of a permissible act.

This may be relevant for those nonconsequentialists who think that constraints on harming persons have thresholds beyond which they may be overridden (so-called threshold deontologists). A way of understanding their views is as follows: Suppose a constraint expresses respect for persons and reveals something about their high moral status. We wrong a person if we violate the constraint, as we owe it to him not to do it. If it is wrong (i.e., impermissible) to do the act that wrongs the person, even as the costs of not doing so go up, then the wrong we would do to him must be very serious. The fact that it would be impermissible to treat him in the prohibited way, as the cost of not doing so goes up, is a further mark of his high status.

Suppose the costs go above some threshold and it becomes permissible—that is, *not wrong*—to override the prohibition. Still, we could be wronging the person in doing the overall right act. What would be the evidence for this? That we had to compensate him or apologize to him? However, might compensation or apology be required even if we overrode a constraint *without* wronging someone in doing so?

For example, when we infringe a right, it is said that we *permissibly* override it (by contrast to violating it, which involves impermissibly overriding it). An example of this might be taking a person's car without his permission to rush someone to the hospital in a grave emergency. In this case, we may still owe an apology or even compensation to the owner. (That there is this negative residue to be made up might, of course, also be an indication of someone's moral status.) Yet, perhaps, we have not *wronged* the owner in permissibly overriding his right. A mark of this might be that it would be morally wrong of him to resist our taking his car simply on the grounds of his property right, even if compensation could not be made.[19]

By contrast, consider the Trolley Case: A runaway trolley is headed toward killing five people. We can redirect it onto another track, but then someone immovably seated there will be hit and killed by the trolley. It is commonly thought by nonconsequentialists to be permissible to do this. However, I would argue, it would not be impermissible for the one person toward whom the trolley is redirected to resist our doing this. For example, if he could press a button and send the trolley back from where it came, even if we or the five originally threatened would be killed, I think this would be permissible. This is true even though he may not, in general, do what harms others to save himself. The permissibility of someone's resisting our permissible act is, I think, evidence for the fact that we still wrong him in acting permissibly and in (permissibly) infringing his right.[20]

The fact that someone could still be wronged even though we act permissibly, and the fact that only a great cost could make it be not wrong to do what wrongs him, are both marks of his high moral status. This status, however, no longer gives rise to the impermissibility of treating him in certain ways. That too is a mark of his status: To what sorts of entities is it possible to owe things or behaviors? Thomas Scanlon has argued that only entities capable of judgment-sensitive attitudes are entities to whom we can owe certain treatment. (Scanlon does not speak of rights as the correlatives of directed duties, but I believe the addition of rights talk in his system would be appropriate.) Entities capable of judgment-sensitive attitudes form attitudes or decide on actions on the basis of evaluating certain factors as reasons—that is, as considerations in favor of some attitude or action. For example, they do not just respond to aspects of their environment (as a cat would); they take these aspects as considerations in favor of or against some action. Scanlon's view seems to be that if some entity can evaluate our conduct toward her so that she can see a reason for us to act or not act in that way, then we may potentially owe it to her to act or not act in that way. He also seems to think that a creature capable of judgment-sensitive attitudes governs herself in the light of reasons, and so it is only to such self-governing creatures that we can owe things. (It is possible, however, to imagine that the capacity for judgment-sensitive attitudes does not go so far as to involve self-governance in the light of reasons. For example, a creature might take certain factors in the environment as reasons to pursue food but not be self-conscious and so not self-governing. I am not sure what Scanlon would say about owing things to such a creature.)

Scanlon thinks that animals count morally in their own right and give us reasons to act for their sake. Hence, our conduct toward them can be right or wrong, independent of further considerations. However, right conduct cannot be owed to them, and they cannot be wronged when we behave wrongly with regard to them. This is because (he assumes) they are not capable of judgment-sensitive attitudes. Furthermore, he thinks that while we have a reason to help an animal in need, we can have the same reason to help a rational being in need plus an additional reason absent in the case of the animal—namely we can owe it to the rational being to help him. On this account (as noted above), the greater moral importance or value of rational and reasonable beings (persons) could get fleshed out (in part) as the additional factor present in our relations with them, namely that we owe things to them or, as I would also say, they have rights against us. But, in addition, the fact that they have reasons for willing one thing rather than another could imply that what we owe them relates to what they will rather than to what is merely good for them. This gives them greater authority over what is owed to them.

If only rational beings can, strictly, be the subjects of directed duties or can have rights, what shall we say of infants or of the severely retarded? Scanlon's view seems to be that, in virtue of their relation to rational beings—that is, they are early or failed members of a type whose norm it is to be rational and reasonable—they too have some rights.[21] Here their extrinsic properties are giving them these rights. Why does this not apply to embryos, too? Scanlon does not say. Perhaps it is because, at least when what is at issue is being destroyed or being kept alive, an entity must be at the stage where it would either have the capacity to get something out of going on living or have the capacity to set itself to achieve a goal by going on. Then we could act for its sake in saving it. Infants and the severely retarded can get something out of going on, as well as have rights in virtue of merely extrinsic properties. As I argued above, even if an embryo would lose out on what would turn out to be a good life, given what it is now, it is hard to see how this loss is bad for it or why it is morally important whether it loses further life.[22]

This leaves it open that we should still react differently to entities at certain stages of development, depending on such extrinsic properties as whether they could or will develop into entities for whose sake we could act, or to whom we might owe certain things. If the entities could but will not in fact develop into such other entities, they may still be more remarkable entities than those that could not. If they will in fact develop into such other entities, then to some degree at least they should be treated so that the later entities do not fail to get what they are owed.[23]

B. THE BEARING OF PERSONAL IDENTITY ON OUR TREATMENT OF PERSONS

Having considered some different types of entities, I now want to consider whether and how we may take account of or ignore the facts of personal identity when we are dealing with persons.[24]

There may be conflicts between satisfying individuals' interests or rights and maximizing satisfaction of interests both intrapersonally and interpersonally. (I shall refer to interpersonally maximizing satisfaction of interests as "producing the greater good.") Consider first the conflict between respecting negative rights and producing a greater good *not* protected by rights.[25]

It is often said that part of the reason why one person's right not to be paralyzed should take precedence over producing the greater good by paralyzing him is that others, not he, will receive the benefit of his sacrifice. However, sometimes it can be a greater wrong to harm a person for his own good when we act against his will than it would be to harm him against his will for the good of others who want to be helped.[26] (The charge of paternalism arises in the former case but not in the latter.) In other cases, it seems that the reason for not imposing harm on one person for the sake of others is not that he will fail to be benefited, but rather that the greater good we produce is of the wrong sort. For example, it may consist in many small goods aggregated over many other persons, rather than in a large benefit to any one other person. Consider a case in which someone has a negative right not to have his car damaged. I might nevertheless permissibly damage his car in the course of using it to rush someone else (who would otherwise die) to the hospital. Suppose it were possible, by doing what will damage the car, to produce the same number of additional years of life as would be gained by the person we helped save by giving an enormous number of people one minute each of additional life. Would doing this also be permissible? It seems not.

However, in this last case and ones like it, is it really the separateness of the person who will suffer a loss and those who will benefit that stands in the way of the action's permissibility? Suppose that each of the beneficiaries of the small benefit faced as bad a prospect as the one person who would die if we did not use someone else's car. (That is, suppose each of them was on the point of death.) Might the small goods to many separate people then justify doing what damages the car as much as saving one person to additional years of life?[27] Suppose we still think that the large, concentrated benefit of the life saved for additional years but not the small benefits to each soon-to-die person justifies the imposition of a loss on another person. It is nevertheless true that aggregating small benefits to people each of whom would be very badly off might sometimes justify imposing a larger loss on a person who would not be as badly off as any of those others.

In the cases just discussed, we have compared individuals one person at a time to see who will wind up worse off and who will get what if we act one way rather than another. This procedure is called "pairwise comparison." A proponent of pairwise comparison claims that the fact that potential recipients are separate persons— not only that the person suffering a loss is separate from anyone benefited—is relevant in deciding whether to perform an action that imposes a loss on one person. By contrast, if we merely aggregate benefits and losses over many people, we ignore the distribution of the benefits over individual persons. (Notice that one person can be worse off than another through *intra*personal aggregation of harms in his life. However, aggregating over one life, even assuming constant personal identity, has problems of its own. For example, suppose one person will suffer a thousand headaches over the course of his life, but he will live seventy years and the headaches are interspersed evenly. He may be better off than someone who will have five hundred headaches over the course of a ten-year life, especially if they are bunched together.)

Arguably, the method of pairwise comparison is not sufficient on its own to provide moral guidance. For sometimes it seems that a loss suffered by someone through our *not aiding* (rather than harming) him can be justified even though the benefit of doing this does not come to him but to others, each of whom would suffer less (if not aided) and benefit less (if aided) than he would. For example, suppose I refuse to save someone from death in order to save ten thousand people from paralysis. If aggregation of the losses to many in this case is permissible even though death is the worst outcome in a pairwise comparison, this seems to diminish the significance of the separateness of persons as emphasized by pairwise comparison. Indeed, if I were to decide it is permissible to kill a person for the sake of saving the lives of a million people—a case in which each person would (if left unaided) suffer no larger a loss than the one who is to be killed—this too would diminish the significance of the separateness of persons, at least as expressed by the requirement of pure pairwise comparison. This is because no one of the million would be any worse off (if not aided) than the one person would be if he died, nor would any one of the million receive a benefit (if aided) greater than the single person would have if he were allowed to live.

So far, we have considered taking account of the separateness of persons either by never allowing a benefit in one person to be treated as compensating for a loss in another (no matter how important the benefit or insignificant the loss) or by pure pairwise comparison. A third way of taking account of the separateness of persons I call "balancing of equals." Imagine cases where there is a conflict of interests and we must decide whether to *aid* a smaller or a larger group (of nonoverlapping persons). A person on one side of a conflict is balanced out against another on the other side, and the side with the greater number is helped, at least when each stands to lose or gain as much and other things are equal. This is a form of substitution of equals, for in a conflict between a group of persons B and C and one other person A, from an impartial point of view, we accomplish as much if we save B as if we save A, and hence we can substitute saving B for saving A so that we can also save C. This is so even though A does not benefit if B is saved (because they are separate persons) and even though, from A's partial perspective, the outcome in which she survives is better than the one in which B (or B and C) survives.

The balancing-of-equals approach can still respect the separateness of persons by not weighing against A's loss of twenty years of life a combination of B's loss of ten years and C's loss of ten years. That is, we can first engage in pairwise comparison to check to see if a person will suffer a greater loss, or receive a greater benefit, or wind up worse off,[28] and only balance out those who stand to fall to as low a level and (perhaps) gain as much. The combination of pairwise comparison and balancing can allow us to justify saving a greater number of people rather than a smaller number of people in a conflict situation. However, suppose we allow an aggregation of losses suffered by several persons to outweigh another individual's greater loss, resulting in his being worse off than anyone else when he otherwise could have been significantly aided. (For example, suppose we save a million people from paralysis rather than one person from death). Then we move beyond what balancing requires.

In cases involving negative rights, balancing is ruled out more frequently even when the greater good we would produce by transgressing one person's negative right involves minimizing violations of comparable negative rights in others (when each person stands to fall to as low a level). For example, we may not kill one person to harvest his organs in order to save ten people from death (the Transplant Case). What is being relied on here to reinforce the moral significance of the separateness of persons and to rule out balancing? It is, I believe, a claim on the part of the person who would be deprived of something to what he would be deprived of (e.g., his property, life, or liberty) that is much stronger than anyone else's claim to it. By contrast, in cases where I must choose whom to aid, each party may have the same (including no) right to my assistance.

In some cases, however, it seems permissible to balance even when we will transgress a negative right. For example, it seems to be permissible to redirect a runaway trolley from killing five people onto a track where it will kill one person instead (the Trolley Case).[29] In my *Intricate Ethics*, I tried to account for the moral distinction between the Transplant Case and the Trolley Case by considering different required causal relations between means, goods, and harms.[30] This led me to suggest that there is a moral distinction between merely *substituting* one person for another and *subordinating* one person to another. The Trolley Case, I argued, involves transgressing a negative right in a way that involves substitution without subordination. The Transplant Case involves subordination, and it is this that makes the killing in that case impermissible. The details of the causal distinctions on which this further distinction seems to supervene are not important here, so long as it is accepted that the permissibility of killing in these cases is different.

Another suggestion has been made to explain cases like Transplant and Trolley that involve transgressing negative rights. It reminds us of yet another way in which the separateness of persons has been thought to play a role in ethics. Some have said that *my* transgressing a right in order to prevent *others* from doing so produces a worse state of affairs from my perspective. The emphasis in this account shifts from the significance of the separateness of the potential victim from the potential beneficiaries to the significance of the separateness of a particular agent from other agents. This suggests that if another agent were to transgress someone's negative right for the sake of minimizing comparable rights violations, I would have no reason to stop him. However, suppose B will violate A's right not to have his arm amputated in order to save many others from having their arms impermissibly amputated. Do I have a reason (even if not a duty) to put aside my activities to stop the violation of A's right rather than let it be the cause of the greater good? I think I do.[31] The greater good does not trump the single person's right merely because I will not be the one transgressing that right. Also, if it were most important from my point of view that *I* not be involved in violating a negative right, should I minimize the number of such acts that I commit? May I kill one person now to stop a threat I started yesterday that will soon kill five other people, thus making me the killer of five people? I think not. These cases suggest that the constraint on transgressing one person's right in order to help others does not fundamentally express an agent's concern with his own agency as a separate person.[32]

So far, I have been characterizing ways in which the separateness of persons is taken account of in certain moral theories. We can summarize some of these ways as follows: (1) not substituting one person for another, period; (2) not substituting one person for another unless there is an equal gain to be gotten by each and/or an equal level to which each would fall through a loss; (3) not substituting one person for another when the person to be substituted for another has an overriding claim to control what would be taken from him by substitution; (4) an agent not substituting for other agents. My discussion has suggested that substitution of persons can sometimes be permissible even within a nonconsequentialist theory, and so (1) is not true, even (2) is too stringent a requirement, and (3) may be true only when subordination occurs. I also argued against a major role for (4) in explaining constraints on harming some for the benefit of others.

C. SUBSTITUTABILITY AND WAYS OF MATTERING MORALLY

Now let us consider, as described in section A, creatures who have a good but are not rights-bearers, and also entities that have value in their own right but are not ones for whose sake we can act. Let us see whether there are any moral principles analogous to those dealing with the separateness of persons that can be applied when dealing with such entities. Would it be permissible to destroy (even in a way involving subordination) one non-rights-bearing animal in order to prevent the destruction of others? Arguably, yes. (Notice that such sacrificeability of one animal for others is consistent with the fact that it is the sort of being that has a life of its own and could have been benefited by continuing to exist if we had not destroyed it.) Does this further imply that we may be utilitarians and simple maximizers with respect to animals? No, because it may still be wrong to aggregate small losses to many animals against a big loss to one animal at least when each of the former would not be as badly off (if not helped) as the latter. It might also be wrong to sacrifice a higher animal (for example, one with a greater degree of intellectual and interactive capacities) to save a greater number of lower ones.

Would it be permissible to destroy, in a manner involving subordination, one embryo to save others from being destroyed, at least when each of the latter will develop into people if saved? I believe so. Would it be permissible to similarly destroy one great artwork to prevent several other comparable artworks from being destroyed? I believe so. Would it be permissible to similarly destroy one human embryo to allow many *monkey* embryos to develop? I believe so.[33] Would it be permissible to destroy one great art work for the sake of several less significant ones? Interestingly, this seems truly misguided.

This broad sacrificeability of one entity, even in a manner involving subordination, for the sake of others is in sharp contrast to the way it is permissible to treat persons. Yet it is also in contrast to the way we should treat some other non-rights-bearing entities. For such sacrificeability is not true of entities whose value is purely symbolic, like flags, or of holy entities. These things have no rights and no good for whose sake we act, yet there are reasons not to destroy one for the sake of others, at least in a manner involving subordination, that are analogous to reasons that apply to persons. For example, sometimes it could make no sense for it to be permissible to burn one flag to prevent many other flags from being burnt impermissibly. This is the case if it is their inviolable status with which we are concerned in trying to save the many flags, for the *permissibility* of burning one to save others denies that very inviolability. (The same is true for persons.) Suppose it makes no sense to destroy one entity whose value resides in its symbolic function to save other entities with the same value, but it makes sense to destroy one human embryo to save other human embryos. This suggests that the value of the embryo does *not* reside merely in its role as a symbol of human life. An embryo may serve merely as a symbol only when we are *not* interested in its future development. Hence, we may think that it makes sense to destroy one embryo for the sake of the *future development* of other embryos, but not for the sake of their survival as embryos in a freezer as mere symbols of life.

In part II, I have considered different types of entities falling into increasingly narrow categories: those that count in their own right, those that have moral status (in the narrow sense), and those to whom we owe things. I have argued that the moral nonsubstitutability of the latter entities is stronger, at least in cases involving their destruction in a way that subordinates, than the nonsubstitutability of those that merely count in their own right or that merely have moral status. This is true even though those who have moral status can have separate points of view and interests of their own. In the next part, I attempt to apply these conclusions about nonsubstitutability to the issue of reproductive cloning.

III. Reproductive Cloning

"Your clone, Melford, has come of work age. You must leave now."
—*New Yorker* cartoon, February 9, 2004

One sheep to another: "Sometimes I worry that I'm a wolf dressed as me."
—*New Yorker* cartoon, February 2, 2004

A. CLONING AND SUBSTITUTABILITY

There are many objections that people raise to reproductive cloning. My primary concern in this context is with the sense that reproductive cloning might be "a threat to one's personal identity" and to the nonsubstitutability of persons that I have discussed above. Let us deal with the substitutability issue first.[34]

As we have seen, nonsubstitutability in a strong sense—for example, not violating, in a manner involving subordination, a strong negative right even to minimize the violation of comparable rights in others—pertains, for the most part, to the sorts of individuals to whom one can owe things: self-conscious, rational beings who have authority over themselves. Such nonsubstitutability seems connected to what we call the dignity of persons. Hence, some may think that cloning is incompatible with the dignity of persons because it would reduce such nonsubstitutability. How could being a person who exists as a result of cloning deprive one of being entitled to such regard? Imagine you are under a massive delusion about the way in which you were actually created. Everything about you remains as you are now except that you are not the product, as you believed, of sexual reproduction, but of mono-parental cloning. Would you think that your rights had changed dramatically? I do not think you would, and I think you would be correct not to. The question of the historical course of events that leads to the existence of a certain sort of being can, for the most part, be distinguished from the value and rights of the entity that is produced and what gives it value and rights.[35] That is one of the most important things to remember in this area.[36]

If a person is genetically identical to someone else (as a result of cloning or otherwise), is she replaceable by that second person? Sometimes people say that your genetic clone will not have the same *phenotype* as you do, and thus is neither going to be you nor be a replacement for you.[37] But we all know that, strictly speaking, the clone will not be you: "numerical nonidentity" dictates that you and she are two different beings; we do not need to point to a difference in phenotype to know that a clone is not you. Indeed, I think that in arguing for nonsubstitutability, it is a mistake to focus on the fact that genotype alone does not lead to the same phenotype. The core point is that, even if there were a clone who was phenotypically identical to you—identical genotypically and phenotypically but numerically nonidentical—that would not mean that you would be replaceable by it. It is tempting to say that this is because you would not be replaceable *to* yourself (that is, from your own perspective). However, if this suggests that someone might not be willing to replace herself with another person (e.g., give up her life so that a new person can exist), that is not necessarily true.[38] The point is that you cannot replace yourself with another and still continue being you, and the clone is another, not you. The other crucial ethical point is that you are still the type of creature who may have a claim to what would be taken from you (life, job) in replacement, and thus it should not be taken from you without your consent.

Suppose someone told me: "If we kill you or fire you, we will also replace you with a clone that is genetically and phenotypically identical to you but, of course, numerically distinct." That would not in any significant way compensate *me* for my loss of life or job, given that I do not care enough about the clone.[39] Now, this raises the question that philosophers often discuss: What is it that we ought to be concerned about in our survival? Is it just the survival of a type of genetic makeup or a phenotype, or the survival of a particular individual? It seems to many that it is the particular individual's survival rather than the survival of his type, either genetic or phenotypic, that is crucial. Now, suppose you were replaceable *to* everybody else—that is, suppose they do not care about you except for your genotype and your phenotype; they do not care about you as a particular person. It would still be the case that your right to life and to respect would be as strong as any other person's, given that you are the sort of creature who has a claim to his life and does not waive it. The crucial foundation for the idea of respect for the person or the right to life would not be changed by cloning someone who is replaceable for you to others.

In literature, the idea of one's double (as in Dostoyevsky's *The Double*)[40] is threatening only in part because others take the double to be entitled to what one would otherwise be entitled. In Dostoyevsky's novel, the double is also threatening because the protagonist seems to lose his sense of himself as himself, actively confusing himself with the other. This is the problem of the sheep in the *New Yorker* cartoon who thinks he might be the wolf (dressed up to look like him). But we laugh at the cartoon and think the person who literally identifies himself with his double is insane, because there is no way for a being with a subjective point of view to correctly think such things. (Notice that the sheep refers to himself as "me" and also worries that he is someone else impersonating "me" [i.e., "dressed as me"]. This is different from worrying that "me" is a wolf dressed as a sheep [i.e., that "I am a wolf in sheep's clothing"].) Hence, there is no way that a still rational being would literally identify his clone as himself.[41]

In sum, it should be emphasized that an argument based on the fact that cloning will not result in the same phenotype, though well-intentioned and probably correct, is misplaced. Respect for persons, entailing whatever nonsubstitutability commits us to now, would still hold even if *everyone* had the same phenotype and genotype. It would be based on each person being self-conscious, capable of responding to reasons, and having a claim to their individual lives greater than anyone else has.

Notice that so far I have been arguing against the view that cloning is inconsistent with the dignity of the person in the sense that one could not be a person with such dignity if one were oneself a clone or if one had a clone in existence. But the view might be interpreted differently: Given that the clone will be a person with dignity, it is wrong to bring such a being into existence by cloning. But why should this be true? If cloning of persons were the natural form of reproduction, would there be a prima facie moral obligation to develop sexual reproduction instead, out of concern to avoid insults to the dignity of persons cloned? And if not, why is it contrary to the dignity of persons to *introduce* reproductive cloning?

It has been argued that a child cloned from an elderly person would tend to think that the type of future it can have has already been lived by the older person from whom it was cloned. But this depends on a mistaken view of genetic determinism. If phenotypes depend on more than genes, the types of futures clones have can differ.

Would there be a prima facie obligation not to clone (or to introduce sexual reproduction if cloning were the natural way to reproduce) if clones were phenotypically the same? Why is it an insult to one's dignity—understood as one's having claims against others related to nonsubstitutability—that others share (and are made to share) the same phenotype? It is inconsistent with respect for persons to force them to adopt traits just because others have these traits, and genetically controlled uniform phenotypes suggest that individuals are allowed no choice in the course of their lives over what to be like. But we do not necessarily object to uniformity with respect to agreed upon *good* traits, or to unforced choice by all people to adopt the same good traits. Furthermore, genetically programming *diverse* phenotypes would involve as little choice by people in the course of their lives over what to be like as programming a uniform phenotype.

Possibly, cloning raises concerns about joint ownership over a type of genetic information when it is shared by several people. Suppose a single parent had cloned his first child from his own cells and the parent decides that he wants to use his own genetic material to make yet another clone. Because the first child would also be a clone of the second child, is the first child's consent required for creating yet another individual with the same genetic makeup? A possible analogy is the sharing of a house—someone we have incorporated into our household should, perhaps, be consulted before another party joins us. Still, I recognize problems with such a requirement of consent, for suppose a child clone of a parent himself comes to the point of wanting to reproduce by cloning. It would be odd to think he must get his parent's permission to do so. Possibly there could be some asymmetry here: A parent's responsibilities to the child are not reflected in the child's responsibilities to the parent. (Nor is there a personal responsibility to any sibling from which one is cloned to get that sibling's permission before one clones one's own child.)

B. CLONING AND HOLISTIC IDENTITY

I have tried to argue that the worth and nonsubstitutability of persons, as we know them, are not incompatible with reproductive cloning, either in the sense that cloning would rob persons of dignity or that it would insult the dignity that they have. I now want to consider the view that cloning is a threat to human identity and personal identification in a less than strict sense. My comments also apply to the cases of human clones that already exist—genetically identical twins—except that I will sometimes imagine (for argument's sake) that twins have an identical phenotype as well as genotype.

There is a sense of "personal identity" that is commonly used by psychologists, doctors, and biologists. It is what I shall call a "holistic sense" of personal identity closely related to one's phenotype—the sense in which I am a philosopher, someone who is interested in art, and someone who makes jokes. All of this is part of my holistic identity, for someone would not be me in the holistic sense if she were not interested in philosophy or art or making jokes.

Consider a way of presenting the views of those who emphasize the importance of differences in actual phenotypes with which, they say, we identify ourselves holistically. Figure 16.1 represents four logical possibilities. (I do not mean to imply that all are physically possible.) In condition A, we have the same genotype and the same holistic phenotype. In condition B, we have the same genotype and different holistic phenotypes. In condition C, we have different genotypes and the same holistic phenotype. In condition D, we have different genotypes and different holistic phenotypes.

	same holistic phenotype	different holistic phenotypes
same genotype	A	B
different genotypes	C	D

FIGURE 16.1 Logically possible genotype/phenotype relations

To those who think that what is worrisome about reproductive cloning is only identical holistic phenotypes, condition A (where, let us assume, there is cloning) is as worrisome as condition C (where there is no cloning), and conditions B and D are equally unworrisome per se. Suppose (contrary to fact) that the only way we could ensure holistic phenotypic *nonidentity* were by ensuring genetic *identity*. Suppose all we should be concerned about is holistic phenotypic nonidentity. Then (supposing genetic identity did not occur naturally) cloning would be the preferred mode of reproduction. This view seems reinforced by the following thought experiment: Suppose that we have all been misled and all our natural genetic makeups are already identical. If our phenotypic differences remain as they are, we would not worry about losing a holistic sense of identity differentiation.

This psychosocial, holistic notion of personal identity is not the ordinary notion of personal identity, however. The ordinary notion of personal identity concerns those properties that are essential to one's nature, such that if they were changed, one would no longer exist in a strict sense.[42] It is a premise in most philosophical arguments about identity or survival that there are many things about you that could be very important facts about your holistic identity, and yet they could have been different and you would have continued to exist. For example, if you suddenly lost twenty points of your IQ, a holder of the holistic notion might say the person in existence was no longer you, but a philosopher (and ordinary people) could say that it was still you in an intellectually reduced state. Indeed, the decrease in your IQ would explain why *you* were much worse off than *you* had been.

Some philosophers claim that if the same sperm and egg from which you arose had been placed in a different environment or had started dividing at a later point in time, it would still have resulted in you.[43] Like most phenotypic properties, many historical properties like the date of your birth or the date of your death are not essential properties. These properties could change and the new ones would still be had by *you*. Some genetic properties are similarly nonessential. Now, the question is: What are the essential properties? There is much debate over this, and I have no answers.

As I have already noted, many people who say that a clone will *not* be you point to the expected phenotypic difference, and they probably do this because they think that holistic phenotypic differentiation among people is very important, even though we would not literally fear we were someone else or fear that moral nonsubstitutability would disappear if there were no phenotypic differences. The fact that it could have been *you* with a different holistic phenotype may make the response to the "threat of cloning" that emphasizes continuation of phenotypic differences seem weaker. For when I consider individuals who are holistically phenotypically different from me but genetically identical, I may think that any one of those individuals is an example of what I phenotypically might have been like, while (to be redundant) still being me. The point is that, though we are holistically phenotypically different, I could have had your holistic phenotype, and thus it is not holistic phenotypes but something else that is crucial to who I am. (Of course, even if we had the same genotype and could have shared holistic phenotypes, I would not *be* you, since we are numerically distinct and *in fact* do not share the same holistic phenotype.)

In addition, consider that there is a tension between the importance of genetic connection with offspring and the idea that holistic phenotype, not genotype, determines who we really are. Suppose someone offers me a genetically unrelated child who is phenotypically very similar to me, having all the same interests and values that I have. Many people think that I still would not have satisfied a supposed intense desire for genetic connection. If genetic connection is so important, this suggests that people think their genes *are* very important to who they are. It is the latter thought that leads people to think that they should project their genes into the future by reproducing. Thus, the idea that passing on his genes is important to a person is at war with the idea that phenotypic difference is enough to distinguish individuals from one another (in a nonphilosophical sense) and that phenotypic similarity is enough to significantly relate individuals to one another.[44]

Perhaps considerations such as these—only partially grasped, not as a full-fledged philosophical theory of identity—underlie some people's sense that it is undesirable to have beings who share their genotype. This would make condition B in figure 16.1 worse than condition D. Here the presupposition is that it is a genotype, or at least part of it, that is essential to me. (Of course, it cannot be the only thing essential to me, since, by hypothesis, someone else has it, too.) This leaves it open that phenotypic nondifferentiation would be too high a price to pay if it alone (hypothetically) were compatible with genetic diversity. (Thus condition A in figure 16.1 could be the worst outcome.)

I do not believe that thinking along these lines would provide a decisive argument against cloning because one's genetically identical natural twin now shares one's genotype as well—and do we think there is a strong reason to prevent natural identical twinning? But perhaps thinking along these lines may provide one with some reason to prefer a world in which there is no natural twinning and a reason not to seek such twins, even with phenotypic diversity.[45]

Genetic twins as we know them now are synchronic (that is, they come into being as conceptuses simultaneously and as infants close to simultaneously and live on at the same times). Clones might come into being diachronically (for example, one conceptus is created later than the original or after the original has ceased to exist). It might be thought that the very thing that makes one uncomfortable with even a phenotypically different clone existing synchronically with oneself could be desirable if the clone existed diachronically after one ceased to exist: if we cannot be immortal, having a successor who is a clone could bring us as close as possible to immortality. (According to at least one philosophical theory of personal identity, a successor to you that had certain very tight causal relations to you might actually be you.[46])

Diachronicity, however, also seems to raise problems not present with synchronicity.[47] Synchronic cloning is in one way less threatening because it seems clearer that an original and a clone are separate individuals when they both exist at the same time. When the original has passed away, however, the possibility that someone else will be identified as the original may seem greater. Suppose we think the identification of such a successor with the original is a mistake. Then if identification takes place, we shall be disturbed by the sense that acts and accomplishments that are someone else's may be added to the account of the original person, making "his life" be beyond his control. Another way of putting this point is that so long as I exist as a token of a type, I am definitely to be distinguished from other tokens. If I cease to be a token of this type (because I cease to be), the fact that another token could "extend" me can become a cause of concern.

IV. When Identity Might Not Matter Morally

A. THE EMBRYO OF A DEFINITE FUTURE PERSON

I have argued that a cloned person could not permissibly be harmed any more than a noncloned person in order to minimize comparable harms to other persons.[48] Now I want to consider whether an embryo that *will in fact* develop into (or give rise to) a person is also protected against less-than-lethal subordinating interventions that will negatively affect the future person it will develop into (or give rise to). In particular, I shall consider cases when these interventions are undertaken for the sake of benefiting other future persons by affecting other embryos that will develop into (or give rise to) the other persons.

Elsewhere, I have argued against what I shall call the View:[49] We have as strong a duty not to do things to an embryo that will result in harm (or failure to prevent harm) to the person that the embryo will definitely develop into (or give rise to) as we have not to harm (or not to fail to prevent harm to) that person when he is already in existence. Notice that the View is compatible with thinking that a pregnant woman is not obligated to do (or refrain from doing) certain things that a woman would have to do (or refrain from doing) for an offspring outside her body. This is because more of an imposition on her may be involved if she must do these things when the embryo is in her body than when it is outside, and the duty she has may not license such an imposition.

One premise in what I shall call the Argument (for the View)[50] is that, if we have duties to an embryo while it is still only an embryo, it is because of the person it will develop into or give rise to. Those who make the Argument think that this premise implies the View—duties that exist while there is only an embryo should be as strong and of the same general type as duties that we have to the person once he has developed—at least if we are certain that the embryo will develop into or give rise to a person, and that what we do to it as an embryo will affect the person in the same way.

Elizabeth Harman has characterized the Argument as follows, speaking of early fetuses. (She claims that early fetuses have no moral status [as she understands the term] but are capable of being harmed. This implies that harm to them does not matter.)

> According to the existing account, we are prohibited from harming those early fetuses that will be carried to term not because of anything constitutive of the harming itself. It is not that these things, these early fetuses, are the kind of things we should not harm. It is merely that there is a bad further consequence of harming these fetuses: in the future, a baby is born who suffers from fetal alcohol syndrome or some other bad effect of the earlier harming. This bad account may fail to address the worry expressed by those who challenge the liberal view [on abortion]. The worry may not simply be that the liberal view is incompatible with prohibitions on harming early fetuses. Rather, it may be that the liberal view is incompatible with its being the case that some early fetuses are the kind of things [we are] prohibited from harming. The worry is that the liberal view cannot appeal to the nature and status of these early fetuses themselves in explaining why we are prohibited from harming them.[51]

In place of the Argument and its crucial premise, Harman offers what she calls the Actual Future Principle: "An early fetus that will become a person has some moral status. An early fetus that will die while it is still an early fetus has no moral status."[52] (I assume Harman would apply the principle to embryos, too.) Notice that Harman's principle takes the view that the fetus does not merely *give rise* to a person. Harman thinks that it *becomes* a person in the sense that there is one human being from conception through personhood—identity of a human being over time—and the fetus that will become a person is that human being's earliest stage. Notice also that, as stated, the Actual Future Principle does not fully support the View. This is because it does not claim that the fetus's moral status is the same as the status of the person it will become and therefore that we have as strong a duty not to do things to an embryo that will result in harm to the person as we have not to harm the person when she is already in existence. Thus, Harman's principle may not strictly imply that the duty not to do things to the fetus that will harm (or not prevent harm to) the person it will become is as strong as the comparable duty to the person when she already exists. Nevertheless, it is not clear why Harman should not hold the View, for she also says: "The Actual Future Principle recognizes the moral status of early fetuses that will become persons; it is precisely these early fetuses in which *persons can be said to be already present.*"[53] [Emphasis added.] If a person is already present, then the fetus's moral status should be the same as the status of the person.

A problem that arises for the Actual Future Principle that does not arise for the Argument is that the former implies (when combined with Harman's view that it is possible to harm early fetuses, and presumably embryos) that we may not do things to a fetus that harm it, even when the harm is short-lived and will not affect the person whom the fetus will definitely become. This is because we have a prima facie duty not to harm a person, even when the harm is short-lived and will not go on to affect the person in the future. The Argument, by contrast, is concerned with what we do to a fetus or embryo only if this will affect the person-to-be. I think it is either (a) not true that it is impermissible to cause a short-lived harm to a fetus or embryo, or (b) if it were impermissible to cause such a short-lived harm, this could sometimes be true even if the embryo/fetus will *not* develop into a person. Consider an example of (a): It seems to be a harm to an embryo per se to remove one of its cells. However, removing one of its cells (for example, for genetic testing) does not (let us assume for argument's sake) badly affect the person that the embryo gives rise to or becomes. Harman should think that removing the cell is wrong, but it does not seem to be wrong. Consider a possible example of (b): Suppose fetuses were capable of feeling pain. It would be (pro tanto) wrong to cause a fetus short-lived, intense pain, even if it would not develop into a person.

I shall put this concern about Harman's view aside, for I am interested to show that the View is incorrect and that if the Actual Future Principle implies the View, it is incorrect for this reason. Hence, either the Actual Future Principle does not imply the View and we need to know why it does not or the Actual Future Principle is incorrect. With respect to the Argument, I claim only to show (as I have tried to do elsewhere) that while its premise may be true, it does not imply the View. That is, we can agree that any duties we have to treat a fetus in a certain way exist only because of the person it will develop into, or give rise to, but this does not imply the View.

Here is an example which, I believe, shows that it is permissible to affect a future person by doing something to the fetus (or to the embryo) from which he develops or arises, though it is not permissible to affect the person in the same way by doing something to him once he exists. Suppose a woman has (via the natural lottery) given a fetus genes that will result in a person with an IQ of 160. She decides this is too smart, not for the good of the person who would have the high IQ, but for the good of the family. As a result, she takes a drug during early pregnancy to reduce the future person's IQ to 140.[54] I shall assume that this is an identity-preserving change and so this is a case of causing a person to be worse off than he would otherwise have been. I believe doing this is permissible (for reasons to be given below). But once her child exists, it would not be similarly permissible for the woman to give it a pill that reduces its IQ from 160 to 140 or that alters its genes so that the child will have an IQ of 140 rather than 160 in the future.

What is the difference between (1) affecting the person by affecting the fetus and (2) affecting the person himself? A fetus is not the sort of being that is entitled to keep a characteristic that it has, such as a genetic makeup that will generate a 160 IQ. This is because it is not the sort of being that can be the bearer of rights (to retain anything). It lacks moral status (as defined in part II) and lacks additional properties that would make it a rights-bearer, in part because it is not sentient or conscious. In addition, the person who will develop from the fetus will not fall below an acceptable level of intelligence if he has only a 140 IQ, so he (as a person) is not owed a 160 IQ by his parent. (An IQ of 140 is already far above the minimal goods that, it might be argued, we owe to the people we create. I shall here merely assume and not argue for the claim that persons do owe their offspring certain things beyond a life that is minimally worth living.[55]) These two facts are crucial to the permissibility of taking back from the fetus IQ points that the parent gave it. But since a child is already a person (I assume), it is usually entitled to keep a beneficial characteristic it has, even if doing so raises the child far beyond the standard it is owed from its creator. Hence, I believe it is impermissible to give the IQ-reducing pill to the child, even if doing so would not cause his IQ to fall below the minimum a creator owes to its child.[56] By contrast, suppose we owe a good chance of an IQ of at least 100 to people we create. In this case, doing something easily avoidable in early pregnancy to a fetus that results in a person who develops with an IQ below 100 may well be as impermissible as doing to the later child something that lowers its IQ to below 100.

Because the fetus is not yet a person (or does not yet have other properties that make it an entity that is entitled to keep what is given to it), the act of taking away characteristics the fetus has (which will impact the person that will be) is no different from not giving the fetus those characteristics to begin with. And one would have a right not to give a fetus or future person that one created genes sufficient for a 160 IQ. Analogously, suppose that a parent puts money she need not give into a bank account that will belong to her child when he exists as an adult. The fact that the child will definitely exist as an adult does not imply by itself that it is impermissible for the parent to take back the money before the person reaches the age at which he can claim his bank account. There is no retroactive claim had by the person who will definitely exist to the good that precedes his appearance. (This is true even if the parent has not earned her own money, but has inherited it from others as people inherit their genes.)

What about the permissibility of a parent not rendering assistance to a fetus to prevent a natural change that will lead the person who develops or arises from the fetus to have a 140 IQ rather than a 160 IQ? If the change would occur in the fetus before it is entitled to keep the traits, I believe that one need not make as great an effort to stop the reduction in IQ as one should make once one is the parent of the child who has the 160 IQ or the genetic traits that will lead to the 160 IQ. It seems to me that a parent's duty to help a child keep a beneficial trait (or genes that will lead to it) that the child already has can be stronger than a parent's duty to see to it that her child comes to have such a trait by helping the embryo retain the genetic material.

Some believe that the early fetus does not merely give rise to the later person but is an early stage of the human being whose later stage is a person. (As noted, Harman holds such a view.) Some who believe this may want to distinguish between the early fetus and the set of sperm and egg before these combine with respect to retroactive claims of the later person. Those who support the View, however, should *not* distinguish our duties to an early embryo from those to a sperm and egg that will be combined. That is, they should hold that if duties we have with respect to a sperm and egg are on account of the person to which they will give rise, then our duties with respect to the sperm and egg should be as strong as duties to the person who will definitely arise from them. For example, they should hold that it is wrong to do certain things to an egg that will not change the identity of the person who will arise from it but will make that person worse off than he would otherwise have been. Hence, I suggest that we can also show that the View is wrong by considering a variant on the 160 IQ Case in which the woman knows that the child created from a particular egg would have an IQ of 160; she takes a drug that alters her egg so that the child will instead develop an IQ of 140. Call this the Egg 160 IQ Case. I believe it is permissible for her to use this means of making a change to a definite future person even though it would be impermissible for her to give an IQ-reducing pill to her child.[57]

But now consider an in-between case called Delayed Change.[58] Suppose the parent is not physically able to remove the genetic material at the fetus or egg stage and (as I have argued) not permitted to take an action that would remove IQ points from the child-person. May she give to the fetus or egg a drug that will have a delayed reaction in childhood (like a slow bomb), eliminating the child's genetic material that would lead it eventually to have a 160 IQ rather than a 140 IQ? I do not believe this is permissible. I also do not believe that anything I have said implies that it is permissible. For it involves doing something at time t_1 that will remove something good at t_2 when there is a person to whom that item belongs.

Recall the View as I set it out at the beginning of this section: We have as strong a duty not to do things to an embryo that will result in harm (or failure to prevent harm) to the person the embryo will definitely develop into (or give rise to) as we have not to harm (or not to fail to prevent harm to) that person when he is already in existence. Suppose that my arguments have shown that the View is incorrect. If the View is implied by Harman's Actual Future Principle, then the latter is also incorrect. It is also incorrect to think that just because we do something to *this same human being* when we do something to a person, and when we do something to an embryo that will (according to Harman) become the person, we may not do the latter if we may not do the former.

Now imagine again that a woman has given a fetus genetic material that would give the person it will develop into a 160 IQ, but that she takes back from the fetus some genetic material and this makes the fetus develop into a person with a 140 IQ instead. This time, however, the woman does this in order to then transfer the material into two other fetuses, thereby raising their IQs from 130 to 140 each. What I have said above, I think, implies that doing this would be permissible. The woman would be morally free to equalize beneficial traits among future persons by affecting their embryos (or the eggs from which they arise), even though she thereby makes some person worse off than he would otherwise be for the sake of other persons. However, I do not think it would be permissible for her to (safely) take from a child (already a person) some characteristic that will or does give him a 160 IQ, leaving him with a 140 IQ, so that she can transfer the material into her two other children, raising their IQs from 130 to 140 each.

When modifying the genetic material of an embryo is contemplated, it is usually in a context where we can improve the life of the person who will develop or arise from the embryo. I have raised the possibility that it might be permissible, for good reason, to alter an embryo in a way that will cause the person who develops or arises to be worse off than he might otherwise be. It might be noted that in the real world, there would be no need to take something from one embryo in order to place it in another embryo (if this were possible) as a means of improving the latter, as was true in my hypothetical case. And while making one person worse off without thereby improving others could increase equality among people, this sort of "leveling down" to achieve equality is often taken to be a counterexample to the value of achieving equality. However, taking something away from one embryo even without transferring anything to others could still improve the lives of persons who will develop from the other embryos. This is because it might make it more likely that they will win their share of competitions with the other person.

Then there could be an increase in their absolute well-being and the charge of "leveling down" to achieve equality would be defeated.

Hence, even if it is wrong to take organs from one person to save others, it could sometimes be permissible to take from a fetus genetic material necessary to form an organ in the person the fetus will give rise to or develop into, in order to generate such organs in other persons who would otherwise lack them. An embryo, even of a person who will definitely come to exist, could be substitutable *and* subordinatable. This will be true when removing the genetic material from the embryo does not make the person into which it will develop fall below the level that a creator is obligated to try to attain in creating a new person.

B. FUTURE GENERATIONS AND THE NON-IDENTITY PROBLEM

These results may bear on our responsibilities to future generations.[59] Take the imaginary case in which we know that certain particular people will definitely exist in a hundred years, though we do not create them and the fetus from which they will arise or develop does not yet exist.[60] Suppose we engage in activities today that will affect the environment in such a way that the air quality will not be as good in one hundred years as it would otherwise have been, though it will still be above the level that we owe to future generations. Suppose, further, that there is no person in existence yet whose environment that future environment is. I believe we may engage in such activities. But if we were (somehow) transported one hundred years hence, it could well be impermissible to engage in the same activities that reduce to the same degree the air quality that the persons then living are already enjoying. In fact, it is not necessary that these people (or the children in my previous cases) actually already be in possession of the better environment (or the more advantageous trait, whether it is the higher IQ or the genetic trait that will lead to it). Given that they are already persons, if their *prospects* as persons are for acquiring such a superior environment (or advantageous trait), it is possible that they should not be deprived of these prospects, at least by certain types of events that would occur once they exist.[61] This means that we are permitted to act in ways that reduce the superior air quality (but not below an acceptable level they are owed) before future persons who will be affected by this exist, even though we know that certain particular people will exist. By contrast, we may not be permitted to have the same effect on the environment somewhat delayed, so that it occurs when the future persons already exist and impacts an environment they can claim as theirs. If we wish to do right by future generations, therefore, it will be very important to know what level of environmental quality they are owed independently of what they will be entitled to keep once they have it, and *when* the alteration to the environment will occur relative to the existence of the persons affected by such an alteration. We cannot merely say that there is a duty not to make any future environment worse than it would otherwise be without our action.

Finally, let us consider the possible bearing of these issues on what is known as the Non-Identity Problem. Derek Parfit famously argued that sometimes, at least, it seems not to matter morally whether we are affecting the same (identical) person for the worse or just making someone worse off than some separate (non-identical) person would have been.[62] Moral principles that tell us not to make persons worse off than *they* would have been or to make persons better off than *they* would have been are called "person-affecting principles." The moral significance of nonidentity is a problem for those who think that all moral principles are person-affecting. Moral principles that tell us not to make there be people who are worse off than *other* people would have been (or to make persons who are better off than other persons would have been) are called "non-person-affecting principles." This is not because there are no effects on persons in the latter cases, but rather because no person is worse or better off than *he* would otherwise have been, given that the worse off or better-off person is someone else. So, for example, suppose that if we behave in a certain way now, we will affect the environment so that future people who would otherwise have existed anyway are worse off than they might have been. In this case, we affect people for the worse. Alternatively, suppose that if we behave in a certain way now, we will affect the world so that different people will exist in the future than would otherwise have existed, and they will live worse lives than those other people would have lived, due to changes our behavior makes to the environment. In this case, we do not affect anyone so that he is worse off than *he* would have been. Parfit claims that at least sometimes, it does not matter morally whether we affect persons for the worse or instead create persons who are worse off than others would have been.

Let us assume that the worse life in these examples is still a life worth living and also that it is a life that is good enough to meet the standards that a responsible creator could be held to in creating new people. Then we cannot argue that people are entitled not to have the worse life because they are entitled not to be in certain states, whether by our making them worse off than they would have otherwise been or by our doing something that leads to the existence of worse-off people than would have otherwise existed. That is, we cannot argue that person-affecting principles do not have special weight because people simply have a right not to be in the particular worse state. It is just the comparative worseness of one set of people that speaks against the act that produces them, just as it is the comparative worseness of the way in which a given person's life will go that speaks against acting in a way that makes him worse off.

I think that what I have said against the View may bear on the Non-Identity Problem because I have argued that sometimes *the way in which* we affect someone for the worse can make a moral difference, not just the fact *that* we affect him for the worse. If we affect him by doing something to him or to some trait or resource to which he is entitled because he has it and it is or would be beneficial to him, this can have greater moral significance than if we affect him similarly by doing something to a trait or resource to which he is not yet entitled because he does not yet exist as a being who can have entitlements. Standard cases in which we affect people for the worse involve the former way of affecting someone. This leaves it open that *person-affecting* cases involving the latter, nonstandard way of affecting people are not morally different from *non-person-affecting* cases, while cases of the former, standard sort *are* morally more significant. Choosing to perform easily avoidable acts that affect an embryo and lead to a given offspring having fewer resources may have the same moral significance as choosing to perform easily avoidable acts that lead to creating a worse-off person rather than a different better-off person. And both sorts of acts may be less morally problematic than performing an act that will take from someone what he is entitled to keep (or not provide him with help he is entitled to get), resulting in his having fewer resources.

If the person-affecting cases that are used to help illustrate the Non-Identity Problem do not involve entitlements based, for example, on personal possession, then they do not compare the strongest form of person-affecting principles with non-person-affecting principles. This means that an argument for the moral equivalence of non-person-affecting and person-affecting actions using the weaker form of person-affecting cases would be crucially incomplete. For example, suppose we compare (1) a case in which someone does something that affects her fetus in a way that results in her child having a 140 rather than a 160 IQ (e.g., she smokes during pregnancy) with (2) a case in which someone does something that creates a 140 IQ child rather than a different 160 IQ child (e.g., she smokes prior to pregnancy). If these cases were morally alike, this would not show that the non-person-affecting case is like (3) a case in which someone does something that affects her child so that his 160 IQ is reduced to 140 (e.g., she smokes in his presence).

We can further see the importance of entitlements in the treatment of future generations by considering the much-discussed question of whether we may "discount" their interests—that is, the question of whether goods and bads that are certain to occur to future generations should be counted for less simply because those goods and bads will occur in the distant future. Some (such as Kenneth Arrow) claim that discounting is a way to express the fact that it is morally permissible for agents to give greater weight to their own interests (e.g., present people) than to the interests of others (e.g., future people), without denying that these interests are equally important from an impartial point of view. When agents do this, it is said that they act on a morally sanctioned "agent-centered prerogative."[63]

A problem with applying the idea of an agent-centered prerogative to our treatment of future generations is that such a prerogative, in general, only seems correctly to apply when agents are deciding how much to do to benefit others by way of positive assistance. It does not correctly apply when agents must impose costs on themselves rather than do what will cause harm to others.[64] For example, I may not be morally required to forgo a big personal gain to help someone else, but I can be morally required to forgo a big personal gain if the means to it will harm others. And in the cases I have been discussing relating to future people, we would be doing things that harm future people, not merely things that do not aid them. Hence, the argument from the agent-centered prerogative for discounting future people's interests is weakened, and it does not show that we need not make large sacrifices rather than set back those people's interests.

However, we are not always morally required to forgo great gains rather than make others worse off. It is only if we would make others worse off by causing them to lose what they are owed or entitled to keep that we must make sacrifices to avoid harming them. This is why I think that knowing what future generations are owed by us, and entitled to keep once they have it, may be crucial to deciding whether and when we may discount the interests of future generations relative to our own as a way of exercising an agent-centered prerogative.

Indeed, the role of such considerations can help us criticize a thought experiment that has been used to argue *against* the policy of discounting the interests of future generations just because they are based in the future. Richard Revesz asks us to imagine the following hypothetical case:[65] There are 100 units of utility to be distributed in a society that will contain A, who will live for fifty years and then be replaced by B, who will live for the subsequent fifty years. How should the utility be distributed? Should A get it all merely because he comes first temporally? Revesz intuitively thinks that an equal division is fair; holding (or investing) 50 units for B until he arrives is what we ought to do. Revesz thinks that this shows that we should not discount the interests of future generations. However, I think that an egalitarian judgment in Revesz's case is compatible with discounting as an expression of the agent-centered prerogative. I think that our egalitarian judgment in his case is due to the fact that the utility to be divided is just there like manna from heaven. Neither we the distributors nor A or B have done anything to produce it. If B is owed (and will be entitled to keep) his equal share on these grounds, we should not do anything to deprive him of it, and we should even bear necessary costs to avoid depriving him of it. But suppose that either through luck or investment, A's equal share grows while B's stays constant. If A is permitted to consume the extra utility without seeing to it that B will have as much as he has, he is being permitted in a way to discount B's interests relative to his own. This seems permissible even if B is entitled to his 50 units. Hence, I believe that the fact that we must respect what is owed to someone and what he is entitled to keep once he has it is consistent with discounting the interests of future generations as an expression of a personal prerogative, at least with respect to things they are not owed or not yet entitled to keep.

V. Conclusion

In part II of this chapter, I argued that even those entities that, in their own right and for their own sake, give us reason not to destroy them (and to help them) are sometimes substitutable in subordinating ways for the good of other entities. In so arguing, I considered the idea of being valuable as an end in virtue of intrinsic and extrinsic properties. I also concluded that entities that have claims to things and against others are especially nonsubstitutable, but that this does not exclude some forms of substitution. In part III, I argued that reproductive cloning poses no threat to the nonsubstitutability, such as it is, of persons (and in this sense, to the dignity of persons). I also considered the relation between cloning and (what I called) holistic identity, and between the latter and genetic identity. In part IV, I tried to distinguish cases where identity over time and person-affecting acts have special moral significance from cases where they do not have as great moral significance. I tried to apply my results to cases involving unfertilized eggs, embryos, and future generations, and to the Non-Identity Problem.

NOTES

1. This chapter is a composite of my "Moral Status and Personal Identity: Clones, Embryos, and Future Generations," *Social Philosophy & Policy* 22(2) (2005): 283–307; "Cloning and Harm to Offspring," *New York University Journal of Legislation and Public Policy* 4(1) (2000); "Genes, Justice, and Obligations to Future People," *Social Philosophy and Policy* 19(2) (July 2002); chapter 7 of *Intricate Ethics* (New York: Oxford University Press, 2007); and "Affecting Definite Future People," *APA Newsletter* 9(2) (Spring 2010).

2. The moral importance of different people being harmed than will benefit is discussed in contexts where there is no special concern had by the person harmed for the other person who will benefit. I shall accept this assumption, unless otherwise noted.

3. See John Rawls, *A Theory of Justice* (Cambridge, MA: Harvard University Press, 1971), p. 29.

4. This section also appears as most of chapter 7 of my *Intricate Ethics*.

5. Seana Shiffrin seems to have a different view, as presented in her "Wrongful Life, Procreative Responsibility, and the Significance of Harm," *Legal Theory* 5(2) (1999): 117–48. She is concerned to avoid unconsented harm to entities who are or will be capable of consent because she thinks greater benefits to them cannot by themselves compensate for lesser harms to them. (Only avoiding greater harms can justify unconsented-to lesser harm to such persons, she thinks.) Suppose we treat coming into existence to a very good human life like a benefit. Shiffrin thinks that even a good life has inescapable harms. Among these, she thinks, are the burdens of moral choice, pain, rights violations, and having to cope with eventual death. Hence, she concludes, even an average parent, in creating a life overall well worth living, is involved in tortious conduct and may owe compensation to his child.

I disagree with Shiffrin's analysis of ordinary creation as wronging and as calling for compensation. (See chapters 12 and 15 this volume for more discussion of this.) Here I am most concerned with her views in relation to status. First, it seems odd to treat as problems with being a person or as harms to a person some of the very things that give value to human life, such as moral choice. However, it is possible that some of the things that give value and meaningfulness to human life and contribute to the status of persons are not best thought of as benefits to the person (in the sense of improving his well-being). Hence, deciding whether creating a human person is right or wrong may require more than weighing what are goods and evils to the person created.

Second, I believe that Shiffrin's argument implies that we should reduce both benefits to, and the importance of, entities in order to avoid harming them. I believe her view implies that creating creatures incapable of moral choice, never in pain, and unaware of upsetting truths such as the prospect of death—for example, creating extremely happy, long-lived rabbits or retarded people who have no other problems—would be preferable to creating human persons as they are now. But I think this is the wrong conclusion. It would be wrong, and would have been wrong at the beginning of (a hypothetical) creation, to substitute such creatures for normal humanity. Suppose it would be wrong to eliminate difficulty in a life at the cost of either reducing the overriding benefits to the entity we create or reducing the importance of the entity we create. Then, arguably, one should not be liable for compensation for certain unavoidable difficulties if one produces the benefits and values that justify doing whatever produces those difficulties on balance. (I raised these issues in my "Baselines and Compensation," *San Diego Law Review* 40 (2004): 1367–86.)

I would now here add the following points I also raised in chapter 15 this volume: Notice that Shiffrin's argument deals with harms that can or will come to people we create as though they were harms we (the creators) cause them. This is suggested by an analogy that she uses. She imagines that a benefactor could drop gold cubes on a population, thus benefiting them. However, there is a risk that some people who get the cubes are also hurt by the cubes falling on them. Even though the injured people would still be overall benefited, she thinks it is wrong to cause them the harm and to risk the harm for the sake of the benefit. However, this case does not seem to be analogous to creating people who will face the sort of harms of life with which Shiffrin is concerned. This is because in creating children, Shiffrin is not imagining that parents directly cause the burden of moral choice, rights violations, pain, and having to cope with eventual death, in the way the person who drops gold cubes causes injury. Rather, Shiffrin is concerned that in creating, parents expose their children to harms that will arise through other events in their life. The appropriate analogy to this would be a case in which a benefactor providing you with gold exposes you to the risk of being robbed and the burden of having to decide how to spend your money. But, presumably it would not be wrong to provide someone with benefits simply because it exposes them to such events, if they will still be overall better off with the benefit than without it. In order to nevertheless claim that creating people is problematic, it seems that Shiffrin would have to show that creating is not to be analogized to benefiting but she does not do this. (I consider these issues in more detail in chapter 15 this volume.)

6. See her "Two Distinctions in Goodness," *Philosophical Review* 2(481) (April 1983): 169–95.

7. So this is not the stronger sense of end-in-itself mentioned in part I, chapters 4 and 5 this volume.

8. Except, perhaps, relations between its parts.

9. See his *Life's Dominion: An Argument about Abortion, Euthanasia, and Individual Freedom* (New York: Knopf, 1993) and my discussion of Dworkin's view in part I, chapter 3 this volume.

10. I also discussed this possibility in part II, chapter 9 this volume.

11. I say "have had" in order to deal with the following sort of case: Suppose someone with the capacity for consciousness goes into a coma and also loses the capacity for future consciousness. Suppose further that somehow we could bring back this capacity in such a way that the *same person* would be conscious in the future. It would then be for the sake of

the person who originally had the capacity for consciousness that we would bring back the capacity and its exercise. By contrast, if an entity had always lacked the capacity for consciousness, it could not be for the entity's sake that we would bring about its capacity for consciousness. See part II, chapter 15, this volume, and part I, chapters 1 and 2, this volume, for some discussion of the sense in which it could be bad to cease to exist.

12. For more on this see part II, chapter 9, this volume, especially note 21.

13. Perhaps this fact is overdetermined. First, the table is not the sort of entity that can be benefited by continuing to exist. Second, it is not benefited by becoming something radically different from what it is now (for an entity is only benefited by future existence if *it* is either what will exist or is closely connected to what will exist). These two factors may also be true of embryos. But there could be entities of whom the first factor is not true, while the second factor is true. Some hold that an embryo *can* be harmed (or at least have something bad happen to it) by not developing into a person, and it could get something out of continuing to exist though it lacks sentience and consciousness. But some supporters of this view also claim that the harm or bad to the embryo has no moral significance because the harm or bad occurs to an entity that lacks moral status. That is, its characteristics give us no reason, in its own right and for its own sake, to prevent harm or bad happening to it. But suppose that an embryo will develop into a mildly retarded person. Will it be harmed or have something bad happen to it if it is prevented from developing into such a person who has a life worth living, in the way that a person would be harmed or have something bad happen to him if he were killed rather than allowed to live on as a mildly retarded person?

14. The discussion in the next two paragraphs derives from my "Using Human Embryos for Biomedical Research," *Boston Review* 27 (October/November 2002), which is the basis for chapter 9 this volume.

15. Though not all entities whose lives we could save (or not destroy) for their own sake are things it would be wrong not to save or to destroy (for example, dangerous dogs).

16. An exception may exist if there are duties to oneself, for one cannot have rights against oneself.

17. In giving his theory of moral wrongness, Thomas Scanlon emphasizes what we owe to others. See his *What We Owe to Each Other* (Cambridge, MA: Harvard University Press, 1999). I have raised some concerns about using the idea of "owing to others" as the basis of an account of what it is for something to be wrong. I suggested that "owing to others" may instead be the basis of an account of "wronging others." I also suggested that Scanlon's theory could be more closely connected to the idea of others having a right. For these views, see my discussion of Scanlon's book, "Owing, Justifying, and Rejecting," *Mind* 111(442) (April 2002), reprinted in my *Intricate Ethics*.

18. There are admittedly alternative views on these matters.

19. However, it could be that the wrong to him is not significant, and this is why he should not resist, given what is at stake.

20. Similarly, if torture of an innocent person were ever justifiable, then this would not mean that the victim would not be within his rights to resist the torture. Permissible resistance is not always a mark of our wronging someone, however. For example, in a boxing match, it is permissible for me to try to knock out my opponent and it is permissible for him to resist me. But I would not wrong him if I knocked him out, because it is the authorized (and, let us assume, morally permissible) point of the activity for each of us to try to do this to the other and to try to resist its being done to us.

21. Notice that basing rights on this relation to a *type* is not the same as basing rights on a relation to particular individuals, such as parents who love the retarded child.

22. As noted above (note 11), this could be both because it is not now the sort of being for whom nonexistence is bad relative to continuing existence and because what would come about from it if its life does not end is radically different from what it is now. It was also noted that others say that the embryo loss is bad for it but, given what it is now, this has no moral significance.

23. For further discussion of this issue, see later in this chapter and chapter 15 this volume.

24. I shall deal only with persons in "nonsplitting" cases. In cases where a person splits, survival can occur seemingly without continuity of personal identity. See Derek Parfit, *Reasons and Persons* (Oxford: Oxford University Press, 1984).

25. Under "goods," I include both benefits and the avoidance of harm.

26. Philippa Foot made this point in her "Euthanasia," *Philosophy & Public Affairs* 6 (Spring 1977).

27. Derek Parfit distinguished between focusing on aggregating small benefits across people and focusing on how badly off these people would otherwise be without the benefit in his *Rediscovering Reasons* (an unpublished version of his *On What Matters* [Oxford: Oxford University Press, 2011]).

28. These dimensions measure three different things, as the following example shows: A could stand to lose a million dollars and B half a million. If we help A, we could prevent $100,000 of his loss; if we help B, we could prevent $200,000 of his loss. So A's loss would be greater than B's, but B's gain would be greater (absolutely and percentage wise) than A's. A is a billionaire and B only has his half a million, so the fact that A would suffer the greater loss and recover a smaller part of his loss if aided does not show that he would be worse off than B whether aided or not.

29. In the published essay which is the basis of this chapter, I did not consider fine points that make it permissible to take something to which someone has a claim if we do it in one way (e.g., redirecting a threat to him) but not if we do it in another way (as in Transplant).

30. Kamm, *Intricate Ethics*.

31. And this is not because I would otherwise be intending the violation by another's arm, for my reason for not interfering need not be my intending the act. For example, I may be a very busy person, and making some effort so that transgression does not occur is an imposition I would like to avoid. Yet, I think, I have a reason to make the effort.

32. I would now add: This is consistent with the separateness of agents sometimes playing a moral role. For example, suppose a villain hurls a bomb at me and the only way to save myself is to redirect the bomb to an area where it will kill many people. Arguably, saving myself would be impermissible. But suppose I could redirect the bomb back to the villain. This would be permissible. Furthermore, doing this could still be permissible even if I foresaw that the villain—a separate intervening agent—would then impermissibly redirect the bomb from himself to the same area where it would kill many people.

33. The argument for this is that even an embryo with the potential to be a person does not have the moral status of a person. Its value as an end (in virtue of its extrinsic properties) may be greater than a monkey embryo; nevertheless, it may not have the value of a monkey. Hence, if for some reason it was good to produce monkeys but not necessary to

produce another person, and the only way to produce monkeys was to sacrifice a human embryo, I think the sacrifice of the embryo could be permissible.

34. Some material in this section is drawn from my essay "Cloning and Harm to Offspring."

35. But this is not always the case, since there are interesting cases in which origins do matter to the value of an entity. For example, that a set of marks on paper is an expression of the artist's view of nature, rather than produced by the random acts of a monkey, can give it value. See Arthur Danto's *The Transfiguration of the Commonplace: A Philosophy of Art* (Cambridge, MA: Harvard University Press, 1981), for more on this.

36. I have criticized Ronald Dworkin for inordinately emphasizing origins in his account of value. See F. M. Kamm, "Abortion and the Value of Life: A Discussion of *Life's Dominion*," *Columbia Law Review* 95 (1995): 160, 164–65 (reviewing Ronald Dworkin, *Life's Dominion: An Argument about Abortion, Euthanasia, and Individual Freedom*) and chapter 11 this volume.

37. See Lee M. Silver, comments at the *New York University Journal of Legislation and Public Policy* symposium "Legislating Morality: The Debate over Human Cloning," November 19, 1999, transcript on file with the *New York University Journal of Legislation and Public Policy*. One's genotype is one's genetic material. One's phenotype is one's characteristics due to both genotype and environmental factors.

38. I owe this point to David Copp. He reminded me that a very altruistic person could be indifferent between his own survival and the survival of another. Also, someone who held an inaccurate metaphysics might not recognize the difference between himself and another and, in that sense, think he was replaceable.

39. Unlike cloning, it is possible that brain splitting leads to two individuals, neither of whom is numerically identical to the person prior to splitting, but each of whom is genotypically and phenotypically identical to her. Our response to the prospect of the two people (or to one who remains after the death of the other) could reasonably be different from our response to a clone as the clone does not actually have half the brain of the person cloned.

40. In this novel, Mr. G, a clerk, is rejected by all who formerly befriended him. It seems that either he has done something extremely objectionable to offend everyone or he is not recognized by those whom he visits. As he wanders along the streets, trying to decide why he is being so badly treated, he encounters a man who looks very like himself and, in fact, calls himself by the same name and was born in the same village. Mr. G welcomes the new Mr. G into his life, sharing everything, including a position at his workplace. The newcomer begins to act outrageously, with the consequences being assigned to the first Mr. G. Life becomes unbearable for the first Mr. G and eventually he is tricked into entering a carriage bound for an insane asylum.

41. This leaves it open that he could care more about his clone than about himself.

42. See Harold W. Noonan, *Personal Identity* (London: Routledge, 1989), pp. 2–3; and Sydney Shoemaker and Richard Swinburne, *Personal Identity* (Oxford: Blackwell, 1984), pp. 4–5.

43. See Thomas Nagel, "Death," in Nagel, *Mortal Questions* (Cambridge: Cambridge University Press, 1979), p. 8.

44. I am aware that the underlying drive to have one's genes pass on may only give rise to a conscious *desire to reproduce*, not a conscious desire to pass on one's genes. One could have the first desire before one knows anything about genes. Once one is genetically literate,

however, a new desire to pass on one's genes may arise. John Robertson believes that many people have a very strong desire to have genetically connected offspring and also a desire to rear these offspring and to have a continuing connection to them. See John A. Robertson, *Liberty, Identity, and Human Cloning, Texas Law Review* 70 (1998): 1371–417; and John A. Robertson, *Two Models of Human Cloning, Hofstra Law Review* 27 (1999): 609–33. Robertson believes that so long as a potential parent is capable of having a genetic connection to her normal offspring through sexual reproduction, her reproductive rights do not entail producing a cloned child that assures a stronger genetic similarity. See Robertson, *Two Models of Human Cloning,* supra note 23 at p. 1403 (suggesting that fertile couples might nevertheless resort to cloning to avoid passing on to their progeny genetic defects or disease). This is an argument that challenges the belief that an assumed strong desire for biological connection justifies a right to move from sexual reproduction to nonsexual reproduction. I am not sure it is correct. Consider this hypothetical: Suppose that it actually takes four people to produce offspring; not couples but quadruples are needed. That means that if you have a child genetically related to you, only 25 percent of the genetic material comes from you. Indeed, we can imagine that ten people are needed to produce a child—a *ménage à dix.* Then only 10 percent of the genetic material comes from you. Could we understand individuals in these worlds seeking to clone, assuming there is a strong desire for genetic connection? They already have some genetic connection, so Robertson should say, "No, they have no reason to seek more." But suppose these people heard the latest news out of labs in their world: the invention of *two-person* offspring. That is, only two people would be needed for sexual reproduction. (This is sexual reproduction as we know it.) Would they have reason, based on the desire for more genetic impact, to introduce this two-person, rather than ten-person, sexual reproduction? If there is a sufficient justification to warrant offspring with a somewhat greater genetic connection, there might be a similar reason for introducing cloning in which there is 100 percent genetic connection. These hypothetical cases show that, given the assumption about the desire for genetic connection, it might not be unreasonable to prefer more genetic connection to less (contrary to Robertson). It is, of course, possible that the ideal number for reproduction is the number of persons who are emotionally involved with each other. Then the desire is for producing a genetically related fusion of emotionally bonded individuals, not just having a strong genetic connection. Producing such a "chimera" of different people could even be preferred to emotionally bonded people having a biological role in helping to produce the clones of each.

45. For purely practical purposes, such as organ transplants, it would be preferable to have a clone, though this would also raise pressures on individuals to donate organs.

46. See Robert Nozick, *Philosophical Explanations* (Cambridge, MA: Harvard University Press, 1981), 34–35. Having a successor is different from merely having offspring in ordinary reproduction. For example, the latter do not usually begin life just as the parent is leaving it and do not bear the appropriate causal relation to their antecedent to be a successor. And offspring fuse genetic material (and perhaps phenotypic properties) of different people.

47. Even if we put aside concerns that the later clone will think this type of life had already been lived.

48. Even in cases that do not involve splitting sufficient for survival of the original entity.

49. See F. M. Kamm, *Creation and Abortion* (New York: Oxford University Press, 1992); Kamm, "Cloning and Harm to Offspring," pp. 65–76; and Kamm, "Genes, Justice, and Obligations to Future People," pp. 360–88, and chapter 15 this volume.

50. Such an argument is made in Allen Buchanan, Dan W. Brock, Norman Daniels, and Daniel Wikler, *From Chance to Choice: Genetics and Justice* (Cambridge: Cambridge University Press, 2000). I also discuss it in "Genes, Justice, and Obligations to Future People" and in chapter 15 this volume.

51. Elizabeth Harman, "Creation Ethics: The Moral Status of Early Fetuses and the Ethics of Abortion," *Philosophy & Public Affairs* 28(4) (1999), p. 315.

52. Harman, "Creation Ethics," p. 311.

53. Harman, "Creation Ethics," p. 312 note 3.

54. I first discussed this case in my book *Creation and Abortion* (New York: Oxford University Press, 1992). It is discussed in more detail in chapter 15 this volume.

55. For discussion of this issue, see my *Creation and Abortion* and chapter 12 this volume.

56. I first presented this argument in *Creation and Abortion* and also discuss it in chapter 15 this volume.

57. This case was first discussed by me in "Affecting Definite Future People."

58. I owe this case to Arthur Applbaum.

59. These points were originally made in my "Genes, Justice, and Obligations to Future People." They were omitted from chapter 15 this volume, based on that article, to avoid repetition with this current, longer discussion.

60. This case is imaginary since many things we do could change the identities of the people who will actually exist in one hundred years. Derek Parfit first noted this. See *Reasons and Persons*, pp. 361–64.

61. It might be said that if we act now so as to worsen the environment in a delayed manner, the future persons could not ever be in possession of *the prospects* for a better environment. But what I have in mind are two different causal routes: one route leads to the prospects and the other would lead to their being undone, and the event of their being undone would occur during the lifetimes of the future persons.

62. See Parfit, *Reasons and Persons*.

63. See Kenneth Arrow, "Intergenerational Equity and the Rate of Discount in Long-Term Social Investment," in *Contemporary Economic Issues: Economic Behavior and Design*, vol. 4, ed. M. Sertel (New York: Basingstoke, and Macmillan and St. Martins, 1999), pp. 89–102. Arrow uses the notion of the prerogative, introduced in Samuel Scheffler's, *The Rejection of Consequentialism* (Oxford: Clarendon Press, 1982).

64. Scheffler's views on the agent-centered prerogative have been criticized on the ground that he incorrectly applied it to both harming and not assisting. See Shelly Kagan, "Does Consequentialism Demand Too Much?" *Philosophy & Public Affairs* 13(3) (1984): 239–54, and my "Supererogation and Obligation," *Journal of Philosophy* 82(3) (1985): 118–38. The criticism is related to the issue of whether there is a moral distinction between harming and not aiding. For more on this issue, see F. M. Kamm, *Morality Mortality*, Vol. 2 (New York: Oxford University Press, 1996).

65. See Richard Revesz, "Environmental Regulation, Cost-Benefit Analysis, and the Discounting of Human Lives," *Columbia Law Review* 99(4) (1999): 941–1017.

17

What Is and Is Not Wrong with Enhancement?

EVALUATING SANDEL'S VIEWS

Should we enhance human performance?[1] There are at least two types of enhancement. In the first, we enhance natural qualities to make more people be above the current norm in ways that many people are already without intervention. For example, we might increase intelligence so that many more people who would otherwise be only moderately intelligent function as well as those few who are geniuses. In the second type of enhancement, we introduce improvements that no human being has yet evidenced—for example, living to be two hundred years old and healthy. The question of whether we should engage in either type of enhancement has arisen recently within the context of human genetics. Here, one generation would probably modify the next. However, enhancement can also occur by way of drugs or intensive training and be done by a person to himself or to another.

Michael Sandel has recently argued that there is a moral problem with both types of enhancement regardless of the way in which they would be brought about, even if there were agreement (which there often is not) that the changes would be improvements, that they would be safe, and that they would be fairly distributed among socioeconomic groups (Sandel 2004). Sandel's discussion is worth significant attention both because he was a member of the President's Council on Bioethics and because his discussion expresses some prominent concerns in a way that is compact and readily available to the general public. In this chapter, I shall present what seem to me to be the important components of Sandel's argument and then evaluate it.

In part I, I briefly describe some of his arguments. In part II, I consider whether, as Sandel claims, the desire for mastery motivates enhancement and whether such a desire could be grounds for its impermissibility. Part III considers how Sandel draws the distinction between treatment and enhancement, and the relation to nature that he thinks each expresses. Part IV examines Sandel's views about parent/child relations and also how enhancement would affect distributive justice and the duty to aid. In conclusion, I briefly offer an alternative suggestion as to why enhancement may be troubling and consider what we could safely enhance.

I. Sandel's Views

Sandel thinks that the deepest objection to enhancement is the desire for mastery that it expresses. He focuses especially (but not exclusively) on the attempt of parents to enhance their children, whether by genetic manipulation, drugs, or extensive training. He says:

> [T]he deepest moral objection to enhancement lies less in the perfection it seeks than the human disposition it expresses and promotes. The problem is not that parents usurp the autonomy of a child they design. The problem is in the hubris of the designing parents, in their drive to master the mystery of birth . . . it would disfigure the relation between parent and child, and deprive the parent of the humility and enlarged human sympathies that an openness to the unbidden can cultivate. (Sandel 2004, 57)

And he thinks: "the promise of mastery is flawed. It threatens to banish our appreciation of life as a gift, and to leave us with nothing to affirm or behold outside our own will" (Sandel 2004, 62). However, he believes this objection is consistent with the permissibility and even the obligation to treat illnesses by genetic modification, drugs, or training. He is, therefore, arguing for a moral distinction between treatment and enhancement. He says: "Medical intervention to cure or prevent illness or restore the injured to health does not desecrate nature but honors it." (Sandel 2004, 57). He also thinks parents must "shape and direct the development of their children" but he thinks there must be an equilibrium between "accepting love" and "transforming love."

Among the bad effects of mastery, he identifies the increasing responsibility that we must bear for the presence or absence of characteristics in ourselves and others and the effects this may have on human solidarity. The first point is concerned with the fact that we will no longer be able to say that lacking a perfection is a matter of luck, something outside our control. We might be blamed for not improving ourselves or others. The second point is (supposedly) related to this. Sandel believes that the more our characteristics are a matter of chance rather than choice, "the more reason we have to share our fate with others" (Sandel 2004, 60). He goes on:

> Consider insurance. Since people do not know whether or when various ills will befall them, they pool their risk . . . insurance markets mimic solidarity only insofar as people do not know or control their own risk factors. . . . Why, after all, do the successful owe anything to the least-advantaged members of society? The best answer to this leans heavily on the idea of giftedness. . . . A lively sense . . . that none of us is wholly responsible for his or her success makes us willing to share the fruits of our talents with the less successful. (Sandel 2004, 60)

II. Desire for Mastery

A

Let us first clarify the nature of Sandel's objection to enhancement based on the desire for mastery over life processes. It implies that if (both types of) enhancements were occurring quite naturally, without our intervention, the "desire for mastery" objection to enhancement would not be pertinent. Indeed, interfering with the natural enhancing changes would itself require mastery over life processes, and so Sandel's objection might pertain to this. It is also important to keep in mind several distinctions. Actual mastery is different from the desire for it. We could achieve and exercise mastery over nature as a side effect of doing other things, without desiring it. This might be more acceptable to Sandel, but it might still raise the issue about responsibility and solidarity. For if we become able to control our natures despite never having wanted mastery and power, the question of how to deal with those who do not exercise the power well will arise.

Suppose we did desire mastery, however. We could desire it as a means to some other end (e.g., achieving such good aims as health or virtue) or we could desire it as an end in itself. So long as we desire it as a means to other things considered good, it is clearly wrong for Sandel to conclude that desire for mastery will "leave us with nothing to affirm or behold outside our own will" (Sandel 2004, 62). Even if mastery were desired as an end in itself, this need not mean that it is our only end, and so we could still continue to affirm other good aims (such as virtue, health, etc.) as ends outside our own will in the sense that their value is independent of what we will.[2] I shall henceforth assume that if we desire mastery, it is as a means to good ends, as this seems most reasonable.

Such a desire for mastery is not inconsistent with an openness to the unbidden that Sandel emphasizes (Sandel 2004, 56), if the unbidden means just "those things that come without our deliberately calling for or causing them."[3] For if many good things were to come without our deliberately intervening to bring them about, presumably we would be happy to have them and not regret that they came about without our deliberately bringing them about. Such a form of openness to the unbidden does not, however, necessarily imply a willingness to accept whatever comes even if it is bad when one could change it.[4] Sometimes people are also unwilling to accept things that merely differ from their preferences or that are not as good as they might be, though the things are not necessarily bad. One or all of these forms of being closed to the unbidden may be what Sandel is concerned with, as he speaks of enlarged human sympathies resulting from an openness to the unbidden.

So far, I have been distinguishing various attitudes and states of mind that might be involved in a desire for mastery. Suppose some form of the desire for mastery and nonopenness to the unbidden were bad. The further question is whether there is any relation between having even a bad desire and the impermissibility of enhancing. As noted above, even Sandel supports the efforts to find certain treatments for illnesses. But seeking treatments for illnesses by manipulating the genome typically involves desiring mastery as a means, not being open to all things unbidden, and attempting to master the mystery of birth. Hence, Sandel may think that while there is something bad per se about desiring mastery even as a means, not being open to the unbidden, and attempting to master the mystery of birth, these bads can be outweighed by the good of curing diseases (if not by the pursuit of enhancements). Alternatively, he may believe that when the unbidden is very horrible—not a gift, even in disguise—not being open to the unbidden is not bad at all. If he believes these things, the question then is why enhancements cannot outweigh or transform the negative value of seeking mastery and not being open to the unbidden in the same way that he thinks treatments outweigh or transform them.[5]

There is a further, deeper problem about the relation between having bad desires and dispositions and the impermissibility of conduct. For suppose that desiring mastery as one's sole end in life is bad. Suppose a scientist who works on finding a cure for congenital blindness is motivated only by such a bad desire for mastery. He seeks a cure but only as a means to achieving the goal of being a master over nature. Does this make his conduct impermissible? Presumably not. The good of treating diseases still justifies the work of the scientist, even when his ultimate aim is not that disease be treated but rather to achieve mastery. This is a case where there may be a duty to do the work. However, even when the act one would do would produce a good that it is not one's duty to produce, I think the act can be permissible independent of one's desires or disposition in doing it. So suppose several people could be saved only if you do an act that has a high probability of killing you. It is not typically your duty to do such an act, though it could be worthwhile to do it. If the only reason you do it is to make those who care about you worry, this alone will not make saving the people impermissible. More generally, it has been argued, the intentions and attitudes of an agent most often reflect on the agent's character or the meaning of his act but do not determine the permissibility of his act (Scanlon 2000; Thomson 1990).[6] People often do permissible acts for bad reasons, not for the sake of factors that justify the act.

If desires and dispositions do not generally affect the permissibility of acts, and if Sandel were right that "the deepest moral problem with enhancement" is "the human disposition it expresses," then the deepest moral problem might provide no ground at all for thinking that acts seeking enhancement are morally impermissible (Sandel 2004, 57). We would have to decide whether particular enhancements are permissible independently of the desires, attitudes, and dispositions of agents who act. Among the factors we might consider are the goods that would be brought about and the bad effects that might also occur. It is true that if these goods outweigh the bad effects, then it is possible for a rational agent to have as his ultimate aim the pursuit of the goods, rather than the (supposedly) bad aim of seeking mastery above all else. But still it is the evaluation of objective goods and bads, rather than the agent's actual aims, dispositions, or desires, that plays a role in accounting for the permissibility of producing the enhancement. If the only possible aim of a rational agent in seeking a particular change were to seek mastery as an end in itself, then presumably this would be an indication that no good effect achieved by the change would be able to justify the act and so the act might be impermissible for that reason.

Furthermore, we need not be restricted to a consequentialist weighing of goods and bads in accounting for the permissibility of an act of enhancement. Individual rights may be at stake and the causal role of bad effects (e.g., whether they are side effects or necessary means to producing good effects) could be morally relevant to the permissibility of an act, even if the agent's intention and disposition are not.

In connection with the effects of enhancing, there is a further point that Sandel makes, for he is concerned not only with the disposition that enhancement expresses but with "the human disposition it . . . promotes" (Sandel 2004, 57). Promoting the disposition to seek mastery could be an effect of seeking enhancements, and we have said that the effects of acts can be relevant to their permissibility even if the attitudes and aims of agents who perform the acts are usually not. Indeed, considering the disposition as an effect helps us understand that when Sandel says that "the deepest moral problem with enhancement is the human disposition it expresses" (Sandel 2004, 57), he may not so much be giving an explanation of the wrongness of acts of enhancement as simply focusing on the bad type of people we will be if we seek mastery.[7] But why would we be bad people if we have the disposition to seek mastery as a means, if this disposition always led to permissible acts, and, furthermore, the disposition always led us to act for the sake of the good effects that make the acts permissible because they make it permissible? (Such persons will be very different from the scientist described above who did not care about the good effect that justified his act [i.e., treating disease] per se but only about mastery.) Sandel's account implies that even people with such a disposition to mastery could be worse people in virtue of having the disposition. I do not believe this is true.

Perhaps even such a disposition, not in itself bad, could be bad to have if it leads us to focus on certain types of acts to the exclusion of other worthwhile activities. Consider an analogy. An artist is always seeking to improve her paintings. She never rests content with just appreciating her own and other people's great works. Hence, other people may have a better appreciation of great masters than she has and her worthwhile aim interferes with other worthwhile aims. However, often it is not possible to achieve all worthwhile aims; one has to choose among them. And it is not clear that her way of responding to value—by trying to create more of it—is inferior to an admittedly good alternative way of responding to value (i.e., appreciating valuable things that already exist). Furthermore, sometimes these two approaches to value may be combined to one degree or another. Similarly, the dispositions to enhance and to appreciate goods already present may be combined.

B

I have considered the relation between the permissibility of acts and the desires and dispositions related to mastery that produce them and that are produced by them. It might be suggested that acts themselves can have meaning as well as being the result of intentions and followed by consequences.[8] Perhaps some reason for an act's being permissible or impermissible is given by what it means or expresses because we should not "say" certain things by our acts. Sometimes, meaning can be due to the intention of the agent, but it has been argued by some that it can also be due to context and to the properties of the act itself. If the meaning of an act can be affected by an agent's intention, and meaning is relevant to permissibility, this still does not show that intention per se is relevant to permissibility, but only that to which the intention gives rise (i.e., the meaning) is relevant to permissibility. Consider a situation in which, it has been said, context and not intention determines meaning. Suppose that in the United States, selecting a male rather than a female child to balance a female child one already has means no more than that one is balancing genders. That is, it has been said, with respect to the act's meaning, the context would "drown out" an agent's intention if the parent is actually choosing to have a male child in order to avoid having what he believes is another inferior female in his family. Is his intention, which we shall suppose no one will ever know of, a reason for his act being impermissible? Those who are concerned with an act's meaning would have no reason to think it is.

Now, suppose that, in a case where intention determines an act's meaning, no one will understand what an act means because no one knows the intention. It is not clear that the act's actual meaning, as opposed to people's interpretation of its meaning, can be a reason for its impermissibility. Where a bad intention determines meaning and people will find out about the intention, this still does not imply that there is good enough reason not to do the act. For example, suppose parents want good educations for their children, but only as a means to their own social climbing. When the children understand this, they will get the message that their parents see them as mere tools. But, of course, despite their parents' beliefs, they are not mere tools, and whatever the parents' intentions, the parents do have a duty to give their children a good education. If it is clear that the children will understand their parents' view of them if and only if the parents give them the education, and this understanding will be psychologically very harmful to them, then this must still be weighed against the good of their being educated.

The specific immoral meaning that some think enhancement has, and the immoral message some think it sends, is that the unenhanced have less intrinsic worth than others, where presumably this implies that they do not have equal moral status just in virtue of being persons. (Call this Message 1. Notice that concern about this message could also apply to nongenetic methods of enhancement, such as education and exercise.) Message 1 is to be distinguished from a message that says that some properties are not as good for people to have as other properties. (Call this

Message 2.) Presumably, expressing Message 2 is not immoral if it is true. This is because we can show our concern for someone of equal intrinsic worth by trying to give him properties that it will be better for him to have.

I think that it is highly unlikely that enhancement could carry the immoral Message 1. This is because enhancement is to be done to individuals who are already within the normal range of properties typical of the species. Such people are far less likely to be thought to lack the equal moral status that persons have just in virtue of being persons.[9] Indeed, those people who would be improved by being given treatments (rather than enhancements) are more likely to be in danger of being mistakenly thought to lack such equal moral status, for they fall below the norm. Yet this is, presumably, not a strong reason against treating them. We should cure blindness by drugs or surgery or genetic means because sightedness is good for persons, and because blind persons as much as any persons are worthy of care.

C

I have been focusing on the desires, intentions, and actions of *individuals* and whether their acts of enhancement could be made impermissible by their desires, intentions, dispositions, and the meanings of their acts. One reason why I have discussed the desires, intentions, and dispositions of individuals is that Sandel seems to be concerned with why individual parents might seek enhancement of their offspring. Furthermore, one way to conceive of the dispositions and aims of a society is as the sum of the dispositions and aims of the majority of people in it or of its typical members.[10] It is possible, however, that one would not be concerned if some individuals did certain types of acts from certain dispositions unless there were collective action, in the sense that a good part of the society were acting in this way, perhaps in unison. Indeed, Sandel has said that he is really concerned with social practices, not individual acts, and that he thinks that these are constituted, in part, by dispositions as well as acts.[11] For example, we now have a valuable social practice of parenthood which is constituted, in part, by a disposition to love whatever child comes unbidden and not to predetermine its properties. We now have valuable competitive sports practices which are constituted, in part, by excellence in the skillful exercise of natural gifts. If we pursue enhancements, Sandel thinks, we will corrupt and even eliminate these valuable practices.

Consider how this might happen. If the current practice of parenthood is conceived of as constituted (in part) by an openness to the unbidden in a sense that is in conflict with predetermining a child's properties,[12] then the desire to seek mastery as a means to goods will indeed eliminate the current practice. The question, however, is whether a new practice—which might include the disposition to seek mastery in order to improve children for the sake of the children themselves— would be an even more valuable social practice than the older one. One measure would be its effects on children's lives, parent-child relations, and so on. (This is an issue I consider in part IV, section A, below.) I have already argued that having the disposition to seek mastery as a means to some good need not be a bad characteristic of persons in itself. Of course, if the means chosen to the good effect, even if prompted by a good disposition, were bad, there would still be a problem. For example, Sandel mentions the possibility that the new practice might involve selecting mates on the basis of their potential for producing children of certain types. But the problem with doing this lies in the inappropriate way it treats potential mates, for relations between adults who seek to be mates should, presumably, be based primarily on love between them, as a response to their noninstrumental personal characteristics. So impermissible behavior between adults could be involved if this particular means to achieve mastery were chosen and the new practice of parenthood should not use it. But that does not mean that other ways of giving children good properties could not be part of the new practice.

In the case of sports, one of Sandel's concerns is that when athletes enhance their physical strength as a way to win competitions, we have a practice that is no longer about exercising skill but about whose body mass can fell an opponent. If this were so, I would say that the problem is that a good aspect of our current practice is not replaced by anything else of equal value in the new practice. But no one is arguing for "body enhancing changes" that have overall bad effects. Sometimes, Sandel claims that athletes' eating large quantities of muscle-building substances as a component of the new practice, while not in itself an impermissible act, is problematic because the focus on body mass eliminates a practice that relies on the use of valuable skills. However, sometimes he claims that in making their bodies massive, athletes are degrading themselves. If this were so, then, I would argue, the new practice would not only be less valuable but also involve acts with significant wrong-making features.

My conclusion is that whether we are concerned with individuals and individual acts or with social practices, we shall have to focus on whether outcomes are valuable and can help justify acts or practices, whether means are permissible or have wrong-making features, and whether a disposition to mastery as a means to goods is inconsistent with being good people. Emphasizing social practices merely because the identity conditions of a social practice (as a matter of definition) include effects, means, and dispositions will not alter the basic terms of our evaluative analysis from what they are when we consider individual acts and individual character.

III. Treatment versus Enhancement

As noted above, Sandel's view is that the desire for mastery, rather than letting nature "give" us whatever "gifts" it will,[13] is bad. However, the goods of treatment do justify seeking mastery. We may resist unbidden disease and disability. Why does treatment justify what enhancement cannot justify?

I suggested above that it may not be true that people's mastering nature, uncovering the secrets of life, and trying to improve what comes in life are bad in themselves. If they are not bad, then we do not have to show that avoiding great harm but not achieving great goods can outweigh the bad in order to permissibly engage in these activities. However, if mastering nature were bad, one would have to show not only that the goods of enhancement are not as important as the goods of treatment but that they are not good enough to outweigh or transform the bad aspects of mastery.

There are several possible routes to showing that the goods of enhancement are not as important as the goods of treatment. One is the idea of diminishing marginal utility, according to which the benefit someone gets out of a given improvement in his condition decreases the better off he is. Hence, we do more good if we help those who are worse off than if we help those who are already better off. A second route is the view that there is greater moral value in helping people the worse off they are in absolute terms, even if we produce a smaller benefit to them than we could to people better off. (This is the view behind the position known as giving priority to the worse off.) A possible third route is to distinguish qualitatively between what some call harmed states and merely not being as well off as one might be but not badly off in absolute terms (Shiffrin 1999). All these routes depend on its being true that those to be treated are worse off than those to be enhanced. However, this may not always be true. For example, some illnesses produce states that are less bad than, or equal to, being at the low end of a normal range for a certain physical property. Furthermore, none of these routes to comparing the ends of enhancement and treatment shows that enhancements are not in themselves great enough goods to justify mastery as a means, even if enhancements are not as important as treatment. They also do not rule out that providing enhancements might be endorsed as a means to achieving some treatments. That is, suppose it is only if we are much smarter than we currently are that we will find a cure for terrible illnesses quickly. Then the importance of finding treatments could be transmitted to the enhancement of intelligence. (Of course, not all means are permitted to even justified ends. So if mastering nature to produce enhancements were sufficiently intrinsically objectionable, it might not be permissible to use the only available means [i.e., enhancement] to acquire treatments.)

At one point, Sandel tries to draw the distinction between treatment and enhancement by claiming that "medical intervention to cure or prevent illness . . . does not desecrate nature but honors it. Healing sickness or injury does not override a child's natural capacities but permits them to flourish" (Sandel 2004, 57). The assumption behind the first sentence is that nature is sacred and should be honored. When Sandel claims that curing and preventing illness do not desecrate nature, he implies that enhancement is a problem because of the sort of relation we should have to nature, as if this could be a source of moral imperatives in addition to our relations to other persons. But should we believe this? Cancer cells, AIDS, and tornadoes are all parts of nature. Are they sacred and to be honored? The natural and the good are distinct conceptual categories and the two can diverge: the natural can fail to be good and the good can be nonnatural (art, dams, etc.).[14]

However, it is an important claim made by some that when there are goods in nature, they can indeed be sources of moral imperatives in addition to our relations to persons. By this they mean that independent of their effects on people, certain natural goods give us reasons to protect or promote them. For example, a great oak or the Grand Canyon may give us reasons to protect it even if no persons were favorably affected by this. Furthermore, recognizing their worth means not supplanting them with some things of inferior worth that may be good for people, such as parking lots.

How does this claim—call it the Independent Worth of Nature Claim—bear on not enhancing people? I do not think it serves as any support for the idea that there is a duty to nature not to engage in enhancement. First, it does not imply that, insofar as a "gift" in a person is a good of nature, what is a "gift" should be determined independently of its effect on people (i.e., independently of what is good for, or what is the good of, the person). (So, if a person were turning into a magnificent oak, this would not be a gift because it is not good for the person, and we should act to prevent this transformation.) Second, the Independent Worth of Nature Claim need not imply that we may not enhance, supplement, or even transform the goods of nature with genuine additional or superior goods.

Now consider the idea embodied in the second sentence of the Sandel quote, that healing honors nature by permitting natural capacities to flourish rather than overriding them. If enhancement involves the opposite, then we would be overriding people's natural capacities if we enhanced their immune system (by genetic means or immunization) so that they were able to resist illnesses that they could not naturally resist. Is doing this impermissible because it does not honor nature? Surely not. Suppose nature were sacred and to be honored. We would clearly be overriding its dictates by making people able to resist (by immunization) illnesses that they could not naturally resist. Is doing this impermissible because it does not honor nature? Surely not.

And indeed, Sandel has said[15] that such enhancement of natural functioning in order to combat illnesses is to be understood as part of treatment and is not the sort of enhancement he opposes. This may be because overriding these natural capacities leads to treatment (or prevention) that does not itself override other natural capacities but permits them to flourish.

The position expressed by this view might be illuminated by the diagram in figure 17.1, where "E" stands for enhancement and "T" for treatment (including prevention).

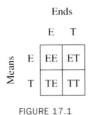

FIGURE 17.1

This figure brings to light a distinction that may be overlooked in most discussions of enhancement: enhancement can be used to refer to an end—enhancing end states; or to a means—enhancing in order to either treat or enhance as ends. In the immune enhancement, we would enhance people as a means to stopping illness that interferes with natural gifts (ET). But a way to treat Alzheimer's disease might also involve increasing general memory power enormously simply as a way to diminish the effects of eventual dementia. Here overriding natural capacities to treat or prevent an illness that interferes with natural capacities does not merely allow those natural capacities to flourish. It overrides by supplementing them. (This is because it does not enhance capacities other than the ones that we seek to protect from the disease.) So Sandel might see this not as a form of ET, but rather as EE. But it is a special form of EE: the alternative to it is not being treated for a disease rather than being in a normal state. Perhaps when EE is the only alternative to disease, Sandel would permit it. (He would presumably object to a more indirect route to stopping Alzheimer's disease, namely increasing the intelligence of scientists so that a cure could more easily be found.) He would object to EE when the alternative is a normal state and also possibly to TE when one treats an illness one would otherwise ignore just because treating it also enhances an end state (in a way that is not intermediate to further treatment).

Treatment, even ET, is commended by Sandel because it permits some natural capacities to flourish by eliminating one impediment to them, namely illness. Why would it not honor nature to interfere with other impediments? That is, might Sandel's view be better expressed as the view that we may permissibly override and not honor nature when we get rid of the things in nature that interfere with the other parts of nature that are its gifts (i.e., good things)? If this is so, then Sandel's position would not rule out dramatically lengthening the human life span and preventing the ageing process. This involves getting rid of things that are normal and not illnesses, but that do impede the exercise of natural gifts that we have had all our lives. Yet most people would consider this a radical enhancement. (And, indeed, life-lengthening seems in some respects like a form of EE [in figure 17.1].) So, Sandel's original objection to enhancement, that it interferes with gifts that nature has given someone rather than allowing them to flourish, is not always true. It is not true in some forms of ET and some forms of EE (such as life-lengthening). But sometimes his original objection is true of treatments, as in enhancing memory power to stop Alzheimer's.

For another example, suppose that a child's natural gifts are those of a Down's Syndrome child and we seek to supplement these and provide greater gifts than nature provided by changing the child's genome. This would change or add to natural capacities, not merely permit them to flourish. Yet, presumably, Sandel would want to classify this with allowable treatment rather than enhancement because it compensates for a genetic defect that caused the Syndrome.[16] This form of treatment, which involves changing and supplementing nature's gifts with new ones, rather than curing or preventing conditions that interfere with gifts already present, raises the more general question of why appreciation of nature's gifts requires limiting ourselves to them. We can appreciate what is given and yet supplement it with something new, even when we are not compensating for a defect.

It is worth contrasting Sandel's views on the treatment/enhancement distinction with those of Allan Buchanan, Dan Brock, Norman Daniels, and Daniel Wikler, as described in their *From Chance to Choice* (hereafter, *CC*).[17] They want to work with the idea of normal species functioning (NSF) (as opposed to enhanced functioning) as an objective baseline that forms an overlapping consensus for political justice purposes in order to decide what obligations the state has, as a matter of justice, to provide health assistance. They, unlike Sandel, do not think the treatment/enhancement distinction has any necessary connection with what it is morally permissible for individuals to do. For example, they say that the "natural baseline has no metaphysical importance: It is not that we must pay some special respect to what is natural . . . rather the natural baseline has become a focal point for convergence in our public conception of what we owe each other" (*CC*, p. 151, to avoid moral hazard, hijacking, etc.). Furthermore, Sandel is concerned with treatments (and enhancements) by drugs, education, therapy, genetics, and so on, but when he says that treatments remove interferences to natural capacities, he may make the mistake that the authors of *CC* say people make when they claim that nongenetic (e.g., environmental) influences do not change a person but only prevent or allow the flourishing of what he is naturally (e.g., what genes make him) (*CC*, p. 160). While on the surface Sandel's view seems to follow *CC*'s idea that treatment of illness eliminates interference with the exercise of one's capacities, Sandel identifies those capacities only with natural gifts rather than with what has also resulted from environmental influences. By contrast, *CC* notes that exercise, food, and exposure to stimulation all play a part in creating parts of one's NSF phenotype, which one thinks are important to who one really is and with whose expression illness might interfere. Given Sandel's focus on treatment as a way to stop interference with natural gifts, his view has the following problematic implication: Suppose neuronal connections that make language use possible only develop if there is environmental stimulation during a certain latency period in early childhood. Then if an illness threatens just these neuronal connections, it would not be interfering with a natural gift and so treatment would not merely allow nature's gifts to flourish. The position put forth in *CC* has no problem with classifying such an illness as interfering with NSF, and the elimination of the illness as treatment, given that they do not conceive of NSF as consisting only of nature's gifts.

There are three primary conclusions to this section so far. First, Sandel's attempt to draw a distinction between treatment and enhancement, based on allowing natural capacities to flourish versus overriding natural capacities, does not seem successful. Second, on one interpretation of how he draws the treatment/enhancement distinction, Sandel's objection to enhancement does not rule out maintaining natural gifts (that would otherwise wither) throughout a greatly extended human life span. Third, we would need much more argument to show that there is some duty owed to nature which we violate when we change natural capacities and that it is our relation to nature rather than to persons that should be a primary source of concern with enhancement.

Consider an alternative way to draw the treatment/enhancement distinction suggested by P. H. Schwartz (2005). We treat when we eliminate a dysfunction, not merely prevent anything that interferes with nature's gifts. Dysfunction is an interference with healthy human life, which involves the normal, proper functioning of the human being. The normal, proper functioning of a human being or its parts is the functioning that contributes to survival and reproduction to a degree that does not fall too far below the mean for individuals of the same age and gender. (Possibly, if we alter a genome to add to a Down's Syndrome child's gifts, we might be seen to compensate for the dysfunction that originally interfered with normal development.) Schwartz thinks that we should value healthy human life and that fixing dysfunction (i.e., treating the failure of a part to contribute to survival and reproduction to a degree that does not fall too far below the mean for individuals of the same age and gender) has "superior moral status" to modifying normal functioning (enhancing), because it alone has "a virtue of accepting the normal" and avoiding the implied rejection of normal human life (Schwartz 2005, 6).

Despite drawing the treatment/enhancement distinction in this way, and identifying treatment as morally superior in at least one way to enhancement, Schwartz thinks there is "no need to treat dysfunctions that are valued by their bearers (such as infertility in some)" and no rule against modifying people so as to produce valued dysfunctions (e.g., infertility by vasectomy). Hence, on his view, the way in which treatment is morally superior to enhancement—by accepting the normal—can be overridden by other ways in which not treating or even producing dysfunction can be morally superior to treatment (e.g., by providing people with things that they reasonably value).[18]

Let me raise the following concerns with Schwartz's analysis of treatment and enhancement.

(a) First, it draws the treatment/enhancement distinction by relativizing the normal to "the mean for one's age and gender." Hence, what would ordinarily be thought of as dysfunctions can be perfectly normal. For example, it is normal for brain cells to die as we age, heart muscle to atrophy, and joints to wear out. So, it turns out on Schwartz's account that common interventions to eliminate such conditions—for example, by providing drugs or doing surgery— is not treatment but rather enhancement. (Only dealing with abnormal dysfunctions would be treatment.) If these are enhancements, then undoing similar normal dysfunctions so that people have radically longer life spans with continuing capacities cannot be distinguished from what we already do by appeal to a treatment/enhancement distinction. (On Sandel's view, I argued earlier, radically longer life spans might turn out to be treatments because they stop impediments to normal gifts. On Schwartz's view, they turn out to be enhancements because they do not deal with abnormal dysfunctions. But neither author's analysis distinguishes such life-lengthening from what they already consider permissible.)

(b) Now consider Schwartz's value analysis. He begins by saying that we should value a life without dysfunction and that it is morally superior not to reject the normal, but he then concludes by saying that it is not unreasonable to sometimes value a life with dysfunction (such as infertility) over a life without it. This, of course, implies that it can be right to reject the normal (either in end state or in mechanism leading to an end state). It seems that this could be true because it could be more important for a life to be good in nonnormal ways than for it to be normal. Hence, as Schwartz recognizes, it remains open that an enhanced life will be a greater good than a normal one, just as a life with a dysfunction can be a greater good than one without it. Furthermore, suppose a very small additional good gotten through abnormality (either dysfunction or enhancement) overrides any merit in normality. This would show that the merit in normality is very weak.[19]

(c) Indeed, it is not clear that there is anything morally preferable about normality at all, or anything morally superior about preserving the normal rather than rejecting it. First, as noted in (a), according to Schwartz's analysis, some dysfunctions (e.g., brain cells not working) will be normal, and if we should value life without dysfunction, this means that sometimes we should not value the normal per se.

Second, recall that on Schwartz's analysis, normal means "functions so as to survive and reproduce at not too far from the mean for one's age and gender." Presumably, survival and reproduction are worth valuing only if there is survival and reproduction of what is good; survival and reproduction of what is bad may be normal but not in any way morally good. Let us assume that what survives and reproduces is good, and this supports the view that survival and reproduction are morally good. Why cannot superior-to-normal performance of these functions be better than normal function? For example, if it were normal for a species to just barely survive and reproduce, could the normal not have less value per se than the supernormal?

In order to see a general problem with using the normal as a basis for deciding when to alter characteristics, it helps to imagine what it would be right to do if, counterfactually, the normal for us were what is, in fact, abnormal. (I shall call this the Shifted Baseline Argument.) So Down's Syndrome is in fact abnormal for humans. But suppose it were normal for our species to have the intelligence of a Down's Syndrome person. Should we think that it would then be wrong for the abnormally intelligent members of our species (who had what is now normal intelligence) to alter the rest of us so that everyone had the sort of intelligence that is now considered normal? Presumably not, unless there were bad side effects of doing this. Those currently opposed to enhanced intelligence or enhanced memory point to the possible problems that might accompany these, such as not being able to forget and noticing too many defects in life. But suppose it were normal for our species to have the same intelligence as a Down's Syndrome person or a weaker memory than we now have. Would we think it wrong for us to be altered so that we had levels of intelligence and memory now considered normal for us, despite some drawbacks relative to the lower states (as those lower states may involve blissful ignorance and a constant pleasant disposition)? Presumably not.

The appeal to the moral value of the normal may just be a hidden way of supposing that there is a delicate balance between all our properties (and between our species and the rest of the world), and that things might go worse overall for people if they made a local improvement to the normal.

I conclude that we have so far not seen why treatment but not enhancement justifies mastery over nature.

IV. Parental and Social Relations

In this part, I shall examine Sandel's views on how enhancement may negatively affect our relations to persons, ourselves or others.

A. ONE'S CHILDREN

As noted above, Sandel paints with a broad brush in condemning enhancements due not only to genomic changes but also to drugs and training. However, he also realizes that much of ordinary good parenting consists of what might ordinarily be called enhancement. Hence, he says the crucial point is to balance accepting love and transformative love. (Perhaps Sandel would want to apply this idea to changes adults seek to make to themselves as well.) But he also seems to think of transformative love as concerned with helping natural gifts to flourish, framing and molding them so that they shine forth. (Similarly, in sport, he thinks that good running shoes help bring out a natural gift by comparison to drugs that would change a gift into something else. Treatment was also said to help natural gifts but only by removing impediments to them.)

Let us first deal with the issue of balance. For all Sandel says, it remains possible that many more enhancements than he considers appropriate are ones that satisfy the balance between accepting and transformative love, even if we expand the latter idea to include adding to natural gifts, for it is not clear what falls under "balancing." For example, suppose my child already has an IQ of 160. Might balancing the two types of love in her case imply that I may (if this will be good for her) increase her IQ another 10 but not 20 points, and that a parent whose child has an IQ of 100 should not change her child as much as to give her a 120 IQ, for this would err on the side of too much transformation?

An alternative to this view of balancing might be called Sufficientarianism. It could imply that there is no need at all to increase the first child's IQ and that in the second child's case much more transformation (in the sense of adding to natural gifts) than acceptance is appropriate—that is, the right balance—in order to reach a sufficient level. (Sufficientarians are not interested in perfection, though they want mastery as a means to getting sufficient goods.)

Let us now restrict ourselves to Sandel's sense of transformation—bringing out natural gifts. One problem, already discussed above, is that it implies that environmental influences only shape and bring forth naturally occurring properties, whereas, in fact, food, exercise, and cognitive stimulation actually produce and change biological properties. Now consider the ways in which natural gifts may be brought out. There may be an enormous range of latent natural capacities in human beings that would not be brought forth without much early intervention. (For example, there is our capacity to easily learn many more languages than we typically do.[20]) Trying to bring these capacities to fruition might involve much more transformation by environmental means than Sandel favors. Such fruition might also be possible only if certain triggering mechanisms were enhanced by biological means.

Furthermore, to the extent that Sandel does allow training and appliances to be used to bring out and shape gifts, nothing in his argument rules out using drugs or genetic manipulation that do exactly the same thing. So suppose that he would allow a certain amount of voice training to strengthen vocal chords. Would a drug or genetic manipulation that could strengthen vocal chords to the same degree also be permissible? If the argument Sandel gives does not alone rule out training, it alone will not rule out transformation by drugs or genetic means because a gift is transformed to the same degree by each method. If appliances such as running shoes are allowed, why not genetically transformed feet that function in the same way? Ordinarily, such genetic changes would be considered enhancements, even if they are only traits in addition to one's natural capacities that allow the other natural capacities to flourish. An argument different from Sandel's, based on the possible moral difference in using different means to transform capacities, would be necessary to rule out drug or genetic means but permit training. As we have noted, Sandel treats training, drugs, and genetic manipulation as on a par. This leaves his position open to endorsing many genetic enhancements (in addition to those that aim at treatment, as discussed in part III).

While Sandel rightly condemns excessive pressure to transform oneself and one's children in a competitive society, especially if the societal values are shallow, he does not condemn moderate training for worthwhile transformation.[21] Unless he emphasizes a difference in means used, he should then permit moderate, worthwhile genetic transformations that bring out natural gifts, even if not excessive ones driven by competitive pressures and/or governed by shallow values. (His argument against giving traits merely to provide one's child a competitive advantage, on the ground that when everyone has the traits no one has gained a competitive advantage, will also fail against traits that are good to have even if everyone gets them.[22] For example, better eyesight or higher intelligence can raise the absolute quality of each person's life even if there is no change in relative advantage.)

Now consider one way in which Sandel may be wrong not to distinguish different ways of either bringing out natural gifts or bringing about more radical enhancement by introducing major new capacities. Perhaps we should separate how we treat changes that are made before a child exists (what I shall call ex-ante changes) from those that are made once a child exists (what I shall call ex-post changes). The former are primarily genetic, while the latter will include drugs and training.

Love, it has been said, is for a particular. Consider love for an adult. Before we love someone, we may be interested in meeting a person who has various properties, such as kindness and intelligence. When we meet such a person, we may be interested in him or her rather than someone else because he or she has these properties. However, though it is through these properties that we may be led to love this particular person, it is the particular person whom we wind up loving, not his or her set of properties. For if another person appears with the same set of properties, that does not mean that we could easily substitute him or her for the person we already love. Even if the person we love loses some of the properties through which we were originally led to love him or her (e.g., his beauty), we would not necessarily stop loving the particular person that we love (Nozick 1977).

It seems then that when we love a particular person, this involves much of what Sandel calls accepting love. If we do seek transformation in the properties of the person we love, this may be because of moral requirements he would fail to meet without the properties, or because we want what is good for the person and can see a way of achieving it that is consistent with what he wants for himself. Indeed, before a particular person whom we love exists (just as before we find someone to love), it is permissible to think more boldly in terms of the characteristics we would like to have in a person and that we think it is excellent for a person to have, at least so long as these characteristics would not be bad for the person who will have them and are consistent with respect for persons.

The latter side-constraint—respect for persons—could even conflict with seeking properties that are good for someone. For example, suppose peace of mind and equanimity are goods for a person. Nevertheless, ensuring their presence by modifying someone so that she is self-deceived about awful truths or about her duties to others would be inconsistent with taking seriously that one is creating a person, an entity worthy of respect. Both the side-constraint of respect and the side-constraint of concern for the person's best interests could conflict with what has been called a "genetic supermarket," wherein parents choose traits for offspring according to their own preferences. I agree with Sandel that such a consumer model is out of place when creating persons. Sandel says, "Not everything in the world is open to whatever use we may desire or devise" (Sandel 2004, 54). This is certainly true of persons.

Still, before the existence of a person, there is no one with certain characteristics that we have to accept, if we love him and do not want to impose undue burdens necessary for changes. Hence, not accepting whatever characteristics nature will bring but altering them ex-ante does not show lack of love. Nor can it insult or psychologically pressure a person at the time changes are made the way ex-post changes might. This is because no conscious being yet exists who has to work hard to achieve new traits or suffer fears of rejection at the idea that they should be changed. Importantly, it is rational and acceptable to seek good characteristics in a new person, even though we know that when the child comes to be and we love him or her, many of these characteristics may come and go and we will continue to love the particular person. This is an instance of what I call the distinction between "caring to have" and "caring about." That is, one can know that one will care about someone just as much whether or not she has certain traits and yet care to have someone, perhaps for their own sake, who has, rather than lacks, those traits (Kamm 2004).[23] Sandel says that "parental love is not contingent on talents and attributes a child happens to have" (Sandel 2004, 55). This is true because love is for a particular about whom one cares, but this is consistent with caring to have, and seeking better attributes in, a person-to-be, at least ex-ante. After all, even though a parent's love is not contingent on whether its child has the attribute of being nonparalyzed, it would not be wrong for a parent to see to it that its child can walk. Hence, it would not be correct for a child to think that just because his parents tried and succeeded in giving him certain good traits, they would not have loved him as much if he had not had these traits.

Applying what I have said to the issue of enhancement suggests that even if transformative and enhancing projects should be based primarily on what is best for the child-to-be, determined independently of mere competitive advantage, this is consistent with trying to achieve ex-ante a child with traits that will be desirable per se, so long as these traits will not be bad for the child and are not inconsistent with respect for persons. By contrast, ex-post enhancement may have to be more constrained, for it could involve psychological pressure on the child and lead to fear of rejection. However, even ex-ante enhancement, given that the child knows about it ex-post, can lead to some forms of psychological pressure. For example, if you know that you have been deliberately given a talent for music, you may feel under pressure to use it, though you would prefer not to.[24] It might be suggested that we could avoid this problem by modifying the person-to-be so that the person would always prefer the traits that we have given him. But doing this would be inconsistent with respect for persons, for the exercise of independent judgment should not be restricted; if anything, it should be enhanced. An alternative way to reduce pressure ex-post is to provide traits that add value either simply in being present (such as better eyesight) or in increasing options for someone (for example, to either play or not play music).

Drawing a distinction between the methods of ex-ante and ex-post "designing" people does not, however, put to rest different sorts of objections to even nonpressuring ex-ante enhancements. Let us consider some.

(1) First, Sandel thinks that people are not products to be designed. I agree that people are not products in the sense that they are not commodities, but rather beings worthy of concern and respect in their own right. But I do not think this implies that it is morally wrong to design them. Consider first if it would be acceptable to redesign oneself. We are accustomed to people having replacement parts, such as knees and transplants. Suppose when our parts wore out, we were offered alternatives among the new ones—for example, teeth of various colors, joints that were more or less flexible, limbs that were longer or shorter; it might well make sense to make selections that involved redesigning ourselves. Similarly, if we could replace brain cells, it might make sense to choose ones that gave us new abilities. This would also be redesigning ourselves.

Now consider creating new people. We already have much greater control over the timing of pregnancy, over whether someone can conceive at all, and over which embryos are chosen (via pre-implantation diagnosis) for development. Rather than humility, we have justifiable pride in these accomplishments. Suppose that we each had been designed in detail by other persons. (We all know that the story about the stork bringing babies is a myth. Just suppose that sexual reproduction and the natural lottery in traits are also myths, and we have really all been designed.) Presumably, we would still be beings of worth and entitled to respect. But might it be that although a being retains its high status despite such an origin, it is inconsistent with respect for persons to choose such a designed origin for them? (Analogously, a person retains his status as a rights-bearer even when his rights are violated, but it is not, therefore, appropriate to violate his rights.[25]) To answer this question, imagine that the natural way of reproducing required that important properties be selected for offspring; otherwise they would be mere lumps of flesh. Surely, selecting properties would then be permissible. If this procedure were working well, would we nevertheless be obligated, out of respect for persons, to introduce a lottery based on chance as a way for definite properties to come about? I do not think so. It is the properties persons have, not how they come to have them, that is crucial for their retaining worth. If this is correct, then the designing of persons is not per se inconsistent with respect for persons and the value of persons.[26]

(2) Some associate designing people with engineering them rather than raising them and letting them grow, and criticize designing for this reason (Ashcroft and Gui 2005). However, I do not think these necessarily are contrasts. One could put together the innate mechanisms that are now present in people at birth (thus engineering them) and then they could grow and be raised as they are now. Some may think that putting together a living being according to a design would threaten our ability to revere and love it; we could not have what might be called the "ooh-response." Worse, the idea of putting something together might suggest that there is nothing wrong with taking it apart (thereby destroying it). But many things we revere and love are created by us, and not just as the result of

acts of inspiration. Works of art and craft, literature, hybrid plants and animals are composed, revised, put together in parts that we can come to understand completely. And yet we can respond to these as more than the sum of their parts, revering and loving them. Of course, such entities are not persons and do not have the moral status of persons. But that is because they do not have the properties of persons. If we gave them such properties (as rationality and emotion), the worth that supervenes on these, and the response to the worth, would be present, too.

Crucially, it is a mistake in criticizing enhancement to focus on its occurring by a mechanical, piecemeal construction process (engineering), for enhancement does not essentially involve it. Consider that parents typically wish and pray that their children be good people, have good judgment and worthwhile capacities. Suppose that wishing made it so and one could be assured that one's prayers would be answered. This would be a means of enhancement. Should parents then not engage in such efficacious wishing and praying, even if they wish and pray for the right things?[27]

(3) A third general objection to ex-ante designing asks, if someone wants to have a child, should she not focus only on the most basic goods, such as having a normal child to love? If so, then if she focuses on achieving many superior qualities, does that not show that she is interested in the wrong things in having a child? To answer this worry, consider an analogy. If the primary concern for a philosopher in getting a job should be that she be able to do philosophy, does that mean that it is wrong to choose between possible jobs that equally satisfy that characteristic on the basis of higher salary? If not, why is the search for properties other than the basic ones in a child wrong, when the basic ones are not thereby put in jeopardy? (Of course, in the case of the child-to-be, unlike the job, the enhanced properties are usually to be for its benefit, not only for those doing the selecting.)

Furthermore, as noted above, searching for more than the basics does not by itself imply that if one could not achieve those enhancements, one would not still happily have a child who had only the basics, and love the particular person she is. In this way, too, seeking enhancement is consistent with being open to the unbidden. What about disappointment? It is true that the more one invests in getting enhancements, the more resources one will have wasted if the enhancements do not come about; the lost resources, rather than the child one has, could be a source of disappointment. There may also be disappointment *for* the child when enhancements fail—that one could not bring about something good for it. But that is different from disappointment *in* the child. Further, while someone who would refuse to have a child without enhancements might thereby show that he did not care about the core reasons for having a child, even this does not show he is unfit to be a parent. For he could still come to love the child if he actually had it, through attachment to it as a particular (as described above).

(4) I have argued that often ex-ante changes would be preferable to ex-post changes because there would be less pressure on, and less opportunity for feelings of rejection by, the child. But a fourth concern about ex-ante enhancements is that a parent will simply have greater control over the child's nature, whether she seeks it or not. (As Sandel agrees, this does not mean that the child will have less control, for it is chance, not the child, that will determine genetic makeup if other persons do not. Nor does it mean that the issues of "designing" children and of parental control are not separable in principle. For if someone other than the parent designed the child, relative to the parent the child would still be part of the unbidden.) Sandel thinks that parents should be open to the unbidden future. By contrast, this fourth concern is that the child has a right to a future that is open, at least in relation to its parents' genetic choices. Is it possible that if we could produce a certain desirable trait in someone equally well and as safely by genetic means or by ex-post drugs or training, we should prefer the latter means because they give the child greater freedom relative to its parent?

Consider the following argument for this position:[28] Suppose a parent is told that its fetus has a gene that will make it aggressive to a degree that is undesirable from the parent's point of view though not outside the normal range. The gene could be altered so that the person who will develop will be less aggressive. Alternatively, the person who will develop could take a drug through her life that will successfully reduce the aggressiveness caused by the gene. The latter course is to be preferred, the argument maintains, because when the child reaches maturity she can decide to stop taking the drug if she decides that she prefers being a more aggressive person. By contrast, if her parents had made the genetic change, the claim is, she would not have this freedom to choose to be more aggressive.

This argument does not succeed, I believe. For it rests on the assumption that a genetic trait for aggression can be altered perfectly well by taking a drug. But if that is so, then it is also possible that the alternative genetic trait for less aggression can be altered by taking a drug that increases aggressiveness. Hence, the child whose parents made the genetic change could have the same freedom to alter her temperament as the child whose parents did not make the genetic change. On the other hand, if drugs could not alter traits as well as genetic modification, this would leave each child with a genetic makeup either given by nature or by a parent; the child would still not be free to modify itself by drugs ex-post.

Suppose parents would have greater control than they now have over their children's characteristics with either ex-ante or ex-post enhancement. In numerous areas of life, persons now justifiably stand in relations of control over other people where once chance ruled. The important thing is that this be done justly and well, keeping in mind that one is creating a free and equal person who has a right to form her or his own conception of the good. Giving the person certain all-purpose enhanced capacities (such as greater intelligence or emotional stability) makes the person better able to find his own way. Hence, if we choose certain characteristics in particular in offspring, the balance of control over the child's life may shift to the child rather than the parent, even if the child does not have the capacity to further alter the characteristic ex-post. What I have in mind is that if we could ensure that a child had such enhancing traits as self-control and good judgment, then the child would be less, not more, likely to be subject to parental control after birth. This is what is most important.

(5) A fifth concern is that if each parent individually tries to do what is best for his child, all parents will end up making the situation worse for all their children. This can come about if we give traits that could benefit a child only by giving her a competitive advantage. If all children are similarly altered, everyone may be overall worse off, in virtue of efforts made that do not alter any individual's benefit. To avoid this prisoner's dilemma situation, I have already suggested that we focus on characteristics that would benefit someone independently of competitive advantage. With respect to other traits some rule that coordinates the choices of parents seems called for.[29]

(6) Of course, many would reject both ex-ante and ex-post genetic and drug modification, whether controlled by parents or by the offspring themselves, rather than modification by effort or exercise. Such opponents try to distinguish means of enhancement that Sandel does not distinguish, but in another way than I have. Sometimes it is said that the struggle involved in effort and exercise has moral value. Or, it is said, that if our performance is not the result of our consciously bringing it about by trying and effort, then there will be no connection that we understand as human agents between our performance and ourselves. There will be no intelligible connection between means and ends. The performance will come about as if by magic.[30] However, these points suggest that it would be better if most members of our species did not have, for example, the genetic tendency that they in fact have toward fellow feeling, but rather, like the few among us who are very aggressive, had to produce fellow feeling in themselves by great effort or through a process that intelligibly led to fellow feeling. But this would not be better. Similarly, consider the following imaginary case. Your high intelligence and natural grace, which in someone else would be due to an enhancement, is your normal luck in life's lottery, and it is largely due to your genetic makeup. Then normal changes in your physical makeup lead to your losing the automatic presence of high intelligence and grace. Would you now be thankful that you had the freedom to decide whether or not to work extra hard and, by a humanly intelligible process, bring these good things about in yourself, or even take many drugs each day to bring them about? Or would you prefer genetic surgery so that your system worked automatically the way it always had? Presumably the latter. Here I have again employed the Shifted Baseline Argument, by imagining that a characteristic that is normally genetically controlled,

either in the species or just in you, is absent. Then we consider whether there is anything offensive per se in introducing a genetic trait to restore or produce the desirable characteristic.

The basic point is that people do not now complain that many good capacities they have come about independently of their will and not through an intelligible process. Indeed, one might analogize genetic changes (or taking drugs) in order to improve performance to maturation. Often, when someone cannot do or appreciate something, we tell her to wait until she matures. This means that no act of will or effort in an intelligible process can substitute for a physical or psychological change that will, as if by magic, make the person capable of doing or appreciating something.[31]

One major conclusion of this section is that Sandel does not show that seeking to enhance children, especially ex-ante, is inconsistent with a proper balance between accepting and transforming love.

B. SOCIAL JUSTICE

Finally, we come to Sandel's views on the connection between enhancement and the twin issues of burdens of responsibility and distributive justice. Consider responsibility first. If people are able to enhance themselves or others, can they not be held responsible in the sense of being blamed for not giving themselves or others desirable characteristics? Not necessarily, for one does not have a duty to do everything that could make oneself or someone else better, and if one has no duty, then one is not at fault in not enhancing and so not to be blamed. Even if one has certain duties—for example, to be the best doctor one can be—and taking certain drugs would help one to perform better, it is not necessarily one's duty to take the drugs. One could retain a right not to alter one's body even in order to better fulfill one's duties as a physician. Hence, one need not be at fault even if one does not do what will help one perform one's duties better. But retaining the right not to alter one's body does not imply that such alterations are impermissible for anyone who wants them. Of course, if the characteristics one will have must be determined by others (for example, one's parents), then one could not be blamed for causing or not causing the characteristics, as one could not have directed one's parents' behavior.

What about cases in which one can be blamed for a choice not to enhance? Thomas Scanlon has emphasized that one can hold someone responsible for an outcome in the sense of blaming him for it without thereby thinking that it is also his responsibility to bear the costs of his choice.[32] These are conceptually two separate issues. For example, suppose someone is at fault for acting carelessly in using his hairdryer. If he suffers severe harm and will die without medical treatment, his being at fault need not mean that he forfeits a claim on others he otherwise had to medical care.

By contrast, Sandel thinks that the issue of responsibility for choosing to have or to lack certain characteristics is intimately related to how much of a claim we have against others for aid. However, he is not always clear in distinguishing the role of choice from the role of mere knowledge of one's characteristics. For example, in discussing why we have insurance schemes, he seems to imply that even if we had no control over our traits but only knew what they were (for example, via genetic testing), we would lose a claim against others to financially share the costs of our fate. For, if people knew they were not at risk, people would not enter into insurance schemes that mimic solidarity. So Sandel's argument against enhancement based on mimicking solidarity seems to be an argument against knowledge of genetic traits as well as against control of them. But those who urge us to use a veil of ignorance in deciding whether and when we should share others' burdens (via allocation of resources) are, in effect, saying that even if we have knowledge of one another's traits, there are sometimes moral reasons for behaving as though we lack this knowledge.

Let us put aside the issue of blameworthiness for, and the effect of mere knowledge of, traits. How should the mere possibility of making responsible choices that determine one's traits affect responsibility for bearing costs for the outcome of choices? Sandel here seems to share with some philosophers (known as luck egalitarians) the view (roughly) that if we have not chosen to have traits but have them as a matter of luck (or other people's choices), the costs of having them should be shared among everyone. However, if we choose the traits (by action or by omitting to change them if we can), then even if we do not in any deep sense deserve to have made this choice, there is no reason for the costs of having the traits to be shared. (According to some luck egalitarians, however, we may choose to buy insurance that will protect us against bad choices.) Sandel says he cannot think of any better reason for the well-off to help those who are not well off except that each is not fully responsible for his situation. (It is important to remember that some do not find lack of responsibility a compelling reason for sharing with others. Robert Nozick, for example, argued that one could be entitled to (or rightfully burdened with) what followed from traits that one was not at all responsible for having.[33])

Contrary to Sandel, it seems that often we want to give people new options without taking away from them help they would have gotten from others when they had no control over their fates. One example given above involved someone whose choice—even a faulty one—to use a hairdryer need not lead to his forfeiting a right to aid to avert a major disaster. Similarly, if someone for reasons of conscience refuses to take advantage of the option to abort a difficult pregnancy, we do not think that she should forfeit medical care simply because she could have avoided the need for it. In many cases, arguments for the duty to aid others seem to have more to do with respect and concern for persons and a willingness to support their having an opportunity for autonomous choice without fear of costs[34] than with whether they have or have not gotten themselves into whatever situation they are in. Of course, in cases I have been considering, someone chooses in a way that leads to a bad outcome he does not per se choose. But recall that Kant thought we had a duty to help people pursue even the ends they themselves had deliberately chosen because people's choices give us reasons to value their ends, rather than because they could not be held responsible for outcomes or because it was only the unwilled consequences of their choices with which we were asked to help.

It may throw further light on the effect on shared responsibility of the option to enhance to consider the effect on shared responsibility of the option to *treat*. Sandel, of course, is not against giving individuals the option to treat or prevent their diseases. This is so despite the fact that one might construct an argument concerning the option to use treatments and preventions parallel to the one he constructs for the option to use enhancements. That is, someone might say that giving the option to use treatments and preventions will destroy the willingness of the healthy to aid the sick who had the option to avoid illness by earlier treatment or prevention but did not, especially when the healthy attribute their own health to their choice to use such earlier interventions. The fact that this is not a successful argument against spreading the option of treatments—presumably because we think many will make use of the treatments and then not need the help of others—should lead us to question its success against enhancements.

Might it be that Sandel also believes that people should be able to call on the assistance of others when they need it, regardless of many individual choices they make? Such a belief might account for the subterfuge of eliminating the possibility of individual choice for enhancement, as a device to sustain a duty to aid. This would be somewhat like the strategy of pretending that one cannot figure out what share of an outcome each person is responsible for producing as a way of ensuring equal shares of a social product. The fact that one seeks such a subterfuge suggests that one simply believes that equal shares are right, regardless of differential input. But it also suggests that one cannot really see how this could be so. One deals with this intellectual conflict by eliminating the factor one is having trouble seeing as consistent with an outcome that one wants.

I think that a good account of the worry that lies behind Sandel's view focuses on a conflict between the right and the good. Here is an analogy that helps make this clearer. From the point of view of considering the good of a person, we may want to be sure that he gets help when he needs it. Suppose someone has the option of declaring himself emancipated. We can see the attraction in this status for him, but if we are concerned about his welfare, we may recommend against it. This is because we take seriously the idea of emancipation as implying that he will have to be self-reliant and can no longer be shielded by his parents from complaints against him. It is not open to us to say, "We care about your good, yet we see the attractions of being emancipated. So, we will combine emancipation with the continued care and protection by a parent when you need it." This would not be taking emancipation as a component of the right seriously; if we take it seriously, we can be constrained from dealing with bad effects to which it leads, even when this is contrary to the good of the person. Hence, one's concern for his good could lead us to urge against emancipation, even though concern for the good is not the only basis for deciding what to do, given that we agree that the good may not override a consideration of the right (e.g., emancipation) when the latter is present.

Hence, eliminating choice (or the ability to determine differential productive input) might indicate that one thinks one should take these factors very seriously if they are present and they could militate against good outcomes. A solution to this quandary is to show that appropriate respect for considerations of the right is often consistent with a duty to help, even when someone has made a choice. (I focused on this in my previous discussion.) Another solution, to which I now turn, is to show that the good would be overall promoted even were the duty to help less strong due to choice.

Let us suppose it were true that to some degree, as we increase the range of individual choice, we limit the claim of a person to the assistance of others. (For example, choosing to be or remain paralyzed, given the option of a cure, because one preferred that sort of life might be considered an "expensive taste," and public assistance to make such a life go as well as an unparalyzed life might justifiably be denied.) Does this mean that we will have lost valuable solidarity? If it is appropriate that people who have equal opportunity to choose enhancements but decline to do so bear more substantive responsibility for their condition, then the moral status of solidarity will have changed; it will no longer be the only correct, valuable, and virtuous response that it is in other circumstances.[35] If so, its absence will not necessarily be bad. Furthermore, it is still true that if having the option to enhance leads many people to improve themselves or others, there will be fewer instances of people who are badly off, hence fewer who require the assistance of others. For example, rather than distributing wealth that only the talented can produce in a certain environment, each might have a relevant talent and so have the opportunity to be more productive in that environment. Most importantly, each person would not only have the material benefits that can be redistributed from some to others. Each person could have the intrinsic rewards of exercising enhanced abilities and talents, rewards that cannot be *redistributed* from some to others.

Let me conclude this section by noting that if Sandel were concerned with the increased burden of responsibility had for one's traits and one's children's traits, not by individuals themselves but by society, there would be no way to completely avoid the burden of increased responsibility. For suppose a society or species knows that it could change traits of its members by using or developing genetic or chemical means. Those who decide that the society will not use these means will be to some degree responsible for the absence of enhanced traits.

(This is so even if some other individuals will not be responsible because others in the society made it impossible for them to have a choice about use of the means at the individual level.) However, society will be to *blame* for failures to improve people only if there were no good reasons not to engage in enhancement. Some, such as Sandel, seem to think that preventing individuals from becoming substantively responsible for individual outcomes could be offered as such a good reason. But can preventing more *social* responsibility for outcomes be offered as a reason, if society already has increased responsibility when it is responsible for denying use or development of enhancement techniques? Possibly this reason would still be available, if a distinction could be drawn between degrees of responsibility, so that there is less social responsibility for genetic traits if society chose to let chance determine them than if society actually selected the traits.

The primary conclusions of this section are that Sandel does not successfully show that we should limit options to enhance ourselves or others as a way of ensuring a right to social assistance.

V. Conclusion

Sandel's objections to enhancement focus on the desire for mastery and the unwillingness to live with what we are "given." (He also focuses on the more contingent issue of the misuse of the ability to enhance ourselves and others that is likely to occur in a competitive environment, especially one governed by shallow values.) I have argued that what is most troubling about enhancement is neither that there will be people who desire to have control over nature, offspring, and themselves, nor that there will be unwillingness to accept what comes unbidden. However, I do think that there are major problems with enhancement. Some are the ones Sandel puts to one side. Given our scarce resources, where should enhancement be on the list of things to do? Will there be a fair distribution of benefits of enhancement? Could we really safely alter a system as complex as a person (by genetic enhancement or treatment) without making disastrous mistakes? Consider the last point further.

It has been pointed out that in a complex system such as a human being, whose parts are densely interdependent, even small alterations can have unexpected bad effects. Extreme caution, at least, seems called for (Coors and Hunter 2005). Genetic manipulation has been contrasted with surgery or taking drugs in this respect. (Sandel's complaint holds equally against all these means of enhancement, and he deliberately puts to one side issues of differential safety to focus on an objection that he thinks would be present even if there were no safety issues.)

In rebuttal, it might be suggested that genetic changes to individuals that would not affect their offspring could be made no less safe for the individual and the species than use of drugs. For in using drugs or even surgery, one usually thinks that one can, at least often, stop a change and revert to one's original condition if things go badly. If genetic changes could also be reversible, or at least counteractable in some way, then the risk of using them would also be diminished.

Further, it might be pointed out that the dense interdependence of the parts of our system also creates great risks even with therapeutic interventions, so it would be good to know specifically why enhancements present greater potential threats than treatments. And then there is the interdependence of human beings with the rest of the world. Is it possible that treating a defect in individuals that eliminates the normal presence of such defects in the human species would upset some delicate balance between our species and the rest of nature? Would we let this possibility interfere with our search for treatments?

Another issue in enhancing, I think, is that *we* will be doing it, and so our lack of imagination as designers may raise problems. That is, most people's conception of the varieties of goods is very limited, and if they designed people their improvements would likely conform to limited, predictable types. But we should know that we are constantly surprised at the great range of good traits in people, and the incredible range of combinations of traits that turn out to be good. For example, could we predict that a very particular degree of irony combined with a certain degree of diffidence would constitute an interesting type of personality? In part IV, section A, I mentioned the view that potential parents should focus on having children with basic good properties rather than seek improvements beyond this. Oddly, the "lack of imagination" objection to enhancement I am now voicing is based on a concern that in seeking enhancements people will focus on too simple and predictable a set of goods.

How does the lack-of-imagination objection relate to Sandel's view that an openness to the unbidden (excluding illnesses) extends the range of our sympathies? One construal of his point is that if we have no control, we are forced to understand and care about people, as we should, even when they are difficult and nonideal. By contrast, the lack-of-imagination objection emphasizes that when creatures of limited imagination do *not* design themselves and others, they are likely to extend the range of their appreciation of great positive goods because the range of such goods is likely to be larger. Seventy years ago, a parent who would have liked to design his child to have the good trait of composing classical music could not have conceived that it would be good to have a child who turned out to be one of the Beatles. (To have conceived it would have involved creating the Beatles' style before the Beatles did.) The lack-of-imagination objection is concerned that too much control will limit the number and combination of goods from what is possible. Hence, at least in those cases where greater goods are more likely to come about if chance rather than unimaginative choice is in control, the desire for enhancement will militate *against* control.

Finally, if the controlled selection of enhanced properties is a morally acceptable means, at least sometimes, what are the good ends to which it could safely be used? Presumably, if it were at all possible, it would be a safe end to enhance our capacities to recognize and fulfill our moral duties, at least if the enhancement involved our appreciating the reasons for these duties and not a purely mechanical response. Recognizing and fulfilling moral duties is a side-constraint on the exercise of any other capacities and the pursuit of any ends. There is no point in worrying that having such moral capacities would interfere with unimagined goods. For if such moral capacities interfere with other goods, this just means that those other goods are not morally permissible options for us.

Notes

1. This chapter is a revised version of "Is There a Problem with Enhancement?," *American Journal of Bioethics* [AJOB], 5(3): 1–10. It also appears (without some minimal changes present here) in *Human Enhancement*, eds. J. Savulescu and N. Bostrom (Oxford: Oxford University Press, 2009). It incorporates some of my responses to the very useful commentaries on the article as it appeared in AJOB. The commentaries appear in the same issue of AJOB, and my complete responses appear at the AJOB website. It also incorporates some of my responses to Sandel's helpful commentary on my presentation of parts of this article at the Inaugural Conference of the University-Wide Program on Ethics and Health, Harvard Medical School, November 19, 2005. I am also grateful for comments to audiences at that conference, at the UCLA Program in Genetics and Society, at Bowdoin College, and at Harvard Law School.

2. Note that some Kantians claim that it has always been true that only what rational beings will determines what is good.

3. Notice that not deliberately causing something is not the same as not causing it. For example, a parent may cause her child's IQ to move down from 160 to 140 by inadvertently eating improperly during pregnancy. This reduction is unbidden, though caused by the parent. It is in part because we might be causally responsible for making things worse than they could naturally be, that some may think that we have a duty to achieve at least the knowledge of life processes that prevents our interfering with naturally occurring goods.

4. When one cannot change bad things that come, one could be open to them in the sense of being accepting of one's fate. This is consistent with desiring mastery so that one could change one's fate. I owe this point to an anonymous reader.

5. I shall return to this point below.

6. Judith Thomson (1990, 1999) has argued that intention never matters to the permissibility of action. Thomas Scanlon (2000) makes a somewhat more limited claim.

Notice that sometimes, we think that an act is permissible only if it aims to satisfy a certain desire in an agent who does the act. For example, suppose we set aside scarce resources for a musical performance in order that those who desire pleasure from music shall have some. But if someone's only desire in going to a concert is to mingle with other people, this is an indication that he has no desire for music per se. Hence, it is an indication that an end (give pleasure from music) which justified the use of scarce resources for musical performances will not be achieved. Hence, if this agent should not go to the concert, it is not because of his having only a desire to mingle per se, but because the desire is an indication that some effect that justifies funding concerts (pleasure from music) will not come about.

Now, suppose someone has a bad motive or further aim (e.g., to show off) in doing something otherwise permissible, such as chewing gum. It might be appropriate for him to, in a sense, be punished for the bad motive with which he would chew the gum, by making it impermissible for him to chew the gum. This, of course, is not just any punishment. It specifically makes it the case that his bad motive is not efficacious. But if the achievement of an important good for others or the performance of a dutiful act (e.g., not harming someone) is at stake and this can justify the act, it would not be appropriate to require someone to forgo the act as a way of making his bad motive inefficacious. That would be to "punish" others for the agent's bad attitude.

7. As emphasized by Paul Litton and Larry Temkin.

8. This was emphasized in Martin and Peerzada (2005). The discussion that follows is my response to their views and some of their cases.

9. Julie Tannenbaum, however, pointed out (in discussion) that the equal moral status of enhanced and nonenhanced persons may depend not only on their shared property as persons but possibly on the fact that the properties of the enhanced would make them different only in degree but not in kind. For suppose we were creating gods. It might then be an open question, she suggests, whether persons would have fewer negative and positive rights in relation to gods than in relation to other nongod persons. I suspect, however, that once persons have the characteristics that give them claims over their own lives, then negative rights, at least, would be assured even against gods.

10. Of course, it is possible that in a society only its leaders have certain particular desires, intentions, or dispositions and they arrange rewards and punishments so that individuals in the society fulfill the leaders' aims without necessarily sharing their desires, intentions, or dispositions. However, I do not think Sandel deals with such a scenario.

11. This was part of his response to me on November 19, 2005. This section C summarizes my understanding of our discussion on that occasion.

12. Recall that earlier I considered senses of "openness to the unbidden" that were not in such conflict.

13. Carson Strong emphasizes that the idea of a gift requires a gift giver and that, therefore, from a secular perspective where we do not assume a God, it is not literally true that children or naturally occurring good properties are gifts, as Sandel speaks of them (Strong 2005). However, Strong himself notes that Sandel might simply emphasize the role of chance and good luck—as in a Rawlsian natural lottery—and use a metaphorical sense of giftedness. Strong also suggests that literal giftedness would come into the world, in the secular point of view, if parents did deliberately give good traits to their offspring. But "gift" has another connotation that militates against this conclusion to some degree, I believe. For a gift suggests some good that one gives beyond the call of duty; the recipient is not entitled to receive it. Children, however, might be entitled to certain enhancements, let alone certain treatments, from their parents and then those would not be gifts in the strict sense.

14. Similarly, the human and the good are distinct conceptual categories. Human traits (such as arrogance) could be bad, and inhuman altruism could be good.

15. In discussion on November 19, 2005.

16. An anonymous reader suggested the following: Suppose that we would permit the person's natural capacities to flourish even if we compensate for a congenital disease by genetic intervention. On this view, the originally present "bad" genes would mask, but not

alter, an individual's natural capacities. So what are natural capacities? Not those likely to exist given an individual's genetic endowment. If, instead, they are those capacities that can be achieved in an individual given practical genetic interventions, then we permit an individual's natural capacities to flourish however we intervene, whether through treatment or enhancement. (Perhaps, the natural capacities would be those given by the idea of the normal capacities for the species?)

17. Allan Buchanan, Dan Brock, Norman Daniels, and Daniel Wikler, *From Chance to Choice: Genetics and Justice* (Cambridge: Cambridge University Press, 2000). See chapter 15 this volume for my discussion of this book. Daniels emphasized the importance of normal species functioning in his earlier book, *Just Health Care* (Cambridge: Cambridge University Press, 1985).

18. Miller and Brody (2005) suggest that induced infertility by contraception is an enhancement. Schwartz thinks of it as an induced dysfunction. This suggests that sometimes dysfunctions are enhancements. Miller and Brody at one point attempt to fit contraception into a narrow notion of medical care by suggesting that even though it is an enhancement, it prevents clear medical risks involved in pregnancy and mental health problems associated with unwanted births. But suppose (counterfactually) that pregnancy had no medical risks and hormonal changes in women made it possible for them to always adjust psychologically to each additional child. It could still be true that a woman could sometimes have a better life if she did something besides have another child, and she should use contraception to achieve that good. Here the provision within medical care of contraception, which itself has some medical risks, would be unrelated to avoiding health risks. Yet it could be appropriate for a doctor to prescribe it.

19. There is also another sense in which enhancement is more important than normality-preserving treatments: We are all willing to risk some illness by spending money on life-enhancing activities (such as education) rather than on cures for disease. I owe this point to Julian Savulescu.

20. I owe this point to Regina Goldman.

21. Hilary Bok emphasized this point.

22. This point was emphasized by Marcia Angell in discussion.

23. I previously argued for this distinction in Kamm (2004) when discussing the compatibility of (a) a disabled person caring about his life as much as a nondisabled person cares about his life, and (b) a disabled person caring to have a nondisabled life rather than a disabled one.

24. I owe this point to Seana Shiffrin.

25. The following reductio argument might be suggested for this conclusion (modeled on one David Velleman offers against suicide in his "A Right of Self-Termination?" *Ethics* 109(3): 606–28; for discussion of his view, see chapter 5 this volume. It is important to seek good enhancements for people only if people matter. If people are products we design, people do not matter. Therefore, it is not important to seek enhancements for people. According to this argument, the permissibility of seeking certain goods for people is incompatible with the importance of pursuing their good.

26. Notice also that there is an alternative of designing the gene pool so that only enhanced options are available and this is compatible with chance determination of the properties of any given individual.

27. It is true that when we pray and wish now, we may hope there is a superior being who will grant our prayers only when they are appropriate. (This is the point of the "if it be

Thy will" part of the prayer.) But this can signal our concern that we may not really be enhancing in getting what we want. I discuss this problem of limited wisdom and imagination in the last part of this chapter.

28. Presented by Anja Karnein and based on one by Jurgen Habermas.

29. Larry Temkin emphasized this problem of a prisoner's dilemma. Another objection to some ex-ante enhancements was raised by Matthew Liao (in Liao 2005). Liao argues that some ex-ante enhancements (which I contrast to ex-post enhancements) are impermissible, even though the person does not yet exist, and this is not because of any property the person eventually comes to have, but because of the morally dubious intention of the enhancer (pp. 2–3). For example, suppose someone sex-selects a female child for the purpose of selling her into prostitution, or (in my own illustration) creates a brain-enhanced child for the purpose of exhibiting her in a zoo. However, each creator then comes to love the child for her own sake and treats her properly. Liao notes that I suggest that characteristics sought ex-ante should not be bad for the person who will have them and should be consistent with respect for persons. But being female or brain-enhanced is not bad for a person or inconsistent with creating a person worthy of respect. Hence, he thinks, it is not because of the properties that would be given, but because of the intentions of the agents that their acts are wrong (p. 5).

He also thinks that I mean to imply that properties that are morally undesirable (such as being subject to self-deception) make persons no longer worthy of respect, but he counters that having a morally dubious property does not do this. Yet, he agrees, it is still wrong ex-ante to do what gives this property to someone. This cannot be, he thinks, because of what the property is in itself, or because the person could have existed without the property and been better. The latter claim, Liao thinks, cannot be true because an individual comes into existence at the same time as his ex-ante chosen properties and the person without that property would have been a different person. Hence, the person now in existence with the property cannot complain that he was harmed by being given the property, assuming his life is worth living. Liao concludes from all this that the wrongness of giving such a property lies in the morally dubious intentions of the agent (p. 6).

I do not think Liao's arguments succeed. First, consider the person who creates either a female child intending to make her a prostitute or a brain-enhanced person intending to exhibit her. I would say that the first creator is attempting to create a prostitute and the second an exhibition animal, and each of these properties is not one that persons should have. But suppose that an agent attempting to create someone with these properties cannot succeed, perhaps because he is bound to love each of the people he creates. Then I would say that his actual act of creating the people is not impermissible, though what he attempts to do (make prostitutes or exhibition animals) is impermissible. I would say that a morally worse event or act has taken place in virtue of the bad intention prompting his act, but this does not mean his act is impermissible.

Second, contrary to Liao, I do not mean to imply that giving a person a morally dubious property makes the person not worthy of respect. The person just remains someone worthy of having properties more appropriate to his respect-worthy status. Similarly, violating someone's rights can be inconsistent with respect for a person without in any way altering his status as a creature worthy of respect. Most disturbing, from the fact that a naturally disabled person remains a person worthy of respect, Liao concludes that the wrongness of deliberately creating a disabled person cannot be due to his winding up with the property of being disabled; the act must rather be wrong because of the motivation or intention of the agent. But surely it can be wrong to do what gives people properties that do not diminish their worth but just make their lives much worse for them to live, regardless of one's motivation or intention (for example, as a mere side effect of some useful act). Now consider Liao's arguments based on identity considerations for the claim that an act creating a person with a certain property cannot be wrong because of the property. First, it is not always true that a person would not have existed at all if he had not existed with a certain property. For not all properties are essential properties (i.e., properties without which that person would not exist), and we could imagine having changed a given embryo for the better by affecting one of its nonessential properties. Then that person could have been better than he actually is. Now consider the cases in which a different person would have been created if a property had been different—perhaps because an essential property is at issue. Liao says that in such a case, the person created with the nonoptimal property cannot complain that he is worse off than he might otherwise have been. But it does not follow from this that we cannot say it is impermissible to have created a person with the property rather than someone else without the property, in virtue of what the property is. Hence, we need not refer to the intentions of the creator in judging the permissibility of his act.

30. This point is especially emphasized by Leon Kass (2007).

31. Asian traditions involve many techniques that produce good results by exercises (such as repetition of a mantra) that do not involve trying or moving by intelligible steps toward a goal.

32. In Scanlon (1999), chapter 6, he distinguishes between responsibility as attributability and as substantive responsibility.

33. See Nozick (1977). Unlike luck egalitarians, Rawlsians may think that what is necessary to justify shared responsibility as a matter of justice is the fact that a particular social structure is, to a large degree, responsible for what sort of fate in life one's genetic properties will yield. By contrast, in the case of bad luck that is the result of socially unmediated natural effects, a Rawlsian might think that shared responsibility is not a matter of justice. Notice that the problem for shared responsibility of outcomes (solidarity) with which Sandel is concerned is different from another problem that concerns J. S. Robert (Robert 2005). Robert is concerned that giving people the choice of enhancement before we take care of the many who lack basic necessities is already to show a lack of solidarity with others (p. 6). The fact that we might have such priorities weakens Sandel's view that we are more likely to help people when our traits are not chosen. For they are not chosen now, and yet, as Robert sees it, we are unwilling to share with the needy now. But does seeking enhancement indicate a lack of solidarity? Robert himself thinks that it is psychologically realistic to demand only moderate self-sacrifice from each of us. But such a degree of self-sacrifice may be consistent with seeking enhancement for oneself while others are in need of basic necessities. Further, if we were trying to provide the autonomous choice of enhancement to everyone, even though this is not what many need most, this itself would be an instance of solidarity, in the sense that we care for others as well as ourselves. And if it were unrealistic to expect—or not morally required of—us to sacrifice a great deal for others, helping them to enhance themselves at small additional cost (if this were possible) may leave them better off overall than if there were no opportunities for enhancements. However, none of this would solve the problem of solidarity with which Sandel is concerned, as that only arises after people have the option of autonomously enhancing themselves, and thus are thought (by Sandel) to both lose a claim to further assistance and to lose the requirement to assist.

34. The latter point in particular is emphasized by Seana Shiffrin.
35. This point was emphasized by Alexander Schwab.

References

Ashcroft, R. E., and Gui, K. 2005. "Ethics and world pictures in Sandel and Kamm." *American Journal of Bioethics* 5(3): 19–20.

Buchanan, Allan, Daniels, N., Wilder, D., Brock, D., and Wilker, D. 2000. *From Chance to Choice: Genetics and Justice*. Cambridge: Cambridge University Press.

Coors, M., and Hunter, L. 2005. "Evaluation of genetic enhancement: Will human wisdom properly acknowledge the value of evolution?," *American Journal of Bioethics* 5(3): 21–22.

Daniels, N. 1985. *Just Health Care*. Cambridge: Cambridge University Press.

Kamm, F. M. 2004. "Deciding whom to help, health-adjusted life years, and disabilities." In S. Anand, F. Peters, and A. Sen (eds.), *Public Health, Ethics, and Equity*. Oxford: Oxford University Press, 225–42.

Kass, L. 2007. "Deeper disquiets with biotechnological enhancement." Paper presented at Harvard Law School, March 19.

Liao, S. M. 2005. "Are "ex ante" enhancements always permissible?" *American Journal of Bioethics* 5(3): 23–25.

Martin, A., and Peerzada, J. 2005. "Impermissible attitudes, impermissible enhancements." *American Journal of Bioethics* 5(3): 25–27.

Miller, F., and Brody, H. 2005. "Professional integrity and enhancement technologies." *American Journal of Bioethics* 5(3): 15–17.

Nozick, R. 1977. *Anarchy, State and Utopia*. New York: Basic Books.

Robert, J. S. 2005. "Human dispossession and human enhancement." *American Journal of Bioethics* 5(3): 27–29.

Sandel, M. 2004. "The case against perfection." *Atlantic Monthly* 293(3): 51–62.

Scanlon, T. M. 1999. *What We Owe to Each Other*. Cambridge, MA: Harvard University Press.

Scanlon, T. M. 2000. "Intention and permissibility I." *Proceedings of the Aristotelian Society* 74 (Suppl.): 301–17.

Scanlon, T. M. n.d. "Blame." Unpublished article.

Schwartz, P. H. 2005. "Defending the distinction between treatment and enhancement." *American Journal of Bioethics* 5(3): 17–19.

Shiffrin, S. 1999. "Wrongful life, procreative responsibility, and the significance of harm." *Legal Theory* 5(2): 117–48.

Strong, C. 2005. "Lost in translation: Religious arguments made secular." *American Journal of Bioethics* 5(3): 29–31.

Thomson, J. J. 1990. *The Realm of Rights* (Cambridge, MA: Harvard University Press).

Thomson, J. J. 1999. "Physician-assisted suicide: Two moral arguments." *Ethics* 109(3): 497–518.

PART FOUR

Allocating Scarce Resources

18

Health and Equity

In this chapter, I shall consider some principles for rationing and resource prioritization in regard to health.[1, 2] I shall also try to suggest some philosophical foundations for these principles, beginning at the most basic level. These issues arise at both a micro level (where we make decisions about particular individuals in particular cases) and a macro level (where we make decisions that will affect many people, perhaps in advance of particular cases). At the micro level, some principles for rationing can fall under what is described as the *responsiveness* of a health-care system; for example, is it procedurally fair between competitors for health care and just in what it gives to each? ("Responsiveness," in the World Health Organization health-system performance framework, is used to refer to respect for autonomy, dignity, and confidentiality and allows for the measurement of the distribution of health care.) To apply what I say about fairness and justice to the macro level, *often* all we have to do is think of cases where how we allocate resources will affect large numbers of people instead of a few. Sometimes, as I shall indicate, there is more to moving from micro to macro.

I shall distinguish between goodness, fairness, and justice. To make one distinction clearer, consider the following case: A doctor must decide whether to stop a severe pain in person A or a minor pain in person B. She thinks, correctly, that she will do more good if she helps A. But she also remembers that yesterday B suffered a much *worse* pain than A will suffer and no one helped B (while A suffered nothing in the past). So she thinks it would be unfair to let B suffer again, even though she will do less good if she helps him. If it is overall right to do this, this means she does the morally better thing in helping him and the state of affairs in which B is helped rather than A is morally better than one in which A is helped. But this is not because it produces more good.

I distinguish justice from fairness as follows: considerations of fairness are essentially relational; that is, how is A treated relative to B? Justice is concerned with someone getting his due. I can make a situation more just but less fair by giving only one of two people his due when otherwise neither would be given his due. Equality is a particular relation between people; sometimes it is fair, but other times, fairness demands inequality—as when one person has morally relevant characteristics in virtue of which he should be treated differently.

Justice and fairness are typically thought to function as "side constraints" on the maximization of the good. That is, unlike the good, they are not treated as goals to be maximized. If they were only goals, it might be morally right to treat someone unfairly in order to maximize fairness overall (or to minimize unfairness). But if fairness is a side constraint, this would account for why such behavior is often ruled out. This distinction may be important to keep in mind when constructing a measure for the health of populations. Some would like to have a measure that assigns grades to end-states of population health that includes considerations of how fairly health is distributed. But this involves treating fairness as a characteristic of an end-state (i.e., as part of a state which it is our goal to achieve) rather than as a side-constraint on bringing about end-states. If we aim to maximize the grade, this may incorrectly lead us to deliberately act unfairly in order to maximize fairness. This is one reason to think of fairness and goodness as separate considerations.[3]

I. Equality, Priority, and the Veil of Ignorance

Some think that providing equal health, understood as equal normal species functioning (NSF), or equal health expectations or opportunities for all persons is a requirement of fairness and, therefore, morally required.[4] This might be denied for several reasons. The first is that if the only way to produce equality of health among people were to *reduce* the health of some without improving that of anyone, then (all other things equal) this would be morally wrong. (This is related to what is known as the "leveling down" objection to equality.) The second reason is that it may be morally most important to raise the health of worse-off people, even if the route to doing this required us to introduce inequality. For example, suppose the Blues are relatively worse off healthwise and in bad health in absolute terms. The Reds are better off healthwise. If the *only* way to help the Blues rise up in absolute terms involved introducing a system that helped the Reds even more than the Blues, it might still be morally desirable.

Giving priority to helping the worse off might be justified from a utilitarian standpoint when we thus produce more good. That is, on account of diminishing marginal utility, each unit of resource devoted to the worse off produces more good than if it were given to those already better off and this may result in more overall good being produced. However, what is known as the Priority View claims that even holding the amount of good we produce constant, it can be morally more important to help those who are worse off. This may be because (other things equal) it is morally more important that a good go to someone who will have had less if not helped. On the Priority View, there is diminishing marginal goodness of utility, since equal benefits do less to make the outcome better when given to those who are better off.[5] If we gave lexical priority to helping the worse off, we would *first compare* people to see who is worse off, but then we would know whether we are satisfying the lexical priority principle just by seeing if the worse off are getting better off; we would not need to compare them to others, except to know when to stop focusing on them because they are no longer worse off than others. The principles I shall be discussing in the rest of this article are consistent with giving *significant but not lexical priority* to those who are worse off in health, since the principles might rule out helping those who are worse off at no matter what cost in improved health to those already better off. Hence, the principles could also require comparing possible health outcomes to better and worse off people.

Of course, it is an empirical question whether doing what creates inequality in health leads to those worse off in health having better health than they would otherwise have. Empirical data may show that what produces inequality in health also makes those with the worse health worse off *in absolute terms* than they would be were there equality of health. (I shall return to this issue below.)

One supposed ground for requiring equal prospects for health is that it is necessary for there to be equal opportunity to develop and use one's talents and abilities. Norman Daniels argues in this way. The first part of Rawls's second principle of justice requires equal opportunity and so, as a Rawlsian, Daniels argues for equal NSF.[6] If all anyone could want in the way of opportunity were equality with others, there would be no point in introducing inequality of opportunity as a means to making the absolute level of opportunity each person had greater, and hence no justification (within a Rawlsian framework) for such inequality. However, suppose everyone were *equally sick*; then everyone could still have equal opportunity, for everyone would be working under an equal burden in exercising their talents and abilities. I assume we think that this is not yet an ideal condition even from the point of view of opportunity (e.g., to use one's talents). Hence we really want *more* than equal opportunity; we want the degree to which people can use their talents not to be negatively affected by sickness (even if this were to occur equally). And it is again at least possible that unequal health could increase the absolute degree to which sickness does not interfere with people's using their talents and abilities. (An easy-to-imagine case is one where doctors are kept healthier than others because this is necessary to maximize the health of other members of the population.)[7] This criticism reminds us that equality is only a comparative notion, but we want a certain absolute level of health to be aimed at as well.

The argument for equal NSF as a precondition for equal opportunity may also face the problem of instability. Suppose talents and abilities are unequal among people and fair incentives to the talented to employ their talents result in their being better off economically than others. If health varies with social class (as some data suggest)[8] and social class varies with economic class, then equal NSF will be short-lived; it will undo itself. But those worse off in health may still do better overall (on other dimensions of well-being) as a result of the economic inequality. (It is even logically possible for them to do better in absolute terms healthwise than with equality, though in fact this may not be true.)[9]

We think that leveling down health so that we make some sicker without thereby improving anyone else's health in order that all can be equally sick is morally problematic. This may bear in an interesting way on a claim made by Christopher Murray and his coauthors.[10] They say, "We propose that the relation 'is healthier than' can be defined such that population A is healthier than population B *if and only if* an individual behind a veil of ignorance would prefer to be one of the existing individuals in population A rather than an existing individual in population B, holding all non-health characteristics of the two populations to be the same."[11] Hence, one population cannot be less healthy than another and yet be preferred, holding all else constant. They also say, "Imagine two populations, A and B, with identical mortality, incidence, and remission for all non-fatal health states, but with a higher prevalence of paraplegia in population A. Behind a veil of ignorance, an individual will prefer to be a member of population B" (p. 987).

As Murray and coauthors note, it is important whether we use a thick veil, as Rawls does, or a thin veil. A veil is thin if it allows people to know a great deal about the different populations, including the differential rates of conditions such as paraplegia. People do not know only who they would be in a community—the person with or without paraplegia. Given knowledge of different rates of illness, they can make probability calculations of getting an illness. Thin veils are involved when people say that the results one gets from using a veil of ignorance can depend on one's risk aversiveness. Rawls uses a thick veil: one does not know about the distribution of various conditions in a society or between societies; one is deliberately hindered by Rawls from using subjective probabilities in decision making. Rawls claims to get his maximin results—make the worst off as well off as possible—not by assuming that people are very risk averse. He denies he needs this assumption. Rather, if one lacks the data to reasonably formulate subjective probabilities, one is deciding on principles that will determine the whole life prospects of people, and one is a head of a family, then one need not be risk averse to favor maximin, he thinks. Why does Rawls use a thick veil instead of a thin veil? I shall return to this question at the very end of this chapter. For now, let us consider the use of the thin veil in Murray et al.'s Paraplegia Case and its relevance to leveling down.

For all that has been said, the higher incidence of paraplegia in population A might result in *greater equality* of health in population A than in population B by leveling down. Hence, if one cared about equality from behind a veil of ignorance, one might prefer to be a member of population B without this implying that population B is healthier than population A. One could avoid this result by insisting that those behind the veil must not care about relational goods such as equality or by insisting that equality not be achieved by leveling down. Without such restrictions on the decision making of those behind the veil, what a person would choose from behind a thin veil of ignorance will not be an adequate test for which is the healthier society. This problem for the criterion of the healthier society that uses choice-behind-a-veil arises because a worsening of health might unavoidably produce a characteristic (e.g., equality) that is of potential interest to choosers behind a thin veil. A less healthy society may also be preferred because it involves more illness overall but distributed in smaller quantities per person by contrast to another society in which there is much less illness overall but a few people are very ill. In this case, the society with more illness could be preferred if we give priority to reducing the degree of illness of the people who would be most ill. It is possible this analysis could even apply in the Paraplegia Case. Suppose the lower prevalence of the paraplegia at any given time resulted from the *same* group of people being paralyzed at different points of time, whereas the higher prevalence involved paraplegia in different groups of people at those times. Then we might prefer the society with higher prevalence because one group would not be paralyzed all the time. That is, no one would be as badly off in the society with greater prevalence as in the society with smaller prevalence.

II. Conflicts with Different Numbers of People

Suppose we are dealing with two-way micro conflict cases between potential recipients of a scarce resource. When there are an equal number of people in conflict who stand to be as badly off if not aided and gain the same if aided (and all other morally relevant factors are the same), and each person prefers that he be one of those who benefit, fairness dictates giving each side an equal chance for the resource by using a random decision procedure. This is so even though the health outcome would be the same even if we were unfair. Concern for each implies that we should give each a maximal equal chance.

But there may be a conflict situation in which *different numbers of* relevantly similar people are on either side and they stand to be as badly off and gain the same thing. (In micro situations, there will be few on either side; in macro, many.) The following Argument for Better Outcomes, applied in a micro context, tells us that it is a better outcome if more are helped: (1) It is worse for both B and C to die than for only B to die; (2) A world in which A dies and B survives is just as bad, from an impartial point of view, as a world in which B dies and A survives. Given (2), we can substitute A for B on one side of the moral equation in (1) and get that it is worse if A and C die than if B dies.

But even if it would be a worse outcome from an impartial perspective that A and C die rather than that B dies, that does not necessarily mean that it is right for us to save A and C rather than B. We cannot automatically assume it is morally permissible to maximize the good, for doing so may violate justice or fairness. (In other cases, seeking the greater good may be correctly constrained by justice. For example, we should not kill one innocent bystander to save five people from death.)

Here is an argument against its being unjust or unfair to save the greater number in the case involving A, B, and C. The Balancing Argument (I) claims that in this conflict, justice demands that each person on one side should have her interests balanced against those of one person on the opposing side; those who are not balanced out in the larger group help determine that the larger group should be saved. If we instead toss a coin between one person and any number on the other side, thereby giving each person an equal chance, we would behave no differently than if it were a contest between one and one. Suppose the presence of each additional person would make no difference to how we reason or to the outcome when his being considered could alter it. This seems to deny the equal significance of each person. Thus, justice and fairness do not here conflict with producing the most good.[12]

How might we extend these principles to conflicts when the individuals are *not* equally needy? Consider a case where the interests of two people (D and E) conflict with the interests of one (C). The position to which C would fall (death) and his potential gain (ten years of life) is matched by D, and they are otherwise equal. The potential loss and gain of E is very small—for example, a sore throat and its cure—and he is otherwise fine. To take away C's 50 percent chance of having ten years of life rather than dying in order to increase the overall good by helping D and E with the marginal benefit of a sore throat cure and satisfaction of E's preference for a minor improvement fails to show adequate respect for the single person who could avoid death and gain the ten years. This is because from her *personal point of view*, she is not indifferent between her being the one who gets something very important (being saved for ten years) and someone else getting it. The form of reasoning I am here using to justify *not* maximizing the good gives consideration from an impartial point of view to each individual's partial point of view, so it combines subjective and objective perspectives. Hence, I call it *Sobjectivity*. It accounts for why we should give fair chances when equal numbers of people compete for a scarce resource. It also implies that certain extra goods (like the throat cure) can be morally irrelevant. That is, it implies what I call the Principle of Irrelevant Goods.[13] Whether a good is irrelevant is context-dependent. Curing a sore throat is morally irrelevant when others' lives are at stake, but not when others' earaches are. (Notice that the ground for ignoring the small extra good in its role in the Sore Throat Case is not that we should not think of such matters in life-and-death situations. It would not be wrong to choose between two decision procedures that give D and E equal chances on the ground that one procedure will magically also cure a sore throat.)

This Sore Throat Case shows that we must refine the claim that what we owe each person is to balance her interests against the equal interests of an opposing person and let the remainder help determine the outcome. Sometimes the remainder is not determinative. Further, so long as what is at stake for C or D is large, it may be that *no number of the small losses occurring in each of many people should be aggregated on D's side* so as to outweigh giving C an equal chance of avoiding the large loss, for none of the many will suffer a significant loss.

The Sore Throat Case also raises the possibility that self-interested reasoning ex-ante behind a veil of ignorance cannot be relied on to give morally correct answers. For, using such reasoning, each person would consider that he maximizes his expected good by there being a procedure, ex-post, which saves one person and also allows us to provide the sore throat cure. Yet endorsing such a procedure seems the wrong conclusion.

But suppose the additional lesser loss in one of the pair is losing a leg. We should save a person's life for ten years rather than save someone else from losing a leg when all else is equal and these are the *only* morally relevant choices. However, perhaps it is correct to together save one person's life for ten years and a second person's leg rather than give a third person an equal chance at having his life saved alone. This might be because one and only one life will be saved no matter what we do and the loss of a leg is a large loss for another person. This would be evidence that giving someone *his equal chance for life* should not receive as much weight from the impartial point of view as saving a life when we would otherwise save no one. We might try to explain why this latter judgment is consistent with our judgment in the Sore Throat Case in the following way: According to most nonconsequentialist views, each of us who is otherwise fine has a duty to suffer (at least) a relatively minimal loss (e.g., a sore throat) in order to save another person's life. So long as suffering the small loss is a duty for any given person, no number of the small losses can be aggregated to outweigh saving the life. Further, if it matters to each person from his partial point of view that his be the life saved in a conflict situation, we each also have a duty to suffer a minimal loss in order to give someone else a significant chance at life. So long as suffering the small loss in order to give someone a significant chance at life is a duty for any given person, no number of the smaller losses can be aggregated and combined with another's life to outweigh someone's significant chance to live. However, when the loss is greater than the loss we each have a duty to suffer in order to save the life (e.g., losing a leg), then we should save the life and leg rather than give someone else an equal chance to have his life saved.[14]

So far, I have been discussing decision procedures that are consistent with what philosophers call "pairwise comparison." That is, we check to see that for everyone who will fall to a certain level on one side if not aided, there is someone who will fall to a very similar level on the other side before we consider those who will not fall to levels anywhere as bad in order to determine which side gets aided. This is one way of being sure we help the worst-off people first. However, I have also attended to how great a gain someone could receive if he is helped. For it is possible that if we cannot give the worst-off person very much, we should give more to those who would not be as badly off if not helped. This approach gives some priority to the worst off, but not lexical priority.

Furthermore, it is possible that principles which involve pairwise comparison to see who will be worse off are requirements of fairness in choosing whom to aid only in micro situations (e.g., in the emergency room, where no number of headaches, each occurring in different people, should be prevented for their own sake rather than certainly saving a few people to live for a considerable period of time).

To make macro decisions—for example, whether to invest in research to cure a disease that will kill a few people, depriving each of them of ten years of life, or in research to cure a disease that will only wither an arm in many—we might have another principle. Such a principle might permit aggregation of significant (though not insignificant) lesser losses (which can be corrected) to many people to outweigh greater losses to a few, even though no individual in the larger group would have as bad a fate as each individual in the smaller group would have. As such, it does not give absolute priority to helping the (even greatly) worst off. Whether a lesser loss is significant and hence may be aggregated over people would be determined by comparing it to the greater loss, and so determining if a lesser loss can be aggregated is context-dependent (as it was for the Principle of Irrelevant Goods). On this view, the important point is that whether a lesser loss should be aggregated over people to weigh against a greater loss in others is *not* merely a function of how many people suffer it, but also of its size relative to the size of the greater loss.

Notice that this may raise what seems to be a problem due to intransitivity: Suppose that relative to n, y is a significant lesser loss. So at the macro level, it may be better to prevent many people from losing y than to save a few from n. But relative to y, z is a significant lesser loss, and so it would be better to save a great many suffering z than a few suffering y. Yet, it may be that relative to n, z is not a significant loss, since "significant" is context-relative (it depends on what we are comparing). What should we do when we must choose among the three options?

My suggestion for dealing with this issue is as follows: If we can save a few suffering from n, we may save many from suffering y instead, but we should not go so far as to save a great many from suffering z. (This is so on the continuing assumption that the people involved are alike in all morally relevant respects besides the size of these losses.) This is true, even though if the few suffering n had never been part of our choice set; we should save a great many from z rather than save many from y. This is because which act is correct can depend on the alternatives we could bring about, even when we do not act on the alternative (save those suffering from n) whose presence helped eliminate an option (save many from z).[15]

Finally, in the micro-level cases involving different numbers of people, suppose we have a choice between helping one person (A) who will be very badly off and much benefited by our aid, or helping a couple of people (B and C) who will each be as badly off as A but not benefited as much by our aid. So long as the lesser benefit is significant, it is morally more important, I think, to distribute our efforts over more people, each of whom will be as badly off as the single person, rather than to provide a bigger benefit concentrated in one person (other things equal). One way to analyze this situation employs what I shall call Balancing Argument (II): We should find the part of the potential large gain to A (part 1) that is balanced by the smaller gain to B. Then we must decide how to break that tie between them. If we care about giving priority to those who are worst off, we will care more about benefiting the next person in the group, C, rather than giving an additional benefit (part 2) to A, who, had he received part 1, would already have more than C. This means that instead of breaking the tie between A-with-part-1 and B by giving A a greater benefit, we break the tie by helping two people, each to a lesser degree.[16]

III. Same Numbers of People in Conflict and Comparing Their Different Features

A theory of the fair distribution of scarce resources should also tell us if certain characteristics that one candidate for a resource has to a greater degree than another are morally relevant to deciding who gets the resource. I call this the problem of interpersonal allocation when there is *intrapersonal aggregation*, because one candidate has characteristics the other has *plus* others that can be relevant to allocation. We have already considered principles that may apply when additional goods we can achieve, if we help one rather than another of the worst-off people, are distributed over several people. The question arises whether we can revise these principles to apply when additional goods we can achieve are *concentrated* in one person rather than another.

A system I suggest for evaluating candidates for a resource who differ intrapersonally starts off with only three factors—need, urgency, and outcome—but other factors could be added. Urgency is defined here (atypically) as how badly someone's life *will* go if he is not helped. "Need" is defined as how badly someone's life *will have gone* if he is not helped. "Outcome" is defined as the difference in expected outcome produced by the resource relative to the expected outcome if someone is not helped—that is, the relative benefit someone will get from the resource.

The neediest people may not be the most urgent. Suppose C will die in a month at age 65 unless helped *now* and D will die in a year at age 20 unless helped *now*. I suggest that often this will mean that D is less urgent but needier, since one's life *often will have gone* much worse if one dies at 20 rather than at 65. (This does not mean we should always help the neediest; for example, if we could only extend the younger life to age 21 but could give the 65-year-old ten years more, this would be a reason to help the 65-year-old.)[17]

Notice that there is an ordinary sense of urgency in which both C and D are equally urgent, namely they require care just as soon—*now*—in order to be helped.[18] Here I have chosen to use "urgent" to refer to how bad one's prospects are; I shall use the term "urgent-care" if necessary to refer to how soon treatment is needed.

In thinking about how urgent or needy someone is, or how good an outcome is, we must think how badly or well life will go or have gone *in what ways?* In microallocation of health services, I believe we should be concerned with the "*health*-way" rather than overall well-being (including economic and cultural factors). This means that at the micro level, health is treated as a separate sphere of

justice.[19] So, if E would be in worse health than F, the fact that F would be economically much worse off than E is not a reason to say F is more urgent than E and treat
F with the health-care resource. But suppose E's health overall has been painlessly
much worse than F's in his life (e.g., limited mobility), but F now faces a lot of pain
and E just a little. It is possible that we should consider all *dissimilar* aspects of ill
health and help E, so that he will not have had to lead a much worse life healthwise
than F. On the other hand, since we can only help E's future in a small way and can
do nothing to undo his past, the much greater good we can do for F's future may
be determinative. (Some may find the judgment that we should help E more convincing when we ignore E's past but decide based on the fact that he but not F *will*
also have limited mobility *in the future*. That is, given that he, but not F, will have
to deal with the problem of limited mobility, should we not take care of E's pain
problem? Some may think it correct to consider only how much pain each will
have in the future or will have had overall, since some part of this pain is the aspect
of well-being we can affect now. I shall not here choose between these conflicting
ways of deciding.[20])

By contrast, at the macro level, when deciding whether to invest in providing one
health service or another, it might be that we should make an *all-things-considered
judgment* about how well off people will have been or will be if aided or not aided.
That is, the way in which people have fared and will fare in health may be considered together with the way they have or will fare economically and culturally. This
means health would not be treated as a *separate sphere of justice* at the macro level.
This has important implications for the very idea of "health equity." Suppose, for
example, that we can invest in curing a disease that causes the poor to die at age 70
or a disease that causes the rich to die at age 60. If we care about equality, we might
chose to invest in the former, since having an economically better life might compensate the rich for having a shorter one; things will be overall more equal if the
poor at least live longer, so long as their lives are worth living. *So, equity of health—
getting the just or fair amount of it—is not inconsistent with inequality of (opportunity for) it.* (We already knew this as a result of the discussion in section 1, for there
the possibility was raised that helping the worst off might, theoretically, require
inequality of prospects for health.) Even those who care about equality may not
care about equality of (opportunity for) health per se but rather equality of a
bundle of goods, including health as one good. It is when those who have less on
one dimension (e.g., health) *also* have less on other important dimensions of value
(e.g., wealth) that egalitarians should be most concerned about equality on a particular dimension.

Notice that if this is so, it alters how we look at such empirical results as the
Whitehall Study.[21] Researchers found a perfect correlation between class and
health in the positive direction. That is, as class went up, health went up; as class
went down, health went down. Concern over the data should not be merely that
there is correlation between wealth and health; presumably, it is the causal direction that is crucial. We should not be as disturbed if greater health *causes* greater

wealth, for that just means that when people are healthier, they are more productive, and that is one of the things we expect and even hope for. (Of course, if this
were the direction of causality, we may still be concerned that some are healthy
and others are not.) We should (plausibly) be more disturbed if the direction of
causality is such that greater wealth causes greater health, so that the poor being
short on money causes their being short on health. If we are disturbed by this data,
assuming the second causal direction, is this best described as concern over inequality of health—that is, concern that all classes do not have the same level of
health? Suppose the data showed a perfect correlation, only negative—that is, as
class goes up, health goes *down*; as class goes down, health goes *up*. I hypothesize
that we would not be as concerned with this second result as we are with the first,
yet there is just as much inequality in health on the basis of class in this second,
hypothetical result as in the first, actual result. I venture that we would be less
concerned because we think that the goods of high social class may compensate
for the poorer health. When there is such compensation, there may be *overall*
equality between classes.

Of course, it may be that overall equality is not the right goal if we can increase
the absolute position of some people further only with overall inequality. Hence,
suppose that wealthier people had better health but the inequalities of wealth were
just (for example, because they were necessary to improve the absolute condition
of the worst off overall, even including their relatively lower health). Then the
resulting inequality of health might not be unjust. On this view, we should be
disturbed by the Whitehall results only because we think the distribution of wealth
is unjust. (It might be unjust, in part, because it results in lower *absolute* health for
the worst off with no adequate compensations, by comparison with a different
distribution of wealth). An alternative view is that it is reasonable to be concerned,
even if the unequal distribution of wealth is *not* unjust, because health simply
should not be a positive function of wealth, at least if the poor would prefer to have
more health and would spend on it if only they had the money. (We might not be
as concerned if we knew that given more money, the poor would not spend it on
what produces health because they have a different reasonable preference ranking.)

This alternative view is based on the idea that we should treat health as a separate sphere, even at the macro level, in the way we treat liberal freedoms. We
would not consider a person who lacks a right that others have to free speech to be
adequately compensated by the fact that he has more money than they have or by
the fact that he has more wealth than he otherwise would have had. This should
also be the position of those who think that equal health is a precondition for
equal opportunity and that equal opportunity has priority over improving the economic or cultural condition of the worst off. If health should be treated as a separate sphere, we would have to compare how people are doing just along the health
dimension separately, even at the macro level. This could lead to even those with
more economic wealth or power than is just being helped to achieve the correct
and equal level of health. This may increase the *overall* unjust inequality between

them and others, for they would have equal health and more of everything else that is good. For this reason we might make getting the correct level of health conditional on unjustly better-off people ceding some of the other (admittedly) non-compensating goods they have in greater abundance than others do. (One way to do this is to require them to pay for more of their health care.) There is an asymmetry here: we cannot deny them their right to certain health prospects because they have other things; but we could deny them other things (e.g., retaining all their wealth) because they get correct health prospects. Of course, if inequality in wealth will always cause inequality in health to return (let alone lower levels of health in absolute terms), we may have to decide whether equalizing health (to the extent this is under our control) is worth imposing equality in wealth. Alternatively, if there is an intervening mechanism through which inequality in wealth produces differential health (such as better food and sanitation), we may be able to just interfere with that mechanism directly.

IV. Weighting of Factors

A. NEED AND URGENCY

Let us return to need in the microallocation context. To consider how much weight to give to need, we hold the two other factors of outcome and urgency constant and imagine two candidates who differ only in neediness. Often those who will have had the worse life healthwise are those who will have had fewer years alive if not helped with a scarce, lifesaving drug. Then one argument for taking differential need into account is fairness: give to those who, if not helped, will have had less of the good (e.g., life) that our resource can provide (at least if they are equal on other health dimensions) before giving to those who will have had more of it even if they are not helped. Fairness is a value that depends on comparisons between people. But even if we do not compare candidates, it can often be of greater moral value to give a certain unit of life to a person the less life he will have had if not helped—that is, the younger someone will die.

But need will matter more the more absolutely and comparatively needy a candidate is. Further, some differences in need may be governed by a Principle of Irrelevant Need, which implies that relative to a context, some differences in need are morally irrelevant. This is especially so when each candidate is absolutely needy, a big gain for each is at stake, and if the needier person is helped, he will wind up having more of the good (e.g., a longer life) than the person who was originally less needy than he. Need may also play a different role depending on whether life is at stake or quality of life is at stake. One reason for this is that a low quality of life can be less bad for someone than his dying. When it is, we deprive the needy of less if we do not give them priority when quality of life is at stake, and of more if we do not give them priority when life is at stake. (For a different view, see note 17.) A further difference between allocating treatments for quality and quantity is that if those who will have had more life are not helped to live, they will die and no longer be members of our society. By contrast, suppose we deny people who will have had qualitatively better lives (in virtue of their better pasts) a quality-improving drug and give it to those who will have had qualitatively worse lives if not helped. Then we create synchronic (i.e., same-time) inequality in quality of life between citizens that might be greater than if we had had the reverse allocation. This may lead to older citizens living on with lower quality of life than younger citizens have, and so lead to much social inequality between living members of society on the basis of age. If we reject this, we shall be insisting that how people compare at any given time may take precedence over whether they would have equal lives *overall*. (Of course, once this becomes policy, each generation will be treated in this way and wind up being equal overall with other generations.)

Returning to lifesaving resources, suppose there is conflict between helping the neediest person and helping the most urgent person (when we can give each the same benefit). I claim that when there is true scarcity, it can be more important to help the neediest than the most urgent. If scarcity is only temporary, the person in need of urgent-care should be helped first, since the others will be helped eventually anyway.[22]

Still, there are further constraints on the relevance of need (one concept of the worst off) in a correct theory of distribution. For example, it may be impermissible to give a resource to the person who will have had a worse life healthwise if he is not aided (because he will have had less overall of the good we can provide) if doing so fails to respect the rights of each person. Consider another context: If two people have a human right to free speech, how long someone's right will have been respected may be irrelevant in deciding whom to help retain free speech. If having health or life for a number of years were a human right, it might not be appropriate to ration resources on the basis of the degree to which people's rights will have been met (or on the basis of whether they will have had more of other goods). On this view, how much life one will have had would not be a reason to ration lifesaving resources on the basis of age, so long as one had not reached the age governed by right. If this is true, it implies that we should be very careful to determine whether people have rights to certain goods (rather than just an interest in having them). For it could have a big impact on which distributive principles we should use.

An additional consideration that militates against helping on the basis of need where this is linked to rationing lifesaving drugs according to age relates to the risks that it may be rational for each individual to take. Suppose the probability of conditions that threaten life is low in youth but high in old age, and there is a fixed total health resource budget/per person to be distributed over the course of her life. Assume also that (for the most part) if one dies as a young person, one will lose out on a longer future than if one dies in old age and one will also have had a *worse* life. Even on the latter assumptions, it would not necessarily make most sense to invest resources so as to insure against the smaller probability of death in youth (when the procedures funded by these resources will probably not be used) and ignore much higher probabilities of death in older age (when procedures would be useful). Suppose it turned out to be rational for people to accept some risk of death when young to ensure care when old. Then each person who is old now will have accepted (and survived) the risk he takes when young. It would be unfair to now deny him treatment to save the young person for whom it too was rational to accept the small risk of death through absence of resources.[23]

B. OUTCOME

Now we come to outcome. Some might think it appropriate to take into account all the effects of a resource in determining the outcome it produces. By contrast, at least in micro contexts, I suggest:

1. Some differences in outcome between candidates may be irrelevant because achieving them is not the goal of the "health sphere," which controls the resource. (For example, that only one potential recipient in the health-care sphere will write a novel if he receives a scarce drug should not count in favor of his getting it. The health-care system is not the National Endowment for the Arts.)

2. Effects on third parties whose health a resource helps only indirectly should be given less weight than direct health effects of the resource. For example, if we face a choice between saving a doctor and a teacher, the fact that the doctor will be irreplaceable in saving lives should not mean that all the lives he will save (an indirect effect of the resource he gets) are counted on his side against the teacher. (Hence, even if only health effects should count, not all health effects should count.[24])

3. Other differences in expected outcome between candidates for our resource may be covered by the Principle of Irrelevant Goods, even if they are part of the health sphere. For example, relative to the fact that each person stands to avoid death and live for ten years, the fact that one person can get a somewhat better quality of life or an additional year of life should not determine who is helped, given that each wants what she can get (and other things are equal). One explanation for this is that *what both are capable of achieving (ten years) is the part of the outcome about which each reasonably cares most in the context*, and each wants to be the one to survive. The extra good is frosting on the cake. The fact that someone might accept an additional risk of death (as in surgery) to achieve the "cake plus frosting" for herself does not necessarily imply that it is correct to impose an additional risk of death on one person so that another person, who stands to get the greater good, has a greater chance to live.[25]

However, it might be suggested that, in life and death decisions, any *significant* difference between two people in expected life years (even if not quality of life) should play a role in selecting whom to help. This result would be analogous to the claim that if we could save x's life or else y's life plus z's leg, we should do the latter. Still, because the large additional benefit would be concentrated in the same person who would already be benefited by having her life saved for at least the same period as the other candidate, the additional good may count for less in determining who gets the resource than it does when the additional benefit is distributed to a third person. This is on account of the greater moral importance of first helping either person avoid the bad fate of dying faced by each, and the diminishing moral value of providing an additional benefit to someone who already stands to gain a big benefit (e.g., ten years of life) that the other candidate can also get. (The same issue arises for large differences in expected quality of life among candidates for a resource in situations where improving quality of life is the point of the resource.[26])

In between the irrelevant differences in outcomes and those that are large enough to outweigh other factors, there might be differences in outcome that should be treated by giving people chances in proportion to the good of the differential outcome.

What if taking care of the neediest or most urgent conflicts with producing the best relevant difference in outcome? Rather than always favoring the worst off, we might assign multiplicative factors in accord with need and urgency by which we multiply the expected outcome of the neediest and urgent. These factors represent the greater moral significance of a given outcome going to the neediest (or most urgent), but the nonneediest could still get a resource if her expected differential outcome was very large. Furthermore, doing a significant amount to raise those who are very badly off in absolute terms to an appropriate minimal level of well-being might have lexical priority over even an enormous improvement in those already much better off.

My views on outcome, need, and urgency can be summarized in what I call an *outcome modification procedure for allocation*. We first assign points for each candidate's differential expected outcome. We then check the absolute level of need and urgency of candidates. If the need or urgency of some puts them below a certain minimal level of well-being (e.g., very needy) and the good we can do would significantly raise them toward the minimal level, they receive the resource. For those above this minimal level of well-being (e.g., not very needy), we assign multiplicative factors for their need and urgency in accordance with the moral importance of those factors relative to each other and relative to outcome. We multiply the outcome points by these factors. The candidate with a sufficiently higher point score gets the resource. If the difference is too small to be morally relevant, we give equal chances. If it is in between, chances in proportion to the score might be suitable. At sufficiently low levels of absolute need, significant differences in outcome alone may be determinative.[27, 28]

V. QALYs and DALYs

Quality-adjusted life years (QALYs) and disability-adjusted life years (DALYs) are used to measure the impact illness has on someone in terms of both morbidity and mortality; they also measure the impact of care on someone in terms of reducing both morbidity and mortality. The theory of outcomes is that we can do more than merely count the number of years that will (we expect) be gained as a result of health intervention—note that even this is a step beyond merely considering whether a life has been saved but not considering *for how long it will be saved*. We also count how good these years will be. So we may multiply the number of years of life by the quality of each year. Alternatively, we may determine how effective aid is by considering how badly someone's life would have gone—or as it is said, how disabled he would have been—without the intervention. In this way, we see how much reduction in such disabled years we produce by the intervention. We aim to increase QALYs and decrease DALYs (though not by eliminating the life).[29]

How do we measure the quality of a life or the degree to which it is disabled? Philosophers have tried to offer hedonistic, desire-satisfaction, and objective list theories of good and bad lives to answer such questions. That is, they have suggested that a life is of higher or lower quality depending on how much pleasure/pain there is in it, how many of one's desires (regardless of the object of desire) are satisfied, or how much of certain objective goods (including but not limited to pleasure/no pain) there are in it. But those who use QALYs and DALYs do not use such philosophical theories. They take surveys of either ordinary people (in QALYs) or experts (in DALYs), asking them to rate the quality of various lives with or without various limitations in them. The aim is to assign numbers to the effects of aid. Two tests are often used in achieving this goal: the tradeoff within one life test and the standard gamble test. (I shall deal separately with the test dealing with tradeoffs between people.) In the first, we are asked how many years with disability x we would trade for how many years of perfect health. So if ten years of life as a paralyzed person would be exchanged for five years as a healthy person (ranked at 1), we know that being paralyzed is to be assigned a 0.5 value. The tradeoff test makes clear that people would exchange some length of life for some increased quality of life (or disability reduction). The standard gamble test asks one to imagine what risk of death one would take (e.g., in surgery) to exchange some length of life at one level of quality/disability for the same length at a higher quality. For example, is a 40 percent chance of death and a 60 percent chance of perfect health equivalent to a 100 percent chance of life with paralysis? The greater the chance of death one would take to achieve perfect health, the worse is the state from which one is escaping, presumably.[30]

Let us consider the DALY, in particular. Suppose perfect health is rated at 1; wearing glasses reduces the quality of the life to 0.999 (and so one is disabled to 0.001); a certain form of paralysis brings one down to 0.5. Having this information can be important in deciding how much good we can do if we aid or how much badness will occur if we do not. It has been argued that it can also help us decide whom to aid when we cannot aid everyone. For example, if we think it just to give priority to helping the worst off (not necessarily overall worst, but perhaps only healthwise worst), it is important to know that paralysis is worse than wearing eyeglasses. If we ranked paralysis no lower than wearing eyeglasses, we could not argue in favor of investing in cures or preventions for paralysis rather than near-sightedness (a macro decision) or treating a person to cure or prevent paralysis in an emergency room rather than to cure or prevent nearsightedness (a micro decision). Of course, even if we would reduce more DALYs if we treated paralysis rather than nearsightedness, the cost of doing so may be much greater, and hence the DALYs reduced per dollar (cost effectiveness of allocating) might be greater if we instead treated nearsightedness. (If this were so, it also implies that for every one paralysis we cure or prevent, we could cure or prevent hundreds of cases of nearsightedness. I shall return to this issue below.)

Notice that I have mentioned both curing and preventing a disability. It seems reasonable to think that one would want to avoid (and hence prevent) a disability in accordance with how bad it would be to have the disability, and hence how much one would want to be cured of it if one had it. If one knew that if one fell into a state x, there would be no good reason to try to leave it, would it be reasonable to want to avoid it? Surprisingly, the answer might be yes, as going into the state might be disruptive of one's current plans but once in it one alters one's plan so that there is no more reason to leave it.[31] Avoiding disruption of current plans might be the only reason to avoid state x. Brock has suggested that this is why nonparalyzed people rank paralysis as worse than people who are already paralyzed. If avoiding disruption of current plans were the only reason, or at least a contributing reason, to avoid paralysis, it would be a reason for society to put a higher value on prevent-ing a nonparalyzed person from becoming paralyzed and a lower value on curing a paralyzed person. (Another less normative and more purely psychological finding might be pointed to in this connection. Psychologists Daniel Kahnemann and Amos Tversky report that subjects ask higher compensation ex-ante than ex-post for an injury.[32] That is, when asked how much they would want in order to go through some loss, they ask for more than they ask as compensation once they have suffered the loss.)

However, suppose that those with disabilities must engage in less intrinsically valuable activities and/or have diminished freedom to choose whether to do some-thing or not (even if their remaining options are good ones). These might be rea-sons, I believe, to rate curing a disability as highly as preventing it. In any case, in what follows, I shall assume this is so.[33]

Some recommend employing DALYs and QALYs in allocating scarce re-sources between people. Some who recommend this also believe that in allocating, we should first help those who would have been worst off if not aided, at least when expense per DALY is the same as it would be if we helped those who would not have been worst off. Indeed, raising QALYS or lowering DALYs and helping the worst off are not incompatible. But even when the choice is between helping two people, helping the worst off need not follow *merely* from trying, for example, to minimize DALYs. This is because in helping the worst off, we might not reduce as many DALYs as in helping someone who would not have been as badly off without aid. Further, if we must choose between helping a greater number of people each avoid a small disability and one person avoid a large disability (when the people are otherwise relevantly similar), total DALYs reduced could be the same. Yet those who think it is right to favor the worst off might still prefer to help that person in these cases. Dan Brock points out that if we just consider people's rankings of various health conditions and 1 represents perfect health for one year while wearing eyeglasses reduced health by 0.001 per year, then we could produce as much good by relieving one thousand people of the need to wear eyeglasses for twenty years as if we save someone's life who would go on to live in perfect health for twenty years.[34] But if we should try to help the person who will have been worst off without aid (still assuming same cost/per DALY reduced), we should save the life nevertheless.

I agree with Brock about this last case. However, notice that preventing the aggregate of small disabilities may not always be the morally wrong answer. For example, suppose that having a sprain for a year reduced one's health to 0.9. Might saving the life of an 80-year-old for one additional year be morally the equivalent of providing (a) ten people with a drug that relieved their sprain for a year, or (b) one person with a drug that relieved his sprain for ten years (Eighty-Year-Old Case)? This case reminds us that saving a life does not always have the same moral significance. The possibility of option (b) should remind us that aggregation can occur intrapersonally—within one life—and that many small losses or gains (in the sense of avoidance of these losses) occurring to one person can have more moral significance than many small losses (or avoidance of these) occurring to many people. Twenty small headaches occurring over a short period in one life can be a much worse outcome than twenty small headaches, each occurring in the lives of twenty people. Notice also that the moral difference between alternatives (a) and (b) decreases depending on whether we conceive of each of the ten people in (a) as either facing one year in his life in which he suffers from a sprain (a year we can improve) or, by contrast, facing the same ten years of sprain as the person in (b), but having only one year of relief from that greater burden. This latter point reminds us that often small disabilities can occur to people who have other major problems. Aggregating the cure of many small disabilities that will occur in the lives of many who each will be among the worst off might have greater significance than helping one person avoid being one of the worst off by improving his condition greatly.

Finally, we have been considering a case in which we might save one person's life for a year, and we probably imagine this as *rescuing* someone from death. We might put the choice differently: we have to decide when someone is 50 whether to give him medical treatment that is good enough to help him live to age 81 or only good enough to help him live to age 80. If we give him the medical care that helps him live to only age 80, we will be able to help someone else not suffer from a sprain for ten years. This case compares intrapersonal aggregation in the latter person and long-term prospects for life (rather than rescue efforts) in the former. In such a case, by contrast with Brock's original case, it may be less clear that we should favor extending the life over avoiding aggregated smaller losses.

What if more DALYs could be reduced if we aid 1,001 people who are otherwise fine so that they no longer need eyeglasses for twenty years, at less cost per DALY reduction than if we save someone's life for twenty years? We might still think it right to help the person have his life saved because he will have been much worse off if not aided than any other person and will be greatly benefited. We could use a method like that embodied in the outcome modification procedure (described above) to represent favoring this person in a DALY system: Multiply the number of DALYs reduced when we help the person who would die by a factor that represents the greater moral value of aiding him. This will also lower the cost/ per DALY reduction in his case, in a sense.

But now consider the following scenario: One person is on island A, and another person is on island B. They share all the same properties, except that one has recently lost a hand and the other has not.[35] We can save the life of either one but not both. Each will be as badly off as the other if we do not help him (dead). But if we help the person without the hand, we cannot reduce DALYs as much. (Call this the Islands Case.) I think it is morally wrong to decide to aid on this ground. We cannot rely on the principle of giving weight to the worst off to account for this conclusion, since each will have been, by hypothesis, as badly off as the other if not aided. However, the Principle of Irrelevant Goods, which I described above, might account for the right decision.

The point in the Islands Case seems to be that the part of what is most important to each person can be had by either—long life saved with good quality of life. Furthermore, we should take seriously from an *objective* point of view the fact that each person, from his *subjective* perspective, wants to be the one to survive. We should, therefore, not deprive either of his equal chance for the great good of extended survival for the sake of producing the additional benefit to one person. This benefit is irrelevant in this context, though perhaps not in another. This is especially true when that one person would be someone who would already be getting the other great benefit of additional life. (That is, it is a case of concentrated rather than dispersed additional good.)

Now consider the Islands Case (2), exactly like the Islands Case, except that there are six people on each island and each person on island A will have recently lost his hand while all on island B will be intact. The additional claim based on the Principle of Irrelevant Goods is that if any individual's having a benefit that is an irrelevant good is not a reason to deprive someone else of an equal chance for a major good, then no number of these benefits aggregated across many people (possibly yielding a large total) should deprive other people of their equal chances for a major good.

On the basis of these cases, we can see that it is compatible with recognizing that not having a hand makes a life worse to think that, relative to the question of whose life we should save, the absence of a hand could be a morally irrelevant consideration. Hence, targeting funds to replace a missing hand seems to be consistent with giving equal weight to saving the lives of the disabled and the nondisabled at least sometimes.[36]

VI. Ex-ante Objections

Here are some objections that may be raised to giving two people equal chances to have their lives saved when saving one will yield a larger benefit or reduction in disability (e.g., cure of paraplegia): (1) The paralyzed person would himself accept some additional risk of death if the treatment we used on him would not only save his life but cure his paralysis. (People do, after all, undergo surgery with risk of death in order to remove their disabilities.) Does this not mean that we should be allowed to impose that greater risk of death on him in order that someone else who is not paralyzed be saved? (2) Ex-ante, behind a veil of ignorance, before we know whether we are paralyzed or not, we should assume that we had an equal probability of being the paralyzed or nonparalyzed person. Hence, we increase our own chances of living a nonparalyzed life—which we prefer—if we agree, ex-ante, to a policy which always saves the nonparalyzed person's life. The conclusions of (1) and (2) differ slightly, since (1) may only require us to give a greater proportional chance of survival to the person who will not be disabled; (2) requires complete preference.

A response to (1) is that being willing to take a risk of death in order to achieve a benefit for oneself is morally different from risking death in order to benefit someone else. A response to (2) is related to the response to (1), since a similar use of ex-ante reasoning in (1) could suggest that one is, in a sense, taking the risk of death for oneself. This is because behind a veil of ignorance, one should think that for all one knows, it is oneself who will be benefited if the odds favor the nondisabled person. A response to this extension of (1), as well as to (2), is that this form of ex-ante reasoning is morally problematic. Thomas Scanlon has argued that it is a mistake to think of people behind the veil of ignorance deciding what is morally correct by each imagining that he might possibly occupy any one of various positions in real life, though, of course, he can occupy only one.[37] Scanlon is concerned that the procedure to be used in deciding on principles—that both do not favor one person over another and that one could accept independently of knowing what one's actual position is or will be—adequately respect the separateness of persons. Scanlon agrees that it can be helpful in finding such principles to use a procedure in which each imagines that he is in every other person's actual position in life (outside the veil of ignorance), having that person's perspective on things, in order to see whether each person in any actual position could approve (or not reject) a proposed principle governing relations between people. While Scanlon does not make use of a veil of ignorance, his interpretation of impartiality implies that (i) if no person in any position outside the veil could reasonably reject a principle on his own behalf, then (ii) any individual behind a veil of ignorance could agree to the principle. If someone from some position beyond the veil could reasonably reject the principle, then it could not be agreed to by any (in the sense of every) person behind the veil of ignorance. The reasonableness of rejection beyond the veil is a function of comparing the possible complaints to different principles of people in different (generic) positions.

Scanlon rejects an alternative interpretation of impartiality according to which it is best exemplified by a single person deciding behind a veil of ignorance on the assumption that he has an equal probability of being in any person's position beyond the veil. The assumption of equal chances of being in any position is supposed to ensure that one does not choose principles that favor one position over another. But there is still no requirement that a decision-maker behind the veil take account of whether each person actually occupying each (generic) position could reasonably reject a principle, before he, behind the veil, decides to accept it. Rather, the order is the reverse of what it is on Scanlon's view (described above): (i)$_a$ if any individual behind the veil of ignorance would choose a principle on his own behalf, then (ii)$_b$ no person in any actual position outside the veil could reasonably reject the principle. It is this Order Reversal, as I shall refer to it, that seems to lie at the heart of Scanlon's concerns, for he thinks it is the wrong way to take account of the points of view of separate persons. He says:

> Whatever rules of rational choice this single individual, concerned to advance his own interests as best he can, is said to employ, this reduction of the problem to the case of a single person's self-interested choice should arouse our suspicion . . . it is important to ask whether this single individual is held to accept a principle because he judges that it is one he could not reasonably reject whatever position he turns out to occupy, or whether, on the contrary, it is supposed to be acceptable to a person in any social position because it would be the rational choice for a single self-interested person behind the veil of ignorance.[38]

In Scanlon's picture, the one person behind the veil would not conceive of the different positions beyond the veil as mere slots into which he might fall. He might imagine them as ones he actually occupies, as if he occupied all simultaneously.[39] In this way, he is forced to think of all the different people who will actually occupy each position, which is what is ultimately important. Indeed, to return to an issue raised at the beginning of this chapter, Scanlon believes that forcing people to identify in this way with each person is why Rawls uses a thick veil (excluding probability calculations). Notice also that on Scanlon's interpretation of impartiality, one does not need to assume that ex-ante one has an equal chance of being in any position in society, for one would have to check whether someone who is in a particular type of position could reasonably agree to or reject a principle even if there were not ex-ante an equal chance of being in that position.

Scanlon also argues by example against the conclusion that an individual's choosing behind the veil of ignorance a principle that maximizes his average expected good bears on the inability to reasonably raise a complaint to an arrangement based on this principle. The example he employs involves ex-ante average good being maximized because a principle will allow many people to receive small benefits when only a few will be very badly off. He thinks that the people who are badly off could reasonably reject the principle because no one of the many stands to gain much individually while others are very badly off, at least when there is an alternative that could greatly improve the worse off at a small cost to each of the many.

One concern with accepting Scanlon's position on impartiality is that even he can accept that oftentimes an individual's actual (rather than hypothetical) choice to take a risk of falling into a disfavored position *does* undermine his complaint if he loses; such a choice can be a substitute for considering his perspective simply as a person in a disfavored position. Scanlon would either have to explain why hypothetical choice is different or in which circumstances taking risks are acceptable and in which not.

Let us consider this and related issues further in the context of whether to employ QALYs and DALYs to allocate resources. Consider that many people might take a 5 percent risk of death (thereby risking losing, let us say, twenty years of life) in order to have a 95 percent chance of being cured of paraplegia. What does this data on intrapersonal risk imply for interpersonal decisions? For example, does this data from the individual case imply that as a society, we can allow five people to die of a disease, thereby robbing them each of twenty years of life, so that ninety-five people can be cured of paralysis, when the one hundred are otherwise relevantly similar for moral purposes? This question might be asked about allocation in a microallocation scheme, where the one hundred people came into the emergency room at the same time, as well as in a macro decision about whether to invest our research funds in a cure for a rare life-threatening disease or in a cure for a more common disease that causes paralysis.

It might be said that when an individual takes a chance, no one may die and he may benefit. Indeed, he takes the risk hoping this is so. And when each person in the society thinks of the gamble in his case, he may also imagine that he will not die and hope to benefit. But *in a large enough group, some people will certainly die* and others will be benefited. Perhaps this is a morally significant reason not to derive the social-welfare function from the combination of individual welfare functions. This conclusion might seem to follow if we think that we will get the morally wrong principle of social justice from ex-ante reasoning behind a veil of ignorance that involves each person's thinking of what probability he has for occupying each outcome-position—for example, ninety-five chances to be one of the cured and five to be one of the dead if we invest in the paralysis cure. Rather, the veil of ignorance should lead each person to take seriously the fates of the separate persons who will actually occupy each of the outcome-positions, including the ones involving death.

However, there might be a less extreme position. Contrast the following two types of cases: (a) Some people each take a small risk of a very bad fate (death) in order to get something good (high chance of cure of paralysis), and there is no way to rescue someone if the bad fate comes to pass. This could occur when they agree that all should invest in a cure for a common paralyzing disease rather than a cure for a rare fatal one. (b) Some people each take the same risk (as in [a]) and there comes to be a way to rescue those who face the bad fate, because it has just been discovered that all the medicine available for curing the paralysis can also save these lives. Suppose that it would be reasonable for each person behind a veil of ignorance and beyond it to take the small risk of death for the sake of the good of a paralysis cure. I do not think this implies that people who would take such a risk should also agree to be left to certainly die (or to leave another to actually die) from a fatal disease when they could be rescued, in the case in (b). Ex-ante, by hypothesis each person's risk of getting the fatal disease and dying was small and his chance of benefit great even if we knew with certainty that someone would actually get the fatal disease. Once a person gets the fatal disease, his risk of death is not small, his death is certain.[40] (Notice also there might be cases in which it would be reasonable to run a considerable risk of death for a benefit, but there could come a point where, though one's risk of death does *not* increase, the chance of a benefit goes away. If it were possible to rescue the person at that point, these cases might sometimes have the same implications as those in which risk of death increases.)

We have supposed that saving the dying persons requires taking away use of all the drug from everyone who had also taken the risk of death and now needs the drug to cure paralysis. Given enough people, we knew ex-ante that some would get the fatal disease. If we should collect all the medicine in order to save the victims of the fatal disease in the emergency room, does this imply that we should never have allowed so many people to take the risk of dying to begin with in order to get a paralysis cure? I do not think that it must have this implication, so long as we keep in mind the distinction between running the risk of dying of the fatal disease at a time in the future when there would be no way to cure it because the drug only cures paralysis and dying at a time in the future when using the paralysis drug could also save lives. At the time when each of many people takes the first risk, the risk of dying is small. Therefore, it might be worth bearing this risk for the paralysis cure even though doing so conflicts with maximin or giving priority to the worst off. At the time that we must decide whether to save some from the fatal disease, they are certain to die without treatment. Saving them could be worth not curing paralysis in many others. This conclusion could be reached by someone like Scanlon, who uses pairwise comparison to decide on distributive justice (even though he is not a maximiner). Scanlon could reach the conclusion that seems correct, namely that willingness to take a small risk of unavoidable death in the future need not be inconsistent with using all the medicine rather than not rescuing people from certain death.[41]

Suppose that one knows ex-ante that the fatal illness will occur and it will be possible to collect all the medicine set aside for paralysis to save a few. Then, indeed, it might not make sense to develop the paralysis cure that will be used to save lives. This has the admittedly odd implication that the better we get at using all sorts of resources to stop immediate death, the fewer risks of death it makes sense for each to take for the sake of creating resources that will produce smaller benefits to many people. However, if one were at least unsure whether death in the future would be avoidable, it remains open whether it could make sense to take the risk. What if some of the medicine will have been consumed before the time that a recall of all medicine would be necessary (and useful) for saving some? If it was not clear that all the medicine would be useful for life saving, it could make sense to prefer using it for other purposes rather than hoarding it for the possibility of lifesaving treatments that might never be needed.[42]

Finally, it is important to realize that the permissibility of investing in cures for a more common but less serious illness, which would make it impossible to save a few people from a fatal illness, also does not imply that it is permissible to deliberately arrange for our being unable to save the smaller number from death rather than the larger number from paralysis in the emergency room, should this be possible. Consider an analogous case that I call the Ambulance Case: Suppose it is morally permissible for a community to use an ambulance because this saves many lives (or saves many from paralysis), though it will, foreseeably, kill a few people as it speeds to the hospital. This need not mean that it is permissible to install a device on the ambulance which makes it impossible for it to stop before fatally hitting someone when stopping means that more people in the ambulance will not reach the hospital in time to be saved.[43]

These cases bear on the treatment/prevention distinction in general.[44] Suppose that investing in preventing a given fatal disease will minimize the number of people (unidentified) who will die of it by comparison to investing in a treatment for the same disease. However, prevention is not perfect and investing in it to minimize deaths also gives each person a small risk of being someone for whom we will have no treatment once he is sick. Given what we have said above, it is arguably reasonable to invest in prevention. However, this need not imply that at the time someone is certain to die without treatment, it would be irrational and morally wrong to use money that had not yet been used for prevention in order to treat. This could be so if the sick person's risk of death once he is sick is much greater than the risk of death of each of those left with reduced prevention.

It might also be argued that just as we should abide by deontological side-constraints against harming people rather than do what maximizes lives saved, there are even reasons to decide against investing in prevention (contrary to what was suggested above). For example, not refraining from treating people when they are desperate (because they are certain to die) might be a morally more important relation in which to stand to people than ensuring that they never get a disease when they are not desperate (because their chance of being among the number of certain-to-occur cases of the fatal disease is relatively small). This could be true even though *more people will actually die* through absence of prevention than will be saved by treatment because we will lack resources to save all people who eventually get ill.[45]

Notes

1. This chapter is based on my chapter "Health and Equity," in *Summary Measures of Population Health*, eds. C. Murray and J. Salomon (Geneva, Switzerland: World Health Organization, 2005), and "To Whom," *Hastings Center Report*, July–August 1994. It adds material from my *Intricate Ethics* (New York: Oxford University Press, 2007) and from unpublished sections of a longer version of my "Should You Save This Child?," published as a response in *Reconciling Our Aims* by Allan Gibbard (New York: Oxford University Press, 2008).

2. I dealt with this issue at length in *Morality, Mortality,* Vol. I: *Death and Whom to Save From It* (New York: Oxford University Press, 1993).

3. However, as Johann Frick has pointed out, we could aim to maximize fairness as a feature of end-states within constraints imposed by fairness as a side-constraint. This is still consistent with fairness being distinguishable from goodness.

4. Equal health, equal prospects of health, and equal opportunity for health are obviously different. To simplify, I will often speak of equal health but much of what is said would apply if the other terms consistently replaced "equal health."

5. See Derek Parfit, "Equality or Priority?," the Lindley Lecture (Lawrence, KS: University Press of Kansas, 1991).

6. Norman Daniels, *Just Health Care* (Cambridge: Cambridge University Press, 1985).

7. Rawls's first principle of justice calls for *maximal* equal liberty. This too means that it is possible that unequal liberty could increase the absolute level of liberty of some from what it would be under maximal equal liberty. (However, Rawls himself does not allow for this, which suggests that he thinks there is a qualitative difference between certain "status goods" and quantifiable goods.) See John Rawls, *A Theory of Justice* (Cambridge, MA: Harvard University Press, 1971).

8. M. Marmot, *Social Causes of Social Inequalities in Health*. Working paper no. 99/01, Harvard Center for Population and Development Studies, 1999.

9. For more on the relation of NSF to equality of opportunity, see chapter 19 this volume.

10. C. J. L. Murray, J. A. Salomon, and C. D. Mathers, "A Critical Examination of Summary Measures of Population Health," In *Summary Measures of Population Health*, eds. C. J. L. Murray and J. A. Salomon (Geneva, Switzerland: World Health Organization *Bulletin of the World Health Organization*, 2002), pp. 13–40.

11. Salomon and Mathers, "A Critical Examination of Summary Measures," p. 24.

12. For more on whether numbers should count, see chapter 20 this volume.

13. In *Morality, Mortality*, Vol. I, I called it the Principle of Irrelevant Utilities.

14. For problems with this approach, see my *Intricate Ethics*, chapter 1, and my *Morality, Mortality,* Vol. I.

15. I argued similarly in proposing a solution to the problem of the Repugnant Conclusion. See *Morality, Mortality*, Vol. II (New York: Oxford University Press, 1996).

16. I developed this additional balancing procedure in responding to Derek Parfit's discussion of cases of this sort in an unpublished manuscript. For more on this, see my *Intricate Ethics*, chapter 2.

17. It is interesting to note that most ordinary people surveyed by Erik Nord et al. disagree that being older makes someone less needy of more life than a younger person. Furthermore, they think that where life is at stake, there should be less distinction between helping young and old, while when quality of life is at stake one might favor the young. Their (unconscious) reasoning seems to be the opposite of the one I would suggest for these two cases. That is, when something they think is very important (life) is at stake, they think we should not distinguish between people; when something they think is less important (quality) is at stake, we may distinguish between young and old. I get the opposite result by taking seriously that having had more life already can make one less needy of more life than someone else, other things equal, even if life remains important to those who have had more of it. See E. Nord, J. Richardson, A. Street, H. Kuhse, and P. Singer, "Maximizing Health Benefits vs. Egalitarianism: An Australian Survey of Health Issues," *Social Science and Medicine* 41(10) (1995): 1429–37. In the case of quality of life, the fact that both young and old will be alive together in the same society suggests that we should promote more equality between them at a given time.

18. As pointed out to me by Derek Parfit.

19. For the idea of separate spheres of justice, see M. Walzer, *Spheres of Justice* (New York: Basic Books, 1983).

20. For more on this, see F. M. Kamm, "Owing, Justifying and Rejecting," *Mind* 111(442) (2002): 323–54, reprinted with revisions in my *Intricate Ethics*; and T. M. Scanlon, *What We Owe to Each Other* (Cambridge, MA: Harvard University Press, 1998).

21. Cited in Marmot, *Social Causes of Social Inequalities in Health*.

22. In *Morality, Mortality*, Vol. I, I did not distinguish urgency from urgent-care and hence mistakenly claimed that in temporary scarcity, the urgent should be treated before the needier.

23. I take this to be the main point of the view Norman Daniels defends in *Am I My Parents' Keeper? An Essay on Justice between the Young and the Old* (New York: Oxford University Press, 1988).

24. It might be suggested that this is true because the person who would *not* be selected for aid is being inappropriately evaluated from only an instrumental point of view. That is, because he is not useful to others, he is rejected. But consider the following case: We have a scarce resource to distribute and if we give it to A, he can then also carry it to another person, C, who needs our resource. B cannot do this. In this case, it is permissible, I think, to select A over B, excluding B since he cannot be instrumentally useful. This is because doing so helps us to better serve those who directly need our resource. Hence (surprisingly), it seems it is not essentially distinguishing persons on the basis of their instrumental role that determines if our behavior is objectionable, but whether we are doing this in order to use our resource for its best *direct* health effects.

25. Again, this conclusion conflicts with the choice that would be made if each person behind a veil of ignorance were trying to maximize his expected good. We consider other possible explanations of better outcomes being irrelevant in chapter 21 this volume.

26. Erik Nord claims that most of the people he surveyed do not care about the length of life that someone will live in deciding whom to help (above a significant

outcome), but they do care about the probability of someone achieving any significant outcome. Presumably, this means they would favor giving a resource to someone who will almost certainly achieve a good outcome, rather than to someone who would have a much lower chance of a good outcome. This could lead to problematic results. For if one is offered certainty of getting two years of extra life with one treatment or a 50 percent chance of twenty years with another treatment, and one is young, it is not unreasonable to think one is doing better to take the latter option. Suppose we combine people's surveyed tendency to discount degree of good outcome (above a significant amount) with the relevance in their mind of probability of good outcome. This combination implies that they could favor giving a scarce lifesaving resource to the young person rather than to someone else when the young person chooses the first treatment but not when he chooses the second. This favors the conservative person over the maximizer, inappropriately it might seem. See Nord et al., "Maximizing Health Benefits vs. Egalitarianism." For more on whether intrapersonally rational choices should bear in interpersonal selection of candidates, see chapter 21 this volume.

27. This procedure can still be only a rough guide where more than two candidates are present. Since what we ought to do is a function of what the alternatives are, it may not always be right to produce what gives the highest score. For example, in the case I discussed above involving one person who will lose n, many who will lose x, and yet more who will lose z, I argue that we should help prevent z rather than x if it were only a choice between x and z, but should help x if it were a choice among all three.

28. Though we sometimes must make choices between different people and different types of losses, an important issue in rationing theory is whether we can avoid someone's getting no benefit because we can in some way help everyone. This is still a form of rationing, I think. For example, if we can find out what the lowest *useful* divisible unit of something is, we may help all. Alternatively, we may reduce the chances of anyone's being helped so as to increase the possibility of all being helped. For example, we might exchange a 100 percent probability of saving ninety-nine people plus definitely losing one person, on the one hand, for a 99 percent chance of saving all one hundred people plus a 1 percent chance of saving no one, on the other hand. We might do this because the possibility of a fate shared by all may be attractive to us for reasons of solidarity. An alternative explanation is that, though the expected utility is the same in both parts of each option, we give more weight to the probability parts of each option—that is, we attach more weight to *certainty* of a small negative factor than to a very small probability of a large negative factor. But notice that at the micro level of individual benefit, we may be reluctant to deprive any one of the ninety-nine people of the certainty of being saved if doing this involved a third alternative, in which we select from all one hundred, one person to die. In this procedure, the one person who will die might be someone who originally would have been saved *instead*. At the micro level, any obligation one has to share one's own decent prospects with others who face a worse fate does not often extend to switching places with the worst off, so that they are now better off and one receives their worst prospects. At the macro level of social benefit, however, we are used to policies which, for example, maximize the number of people who are helped, although this also involves switching the people who occupy the positions of have and have-not.

29. For more on tests used to determine QALYs and DALYs rankings of life with different conditions, see chapter 21 this volume.

30. Is it possible that state A could be worse than state B and yet we would take a greater risk of death to avoid B than A? Yes, if there were some reason why it would be inappropriate to risk death to avoid A in particular (e.g., because one deserved A). Certainly, we could take an equal risk of death to avoid state A and state B, even if one of the states is worse than the other, if the less bad one is already bad enough to make a maximal risk worthwhile. The validity of the gamble test is threatened by these possibilities. Notice also that results might differ for (i) a test that involves risking earlier death in the *near future* for a better life henceforth and (ii) a test that involves risking earlier death much further in the future for a better life henceforth.

31. See D. W. Brock, "Ethical Issues in the Use of Cost Effectiveness Analysis for the Prioritization of Health Care Resources," in *Bioethics: A Philosophical Overview*, ed. George Khusfh (Dordrecht: Kluwer, 2004).

32. D. Kahneman, "The Cognitive Psychology of Consequences and Moral Intuition," Tanner Lectures in Human Values, University of Michigan. Unpublished work, 1994.

33. Wanting a cure for a longstanding condition could be an indication that the cured life is thought to be better even by the disabled person, though it might just indicate a desire to be like the majority. If the majority had a longstanding disability and they desired a cure, however, this would be stronger evidence that the condition is worse than the nondisabled one.

34. Brock, "Ethical Issues," note 28.

35. I say "recently" to hold their pasts equal.

36. For more about disabilities and the equitable distribution of scarce resources, see chapter 21 this volume.

37. T. M. Scanlon, "Contractualism and Utilitarianism," in *Utilitarianism and Beyond*, eds. A. Sen and B. Williams (Cambridge: Cambridge University Press, 1982).

38. Scanlon, "Contractualism and Utilitarianism," note 34, pp. 124–25.

39. This is an idea suggested by Thomas Nagel.

40. I described a similar contrast in my *Intricate Ethics*, p. 36. I there said:

> Suppose that we did argue even for the permissibility of investing in cures for truly minor problems affecting many, such as headaches, rather than in a cure of a rare fatal disease, on the ground that it is reasonable for each person to take a small risk of being the one who will die in order to have headache cures at hand for his many, certain-to-occur headaches. This does not imply that here and now we should not save someone from dying from the rare fatal disease if we could, rather than cure millions of headaches. For example, suppose that, surprisingly, giving someone who develops the fatal disease all of the aspirin that has been produced to cure headaches could still now save him. It could be wrong to leave him to die on the grounds that it was reasonable ex-ante, in order to produce the aspirin for headaches, for each person to take a small risk of dying because no help for him would be available when he fell fatally ill. It is here and now that the irrelevant utilities of headache cures do not aggregate to override saving the life.

I there criticized John Broome for failing to take this into account when he argues for aggregating small benefits in all circumstances on the basis of macroallocation decisions such as are involved in investing in cures for a prevalent, less harmful disease rather than a rare, more harmful one. See his "All Goods Are Relevant," in Murray and Salomon, *Summary Measures of Population Health*, pp. 727–29. I also discussed these issues in commentary on

Allan Gibbard's Tanner Lectures (via discussion of what I called the Chocolate Case), in Gibbard's *Reconciling Our Aims* (pp. 132–35) and in a longer unpublished version of those comments (on which this chapter draws).

41. However, this conclusion would not be reached by those who sum costs and benefits across people. For both in the case where some will avoidably die in the future and in the case where it becomes possible to save some from death in the future, the sum of goods (many saved from paralysis) and bads (some dying) would be the same.

42. In *Morality, Mortality*, Vol. I, I also argued that we might morally distinguish between (1) a procedure for choosing whom to help of those people before us here and now, as in an emergency room (microallocation), and (2) a procedure for deciding how to invest funds for research and facilities to cope with various illnesses (macroallocation). Dan Brock objected to this. He argued that if we must act according to procedure (1) when people come to us, then we will be obligated to do research and develop facilities so that we can best behave as procedure (1) tells us when the time comes. This amounts to the view that we had a duty at t_1 (when doing research and development) to make it possible for use to fulfill the duties we will have at t_2 (in the emergency room). On the other hand, he claims that if we are permitted to fund research and development in manner (2), this must be because we may or must distribute among those before us by using procedure (2). (See his "Aggregating Costs and Benefits," *Philosophy and Phenomenological Research* 51 [1998]: 963–67, which was his discussion of my *Morality, Mortality*, Vol. I.)

I disagreed with both of his claims and responded to his discussion in my "Response to my Critics" in the same issue of *Philosophy and Phenomenological Research*. I said:

> Suppose that I have a car, and a seriously ill person asks me to take him to the hospital. I have a duty to do so. But I do not have a duty to buy a car so that when I face a seriously ill person, I will be able to take him to the hospital. (Indeed, I might permissibly refrain from buying a car just so that I will not be put in the position of having to take people to the hospital when they confront me.) Likewise, I believe that we may have a duty to behave in a certain way if we have a resource, but not necessarily to see to it that we have that resource. Furthermore, it might be permissible (or even required) that we invest our money so as to favor people A over people B, but when . . . people B confront us, we might have a duty to help them rather than people A. For example, I might have to invest in music CDs to keep my friends happy rather than in a car that could take a stranger to the hospital. Yet, if I wind up with some money and confront a poor stranger who needs it to go to the hospital, I should give it to him rather than to my friends who want more CDs.
>
> What I would like to insist on is that even if one principle represents the principle of public investment, it would not on that account be the principle that should govern how we distribute aid in an emergency room, for example, if 100 people come in with arms falling off at the same time as one person comes in with a fatal condition. In part, this is because if a policy allocates some money to an institution like an emergency room, this might just be a way of saying that in some areas of life, however small, a different principle than is involved elsewhere governs distribution.

(This discussion of Brock may also be found in *Intricate Ethics*, p. 46.)

43. I discussed the Ambulance Case in my *Morality, Mortality*, Vol. II: *Rights, Duties and Status* (New York: Oxford University Press, 1996).

44. I noted this in the longer unpublished version of my comments on Gibbard's *Reconciling Our Aims*. On these issues, see also unpublished work on risk by Johann Frick.

45. In *Morality, Mortality*, Vol. I, I attempted to explain prioritizing treatment for people currently ill over being able to treat people who will be ill in the future. I distinguished between intentionally refraining from aid when we could aid currently and being unable to aid in the future because we had used up our resources on earlier cases.

19

Health and Equality of Opportunity

Norman Daniels raises three questions:[1,2] Is healthcare special? When are health inequalities unjust? And: How can we meet competing healthcare needs fairly under resource constraints? In this chapter, I shall focus on Daniels's treatment of the first two questions. (I have written extensively on the third elsewhere.[3])

Daniels argues that a Rawlsian theory of justice must include health, understood as normal species functioning (NSF), since health is a precondition for fair equality of opportunity (FEO), the first part of Rawls's second principle of justice.[4] My understanding is that Rawls takes it to be a mark of FEO that those of equal talents and motivation will fare equally well in a society.[5] FEO in this sense is given lexical priority over the Difference Principle (DP), which allows incentives (and hence inequality) for the more talented if they are necessary to improve the absolute condition of those who would wind up worst off in the society. Hence, Daniels's view, as I understand it, is that without equal NSF, those of equal talent and motivation would not fare equally, since some would be held back by worse health.

Daniels's view seems to imply that if people had equal opportunity despite the fact that some were in worse health than others, the sicker ones would have no right to healthcare as a matter of justice, unless the view allowed some leftover health problems to be dealt with by the DP. Furthermore, if someone (e.g., a prisoner) were justly denied opportunities to develop his talents, pursue life plans, or participate equally as a citizen, Daniels's theory seems to imply that justice would not require that his health be attended to equally with others'. It implies that he would have less of a claim to healthcare and that its source would be different from the claims of others not in his situation. I find these implications problematic, but I shall put them to one side in order to focus on other issues.

I

I have several questions about Daniels's views on the relation of health and equal opportunity.[6] First, is equal NSF really necessary to ensure FEO as Rawls understands it? Equal *unhealth* among all people would be consistent with equal opportunity as well. (This is a form of leveling down.) Indeed, strictly speaking, levels of health that varied with levels of talent and motivation, but that involved equal health among those who occupied any given level of talent and motivation, would be consistent with equal opportunity, as Rawls describes it. This is because those at any given level of talent and motivation would fare equally well given that they all had equal health or unhealth.

Daniels points to empirical data that show that health varies positively with social class. (The direction of causation is important in understanding concern about this data. It might not necessarily be bad if better health caused an improvement in one's social class—through one's greater ability to work, for example. The concern must be that the data show that higher social class [its components or what causes it] is necessary for better health. In particular, higher social class causes better health, rather than just providing greater means for correcting illness. This is how I shall understand the concern.) Daniels takes this variation to imply that FEO is missing. But, as noted, if health varied with social class and social class varied with talent and motivation, it could still be true that those of equal talent and motivation fared equally well overall. Strictly speaking, this seems to satisfy Rawlsian FEO.[7]

If we still find this state of affairs unsatisfactory from the point of view of justice in opportunity, it must be because the mark Rawls uses for FEO (i.e., that those of equal talents and motivation will fare equally well in society) is not satisfactory. We will be concerned that those with fewer talents and/or lesser motivation did not have a full range of opportunities due to ill health, even if they all had the same opportunities and all fared equally well. I believe we can avoid this problem by reconceiving equal opportunity so that we put the emphasis on opportunity rather than merely on equality. A justification for equal NSF as a requirement of justice in opportunity could stem, I believe, from a requirement that people's fates be a positive function only of their talents and motivations, or at least a requirement that their fates not be a function of (i.e., not have as a cause) ill health. This is a noncomparative notion of opportunity. That is, it is not essentially concerned with equal levels of health (which is satisfied by equal unhealth) or with similar fates for those of a given talent/motivation level. It is foremost concerned that each person's fate in terms of opportunity range be a function of certain factors (e.g., talents) and not of others (e.g., poor health); equality on the NSF dimension is a mere byproduct of that requirement, since each person turns out to be owed NSF in order that his or her opportunity range not be a function of poor health. I shall refer to this idea of fair opportunity as FEO*. If FEO* were a requirement of justice, then empirical data linking increasing social class with increasing health as an effect would be a source of concern.

That concern could be alleviated in at least two ways: First, the concern could be alleviated if unequal health raised the absolute level of health of those in worst health. That is, if we want the degree to which people can use their talents not to be negatively affected by sickness, we are interested in how absolutely healthy people are (not merely whether they are at an equal health level). If we cannot automatically achieve the desired absolute level (NSF), we might try to achieve as much of it as possible. It is at least theoretically possible that unequal health could increase the absolute level of health and the degree to which sickness does not interfere with people's use of their talents. (An easy-to-imagine case is one in which doctors are kept healthier than others because this is necessary to maximize the health of other members of the population.) However, Daniels reports, empirical data do not support the view that the social inequality that produces unequal health is associated with higher absolute levels of health among the least healthy. Rather, absolute levels of health seem to go down for many—in particular, the worst off and even the middle classes—with social inequality.

There is a second way to alleviate the concern that FEO* will suffer under social inequality. FEO* depends on other factors besides health. Hence it is theoretically possible for FEO* to increase overall in absolute terms, even if health goes down for many. This could be so, for example, if social inequality improves other factors needed for FEO*, such as education. Strictly speaking, one needs the data on this question before being able to conclude that FEO* is threatened by social inequalities that reduce health in many social levels. However, Daniels presents data showing that these other factors fare no differently from health when there is social inequality. Indeed, he argues that differential social class, which leads to unequal health, leads to less investment in education for the poor, not more.[8]

So now, we should ask whether our concern with unequal health (and unequal FEO*) is such that the absence of FEO* is an isolatable concern. That is, suppose that, contrary to fact, degree of health varied inversely with social class, so that those of higher social class had worse health and those of lower social class were spared ill health. (After all, there once was a respectable theory that those in more responsible positions developed stress-related illness to a greater degree.) There could then be just as much absence of equal health and FEO* as when health varied positively with social class, but I suspect we would not be as concerned. This suggests that it is not inequality of health status (impinging on FEO*) that is our concern, per se. It is when negatives are piled on those in a particular social class that we are most concerned. When there is close to overall equality—those who benefit in one way (financially) suffer in another way—we are less concerned. Even if the opportunity range of the rich with poor health were not as large as with NSF, it still would probably be a bigger opportunity range than that afforded the poor who have better health. Indeed, if those who were most talented had more ill health, they might be inhibited from exercising their greater talents, and so social classes might be leveled. If coming closer to such overall equality compensated for the absence of FEO* (though I am not suggesting it does), this would imply that FEO* did not have the lexical priority that Rawls claims.[9]

II

My second set of questions about treating NSF as a matter of justice implied by the requirement of equal opportunity is suggested by Thomas Nagel's discussion of justice and nature.[10] He argues that Rawlsian FEO is meant to undo certain socially caused inequalities, even if they are the result of other inequalities in society that are in accord with the DP and which, therefore, are not unjust in themselves. For example, consider a hypothetical case in which some are poorer than others because of the way society is organized, but not unjustly poorer since the DP governs social distribution. As a matter of FEO, they might claim access to education they cannot afford but the rich can. On Nagel's view, FEO is not intended to deal with the inequalities caused primarily by nature. For example, Nagel claims that someone born with a disability is not entitled as a matter of FEO to have this corrected, even if it interferes with his using his talents. Rather, correction or compensation for natural inequalities (e.g., whether natural difference in talents or in illnesses that interfere with exercising talents) is captured by the DP. This suggests that correction or compensation for ill health that society is not responsible for causing falls under the DP, and in Rawls's view the DP is subordinate to FEO. This implies that on Nagel's view, as a matter of justice, providing equal educational opportunities will take precedence over compensation for natural inequalities that can have much larger effects on well-being, including naturally caused ill health. (Daniels reports that Rawls's contractors would choose FEO and give it lexical priority. Nagel denies that self-interested individuals behind a veil of ignorance would choose such a principle, since it can interfere with promoting the more pressing interests of the worst off. He thinks that FEO can be defended, but not by veil-of-ignorance reasoning.)

But now notice that even if Nagel's (as opposed to Daniels's) interpretation of Rawlsian FEO were correct, correcting or compensating for ill health that is caused by social class could be covered by FEO. Further, it might also be that if natural ill health continues only in low social classes because they cannot afford treatment that upper classes can afford, FEO would mandate treatment. This is on the model of providing education for the poor that matches what the rich can afford. Empirical data of a special sort linking health and social class would be important, in part because they would allow us to include at least some healthcare under FEO even before considering the DP, whichever interpretation (Daniels's or Nagel's) of Rawls we accept.

III

My third set of questions about equal NSF as a requirement of FEO or FEO* concerns its instability. Suppose there is equal NSF, but talents and motivation differ among people, and incentives to the more talented are permitted if this is in the best interest of the worst off. Given these unequal talents and motivations, if opportunities are really equal and incentives are allowed, there will shortly be no social equality. Further, if health varies positively with social class, then equal NSF will be short-lived; it will undo itself. Daniels originally seemed to assume that one could provide equal NSF without requiring overall equality of other goods. If the empirical data are correct, it now turns out that one will have to argue for social equality in order to get equal NSF; either the DP (which allows inequalities) will have to go or FEO* will have to go. (It is also odd to argue for equal NSF as a condition of the arguably weaker requirement of FEO* when one needs the stronger requirement of social equality to get NSF. And if people would only seek to develop their talents on account of incentives, providing them with NSF so that they may develop their talents by way of a system without incentives would be self-defeating.)

Remember that the problem is not merely that there will be no equality of opportunity if health is influenced by permissible differences in social class and equal NSF is required for FEO*. Theoretically, inequality of opportunity is compatible with those who wind up having less opportunity still having more of it in absolute terms than they would have had if opportunity were equal. It is rather that a crucial component of opportunity—health—will (we are told) get worse in absolute terms if there is social inequality. (We are assuming, for the sake of argument, that no other factors relevant to FEO* improve.)

Daniels notes that those who would wind up worse off in health, not merely relatively but in absolute terms, might reasonably decide to exchange health for greater amounts of other (presumably economic) goods, if inequalities of social class caused by incentives are necessary for those other goods. Indeed, only if the trade were worth making would inequalities of social class really satisfy the DP and be in the interest of the worst off. This, however, implies that it is permissible to trade FEO or FEO* for other goods, and it does away with the lexical priority of FEO* over the DP, on the assumption that NSF is associated with FEO*.[11] Insofar as opportunity is important only for the outcomes it brings, it may make sense to trade. However, this may involve trading one's ability to do something (being a fully functioning agent) for being provided with some things by others.

What if we were unwilling to settle for lower health for some? If the data are correct, we could increase the health of some classes simply by leveling down higher classes, thus producing more equality without engaging in redistribution of wealth for economic change in the lower classes. (Would this reduce the health of the upper classes, however? Perhaps not, if better health in the lower classes [or institutions that caused it] also contributed to the health of the former upper classes.) The benefit of redistributing wealth, rather than just taking it away from the wealthy by leveling down, is that social equality can be achieved at a higher absolute economic level.

Assume that there is a degree of social inequality that undoes any improvement in health resulting from economic improvement in absolute terms. Presumably there is also some point where the two just balance out (i.e., where the health we would gain by social equality is no more than the health we would gain by economic growth associated with social inequality), and presumably there is also a point where more equality results in such bad economic conditions that health suffers. If there is a point where more social equality does not result in better health, at that point we would not face the choice of less health versus more of other goods produced by incentive-driven social inequality.

Some may be pleased if it is true that social equality is good for health. This is, in part, because they then have new knowledge about how to improve health. It is also, in part, because they believe that people's concern to achieve good health will serve as a means to achieve social equality. There is an alternative point of view that is worth considering. Excellence, creativity, and dynamism in a social structure are often fueled by different incentives that result in social inequality. Hence, it might be preferable to some degree to directly treat those with ill health (whatever their social class) rather than eliminate the inequalities that cause the ill health. To some degree, this would involve de-emphasizing social equality as a means of preventive medicine and reemphasizing medical care. We would use what Daniels calls the ambulance that rescues us when we fall off the cliff, rather than preventing the fall in the first place.

Notes

1. This chapter is a revised version of "Health and Equality of Opportunity," *American Journal of Bioethics* 1(2) (Spring 2001): 17–19.

2. Norman Daniels, "Justice, Health, and Healthcare," *American Journal of Bioethics* 1(2) (2001): 2–16.

3. For example, see F. M. Kamm, *Morality, Mortality, Vol. 1: Death and Whom to Save from It* (New York: Oxford University Press, 1993). A brief summary of major points of that book can be found in the second part of Kamm, "Nonconsequentialism," in *Blackwell's Guide to Ethical Theory*, ed. H. LaFollette (Oxford: Blackwell, 2000), pp. 205–26, reprinted with revisions as chapter 1 of Kamm, *Intricate Ethics* (New York: Oxford University Press, 2007). See also chapter 18 this volume.

4. In his article, Daniels says "any theory of justice that supports a principle assuring equal opportunity (or giving priority to improving the opportunities of those who have the least opportunity) could thus be extended to healthcare" (p. 3).

5. John Rawls, *A Theory of Justice* (Cambridge, MA: Harvard University Press, 1971).

6. Some of these were also raised in chapter 18 this volume. As I noted there, equal health, equal prospects of health, and equal opportunity for health are different. To simplify, I will speak of equal NSF, but much of what is said could be put in terms of opportunity or prospects for NSF.

7. Problems could arise on this view if, for example, offspring of those in a lower social class were more talented and yet did not have the health associated with the talented class because of their parents' social level.

8. Daniels, "Justice, Health, and Healthcare," pp. 7–8.

9. For additional discussion of considering benefits from different "spheres" simultaneously, rather than considering separate spheres (e.g., money, education, health) separately at the macro policy level, see chapter 18 this volume.

10. Thomas Nagel, "Justice and Nature," *Oxford Journal of Legal Studies* 17(2) (1997): 303–21.

11. This bears on one of the big differences between Daniels's approach to what is just in health when he speaks as a Rawlsian and Ronald Dworkin's approach. In his "Will Clinton's Health Plan Be Fair?" (*New York Review of Books* 41 [January 13,1994], Vol. 41, no. 1–2) Dworkin recommends that we decide what healthcare a state owes its citizens by considering what health plan the average citizen would choose from behind a type of veil of ignorance. He considers the tradeoffs that such people would make between healthcare (and whatever else promotes health) and other goods. This broad willingness to allow tradeoffs contrasts with Daniels's approach when he speaks as a Rawlsian, insofar as concern for health is a matter of FEO and FEO is a matter of justice, and so cannot be traded away for economic well-being unrelated to promoting FEO.

20

Is It Morally Permissible to Discontinue *Non*futile Use of a Scarce Resource?

In this chapter I consider some of the ethical problems presented by the desire to discontinue the *non*futile use of a resource because it is scarce.[1] By "nonfutile" I mean that a resource can still help in a significant way a patient who receives it. It might be said that doctors should not do "rationing at the bedside" with patients. Rather, rationing should result from a systemwide macro policy that ties doctors' hands and prevents them from allocating resources as they wish. One point for which I shall argue is that there may be an in-between case: When individuals are involved in a trial to see how well they respond to a drug, treatment to them might be discontinued because they do not do well enough, if and only if treating those who do better makes it possible to treat more candidates who are equally worthy.[2] The drug clozapine, uniquely useful for treating schizophrenia, is taken as an example of such a resource made scarce because of its costliness. Other drugs may come to supplant clozapine for treatment of schizophrenia. That will not affect the relevance of my discussion, because I take clozapine only as an example of a scarce resource. Indeed, one part of my discussion will focus on the issue of terminating nonfutile treatments in general. This can involve use of intensive-care units, dialysis, and other scarce resources.[3]

In the first part of the chapter, I consider relevant available medical data on clozapine and I review treatment policy (that was current in 1994) involving clozapine. In subsequent parts, I isolate three major issues that arise in the morality of discontinuing aid in general (not just in trials): regression, doctors' commitments to patients, and the temporal gap between denying aid to one person and providing better aid to someone else. I also deal with whether differential outcome should affect who gets helped. To examine this topic, I present, in outline, some general principles for the distribution of scarce resources,[4] and then begin to make clear what these principles might imply for the case of differential outcomes with clozapine. The concluding parts consider the role of differential numbers of people who might be helped and the significance of urgency relative to outcome. I attempt to provide a morally justified principle that tells us how to relate the *outcome* we expect in treating patients to the *urgency* of patient condition and the *number* of potential recipients of treatment. The final part of the chapter considers the fate of those individuals who are only moderately ill and suggests a possible change in policy that might be of benefit in achieving just distribution to them.

I. Background on Clozapine

Suppose that clozapine is the most effective treatment for schizophrenia, helping people who would not otherwise be helped, helping them more than alternative treatments, and causing fewer side effects. However, suppose it is more expensive than other treatments, at least in the short run. Whether it is more expensive in the long run than other treatments depends on the outcomes it produces.

Suppose that in some people, clozapine treatment essentially results in a return to normality. These people can leave hospitals, so hospital beds can be freed for other use or eliminated. Such patients must continue to take medication costing about $5,500 per year. But they can become self-supporting, returning to work and family. Possibly this implies they themselves could fund their medication. In this population, clozapine is overall less expensive than other treatments.

Suppose that other people show only moderate improvement, both in the sense that the difference between their condition with clozapine and without it is not great and in the sense that when taking the drug they do not return to normality. These individuals must continue the drug in order to get benefits that only clozapine can provide to them, but they cannot live independently. They may move to outpatient facilities, supported by both state and federal funds, or they may have to remain in state-run hospitals. In this population, clozapine use is overall more expensive than other treatments.

Suppose that in a third group, clozapine produces no differential benefits over other drugs. However, the possibility that it produces fewer side effects, even if it is no more effective than other treatments, raises the question of whether its use is nonetheless indicated.

Suppose that there is no way to tell before treatment into which of these three groups a person will fall. For example, there is an equal distribution of big successes (normality) in severe and nonsevere patients. However, once someone is on treatment, one can tell within six months whether that person will respond, and to what degree.

Assume that when clozapine must be provided at public expense, it is a scarce resource owing to its costliness. A significant ethical problem that arises is whether to continue treating those who cannot pay for their own treatment and who make only moderate gains that do not lift them to normality. This is one of the most expensive groups to treat, and discontinuing their treatment would allow us to help more people become normal. In other words, should the maintenance of someone on the scarce resource depend on the outcome it produces?

In 1994, it was said,[5] the publicly-funded treatment policy was essentially two-fold: (1) Keep on treating all those who achieve normality on the drug (indeed, this is taken for granted); (2) Give medication in accordance with the severity of the illness and *keep on* treating even those who improve only to a subnormal level. This means that others who, at the start, are not so severely ill but who might achieve normality are not treated. For prongs (1) and (2) of this policy to be consistent, it must be assumed that most of the normals who are continued on treatment would be severely ill without treatment, even if not all the severely ill who are treated attain normality.

II. Issues Relating to Discontinuing Treatment in General

The decision to stop treating those who are achieving a moderate level of well-being—the rejection of prong (2)—in order to try to increase the number who can achieve normality raises several ethical questions. The first asks: Is there a moral difference between (a) not beginning treatment that would help someone significantly in order to help others more, and (b) terminating such treatment once it has begun, when it can still help someone significantly, in order to help others more? (In the clozapine case, in particular, the question is whether there is a moral difference between not beginning treatment that would help someone achieve only a moderate level of well-being and terminating such treatment once it has begun.) All the issues (for example, concerning action versus omission) that are familiar from the discussion of discontinuing life-sustaining treatment might be thought to arise in dealing with this question. It could be said, however, that *not* giving yet another dose of a drug or more time on dialysis is not the same as terminating (by action) a life-support system. At most, it is like a case involving a life-support machine that needs to be reset every day that we would not reset after a certain point. Then the analogous issue is whether it is permissible to omit resetting the machine.

Whatever the philosophically best way to treat the issue of terminating versus not beginning treatment may be,[6] psychological studies seem to support the view that if people form *expectations* about future treatment on the basis of past treatment, this will set a baseline from which noncontinuation of treatment, even by failure to give another dose, will be perceived as a loss by those people.[7] For those who have not yet received treatment and have not formed expectations about getting treatment, not being treated may be perceived as a no-gain situation. Psychologists tell us that losses tend to be rated more negatively than no-gains, even when they both leave the patient at the same absolute level of well-being. Would this be a reason not to terminate drug use or dialysis, even when we may refuse to begin it? It is possible that one could prevent the development of (reasonable) expectations concerning further treatment by explicitly warning people that beginning treatment does not guarantee that treatment will continue. If expectations do not form, the expectation of treatment could not be a reason to continue. Furthermore, ceasing treatment should then be seen as a no-gain rather than as a loss. Deliberately characterizing the first six months of use of the drug as a *trial* may, for example, succeed in stemming expectations. If expectations form that are unreasonable, these should not bind us.

However, there might be other reasons not to stop treatment that also seem related to the loss/no-gain distinction. For example, if we are clear about what will happen to a patient when treatment ends, we may see another ground for objecting to ending it. To see this, consider that, theoretically (even if not in reality), there are several possibilities in the trial with clozapine: (a) treatment must be continued for up to six months in order for us to know (by some sign) whether someone will become normal on a drug, but there is no change in the patient's condition during that time period; (b) treatment must be continued for up to six months in order for us to know whether someone will become normal and there is an improvement in the patient's condition during that time period, though it does not reach normality; (c) treatment must be continued for up to six months in order for us to know whether someone will become normal and they do achieve normality during that period. I believe it is (b) and (c) rather than (a) that raise a moral problem for terminating treatment. This is so because in (b) and (c), terminating treatment does not merely stop a patient from achieving further progress (as it may in [a] and [b]); it allows or causes the patient to *regress*, to fall back down to the level from which he was already lifted. It is not stopping treatment per se, even when we know this will prevent some future improvement, that seems morally significant relative to not starting treatment. What seems morally significant is (1) *stopping an improvement in the patient's condition that has already occurred by* (2) *stopping what was already being done to achieve the improvement.* (It is important to emphasize that (1) and (2) are not limited to cases where a patient will die if treatment does not continue. The point is more general.)

Consider (1). In (a) we could know that someone would become normal if treatment continued once the sign was present, and in (b) we could know that someone would improve to normality if treatment continued. But in (a), the patient has not yet improved at all, so when we stop treatment, he does not become worse off than when treatment was being provided. In (b), if a patient were to remain at the *improved* but subnormal level once treatment is stopped, I do not think there would be an objection to stopping treatment (by contrast to not starting it), even though he could improve further if kept on the same treatment. However, if the patient will lose the gain she has made (regress), it seems problematic to discontinue treatment relative to not starting it. Similarly for (c).

Now consider (2). Suppose a regression will occur unless we increase the dosage already being given. I do not believe that refusing to prevent the regression in order to help others instead would raise the same concern as in (b) or (c). Hence, it is not even the regression per se but its occurrence as a result of not continuing to do what was already being done that may be more problematic than not starting treatment. (I shall call this regression*.) Regression*, however, does not imply that there is something wrong with depriving a patient of the level of treatment that he has so far been getting when a reduced level of treatment will be at least as useful as the higher level has been in the past. For suppose (i) a lower level of treatment gave the same outcome as the past level had previously, and (ii) the past level of treatment if continued would lead to a better outcome than the patient has already achieved. Intuitively, it seems that it is regressing from the *outcome* already achieved, not losing the level of *treatment* already received per se, that is problematic relative to not starting treatment.

The concern with regression* in (b) assumes that improvement to a point below normality is still better than being at a point further from normality. Some may challenge this assumption in the case of mental illness in particular. They might point out that individuals who are severely mentally ill may live in a world of pleasant delusions. When patients recover partially, they become aware of their problems and for the first time experience misery. Several points can be made in response to this challenge. First, if severely ill schizophrenics are already very miserable, the challenge does not apply to them. Second, the challenge depends on a completely experiential conception of the good life: What you do not experience as bad is not bad for you and there are no nonexperiential goods that compensate for experiential harms. If this were a correct conception of the good life, it would imply that a good life could be had by taking drugs that give one pleasant experiences and only the illusion of living a productive life. And this does not seem true. Such a conception of the good life also denies that pain experienced in coming into contact with reality can be compensated for by the mere fact that one is in contact with reality. There is much to be said against the purely experiential conception of the good life.

I have said that regression* might make discontinuing nonfutile treatment morally problematic relative to not starting it. Yet, a philosopher might reasonably respond that it is as permissible (or impermissible) not to continue aid that one has been providing as it is not to start aid, even if the patient declines, as long as he or she declines to a state that is no worse than the patient would have been in had aid not begun. This assumes that there is no independent commitment (e.g., a promise) to continue aid once started. Is one worse off if one improves for a few months and then declines than if one had never improved at all? I do not believe so, for if all we could ever do for any patient was improve him for a few months before an inevitable decline, I do not think that we should refuse to do so on the ground that it is bad for him.

Admittedly, a doctor has a duty to aid (unlike an ordinary bystander), but even with this duty, a doctor may sometimes refuse *to start* helping one patient in order to help a greater number of other patients. Why then may she not sometimes stop the aid once started, if helping someone else more is what will allow her to help a greater number of patients, given that the patient no longer aided will be no worse off overall? Must the fact that the patient gets worse again through failure to continue what has already been done be definitive because it is thought to involve the doctor harming the patient?

It is inappropriate to apply the doctor's Hippocratic concern with not doing harm above all else to the case of the patient's decline. First, the doctor would be refusing to continue aid and not, strictly, harming. Second, looking only at what happens if we do not continue aid relative to the patient's improved condition considers too narrow a time period; it fails to consider the overall period from before the doctor intervened. The doctor produced the improvement and would not have been duty bound to do so if she could alternatively have helped more people at the earlier point in time. Not helping someone *retain* an improvement and instead beginning to help others may be less pleasing than not helping to start with—as decline to a level may be less pleasing than maintenance of a status quo at the same level—but it is not clear that this makes a moral difference.

This brings us to another objection to terminating treatment based on the idea that a doctor might simply become committed to a specific patient once treatment starts. I do not believe that this consideration gives rise to an obligation to continue aid in all cases. Commitments may be overridden, for example, by the attempt to help greater numbers of people, especially if these are also one's patients already. (Admittedly, it would be no commitment at all if it could be overridden by doing just any additional amount of good for someone else.) In addition, commitments might be undertaken by doctors in an explicitly conditional form—for example, "You will be provided with a drug on condition no one else needs it much more." It may be part of the *responsibility of patients* to accept that their useful treatment may be stopped for morally legitimate reasons.

Most importantly, the idea of a commitment to a patient suggests that a doctor would be wrong to stop treatment that had not yet had *any* good effect, or had not had all possible good effects, on the patient whenever the doctor knows that continuing treatment will lead to some significant improvement in the future. But if what was said above concerning the role of regression* is correct, it helps to undermine or weaken the argument for a doctor's commitment to a patient already being treated, as much as it undermines the idea of a patient's entitlement to continuation of treatment per se (rather than to the effect treatment has already produced). For it does not seem as problematic for a doctor to stop treatment either in a patient who has not yet improved or in a patient who could further improve but who will retain the benefit he has already achieved. (This is, of course, on the assumption that stopping treatment for such a patient in order to offer it to others will result in helping more equally needy people as much.)

All this suggests that it is regression* that raises the moral problem, not simple failure of commitment or simple termination of treatment.

It is true, however, that playing down a doctor's commitment to individual patients makes affirming the establishment of special bonds (comparable to the ones we form with friends or family members) impossible. Such special bonds in the case of family and friends are thought to sometimes legitimately impede meeting even the more pressing needs of other people and/or a greater number of other people. Should we exchange the possibility of such bonds between doctor and patient for fairer treatment? The suggestion is that we could morally afford to do so sometimes.

Nevertheless, there are facts special to the clozapine case that illustrate how there can be further complications to the decision not to continue aid to someone in order to help others more. Terminating aid so as to *definitely help* others more is different from terminating aid to *go searching* for others whom we could help more. In the latter case, we cannot be sure that we will be helping the next person more than we are helping the person already being treated, and it will take up to six months to find out. The person on whom we try our drug next may do no better, and possibly worse, than the person we stopped treating. If he does worse, this means that we could have been doing more good by having continued treatment for the first patient.

What if he and subsequent trial subjects do only as well as the original patient? It might be argued that this is still a better outcome, for there is a fairer distribution of temporary moderate improvements. For example, instead of n months of moderate improvement going to one patient, m patients each get n/m months of moderate improvement. If what we had to distribute to begin with was the good of moderate improvement, we might well have divided it over several people rather than concentrate its duration in one person, as long as what we distribute is still a significant good. (Notice that this is not the same as saying that we would deny normality to someone by dividing a normality-producing dose so as to produce only moderate well-being in many.) Regression*, admittedly, poses the dominant countervailing consideration to such a fairer distribution of even moderate improvement by terminating treatment already started.

In addition, there is at least a chance that the drug will prove *very* successful in the next person, and this is no longer true of the original patient. The probability of finding people who will do much better is an empirical question, and we may be reluctant to stop helping one person unless there is a sufficiently high probability of helping others much more in the *near future*.

This last point makes salient the time gap that can exist between stopping aid to one person and finding another person whom we can help to reach normality. At worst, it is possible that by the time we find someone who will do better and help him, we may no longer be helping someone who was suffering at the same time as the person we originally stopped treating. If this is so, we will have put off helping someone who is suffering *now* with the consequence that will we help others more who will suffer *in the future*. This raises the question of whether we should adopt an attitude of *temporal neutrality*, not distinguishing between those who need help now and those who will come with need later. (I shall return to a related issue below.)

III. Severity, Outcome, and a General Theory of Allocation

There are other questions concerning allocation of clozapine that arise independently of the possible moral problem of stopping treatment, for theoretically they
could also arise in cases where we must just decide whom to start aiding. One such
question is whether the attempt to achieve best outcomes—in the clozapine case
this is mental normality—for some should lead us to deprive others of their chance
for moderate improvement, even if these others are more severely ill than those
who would be substituted for them in drug trials. This question has two subparts:
(a) Should better outcomes dominate equal chances for help? (b) Should better
outcomes dominate greater severity?

Before dealing with these questions, it will be useful to first present some general principles for distributing scarce resources.[8] I have elsewhere attempted to
describe a distribution procedure that takes account of four factors: need (N), urgency (U), outcome (O), and waiting time (WT).[9] Factors besides these four may
be relevant; however, I believe one should not start by cluttering the picture. In
general, the method is to begin with two factors, holding the others constant in the
background, and to see what the relation is between these two factors—for example, which takes precedence over the other. Then we introduce a third factor to
see whether it makes a difference to the relationship between the first two factors
as well as how the third relates to each of the two others. If we follow this procedure patiently, adding additional factors in an orderly way, we have some hope of
making progress.

Let me first describe three of the four factors, N, U, and O. A patient's *urgency*
(U), as I have used the term, is a measure of how severe his illness is insofar as this
tells us how bad his future prospects are if he is not treated; the latter is a function
of how bad his future will be and the likelihood it will come about. (This is not the
ordinary notion of urgency, which focuses on how soon treatment is needed.
Someone could face very bad prospects but not need treatment to avoid such prospects as soon as someone else, in which case the ordinary notion of urgency says
he is not as urgent. I shall refer to the ordinary use as urgent-care.) *Need* (N), as I
use the term, connotes how badly someone's life will have gone healthwise if that
person is not treated. Unlike urgency, need is not merely a forward-looking concept; it takes someone's whole life into consideration. Person A could be more
urgent (in my sense) *than* B, in that A will die in a month if he is not treated now
and B will die in a year if he is not treated now, and yet B could be more in need (of
life-giving treatment) because he would die at age 20 whereas A would die at age
60. This assumes that one will have had a worse life if one dies at 20 than if one dies
at 60 (other things equal). Because need takes into account someone's past, about
which one can no longer do anything, it implies that how we treat someone in the
future could at least compensate her for the past, and that such compensation
could be as morally important as preventions of harm in the future. (This may be
a contentious assumption.)

Outcome (O) refers to the expected difference that treatment will make by comparison with what would have happened without it. In cases where life and death are at issue, I believe that, for the most part, the relevant measure of outcome is additional time alive independent of quality, above a certain minimum, as long as the patient would find the quality of life acceptable. This means that in life-and-death cases, for the most part, we should not use QALYs (quality-adjusted life years) in evaluating different possible outcomes. In cases where life and death are *not* at issue, outcome is appropriately measured in terms of (some types of) quality-of-life differences, such as relative freedom from the symptoms of schizophrenia.[10]

What are some of the things we can say about the relative weights of need, urgency, and outcome? First, let us consider distribution of a scarce, *lifesaving* resource between A and B, holding need, urgency, and outcome (as well as any other factor) equal in the two. Fairness requires giving each an equal chance. It is important to understand that giving equal chances is *not* a symptom of the desire not to be responsible for making a choice. It is, rather, the fair way to choose when there is no morally relevant difference between potential recipients, given that each wants to be the one to be aided.

Now add a third person, C, whose need, urgency, and outcome are the same and who can also be saved only if we save B. What I call the Balancing Argument claims that in such a case, justice demands that each person on one side should have her interests balanced against those of one person on the opposing side; those who are not balanced out in the larger group help determine that the larger group should be saved. Hence, the number of people saved counts morally.

Now consider conflicts when the individuals are not equally urgent. Figure 20.1 represents a choice between saving A, on the one hand, and on the other hand, saving B *and* curing C's sore throat with leftover medicine. The overall outcomes will be different depending on whom we save, as more good, spread over two people, will occur if we save B and C. My claim is that we should treat the difference in outcome as morally *irrelevant*.

The reasoning behind this is as follows: From an impartial view, we should not favor A over B per se (given that they are assumed to be alike *in themselves* in all

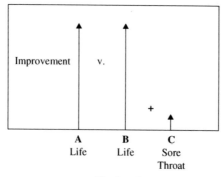

FIGURE 20.1 The Sore Throat Case

morally relevant respects). If they were alone (independent of C), we should give them equal chances. From the impartial perspective, we also see that A and B each has his own partial point of view; A prefers his own survival to that of B, and vice versa. It is important to each, therefore, that he retain his equal chance to survive. The fact that we could save C from a sore throat is a matter of minor importance to him; he is not very needy or urgent and, in addition, the difference in outcome achieved by helping him is small. These three points support the conclusion that we should not deprive A of his 50 percent chance of survival merely to also help C. Hence, in this case, C's cure should be a morally irrelevant good in choosing between these people. (This contrasts with the view that we should *aggregate* the gains to B and C and help them because we would produce a benefit that is larger than the benefit possible to A alone.)

This form of reasoning gives equal consideration to each individual's partial point of view from an impartial point of view, so it combines subjective and objective perspectives. Hence, I call it *Sobjectivity*. It implies that certain extra goods (like the throat cure) can be morally irrelevant; I call this the Principle of Irrelevant Goods.[11] Whether a good is irrelevant is context-dependent. Curing a sore throat is morally irrelevant when others' lives are at stake, but not when others' earaches are. (Notice that the ground for ignoring the small extra good in its role in the Sore Throat Case is not that we should not think of such matters in life-and-death situations. It would not be wrong to choose between two decision procedures that give A and B equal chances on the ground that one procedure will magically also cure a sore throat.) The Sore Throat Case shows that we must refine the claim that what we owe each person is to balance her interests against the equal interests of an opposing person and let the remainder help determine the outcome.

If small increases in good to a person are sometimes morally irrelevant, this can help provide one reason why someone who has a big and even irreplaceable effect on society *in aggregate* should not necessarily be favored in the distribution of a scarce lifesaving resource over someone else. If the big effect amounts to only small effects on the lives of many people, then these effects should not, I believe, be aggregated so as to help outweigh the claim of someone else to have 50 percent chance to have his life saved.

Aggregating small benefits to many people, *none* of whom are very needy or urgent, to outweigh the grave need of a single person can be even more problematic than aggregating saving a life and providing such small benefits in order to outweigh someone else's equal chance to live. Such a problematic procedure would be exemplified by public policies that, for example, provide tooth capping to the great number of people who will need it rather than provide care for a far smaller number of the severely schizophrenic.

Suppose (as in figure 20.2) that if we save B, we can also save C's arm. This is the prevention of a large loss to C. I believe that when the loss to C becomes so significant, it is no longer an irrelevant good, given that we can only save one life no matter what we do. This is true even though C does not stand to lose as much

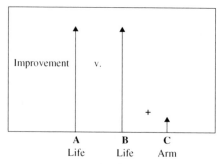

FIGURE 20.2 The Extra Arm Case

as A or B and so is not as needy or urgent as each of them. Explaining why this moral shift occurs is not easy, and I shall not attempt it here. This shift would mean that we should give the treatment outright to B and C. (Some might argue that we should give them a greater proportional chance of getting the treatment.)

What if the extra good is concentrated in the person whose life would be saved? For example, suppose we could save A's or B's life. If we save B, this could also save him from having a sore throat, but if we save A we cannot prevent her from having a sore throat. Here the need and urgency of A and B are the same, but the outcome each presents is different. My claim is that the sore throat is an irrelevant difference in a decision of life and death, and we should not deprive A of her chance to live because of it, even though no more than one person can be saved.

Suppose we could save A or B, but if we save B, this will also prevent his arm from falling off, whereas A's arm would fall off anyway. Is the saving of an arm here a morally relevant good that should incline us to save B rather than A?[12] (See figure 20.3.)

I believe that B's arm is morally irrelevant. Further, I believe this is consistent with my conclusion earlier that C's arm is relevant in figure 20.2. When the improvement in quality of life would occur to the very same person for whom the primary good at stake is life itself—that is, when the good would be concentrated

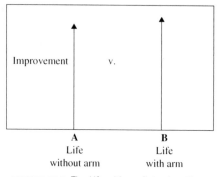

FIGURE 20.3 The Life-with-an-Extra-Arm Case

rather than distributed—I believe the additional good we can do him should not necessarily lead us to deprive A of her chance at a life that she reasonably finds acceptable. Three principles underlie this conclusion. First, *we are more concerned with helping someone avoid a very bad condition than with providing the very same person whom we help in that way with an additional improvement.* Second, *each person wants to be the one who avoids the very bad condition and come close to being normal.* (The fact that A might be willing to run a risk of death [in surgery] to be saved without the loss of an arm does not imply that he must run a greater risk of death so that B can have a greater chance at being saved with both arms.[13]) Third, *when an extra good is distributed over another person rather than concentrated, we positively affect a greater number of people.* This is a right-making feature not present when B receives an extra good.

Finally, suppose we have a choice between helping one person, A, who will be very badly off and much benefited by our aid, or helping a couple of people, B and C, each of whom will be as badly off as A but not benefited as much by our aid. As long as the lesser benefit is significant, it is morally more important, I think, to distribute our efforts over more people, each of whom would be as badly off as the single person, rather than to provide a bigger benefit concentrated in one person (other things being equal). One way to analyze this situation employs what I shall call the Balancing Argument (II): Find the part of the potential large gain to A (part 1) that is balanced by the smaller gain to B. Now we must decide how to break that tie between them. If we care about giving priority to those who are worst off, we will care more about benefiting the next person in the group, C, rather than giving an additional benefit (part 2) to A, who, having received part 1, would already have more than C. This means that instead of breaking the tie between A-with-part-1 and B by giving A a greater benefit (adding part 2 to part 1), we break the tie by helping B and C, each to a lesser degree.

IV. Clozapine and Differences in Outcome in a Two-Person Choice

In this part, I shall begin dealing with question (a) in regard to clozapine: Should better outcomes dominate equal chances for help? In the case of clozapine, we are considering whose quality of life to improve, not whose life to save. Let us assume at this point that need and urgency are great and equal between people, but that outcomes will be different. Also let us assume for the time being that the only two people affected by our choices are A and B, and they can both be improved only by clozapine (figure 20.4).

Assume B will be improved *slightly* beyond A, to the point of normality. The view most clearly implied by my previous discussion is that in this case we should not deprive A of his equal chance to make a critical change from a very bad condition to close to normal, just in order to bring B first close to normal and then (less critically) to normal. The principles that underlie this conclusion are: (1) we are

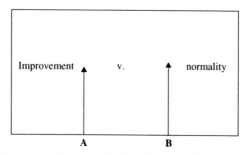

FIGURE 20.4 Two-Person Choices: The Normal Person Case

more concerned with helping someone avoid a very bad condition than with providing him with an additional improvement; and (2) each person wants to be the one who avoids the very bad condition.

Here is an alternative view: Normal mental health (which does not mean perfect mental health) is a unique kind of good. It is closely associated with the characteristics that are commonly thought to account for the moral importance of being a person at all: rationality, self-control, capacity for responsible action, and so forth. The difference between normality and its absence is not just a matter of degree, like the difference between perfect pain relief and some degree of pain.[14] Here is a possible explanation of this: Improvement to a moderate level of mental health is a good for the person who is ill, as is improvement to normality. But normality is also more than a good *for* the person; it helps account for the good *of* being a person. Being in normal physical condition does not have a comparable role. We might, therefore, see achieving mental normality as an especially important goal that represents more than just an additional benefit to someone who already will have achieved the most important part of what is good for him. Call this the Mental-Special View.

Here is a possible position that incorporates an implication of this view: Avoiding a truly horrifying mental condition could be so important that we should not deprive A of his equal chance to avoid it and improve to a substantial degree just so that B can achieve normality. But if A and B are moderately ill, the good of B's becoming normal could override A's having a chance. This position comes close to a guarantee that we will focus on rescuing someone from a very bad fate if we can bring him up to a minimally adequate level. Having done that, we will maximize outcome so as to produce normality where we can, as the Mental-Special View implies. Here is another implication of the view: Suppose we could improve many moderately ill people a significant amount but not to normality by dividing a dose that would produce normality if given to one person. We should not divide the dose. (Here is an analogy within another domain: We can improve to some degree the artistic abilities of many people who are already moderately good at art or we can produce one great artist. We should do the latter, not necessarily because it is good *for* the person who becomes a great artist [or for those who benefit from the art] but just because we produce a great artist who creates great art.)

Whether or not we accept the Mental-Special View as presented, there is yet an additional factor to be considered in the case represented in figure 20.4. Having achieved normality, B may become self-sufficient, thus freeing up money to provide A with clozapine as well. Then the issue becomes one of whether we require A to wait for B's recovery before himself undergoing treatment, losing his chance for earlier treatment. The answer may depend on how badly off each person is.

But now imagine another case. Suppose that with clozapine, we can improve B's condition greatly and improve A's not very much. (We might imagine two different variations: [1] B is still not normal, and [2] B is normal. For present purposes, we need not worry about this distinction. I shall not consider the possibility that we could make someone superior to normal.) (See figure 20.5.)

Even someone who rejects the Mental-Special View could believe that when the difference in mental condition that we can produce becomes quite great in this way, it may be morally appropriate to favor the person in whom we can produce more good, given equal need and urgency in both. This means that while helping someone avoid a very bad fate is a greater concern than providing additional improvement, avoiding the worst fate is not the only thing with which we are concerned. At least when we are also helping someone avoid the same very bad fate, our greater concern is combined with a lesser concern to produce additional significant improvement, and this may override concern for equal chances to avoid the very bad fate. Hence, not all cases of differential outcomes need be like that represented in figure 20.3. However, the worse A's and B's conditions are in absolute terms without the drug, the harder it is for extra good in B to overcome A's claim to an equal chance for significant improvement. The fact that the better A's and B's conditions are in absolute terms, the easier it is to override equal chances by a great good, makes this position close to a position requiring that we be concerned with a guaranteed minimum beyond which we may be free to produce significant differences, regardless of whether anyone achieves normality. (Notice that we can favor the person in whom we can produce much better quality-of-life in non-life-and-death cases, even if the same sort of quality-of-life distinction did not count in life-and-death cases.)

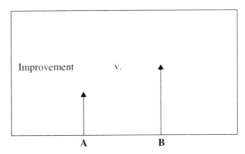

FIGURE 20.5 Two Person Choices: The Below Normal Case

Let us change one of our assumptions and imagine that candidate B, but not A, is susceptible to moderate improvement with a drug other than clozapine—call it mozapine—that is inexpensive and not scarce. Candidate B will not improve on mozapine as much as on clozapine, but he will improve as much as A would improve on clozapine. Suppose one of our principles is that we are more concerned with helping someone avoid a very bad fate than with providing additional improvement. Does this imply that we should make B ineligible to receive clozapine, for we can then treat both A and B, moving each away from a very bad fate? Not necessarily, for suppose that if we treat B with clozapine *he would attain normality* and self-sufficiency, and be able to pay for his own maintenance on clozapine. We (i.e., public institutions) will then have money with which to treat A with clozapine as well. The trouble is that we may have to wait at least six months before we can treat A in this way, whereas if we keep B on mozapine, we can treat A right away. The question is whether some extra months of suffering on A's part are worth the goal of producing normality in B. The answer may vary depending on how bad A's condition is in absolute terms.

V. Helping More People

The last case again reminds us of the additional crucial factor in the clozapine case: more people can be helped if some rather than others are helped.[15] Now suppose that if and only if B is treated rather than A will money be freed up from his care so that someone else, C, can be treated as well. This is because only B achieves normality and once he does, it will be too late to treat A.

Suppose that all those who might be treated have the same need and urgency, and these are great. Then only if we treat B can we treat another person, C, who is as needy and urgent as A is (by hypothesis). This is a determinative reason for treating B rather than A, at least if the improvement in C is significant. But now suppose that we had to choose whether (1) to help B and C, or (2) to help B and D, when D is as needy and urgent as C but D will achieve normality while C will improve to a moderate level only. If money is freed up only if we help someone who becomes normal, and E (with the same need and urgency as C and a possibility for a significant outcome) is also waiting, then we should treat B and D, rather than B and C (or A), for we can then treat E as well, given that it is too late to treat C. (See figure 20.6.)

The principle that accounts for these judgments is that when need and urgency are constant among people, we ought to treat whomever allows us to treat as many people as possible, at least when the greater number of people will be helped significantly. Earlier, I argued that we should not always choose B over A when only these two people are in great need of help just because B will do better. Hence, if we should always help B when other people's welfare is at stake, this implies we are treating B as a means to the good of others, though not as a mere means since he also benefits.

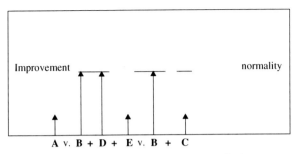

FIGURE 20.6 The Case of Multiple Persons Choices

Several objections can be raised to this analysis. The first objection is connected to the last point: The problem, it may be said, is not that we choose to help one person in part because this is a means to helping others. The problem is that the person who is *not helped* is evaluated solely from an instrumental point of view. (It might even be said that he is "treated as mere means," even though he is not causally useful in furthering our goal.) This is because he is eliminated solely because he is not useful to helping others. To make this clearer, consider the following example (called the Doctor Case): If we face a choice between saving a doctor or a teacher, the fact that the doctor will be irreplaceable in saving lives should not mean that all the lives he will save (which are indirect effects of the scarce resource he would get) are counted on his side against the teacher. It might be suggested that this is true because the teacher who would then not be selected for aid would be inappropriately evaluated from too instrumental a point of view, and not sufficiently as an end in himself. That is, it is only because he is *not* useful as a means in saving others that he is not given an equal chance for treatment. Is this not how the person who only improves moderately on clozapine is evaluated?

But now consider the following case: We have a scarce resource to distribute, and if we give it to A, he can then also carry it to another person, C, who needs our resource as much as A and B do. Person B cannot do this. In this case, it is permissible, I think, to select A over B, excluding B merely because he cannot be instrumentally useful. This is because doing this helps us to better serve those who directly need our resource. This contrasts with the previous case in which the doctor would save others who do not need our resource but only need his skills. Hence (surprisingly), it is not distinguishing people on the basis of whether they have an instrumental role that determines if our behavior is objectionable, but rather whether our choice leads us to use our resource for its best *direct* effect (rather than indirect effect as in the Doctor Case). In the case of clozapine, we select someone who will allow for the best direct use of our supply of clozapine; hence the "treating as a mere means" objection need not, I suggest, defeat the strategy.[16]

A second objection to the analysis that allows us to help more people points to the difference between (a) denying someone treatment (either by not starting it, or by terminating a trial) in order to treat a greater number of other people *here and now*, and (b) denying someone treatment in order to treat a greater number of people *later*. Suppose we should give preference to the *here and now*. By hypothesis, we cannot treat B, D, and E simultaneously, for we must wait for B to recover in order for money to be freed up to treat D, and for the same reason we must wait for D to recover before we treat E. Theoretically, it could be a year before we get to helping E, if it takes six months for B and D to reach normality. Hence, here and now, it is a choice between A and B, and so, it might be said, we should toss a coin between them. However, even if we accept the correctness of giving preference to the here and now, we can answer this objection by noting that D and E do *here and now need to be treated*, even if we cannot treat them until later. Therefore, their case is different from the case of persons (statistical or even identifiable) whom we predict will need care in the future.

However, a third objection is waiting. We have assumed that we *know* that B and D will achieve normality, but in reality the problem is that we do not know who will achieve normality. So, at the time we must choose between A and B, we have no reason to believe B will do better. Still, suppose we have already treated A for six months and he only improves moderately. Then there is at least a chance that B will achieve normality, but none that A will. If we drop A, we would do so in order to *go searching* for someone who will achieve normality so that we may help a greater number of people.

Therefore, even if the number of those we can help matters morally, we must decide whether it matters more than (a) dropping someone after we have started treatment, in order to (b) only *possibly* help someone else more, in order to (c) only eventually help a greater number. I suggest that *at least when there is as yet no positive change in the patient's condition* (and so no regression* if we end treatment), the moral appropriateness of dropping the patient depends on how long it will take to find someone who will achieve normality, and whether we are doing as much good in the interval as we would have done with the person dropped. Suppose that instead of six months, it took only one day to find out who would be normal (call this the One Day Case). I suggest that objections arising from (a), (b), and (c) would then not be weighty, and we could morally afford to go searching for those who will allow us to treat the greater number. This suggests that what is problematic in the real case, where we must wait up to six months before we know if someone will be normal, is not (a), (b), or (c). Rather, it is (in addition to regression*) the possibility of a lengthy time during which no one who is being helped will increase the numbers helped as much as or more than A can.

Notice, however, that what happens in one day in the One Day Case could be our *knowing* in one day that someone will achieve normality, without his achieving it for six months. So we may still have to wait six months before treating someone else. When the *payoff* of treating more people is not achieved quickly, do factors (a), (b), and (c) loom large again? I suggest not. This implies that it is morally more important, at least when the person dropped has not yet improved, how long the gap is between dropping him and beginning treatment for someone else whom we know will achieve normality, rather than how long the gap is between dropping him and treating a greater number of people.

What if A has already improved before we contemplate dropping him? Does the speed with which we can identify and begin treatment of someone who can become normal affect the permissibility of dropping A? If doing what leads to a patient's regression* were impermissible, the speed with which we find others to treat more successfully will not affect the impermissibility of dropping A. If regression* is not an absolute barrier to helping a greater number of other people, the speed with which we can identify a candidate whom we know will be normal and produce sufficient good should increase the permissibility of dropping someone.

VI. Conflicts of Urgency and Outcome in Two-Person Choices

We have been assuming that all candidates for clozapine have the same need and urgency, and only varying outcomes. Now we come to deal with whether outcome dominates difference in severity. But degree of need and degree of urgency may themselves differ in the candidates. For example, there may be unequal need (as I have defined it) but equal urgency (as I have defined it). Suppose A is 20 years old, has had ten years of severe mental illness, and faces a bad future. Suppose B is 20 years old, has experienced moderate mental illness for the last year, and faces as bad a future as A. There is unequal need here, as A's life will have gone worse overall if he is not treated than B's life will have gone if he is not treated. However, there is equal urgency in the sense that A's and B's futures without treatment will be as bad. (There could also be equal urgency in the sense of how soon they need treatment to avoid the bad futures.)

The type of case I wish to deal with in detail involves holding pasts equal, but varying urgency in the sense of how bad a future will occur without treatment. How do we deal with differences in outcomes when some will be worse off than others if not treated? Let us start with two-person cases.

An easy case of this type is represented in figure 20.7, where "U" stands for urgency, "O" for outcome, and the numbers indicate the degree of each.

Here A is both more urgent *and* promises a better outcome (normality) if treated. Here there is no conflict between taking care of the person who would be

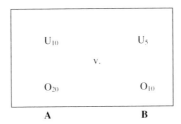

FIGURE 20.7 The Case of Greater Urgency and Outcome Coinciding

worse off and treating the one who will produce the best outcome, at least if the difference in urgency between the two people is significant. But, in another case, a conflict could arise between helping the person who would be worse off if not treated and producing the best outcome (normality). For example, see figure 20.8.

Suppose U_{10} is a very bad prospect and O_5 is a significant outcome that would improve A's condition to the point that he will be only as urgent as B is already. Then it might be argued that we should first improve the condition of the worst-off person, A, before producing a bigger benefit that goes to someone, B, who is already better off. This follows from *maximin*, which is based both on a principle of fairness between people and the idea that we produce a morally more valuable outcome if we give even a smaller improvement in outcome to the worst-off person. This conclusion even follows from nonmaximin principles, such as trying to bring those very badly off in an absolute sense to a minimal level of well-being, even if not always favoring the worst-off person.

An alternative position argues that we need not always favor the worst-off person, even when she is very badly off and we could make a significant improvement to a minimal level, if we can instead produce a much greater benefit in the life of someone else who is badly off. According to this position, helping the worst off counts for somewhat more than merely producing the best outcome, so we should assign a factor with which we can multiply the outcome score of the worst off, in accord with the absolute (and relative) badness of her condition, thus giving some priority to helping the worst off. This means that we give the worst off an edge, but someone less badly off and with a better outcome could always win out. (Presumably, it would take a bigger outcome in the less urgent person to override the weight of urgency in the worst-off person by comparison to the outcome it takes in someone equally urgent to override the tendency to give the two equal chances.)

All these policies on how to deal with conflicts between urgency and outcome conflict with certain claims made about clozapine policy as of 1994.[17] For example, that policy held that treating in accord with urgency and jeopardizing better outcomes is "against intuition." However, policies I have described favoring the worst-off individuals assume that it is not against intuition to do so. (Of course, given that urgency is no indication that clozapine will not lead to normality, sometimes there will be no conflict between favoring the urgent and producing the best outcome.)

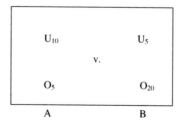

FIGURE 20.8 The Case of Urgency and Outcome Not Coinciding

It is also said that "no one argues against treatment where there is a dramatic response"—that is, marked reduction of symptoms and restoration of normality. If this means that no one could reasonably argue against treating the most urgent (in my sense) who would become normal, then that should be true. But if it means that no one could reasonably argue against treating those who would *not* be the worst off without treatment but who can achieve normality, then that is not true, at least in the two-person case.

VII. Helping More People and Helping More Urgent People

Let us expand our conclusions about conflicts between urgency and outcome to deal with the additional crucial factor in the clozapine case, namely that the number of people we can help may depend upon whom we help. Suppose A is more urgent than B but only B can achieve normality. (This assumes, hypothetically, that we could know before treatment who will become normal.) Suppose C is as urgent as A is and will produce as good an outcome. We free up money to help C only if we help B. So, should we help B and then C rather than A? (See figure 20.9.)

That choice seems peculiar. For if C is already in need now, why would we not choose to help him immediately? That is, why is it not just a contest between A and C? The only answer available is that if we treat A or C first, we will never get to treat B, for A or C will not free up money for another patient. Here we are asked to consider letting a more severe patient suffer for some months while we treat a less severe patient simply because this allows us to treat both.

Suppose we can help B and C *or* B and D but not both sets. Patient D is as urgent as C (and A), but D and not C will achieve a normal outcome. Suppose E, who is as urgent as C but cannot achieve normality, is also waiting to be treated. Only if we help D can we also help E, and so we should help B and D rather than helping B and C. We can then help two people who are as urgent as A instead of one person (see figure 20.10).

One way of interpreting the general principle at play here is as follows: Pay attention to better outcomes when doing so conflicts with taking care of the more urgent only if this makes it possible to significantly help more of those who are as urgent as those we might otherwise have helped. We do not heavily favor those

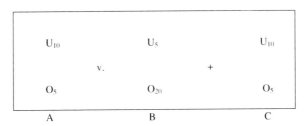

FIGURE 20.9 The Case of Helping More People

U_{10}		U_5		U_{10}		U_{10}		U_{10}
	v.		+		+		v.	
O_5		O_{20}		O_{20}		O_5		O_5

A	B	D	E	C

FIGURE 20.10 The Case of Producing More Normal People

who give better outcomes per se; we favor them so heavily only when it helps us treat more who are urgent.

In the clozapine case, however, we are told that there will be no reason to think, at the time we make a choice, that someone as urgent as A will not have as good a chance of reaching normality as B and, hence, freeing up resources. It is also more important to treat the most urgent. Thus, it seems unlikely that it ever makes sense to treat the moderately ill B with clozapine instead of someone more urgent. This means we should look for those who can produce normal outcomes among the urgent people only. (For one radical alternative to this, see the next part.) (In many medical cases, urgency—in the sense of a worse prognosis without treatment and also in the sense of needing treatment immediately—increases the chance of a poor outcome with treatment. Then the conflict still exists between attending to urgency and attending to best outcomes.)

Also, in the clozapine case, we cannot know that A will not produce a normal outcome until we treat for six months. On the basis of our previous discussion, we can see that two issues then arise. First, may we stop treating A after six months to test another urgent person for restored normality or does regression* matter morally? Second, does it matter how long it is expected to take to find someone who will respond better than A and how much good we produce in the interval? On the assumption that there are now always additional urgent cases who could reach normality, and that it is not always wrong to stop or not start treating some of the most urgent who confront us, we should drop those who are urgent but have only moderate outcomes after six months of treatment, so as to search for those who are now urgent and who will achieve normality (as long as the probability of finding these is sufficiently high and sufficient good is done in the interval of the search).

This policy, however, gives lexical priority to helping significantly as many of the worst-off individuals as we can. As noted above, an alternative is to give only somewhat greater weight to claims of the worst off or focus on them only if they are below a minimal state. On this alternative, we would neither ignore the possibility of achieving normality in the less urgent nor try to maximize the number of most urgent people treated. This might mean also taking care of moderately ill people who will achieve normality in order to increase the number of people who achieve normality.

VIII. The Moderately Ill

If there were no more urgent cases to treat who could achieve normality, would a maximin policy say that those urgent individuals who could only achieve moderate outcomes should be favored over other patients who were already only moderately ill regardless of the outcomes that the latter would produce? If so, then concern for treating the worst off would come into real conflict with the desire to produce good outcomes and with the desire to treat as many patients as possible. For if we treated "moderates" rather than those "urgents" whom we know cannot achieve normality, we might achieve more cases of normality (albeit in those only moderately ill). However, if a policy of treating moderates who become normal freed up enough money to bring more urgents up to the level of moderate well-being in a reasonable time, we would get the benefits to moderates without too great a sacrifice to urgents. Even maximin could then recommend such a policy.

A radical alternative that opens up more possibilities for treating the moderately ill suggests itself. Consider that if we continue treating only those urgents who will become normal, they will wind up *better off* than those who were moderately ill to begin with. Out of fairness, we might stop fully treating the urgents at the point where they become moderately well—assuming we could maintain them at that degree of moderate well-being if full treatment did not continue—and then decide whether to bring them or those who are already moderately ill independent of clozapine use up to normality.

This proposal may strike many doctors as morally problematic: It would have them stop treatment although more good for a patient could be achieved. However, it is not problematic in the way regression* is, and I have already argued that commitment to one patient is not necessarily a strong enough consideration to override concern for other patients. Of course, in this situation, it is just a concern for fairness rather than better outcomes that is driving the proposal, since either patient (it is being hypothesized) could become normal.

A problem with this proposal is that we lose cost-effectiveness, for we would have to use some of our clozapine resources to keep some people who would otherwise be urgent at the level of moderate well-being. Those who survive at a moderate level without clozapine are costly because they require institutionalization, but they are not as costly as those who require institutionalization *and* also require clozapine treatment to achieve a moderate level. Furthermore, when we only partially treat an urgent patient who can become normal in order to *search* for a moderate who can also be normal, we trade a sure bet for many possible failures followed by a random choice.

Notes

1. This chapter was originally conceived in 1994 as part of a Hastings Center Project on Mental Health. The version on which this chapter is based, titled "Whether to Discontinue Nonfutile Use of a Scarce Resource," appeared in *Rationing Sanity: Ethical Issues in*

Managed Mental Health Care, ed. J. L. Nelson (Washington, DC: Georgetown University Press, 2003). That essay was only slightly modified from the version that previously appeared in *Medicine and Social Justice*, eds. M. Battin, R. Rhodes, and A. Silvers (New York: Oxford University Press, 2002). I am grateful for comments from members of the Hastings Center Project, from audiences at Stanford University Medical School and the Bioethics Institute at the Johns Hopkins University, and from Ruth Faden and John Oberdick.

2. This type of trial should be distinguished from trials needed in order to get a drug approved for the market in the first place.

3. However, the method I employ in this discussion may lead to different results where scarce resources other than clozapine are involved because they do not share a particular characteristic assumed to be true of clozapine: the severely ill (what I call the most urgent cases) have as good a chance of attaining normality as those not already severely ill. In other situations (e.g., involving scarce organs for transplantation), severity of illness tends to be correlated with worse outcomes.

4. These are principles I have (for the most part) discussed in detail in my *Morality Mortality*, Vol. I: *Death and Whom to Save from It* (New York: Oxford University Press, 1993), and summarized in my "Nonconsequentialism," in *Blackwell's Guide to Ethical Theory*, ed. H. LaFollette (Oxford: Blackwell, 2000), pp. 205–26, and chapter 1 of my *Intricate Ethics* (New York: Oxford University Press, 2007). These principles are also discussed in chapters 18 and 21 this volume. I present a modified view on the use of QALYs in life-and-death decisions in chapter 21 this volume.

5. In "Mental Health Services: Ethics of Resource Utilization," Hastings Center Background Document, 1994, unpublished.

6. For more on this, see chapters 2–4 this volume and my *Morality, Mortality*, Vol. II (New York: Oxford University Press, 1996).

7. I here make use of Prospect Theory developed by Daniel Kahneman and Amos Tversky. For more discussion of this theory, see my "Moral Intuitions, Cognitive Psychology, and the Harming versus Not Aiding Distinction," *Ethics* 108 (April 1998): 463–88, reprinted as chapter 14 in *Intricate Ethics*.

8. This discussion repeats some of what was said in chapter 18 this volume, in order to make it possible for one to read these chapters independently of each other.

9. See my *Morality; Mortality*, Vol. I.

10. These claims are discussed in more detail in my *Morality, Mortality*, Vol. I. For some modifications of this view, see chapter 21 this volume.

11. In *Morality, Mortality*, Vol. I, I called it the Principle of Irrelevant Utilities.

12. Notice that I have constructed this case and the one in which B would not have a sore throat as ones in which we do something to make a good occur. This is parallel to our doing something to make a good occur in the case where C receives a benefit. By this, I mean that we do not just save someone who would not have a sore throat, or would have two arms if he survives because of his own prior condition or nature. I believe the additional good would also be irrelevant in the latter cases. The distinction between these types of cases plays a more important role in chapter 21 this volume.

13. For reasons I shall not go into here (but discuss a bit in chapter 18 this volume), I do not believe that a correct use of an ex-ante perspective on the issue yields a different result.

14. This was suggested by Ruth Faden.

15. Previously I have considered another real-life case in which the numbers of people we can save matter. That case centered on whether one patient who needs multiple organs should be transplanted with them or whether each of the organs should be given to a different individual so that more people will be saved. I distinguished between (1) what I called synchronic cases, in which at t_1 we either give all the organs to one person or distribute them among others; and (2) what I called diachronic cases, in which at any given time the contest for the organ is between only two people, but the person saved at t_1 will need another life-saving organ at t_2 and at that time compete with a different person. (The contests with others repeat several more times.) The question is whether a person who has already had one organ should not be helped before treating someone who has not yet had an organ. For my discussion of these cases, see *Morality, Mortality*, Vol. I, pp. 324–29.

16. I point out the distinction between direct and indirect use of our resources in *Morality, Mortality*, Vol. 1. I believe there is a striking similarity—indicating that the same underlying principle is at work—between (i) what distinguishes the Doctor Case from the clozapine case and (ii) what distinguishes cases in which it is and is not impermissible to use scarce lifesaving resources on a candidate because he is nondisabled rather than disabled. In the contrasts in (ii), we may favor a candidate whose makeup allows us to use our resources also to cure his disability but not to favor a candidate merely because he is already not disabled. (The latter is like what happens in the Doctor Case when we "piggyback" on the doctor's skills rather than treating more people with our drug.) For more on this, see chapter 21 this volume.

17. As reported in "Mental Health Services: Ethics of Resource Utilization."

21

Aggregation, Allocating Scarce Resources, and Discrimination against the Disabled

I. Introduction

In this chapter,[1] I first re-present certain claims that I have made in past work in which I distinguish between the moral significance of intrapersonal and interpersonal aggregation of (1) life years, (2) need, and (3) quality of life, for the purpose of making decisions about the allocation of scarce lifesaving resources among different people. (I call the latter interpersonal allocation.) Then I consider some partially contrasting views of Peter Singer on these matters. Finally, I present some new views—which contrast with both my earlier views and Singer's—on the role of quality and quantity of life in nondiscriminatorily allocating lifesaving and non-lifesaving resources between disabled and nondisabled individuals. I also examine how ex-ante reasoning behind a veil of ignorance bears on these issues.

The issues I discuss in this chapter, often using hypothetical cases, have relevance to many real-life cases in which lifesaving resources are scarce. Often, we cannot help everyone who needs and could benefit from these resources, and so we must choose whom to help. For example, flu vaccine, ICU beds, and organs for transplantation are often scarce. The focus of most of this chapter is on theoretical issues, especially in relation to aggregation, rather than on their application to these particular cases. However, the theoretical issues do bear on the real-life cases. For example, we shall consider whether how old someone is, or how good an outcome she will have, or how her outcome comes about, matters in determining whom we should help.

II. My Views in Past Work on the Significance of Intrapersonal versus Interpersonal Aggregation for Allocating Scarce Resources Among Different People

A. THE PRINCIPLE OF IRRELEVANT GOODS

In the course of earlier work on moral issues in the allocation of scarce lifesaving resources,[2] I sometimes distinguished between interpersonal and intrapersonal aggregation. I shall here try to make this distinction salient and bring together, in

A		B	E		F		G
↓	vs.	↓	↓	vs.	↓	+	↓
10 yrs		15 yrs	10 yrs		10 yrs		5 yrs
	Case 1				Case 2		

FIGURE 21.1

a way I have not before, cases that show the difference between interpersonal and intrapersonal aggregation. By aggregation, I mean any way of combining goods, bads, values, and rights. In interpersonal aggregation, these things are distributed over different individuals, while in intrapersonal aggregation, these things are concentrated within the life of one individual. In both types of cases, what is to be aggregated (let us say goods and bads, for short) may occur at one time or over a temporal span. As an example of how the difference between interpersonal and intrapersonal aggregation might affect decisions about the interpersonal alloca-tion of scarce resources, I have in the past employed cases such as the following, represented in figure 21.1.

Case 1 represents the choice of saving person A for ten years or saving B for fifteen years, all other things being equal between them. Case 2 represents the choice of saving E for ten years or saving F for ten years plus saving G for five years, all other things being equal between them. My sense was that in Case 1, the extra five years for B intrapersonally aggregated with the ten years that he as well as A could achieve might reasonably not make a difference to whether we decide to save A or B. That is, perhaps we should continue to give each an equal chance. If so, this means that the extra five years for B is what I call a *morally irrelevant good* in this interpersonal allocation. The decision-making principle illustrated here is what I call the Principle of Irrelevant Goods, which says that sometimes the fact that we can produce an additional good if we choose to perform one act rather than an-other is morally irrelevant.[3] This is not because that extra good is always irrelevant. It is possible that a good which is irrelevant to a choice in one context could be relevant to a choice in a different context. Hence, the Principle of Irrelevant Goods is consistent with its being preferable for B to live fifteen years rather than ten years; five years is not an irrelevant good from his intrapersonal point of view. And in the context where the only question is whether to (1) save B to live another ten years or (2) save B to live another fifteen years, we should choose the latter. Also, when pro-ducing the extra five years involves saving a third person (G), as in Case 2, then the five years, I believe, should be interpersonally aggregated with saving F for ten years to determine that we should save F and G rather than E. The fact that we could significantly affect another person (G), equal in all other respects to others, counts morally in a way that benefiting one person (B) to an additional degree does not.[4]

I believe that this is true even independent of any effects of diminishing mar-ginal utility that might be thought to account for the difference in the significance of an extra five years for B rather than for G. (That is, if G will die if he does not

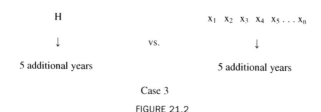

Case 3

FIGURE 21.2

receive our aid but will live another five years if he does, then five years can mean more to him than it does to B, who will be saved for ten years anyway.) For suppose that G, unlike the others, will live for ten years regardless of what we do, but we can also extend his life for another five years if we save F rather than E. I suggest that this might determine that we should save F and G rather than E, even if we should give A and B equal chances. This is because we can give an additional five years to a second person if we help F and G rather than E, thus interpersonally aggregating the five years. This is in contrast to giving an additional five years to B, the same person who already will be getting ten if we help B rather than A, thus intrapersonally aggregating the five years.

There could also be cases where intrapersonal aggregation affects interpersonal allocation decisions but interpersonal aggregation does not. Consider Case 3 (see figure 21.2): We have to go either to one island to allocate a resource to H (who will then live fifteen more years instead of the ten more years he would live without the resource) or to another island to allocate the resource to an enormous number of people, equal in other respects to H, who will be saved for one extra minute of life over and above the ten years they would each live without the resource. I do not think that the interpersonal aggregation of the very small benefit to each person, though it amounts to five years or more in total, should weigh against the significant benefit we can produce for H in allocating to him.

B. NEED

In earlier work, I also argued that the need for a resource that provides additional life could be a function of how much (adequate conscious life) someone will have had if he is not given the resource. How much he will have had without aid is a function of how much he has had up to the point at which he needs aid and how much he will have in the future, even if he is not aided. I said that the person who would die having had the least amount of adequate conscious life was neediest for additional life, and he would be the person who would be worst off without additional life, other things equal. This means that intrapersonal aggregation of past years of life can help diminish the need for additional life. Note that if at the time we must distribute a scarce resource, one person has had only twenty years of life and another has had forty, this will not necessarily mean that the first person is neediest. For if he would live on for twenty-five years even without the resource, but the second person would die in a year without it, it is the second person who is the neediest candidate. This is because the second person will die having had forty-one years of life while the first will die having had forty-five. (The second person is not neediest merely because he will die in a year, whereas the other person will die after many more years. If the twenty-year-old would live for only ten years without the medicine and the forty-year-old would die in one year without the medicine, the first person would still be neediest—as I have defined the term.)

C. OUTCOME

Expected outcome, in terms of future life years, also seemed morally relevant to me in deciding whom to help. If one person could only live another day with the resource and another could live five years, and other things were equal between them, then it seemed right to give the resource to the second person. Because both (1) expected future life years and (2) need (as explicated above) could matter in making interpersonal allocation decisions, we need to aggregate (i.e., combine) these two dimensions. I thought that sometimes a person with greater need should get a resource even though his expected outcome in life years would be worse, when all other factors were equal (including how good the additional years would be). For example, in Case 4 (not represented in a figure), person I is someone who, if he is not saved, will die having had twenty years of life, and person J is someone who, if not saved, will die having had fifty years of life. If person I is saved, however, he will get only ten years of life, while if J is saved, he will get twenty, and all other things are equal between them (e.g., quality of past and future life). My view was that person I should get the resource because his need is great (in absolute terms) and significantly greater than J's, and he would have a significant outcome (even if not as good as J's). This means that being older can be relevant to being denied a resource even if it is not linked to a worse outcome. I called this an Outcome Modification Procedure.

A way to capture this conclusion is to aggregate need and outcome by assigning a multiplicative factor greater than 1 to need above a certain amount, varying the multiplicative factor according to degree of need, and multiplying the absolute value of outcome (in years, for example) by the multiplicative factors.

D. QUALITY OF LIFE

I also claimed that in making life-and-death allocation decisions, while differential lengths of future expected life in different candidates could sometimes be morally relevant, the expected quality of this life was not relevant, so long as it was minimally adequate conscious life (versus, for example, life in a coma) and was desired by the person who would live it. The same would hold true for past life used to evaluate degree of need. To illustrate this, consider Cases 5 and 6. (See figure 21.3.)

K		L	M		N
↓		↓	↑		↑
20 yrs	vs.	20 yrs	20 yrs	vs.	20 yrs
excellent quality		mediocre quality	excellent quality		mediocre quality
			↓		↓
			5 yrs		5 yrs
			excellent quality		excellent quality

Case 5   Case 6

FIGURE 21.3

In Case 5, the fact that K will have excellent quality of life in his expected future twenty years of life and L will not, when all other things (including their pasts) are equal, should not, I think, lead us to deny each of them an equal chance for the lifesaving resource, given that they each want to live on. In Case 6, the fact that M has had twenty past years that were better than N's should not, I think, lead us to favor N for the future five years of life, when all other things are equal between them. These views could be the result of just considering how many years of adequate conscious life someone will have had if we do not aid him and how many additional years of such life (that he wants) our resource can provide.

E. DALYS AND QALYS

This result conflicts with the use of QALYs (Quality Adjusted Life Years) and DALYs (Disability Adjusted Life Years), at least for purposes of deciding how to allocate a lifesaving resource among different people. The principle behind QALYs is to aggregate years of life and degree of good quality of life by multiplying a number for quantity times a number for quality in order to determine aggregate good, either in past years or in future years. The principle behind DALYs is to aggregate years of life and degree of disability of life by multiplying a number for quantity times a number for degree of disability in order to determine aggregate bad, either in past years or in future years.[5] If we were to use these devices to decide how to allocate a scarce resource between people, we could choose whoever will maximize future QALYs or have minimum future DALYs. Alternatively, we might give to the person who will be neediest if not given the resource, in terms of either lowest QALYs or highest DALYs. Another alternative would be to combine consideration of need with consideration of expected outcome. I took my conclusions about cases like 5 and 6 to imply that we should not use calculations of QALYs and DALYs in deciding who lives and dies. This meant that certain sorts of intrapersonal aggregation (e.g., the aggregate of years and quality) should not matter in the interpersonal allocation of lifesaving resources.

III. Peter Singer's Views on the Significance of Intrapersonal and Interpersonal Aggregation for Allocating Scarce Resources Among Different People

A. FUTURE QUALITY OF LIFE

Now let us consider some views of Peter Singer. Singer has argued that in making life-and-death allocation decisions, there is no injustice or unfairness in deciding on the basis of future quality of life.[6] For example, whether someone will be disabled if he survives could make a difference to whom we choose to aid, without this involving unfairness.[7] I shall focus on three types of arguments for this conclusion that can be discerned in Singer's work, though I shall present them in my own way.

(S1) Someone's quality of life is worse if he is disabled than if he is not, other things equal. Evidence for this is that we try to cure or prevent disabilities if we can. We should maximize the good, and this implies saving the nondisabled person, other things equal. Suppose that one of two people (who would have the same quality of life) would live much longer than the other if he received a scarce treatment. It would not be problematic to choose to aid him: "For those who count only QALYs, it makes no difference whether the smaller number of QALYs gained comes from a lower quality of life or from a shorter expected life span."[8]

(S2) One would prefer to live a nondisabled life of a given length rather than a disabled life of the same length, given the choice. Furthermore, people do sometimes trade length of life for quality of life. We can find out how to rank the quality of the disabled life by assigning 1 to a normal life and then seeing how many years of a life with the disability would be traded for normal years. If a person would trade two disabled years for one normal one, then the quality of the disabled year is 0.5. The application of QALYs calculation to one person's life tells us which life for himself a person can reasonably prefer.[9] If someone can live either ten years at 1 or ten years at 0.5, it is only rational for him to prefer an outcome with a QALY rating of 10 (10×1) to one with a QALY rating of 5 ($10 \times .5$). Indeed, as shown by the time tradeoff test, it is also intrapersonally rational for someone to be indifferent between one year without a disability and two years with such a disability that reduces the value of a year to 0.5.

One could add the following point: One would prefer a more cost-effective outcome in one's own case over a less cost-effective one. For example, for a given expense, one would prefer to be nondisabled rather than disabled.

If these are the outcomes that should be chosen *intra*personally, Singer believes that they should be chosen *inter*personally as well, other things equal. For example, we should save someone with a higher QALY outcome, at least when other things are equal. We should give equal chances to live to someone who will live for five normal years and someone who will live for ten years with a 0.5 disability, or twenty years with a disability rated 0.25. We should choose the most cost-effective outcome. Support for this conclusion, Singer thinks, comes from (S3).

(S3) Suppose one is behind a veil of ignorance and does not know whether one will be disabled or nondisabled. Singer describes the person who will be non-disabled as having "a stronger interest in continuing to live" than the disabled person, and as someone for whom continued life holds greater value. He says, "To maximize the satisfaction of their own interests, rational egoists would have to choose a system that gives preference to saving life when it is most in the interests of the person whose life is saved."[10] Another way to put his point is as follows: Ex-ante, one maximizes one's expected average utility by agreeing to a policy that will save the life of the nondisabled person, rather than give an equal chance of survival to disabled and nondisabled, if one assumes one has an equal chance of being either person. For example, if we assign a probability of 1 (certainty) to ten years ranked at quality 1 and a probability of zero to ten years ranked at quality 0.5 (i.e., $(1)(10)(1) + (0)(10)(.5) = 10$), we get a higher sum than if we assign a probability of 0.5 to both ten years at quality 1 and ten years at quality 0.5 (i.e., $(.5)(10)(1) + (.5)(10)(.5) = 7.5$). Singer concludes that if the just and fair principle of allocation between people is the one that they would choose in conditions of ignorance about who they will be, while trying to maximize self-interest, then the principle of saving the nondisabled person is fair and just, not merely maximizing of the good.

As Carlos Soto points out,[11] these arguments from Singer should apply when disability, strictly speaking, is not in question, but when the interpersonal choice is between saving a life of intelligence and happiness versus a life of boredom and dullness. For why, Soto asks, would rational egoists behind a veil of ignorance choose to make health a "separate sphere," where only effects on health and not effects on other goods (such as intelligence, wealth, etc.) are counted in a QALY calculation? Singer's arguments should also make every small difference in QALYs relevant to interpersonal choice; there should be no irrelevant goods or bads.

B. AGGREGATION

Singer says that he is a straightforward aggregationist.[12] That is, whether goods or bads are aggregated intrapersonally or interpersonally is irrelevant to a moral decision, in his view. Apart from cases where diminishing marginal utility is at issue (when we give one person more of a good rather than spreading it around), the distribution of goods and bads between people is irrelevant. Hence, he would disagree with my conclusion concerning Case 3 (in figure 21.2). His view, however, also implies that if many disabled people can be saved rather than just one nondisabled person, the interpersonal aggregation of their QALYs could exceed *one* individual's better outcome.

Singer is known as a supporter of famine relief. Yet as a strict aggregationist, if he had a choice between saving a few thousand people dying of starvation or curing the headaches of each of a sufficiently enormous number of people, he should do the latter. Hence, despite his fame as an advocate of famine relief, Singer's theoretical position does not offer as strong a defense of such aid as does a position that emphasizes giving priority to satisfying the needs of the worst off even if this interferes with maximal aggregate benefits.

It is not clear, however, that Singer consistently adheres to his aggregationist doctrine. For example, he claims that he supports the following principle governing aid: Unless something of *comparable* moral significance is at stake, we should relieve suffering.[13] Singer thinks that this principle implies that one must bring oneself and one's family down to a level such that if one did any more in order to aid, one would be worse off than those whom one is trying to help. But this does not seem to be the correct limit, for it calls for something like a pairwise comparison of oneself and any given individual one might help, to see if anyone one might help is worse off than one would be if one helped him. But Singer supposedly supports aggregation, not pairwise comparison, and it is possible that making oneself and the few people in one's family *worse off* as individuals than those whom one is trying to help might still prevent great suffering in each of many individuals and might prevent more suffering *in aggregate* when we total prevention of even minor losses in the many people whom one's sacrifice helps. (This is especially likely to be true, given the relative costs to feed people in different countries; the money that comes from my depriving myself of food in the United States, even if I let myself starve, can be used to buy meals for hundreds of people in Africa.) For example, I think that, considered impartially, the death of me and my family at a young age is not of comparable moral significance to the avoidable deaths of thousands of others at even a slightly greater age. Hence, Singer's principle, when combined with a commitment to aggregation of equal or even lesser losses, demands more than he says it does.[14]

C. THE WORST OFF

Singer also gives no priority to helping those who will have been worst off if not aided (the neediest, as I am using the term). Hence, aside from the issue of diminishing marginal utility, the fact that someone will have had many more years of life even if he is not aided does not (in Singer's view) weigh against him in competition with a person who will die at a much younger age if not aided, so long as the first person would offer more additional QALYs in the future if he is aided than the second person would if he is aided.

Singer discusses selecting for a lifesaving procedure either someone who has had a poor-quality past life through being paralyzed or someone who has been normal, when either could live for forty more years. He objects to the view that the disabled person should be saved as a way of compensating her for her worse past. This is another way of objecting to focusing on who will have been the worst off if not aided, when both quality and quantity judgments are used in deciding who will have been worst off.[15] He claims, "To the extent that the purpose of health care is to lessen pain and suffering, and to the extent that nothing humanly possible can be done to lessen past pain and suffering, it would seem more reasonable to treat the person who is presently suffering more, since at least this person's suffering can be lessened. Nothing can be done about past suffering, whereas (often) something can be done about present and future suffering."[16] One might object to this that, if one allocates with an eye to the past, something can still be done about how much someone will have suffered in his life overall, and this seems important. Focusing on past pain, furthermore, may be misleading in several ways. When pain occurs, we think it is the intrinsic quality of the experience that is bad, rather than the fact that it interferes with having other good things. But if someone was disabled in the past, he may not have been able to do as much as a normal person in the same period of time, and the things he did not do in the past (that the nondisabled person did) could be done in the future if he stays alive.[17] Similarly, if someone would die not having lived very long, this would interfere with his having more life in the future, and this future can still be given to him.

By contrast to Singer, even someone who thought it right to consider every difference in quality and quantity in life-and-death choices and equated interpersonal and intrapersonal aggregation might still give weight to need. Thus, she might choose to save a person who will have had a short life if he is not aided, even though the difference the aid makes to his future outcome will not be as great as the difference it could make to someone who will have lived a long life even without aid. She would do this because the first person will have been the worst off if not aided. Similarly, someone who relied on choice from behind a veil of ignorance might choose the maximin solution or some other form of priority to the worst off, even if this did not yield the best outcome.

D. FURTHER EFFECTS ON OVERALL GOOD

Despite his views supporting the allocation of scarce lifesaving resources to the nondisabled rather than to the disabled, Singer suggests a reason for treating them equally. He says,

> We have rejected the claim that QALYs are unjust or unfair. . . . This does not necessarily mean that we think that health care should always be distributed so as to produce the largest possible number of health-related QALYs. There is more to overall utility than health-related QALYs, and it is plausible to suppose that tilting the balance of health care towards the more disadvantaged members of society will reinforce feelings of concern and sympathy and lead to a more compassionate society. This, in turn, may be a society with more community feeling and therefore one that provides a higher level of general welfare than a less compassionate society.[18]

The point is that Singer thinks the right acts or policies are the ones that maximize welfare overall. For someone who thinks this, it may make sense to perform an act or accept a policy that produces less than maximal welfare directly because it leads to greater welfare down the road than any other act or policy. He suggests that one could recommend a policy allowing compassion for the worse off to override maximizing good outcomes, if this leads to more compassion in general and if more compassion in general leads to maximizing welfare.

One problem with this proposal from the point of view of someone trying to maximize welfare is that more compassion may just continue to lead to choices that do not produce maximal welfare. And so compassion can produce no more welfare than continually doing what directly maximizes welfare. Hence, it seems hard for a maximizer to opt for relying on compassion as an indirect way to increase welfare rather than encouraging more direct maximization continually.

Singer not only considers whether compassion for the worse off could increase welfare; he also suggests that people's decisions not to maximize good outcomes in particular interpersonal allocation cases (as shown in surveys) might be explained by either (1) their "concern for the effects that a direct maximization approach has on the kind of society we are,"[19] or (2) their view that it is important to "go beyond abstract justice or fairness," favoring "those who would otherwise feel themselves arbitrarily disadvantaged."[20]

Singer would no doubt prefer to interpret people's concern with the effects of a society of direct maximizers in (1) as a concern that the absence of compassion in some cases will reduce overall social welfare. However, there is another interpretation available: People may be concerned with a society of direct maximizers even if it leads to maximizing welfare, because they do not think that maximizing welfare is the correct standard for right action. With regard to proposal (2), Singer is suggesting that candidates for a scarce resource who will not have the best outcomes may incorrectly believe ("feel") themselves arbitrarily disadvantaged by a rule that selects according to best outcome, and people surveyed may believe that one way to maximize welfare in the face of such an incorrect belief is to go beyond justice and fairness. But an alternative interpretation is that the people surveyed think that always deciding on the basis of maximizing welfare is not what justice or fairness permits or requires. For ordinarily, when beliefs about arbitrary disadvantage are incorrect, we should seek to change them rather than cater to them.

IV. The Allocation of Lifesaving Resources Between the Disabled and the Nondisabled

Having laid out in parts II and III some general positions (my own in past work, and Singer's) on aggregation and allocation, the rest of this chapter will further examine the issues of intrapersonal versus interpersonal aggregation, the quality and quantity distinction, and the relevance of ex-ante decision making to the allocation of scarce resources between disabled and nondisabled persons.[21]

How would the use of DALYs bear on the health of disabled people (who, I shall assume, have physical impairments)? DALYs evaluation of their lives could make it clear that their lives are more physically impaired than the lives of the nondisabled, and so health resources should be directed to curing or compensating for their impairment. But suppose we cannot cure or compensate for their disabilities so that their lives are still higher on DALYs ratings.[22] How will they fare in the competition with the nondisabled for other health-care resources? Even if we cure their other illnesses or save their lives, we often cannot thereby produce a person with as low a rating for DALYs as if we treat the nondisabled. Our outcomes will often not be as good. If it is not, in general, unfair to consider how good an outcome will be in deciding where to use monetary and health resources, then is it not unfair in such decisions to count their disability against the disabled? This is the issue with which I shall be concerned.

We can refer to the issue as The Problem. One way it can arise is from the following argument embedded in (S1) above: Disabilities make life worse for the person whose life it is, other things equal. That is why we try to prevent or correct them (Premise 1). Hence, we will get a worse state of affairs if we help a disabled person whose disability we cannot correct rather than help someone else equal in all respects except that he lacks the disability (Premise 2). In deciding whom to help with a scarce resource, we should try to produce the best outcome (Premise 3). Hence, we should help the nondisabled, other things equal (Conclusion).[23] This conclusion is meant to apply to cases in which we must choose whose life to save, as well as cases in which we must decide whose illness to treat when no one's life is at stake. If we deny the conclusion, it seems that we must reject or modify one of the premises.

In what follows, I shall discuss different approaches to The Problem and the argument from which it can arise. The first approach focuses on the third premise. The second approach, taken up in the last section, focuses on the first and second premises. I shall focus on life-and-death cases but also discuss cases in which non-life-threatening illnesses must be treated.

A. ARGUMENTS FOR TREATING NONDISABLED AND DISABLED ALIKE

The Major Part Argument

Consider the following scenario: One person is on island A, and another is on island B. They share all the same properties, except that one has recently lost a hand and the other has not. Because the loss to one person is so recent, the two people share equally good pasts. We can save the life of either one but not both. Arguably, each will be as badly off as the other if we do not help him, for each will be dead, having had the same length and quality of life.[24] But if we help the person who lost a hand, we do not produce an outcome with as few DALYs as we would produce if we saved the other person. (Call this the Islands Case.) I think it is morally wrong to decide whom to aid on this ground. We cannot rely on the principle of giving priority to the worse off to account for this conclusion, since each would, arguably, be as badly off as the other if not aided.

The Principle of Irrelevant Goods, however, might account for the right decision, for the following reason: In the Islands Case, what each person is capable of achieving is the part of the outcome about which each reasonably cares most, especially given the potential loss that is at stake for each. Put differently, what is reasonably held to be most important to each person can be had by either—long life saved with good quality of life. Furthermore, we should take seriously from an impartial point of view the fact that each person, from his subjective perspective, wants to be the one to survive. Given these facts, the additional benefit of a hand in one person's case can be seen as an irrelevant good in the competition to be saved. Fairness may require, therefore, that we not deprive either person of his equal chance for the great good of lengthy survival for the sake of the additional benefit of a hand in one person's case. This is especially true when that one person who would get the additional benefit is someone who would already be getting the other great benefit of additional life. That is, it is a case of an additional good concentrated in one of the two rather than dispersed over a third person.[25] I shall call this the Major Part Argument, for the irrelevance of some good means that either person can get the major part of what stands to be gotten, and this is all that is relevant to interpersonal allocation.

An analogy to this case is one in which only one of two people can be chosen to avoid extreme poverty. Each could reach a high income, but one could be somewhat richer than the other. One might argue that avoiding very bad poverty by achieving considerable wealth is the major part of what is at stake for each, and each person understandably wants to be the one to be helped; thus, the additional wealth that only one can achieve becomes an irrelevant good for purposes of choosing whom to help, at least when we are only concerned with these two people.

This last case, of course, is disanalogous in that it does not involve a life-and-death choice. However, it reminds us that the Principle of Irrelevant Goods could also be applied to a non-life-and-death case in which we must choose whether to treat a non-life-threatening illness, such as gastritis, in a disabled person or a non-disabled person. (We are supposing that the drug to treat gastritis is scarce and we cannot treat both patients.) Suppose we could cure this illness as well in the person who lacks a hand as in the person who has two hands. One way to apply the Major Part Argument to this case leads to the conclusion that so long as each will have a life with the major part of what it is reasonable for each to want in life, each should get an equal chance for the treatment.

However, the non-life-and-death cases also raise other issues. For example, the person who recently lost a hand might be worse off without treatment for gastritis (given that he will then have to deal with *two* problems) than the person with two hands would be.[26] This, it might be suggested, could give one a reason to favor treating the disabled person, even though we could cure the gastritis equally well in both.[27] However, as the disabled person might still have the major part of what each person wants in life, favoring the worse-off person for treatment seems to go beyond the Major Part Argument per se.

Most importantly, when we can treat non-life-threatening illness equally well in a disabled and a nondisabled person, the overall outcome with treatment will differ by just as much, relative to what the outcome would be without treatment, whomever we treat. To make this clear we can lay things out as follows, where "UD" is undisabled person, "D" is disabled person, and "GC" is the gastritis cure: $(UD + GC) + D = UD + (GC + D)$. It is true that if we treat the nondisabled person, a person with a 1 QALY ranking may result, and if we treat the disabled person instead, a person with no more than a 0.9 may result. But if we do not treat the nondisabled person, he will be alive with close to a 1 ranking anyway.[28] And if we do not treat the disabled person, we are left with someone alive with the lower QALY-rated life (at an even lower level than it would be with gastritis treatment). Only if treating the nondisabled person, for example, led to other good effects (healthwise or nonhealthwise) that would not occur if the disabled person were treated would there be a difference in overall outcome.

At least in the Islands Case, we can acknowledge that not having a hand makes life worse, other things equal, yet this acknowledgment is compatible with the view that relative to the question of whose life we should save, the missing hand could be a morally irrelevant consideration. Hence, targeting funds to replace a missing hand in one person because life without it is worse (e.g., harder) than life with it, other things equal, is not inconsistent with giving equal weight to saving the lives of the disabled and the nondisabled. This is contrary to what a simple use of QALYs in distributing scarce resources would predict, and it is a reason for rejecting the latter approach.

This way of dealing with The Problem (above) accepts the first premise in the argument that gives rise to The Problem, and even the second premise. It rejects the conclusion because it rejects the third premise, as it claims that differences in outcome are not always morally relevant to how we should decide to distribute a scarce resource. Hence, it is part of a nonconsequentialist moral theory that tells us that the right act or right policy is not necessarily the one that maximizes good consequences.

The Moral Importance Argument

Consider a case involving a larger disability. We must choose between saving the life of someone who has recently become paraplegic (where paraplegia is assumed, for the sake of argument, to be rated at 0.5 on a QALY scale, on the basis of a time-tradeoff argument) and a person who would be saved to live a perfectly healthy life (a QALY rating of 1). They have identical pasts and can live an equal number of future years. It might be said that when the prospect each faces is to fall to zero on a QALY scale (death), it is a significant good merely to achieve 0.5, and a person should not be deprived of the equal chance he wants to get that good merely because someone else could achieve that good plus an additional benefit that brings him to a QALY rating of 1.

Why might this be so? We cannot say, in this case, as we could in the Islands Case, that what each would get is at least the major part of what stands to be gotten and the difference is frosting on the cake. If one person can be saved to a life of perfect health (rated 1), this is assumed to be equivalent to an extra 0.5 beyond the 0.5 level of a paraplegic life. We can imagine each individual's getting at least up to 0.5 on a QALY scale but only one person's getting the 0.5 increase to 1 on the scale. But reaching 0.5 on the scale, achievable by each, is not the major part of 1; it is half of 1.

In response, it might be said that it may be morally more important to give someone the basic goods that help him avoid the worst evil and *make his life one worth living* than to give him the goods which admittedly double the overall value of his life. Hence, without claiming that a life QALY-rated at 1 provides less than twice the good as one rated at 0.5, we can claim that *moving someone from 0 to 0.5 is morally more important than moving him from 0.5 to 1*. Another way of putting this point might be that it is having a life worth living that is of crucial significance, and if paraplegics can have this, they have what is relevant to deciding to give equal chances for life, given that each individual (the paraplegic and the nondisabled person), from his personal point of view, wants to be the one to have a life worth living. I call this argument for giving the disabled and the nondisabled equal chances the Moral Importance Argument, because it emphasizes the moral importance of giving people equal chances at what is most important in life.

The analogous argument in the case of income would claim that avoiding extreme poverty and having a reasonable income is what is most important. Hence, we should give equal chances to escape extreme poverty to someone who will achieve middle-class income and to someone who will (with a combination of what we provide and his superior luck or talent) become a millionaire. This assumes that each wants to be the person chosen and that we are only concerned with these two people. As this is not a life-and-death case, it reminds us of the case of choosing whether to treat a non-life-threatening illness, such as gastritis, in someone who has recently become paraplegic or to treat the same illness equally successfully in a nondisabled person. One way to apply the Moral Importance Argument to this case implies that, as the paraplegic whose illness is treated would have as much of those things that it is most important to have as a nondisabled person whose illness is treated would, each should be given an equal chance.

It is beyond the scope of the Moral Importance Argument to take account of the possibility that someone who will also have to cope with paraplegia should be given priority over a nondisabled person in avoiding the additional burden of the gastritis. Taking account of who will be worse off, however, might well be a relevant consideration in deciding whom to aid in this non-life-and-death case. Again, a very important point in non-life-and-death (by contrast to life-and-death) situations is that if we can treat the gastritis as successfully and there are no further differential effects of nongastritis in the disabled and the nondisabled, the overall outcome with treatment would differ by as much relative to what the outcome would have been without treatment, whomever we treat.

The Sufficiently Good Only Option Argument

Another argument for sometimes ignoring the difference between a QALY rating of 0.5 and a rating of 1 in lifesaving cases is as follows. Suppose one can only have a life rated at 0.5 and not 1, and the alternative is zero (death), which is very bad. One may reasonably want 0.5 as much as one would want 1 if one could have it. So, for example, given that 0.5 is all that one can have and zero is very bad, one might reasonably do as much to achieve 0.5 (e.g., spend as much money, suffer as much) as one would do to achieve 1 if one could have it. This is consistent with the willingness even to risk losing 0.5 and falling to zero for a chance at 1, as would happen if someone who is a paraplegic decides to have surgery that could cure his paraplegia, even though he might die in the surgery. (What is known as the *standard gamble test* examines how bad paraplegia is by considering how big a risk of death one would take to avoid it or cure it.) That is, the fact that one would risk falling to zero in order to get 1 instead of 0.5 does not show that one would be more likely to risk falling to zero in other pursuits (e.g., risky leisure activities) simply because one would only be losing a life rated 0.5 instead of 1. Hence, a paraplegic might reasonably choose to risk death in order to get a better life for himself as a non-paralyzed person because he *cares more for* (in the sense of *prefers*) the nonparalyzed life, though he *will reasonably not care more about* this nonparalyzed life, if he gets it, than he cares about the life he already has (were it all he could have). This shows that "if one can have only *x*, one cares about it as much as one would care about *y*, if one had it" is not equivalent to "one cares to have *x* as much as one cares to have *y*."[29] It suggests that the only external measure for 1 being worth more than 0.5 to someone is the willingness to exchange 0.5 for 1 but not vice versa, or to risk falling below 0.5 to go from 0.5 to 1 but not vice versa. The difference in worth between 1 and 0.5 need not show up in a difference in the other goods that one would give up to get or keep 1 or 0.5, if either were one's only option. All this may seem paradoxical, yet I think it is true.[30]

What I have said conflicts with Singer's view, described in (S2) and (S3) in part III above, that the nondisabled person has a stronger interest in going on living than the disabled person has. Singer concludes this on the basis of the time-tradeoff argument (rather than the standard gamble argument). He describes someone with a severe disability who would (let us assume, reasonably) exchange forty years with the disability for four years without it.[31] He concludes that her interest in living forty years with the disability is less than a nondisabled person's interest in living forty years. But what I have said implies that the fact that someone reasonably *cares for* a shorter life with higher quality need not imply that she reasonably *cares about* her only option of the longer life with lower quality less than a nondisabled person cares about the same length of life.

What I have said also supports my view that willingness to take an *intrapersonal* risk of death in order to achieve a better life for oneself does *not* translate into the permissibility of imposing the same risk of death interpersonally on someone whose own life cannot be improved by the risk, if imposing that risk will result in a better life for another person.[32] It supports my view that an intrapersonal preference for a life rated at 1 over a life rated at 0.5, and thus the relevance of the aggregation of 0.5 and 0.5 intrapersonally, does not translate into the importance for interpersonal allocation of a difference between 1 and 0.5 in two different persons.

These results are contrary to the results implied by Singer's arguments (S2) and (S3). For argument (S2) implies that whatever chance of death it would be reasonable to take to avoid one's own disability is the same chance of death it is reasonable to impose on one person so that someone else will live a nondisabled life.[33] ([S3] implies even more: certain death for the disabled so that the nondisabled live.)

To make my point even more graphically, consider the following two cases. First, suppose that someone could undergo surgery that has an equal chance of (a) curing his disability or (b) definitely killing him if he remains disabled. In this case, if the person cannot be rendered nondisabled, he will definitely die. It could be reasonable for someone to choose such surgery if the disability is bad enough. In the second case, someone will definitely die in the case where the surgery fails and he is still disabled only if the single life-support machine in the hospital is not available to him. If he is cured of disability, he will also need life support immediately after surgery if he is to survive. If the surgery cures his disability, he must be taken to one postoperative room; if it does not, he must be taken to another room. The rooms are far apart and the life-support machine must be placed in one room or another before surgery in order to work afterwards. It could be reasonable for the patient to decide to have the machine placed in the room he will be in if he is cured, thus planning to leave himself to die if he is disabled.

These conclusions in the intrapersonal cases do not imply that it is reasonable to definitely let a person die who will be disabled in order to be able to save *another person* who will be nondisabled. This is true even though, ex-ante, the probability of being a disabled person or a nondisabled person is the same in the intrapersonal and interpersonal scenarios, and the ex-ante chance of death is also the same. It could even be true when the intrapersonal chance of death that it is not unreasonable to take in order to be nondisabled is greater than the ex-ante chance of death one would run if the nondisabled person is automatically helped relative to the different disabled person.[34]

The failure to appreciate the difference between "caring for" and "caring about" may be the result of not distinguishing two different notions of the worth of life. First is the notion that involves evaluating lives as better or worse, where all properties of the life are included in this evaluation. (When Singer speaks of those whose continued life holds greater value, he may have this in mind.) Second is the notion of the worth of life, or going on living, to someone. On this second notion, the quality of the person's life—thought of as a set of synchronic properties that modify any period of her life—is treated as a background condition, and we ask whether going on living for a certain quantity of time—thought of as a diachronic property—is worth as much to her as it would be to someone who had different synchronic properties.[35] The view I am proposing is that going on living could reasonably be worth just as much to someone who has a less favorable set of synchronic/quality properties as to someone who has a more favorable set.[36] (If so, we cannot conclude that a life that holds greater value is also, as Singer claims, the life that a person has a "greater interest in continuing to live."[37]) This implies that going on living, at least as a self-conscious person with a certain amount of good in his life, is a separate good for someone, to be distinguished from other quality-of-life goods that his life may be instrumental to achieving.

Nonetheless, there are such other quality-of-life goods, and someone who lacks them might exchange some quantity of life (or risk losing all quantity of life) in order to get the other goods. This does not mean that if he is reasonable, he should care less for continuing life per se if he cannot have these other quality-of-life goods, as compared to someone who can have these quality-of-life goods. (Of course, there may also be some conditions, such as extreme unending suffering, that negate or override the value of continuing to live.) The person with life of higher quality has what is more in any person's interest to have by comparison with a lower quality of life. But the fact that one person will get more of what is in anyone's interest to have if he goes on living need not imply, I suggest, that it is more in his interest to go on living rather than to die than it is in the interest of another person to go on living rather than to die.

Notice that some future life could be worth living (e.g., an additional three happy months of life) but it might not be reasonable for the person for whom this was the only option to sacrifice as much to gain this additional three months of life as to gain a much longer period of life with a QALY rating of 1 (were this possible).[38] Hence, it is not always reasonable to do as much to get one type of life worth living, even if it is all one can get, as it would be reasonable to do to get a better type of life worth living. This implies that in the argument I am now considering, it is not merely having a life worth living that is crucial. On account of this, I shall call the additional argument I have now given the Sufficiently Good Only Option Argument.

If either the Sufficiently Good Only Option Argument or the Moral Importance Argument is correct, it helps expand the reach of the Principle of Irrelevant Goods. This is because these arguments suggest how the irrelevance of certain additional goods can be used to argue for treating equally the nondisabled and those with large disabilities, even when the Major Part Argument cannot be used to support the Principle of Irrelevant Goods.

What does the Sufficiently Good Only Option Argument imply for cases in which we must decide whether to treat non-life-threatening gastritis in someone who is recently paraplegic or in someone who is nondisabled, other things equal? One way to apply the argument implies that if life as a paraplegic without gastritis is a sufficiently good only option, then we should give equal chances to this person and to the nondisabled person. It might also be argued that since the paraplegic would have to cope with two problems if he also had gastritis, but the nondisabled person would have to deal only with gastritis, we should favor the disabled person when deciding whom to treat. This view, however, goes beyond what the Sufficiently Good Only Option Argument itself implies. Again, in non-life-and-death cases, a very important point is that if we can treat the gastritis as successfully and there are no further differential effects of nongastritis in the disabled person and the nondisabled person, the overall outcome would differ by just as much, relative to what the outcome would be without treatment, whomever we treat. This is because both disabled and nondisabled live on.

Being on a Par

It is worth noting that the three arguments just discussed, which support the irrelevance for interpersonal choice of a good that is relevant for intrapersonal choice, seem to be similar to arguments about values that are "on a par." If x and y are of equal worth, and $x + n$ is of greater worth than x, then $x + n$ should be of greater worth than y. But, it has been said, if x and y are merely "on a par," then $x + n$ may not be worth more than y, even if it is worth more than x. An example that can be used to illustrate this point is as follows: Medium good baroque music is on a par with medium good romantic music; slightly better baroque music is clearly better than medium good baroque music, but it is not necessarily better than medium good romantic music; the two can remain on a par.[39]

This might be analogous to saying that while in the life of person A, it is better to have a QALY rating of 1 than a rating of 0.5, a rating of 0.5 in the life of person A can remain on a par with a rating of 1 in the life of person B. A clearly preferable outcome, which should be selected in an intrapersonal choice, remains on a par for purpose of interpersonal choice. What could make them be on a par is that they are being considered relative to death as the alternative, and each person wants to be the one to live. Each person functions like a separate category, the way baroque and romantic music do, and those categories provide insulation from intrapersonal (intracategory) changes having an effect on interpersonal (intercategory) choices. On this view, the separateness of persons can make changes that are relevant intrapersonally irrelevant to the interpersonal choice.[40]

B. A PROBLEM WITH THE ARGUMENTS: DIFFERENCES IN QUANTITY OF TIME

Now consider what I think is a problematic implication of the Major Part Argument, the Moral Importance Argument, and the Sufficiently Good Only Option Argument in life-and-death cases. They would seem to imply that we should treat sufficiently good only options that involve *quantity* of life in the same way as we treat sufficiently good only options that involve *quality* of life. That is, large differences in how long someone can live if we save him should make no more difference to whom we save than large differences in quality of life do, other things equal. (This is the concern raised by Singer that I describe in [S1]: How can we distinguish quality and quantity of life in allocation decisions?) For example, suppose one person can be saved to live for five years and another for fifty years, and everything else is equal between them. Five years is a very significant good, and given that it is someone's only option, she might reasonably do everything to get it that someone who could live for fifty years would do to get that. If there is a moral difference between taking account of expected length of life (both in the future and in how long someone will have lived if not aided) and taking account of disability or some other quality-of-life factor (both in the future and in the life someone will have lived if not aided), then another argument apart from those we have considered is needed to justify this.

Notice also that in previous sections, we have been led to focus on and argue for a difference between intra- and interpersonal decision making. It is this difference between intra- and interpersonal contexts that was supposed to explain why sometimes producing more QALYs would not be a morally correct decision. By contrast, the problem raised by a possible moral difference in counting quantity of time as opposed to quality of time in an outcome does not depend on a jump from the intrapersonal to the interpersonal context. For this problem already assumes that even in an *interpersonal* context, it can be morally right to decide on the basis of big differences in quantity of time, other things equal. So we start with something that it seems permissible to do in an interpersonal context and then the question is why something else (i.e., using another measure—quality—of better outcome) is not also permitted in the interpersonal context.

Here is one possible answer. Each person is entitled to equal respect and (at least for purposes of an impartial distribution of scarce resources) equal concern. That may mean that (at least certain) synchronic properties, such as whether one is or will be paralyzed, even assuming that they significantly affect quality of life, should not bear on selection for scarce resources. If these synchronic properties are appropriately thought of as determining one's type identity, one might say that equal respect makes type identity (in many cases) irrelevant for purposes of allocation. (Call this the Principle of Irrelevant Type Identity.) However, taking into account, for example, how long a person can live if he gets a scarce resource is not treating someone differently because of the type of person he is or will be qualitatively; the latter (it is being suggested) is done only if we consider someone's synchronic properties (properties that determine the character of his time alive). Theoretically, it is compatible with each synchronic type that a person could be, that he could be that type for longer or shorter amounts of time.

However, this does not rule out that having a certain synchronic property could *cause* longer or shorter life. For example, having a disability might make impossible doing exercises necessary for longevity. This is what I call linkage—a causal relation between a disability (or any other property) and other effects that might be morally relevant to allocation. One does not, I think, hold against someone his synchronic property per se in taking account of its causal links. Hence, it may not violate equal respect and concern for different types of persons to consider how long they will have lived or will live even if this is due to their type.

This argument offers an interpretation of meeting the requirements of equal respect and concern, so I shall call it the Equal Respect Argument. In another way, it attempts to extend the Principle of Irrelevant Goods while distinguishing quality and quantity considerations. It suggests that we may take account of large differences in outcome when this does not deny equal respect and concern to people in virtue of synchronic properties they have or will have. Thus, if we had a choice between saving a paralyzed person (with a quality rating of 0.25) who could live for twenty years or an unparalyzed person (with a rating of 1) who could live for six years, the Equal Respect Argument would recommend saving the paralyzed person. This is so even though, in an *intra*personal choice, the aggregation of quality and quantity could make it reasonable for someone to choose six normal years over twenty years with a quality as low as 0.25.[41]

Does the Equal Respect Argument have implications for cases where we must decide whose non-life-threatening illness should be treated? One possibility is that equal respect and concern for different types of people implies giving equal chances for treatment of gastritis to the disabled and to the nondisabled person. However, equal respect and concern need not entail equal treatment, even if they do entail treatment as an equal. Suppose the disabled person who is to be treated as an equal would suffer more healthwise overall if he has gastritis than a nondisabled person would because the former also must deal with a disability. Possibly equal respect and concern *itself* implies that the disabled person should be given priority for treatment. Again, it is also important to remember that in non-life-and-death cases, the difference in overall outcome with treatment *relative* to outcome without treatment can be the same, whomever we successfully treat.

Another possible approach to the problem of treating quality and quantity differently that does not seem to rely on notions of respect can be clarified by extending the analogy involving income that was used earlier.[42] Suppose we must decide whom to help overcome poverty in the following two-choice sets: (1) One person will avoid extreme poverty by having $50,000 a year and another by having $1 million a year; (2) One person will avoid extreme poverty for five years and another for fifty years (whether by having $50,000 a year or $1 million). Intuitively, I think that it could be reasonable to help the second person in (2) (without giving an equal chance to each) even if each should have an equal chance in (1). In these cases, the value of having a certain type of life—in terms of its synchronic properties—need only be sufficiently good in order to be given equal chances with a better type of life. But how long one will retain any type of life that is sufficiently good can be a morally important difference. However, it does not seem that we need to bring in the idea of equal concern and respect for people with different type identities in this discussion of income levels. It is sufficient to say that the types of lives they will lead (in terms of synchronic properties) are sufficiently good or provide them with what is most important (significantly avoiding extreme poverty) and each wants to be the one helped. Once that is settled, it is a question of how long that good will last that is important in an interpersonal choice.

This argument builds on the Moral Importance Argument and the Sufficiently Good Only Option Argument but restricts their scope to types of lives independent of length. Hence it supports the Principle of Irrelevant Type Identity. Once again, this principle does not rule out considering the effect of a type on how long a sufficiently good condition will last. So if having only $50,000 a year meant that one could not sustain a sufficiently good income condition for long, it would be a reason to help the person who would have the type of income level that would sustain a sufficiently good condition for a much longer period of time. Since this argument does not focus on respect, I shall refer to it as the Irrelevant Type Argument.

C. THE TREATMENT AIM PRINCIPLE

Are the results of the Major Part, Moral Importance, Sufficiently Good Only Option, Equal Respect, and Irrelevant Type Arguments, and the Principle of Irrelevant Goods that they support, consistent with what is standardly understood to be the correct account of a nondiscriminatory policy in treating the disabled and the nondisabled? This account says that if a treatment aims to correct a particular problem (e.g., gastritis, or upcoming death due to kidney failure) and is equally successful in achieving that aim in a disabled and a nondisabled person, the difference in outcome represented by the continuing presence of the disability in one person is irrelevant. I shall call this the Treatment Aim Principle. It is one way to capture the result noted above that in non-life-and-death cases, the overall outcome with treatment would differ by just as much, relative to the outcome without treatment, whomever we treat.

However, for various reasons, the Treatment Aim Principle differs from the other principles so far considered. First, the Principle of Irrelevant Goods could imply treating candidates equally when the Treatment Aim Principle would distinguish between them. This is because even if the aim of treatment is to correct a particular problem, the Principle of Irrelevant Goods would imply that some differences in the degree to which *that* particular problem is successfully treated could also be morally irrelevant in deciding whom to treat. So, if one person's gastritis could be treated slightly less successfully than another's, this might be morally irrelevant to who gets the treatment. Alternatively, another way to apply the Moral Importance Argument and the Sufficiently Good Only Option Argument is to argue that if the most important part of the good of treatment is possible in either candidate, or if each could get a sufficiently good improvement due to treatment, we should not select on grounds of different success in treating. If this were true of a difference in treatment outcome between two nondisabled candidates, it should also be true that the difference is not what determines a selection between a disabled and a nondisabled candidate. A similar conclusion could be drawn about life-and-death cases where one candidate would go on to live somewhat, rather than much, longer than another.

What if we could treat a fatal or nonfatal illness *much more* successfully in one person than in another? The Treatment Aim Principle should favor the person in whom treatment is much more successful. For example, suppose that someone's disability interfered with his doing exercises that should accompany a drug that treats gastritis, and so his treatment would not be as successful. The principle takes this as a conclusive reason to help the nondisabled person. The other principles I have considered need not lead to this result, if they are combined with giving priority to the worse-off person. But the Treatment Aim Principle is inherently in tension with an argument based on the importance of need (i.e., priority to the worse off) in deciding whom to aid when treatment is less successful. In the case of lifesaving treatment, giving priority to the worse off could direct us to give a successful lifesaving treatment, or even one that is significantly less successful, to the person who will have been overall worse off if he did not get it (in terms of years lived) rather than to someone else (who would die at an advanced age, for example). By contrast, the Treatment Aim Principle by itself not only ignores this other consideration but seems to exclude it. It implies that we should just consider what our treatment itself can do for people, rather than considering additional problems (e.g., dying much younger or having an additional problem with which to cope) that one person would have rather than another.

Putting to one side the issue of helping the neediest (and continuing our assumption that the disability is recent), let us consider other cases in which treatment of fatal or nonfatal illnesses will be much more successful in the nondisabled person than in the disabled person. In these cases, both the Treatment Aim Principle and the other principles I have considered could favor the person in whom treatment is most successful, even if it is due to his disability that the treatment is much less successful in the disabled person. This is an example of linkage—a causal relation between a disability and other effects that are relevant to allocation decisions. Consider, first, life-and-death cases. Suppose that if we give a scarce, lifesaving organ to a nondisabled person, he will live twenty years. If we give it to a disabled person, he will live five years because his disability makes it impossible to do comparably good surgery on him. In this case, the Treatment Aim Principle might take the aim of surgery narrowly construed (i.e., implanting the new organ successfully) not to have been equally achieved in the disabled and nondisabled, and so can recommend giving the organ to the nondisabled. Hence it, as well as the Equal Respect and Irrelevant Type Arguments, can recommend giving the organ to the nondisabled person. In this sort of linkage case, we are not holding the disabled person's disability against him as a lived component of his life but rather considering its causal effects on treatment success. But suppose the disabled person will live for only five years because, though the organ is implanted successfully, he cannot do certain exercises subsequent to surgery that help maintain the organ well. It is not clear that the Treatment Aim Principle should count the fewer years that he will live against him. By contrast, the Equal Respect and Irrelevant Type Arguments can consider how many years he will live if he is treated. This is no different from considering the causal effects of being *non*disabled—a state which is considered preferable to disability in itself—if it were imagined to cause far fewer years to result from lifesaving surgery. In the latter case, according to the Equal Respect and Irrelevant Type Arguments, the surgery should be performed on the disabled person.

Consider a nonfatal illness. Suppose that someone's disability prevents a successful surgery to correct gastritis. Then the Treatment Aim Principle could recommend allocating the scarce surgery to the nondisabled person. The same conclusion might be yielded by one way of applying the Sufficiently Good Only Option Argument if the outcome of treatment did not make a sufficiently good improvement in the disabled person due to his disability.

There is another way that linkage can occur and be relevant to the allocation of scarce resources that the Treatment Aim Principle does not capture. Suppose that a disabled person and a nondisabled person each have a fatal disease X and can be treated equally well for it, so that X does not lead to a shorter life in one person than in another. However, the disability on its own, not even because it interferes with proper maintenance of results of treatment for X, will result in death shortly after disease X is cured. Strictly speaking, treatment of disease X is equally good in either patient, and so the Treatment Aim Principle should be neutral as to whom we treat. But, presumably, it is wrong not to take account of the fact that the very same negative factor that our treatment seeks to avoid—namely death soon—will occur anyway, though an entirely different cause. The Treatment Aim Principle by itself does not distinguish between helping someone who will succumb in a few weeks to another illness and helping someone whose successful treatment implies that he will live for twenty years. By contrast, the other principles that I have discussed can recommend that the nondisabled person get the scarce resource in such a case.

What if a scarce treatment for a non-life-threatening illness that causes a lot of pain can work equally well in a disabled and a nondisabled person, but the disabled person will end up with the same degree of pain caused by his disability alone? Again, the Treatment Aim Principle, strictly speaking, would recommend not distinguishing between the two candidates, but the principles that I have discussed need not do this.

To avoid these problems, we would have to modify the Treatment Aim Principle to take account of what I call condition similarity, in which conditions similar to the ones we aim to treat will occur in any case in the patient. A Condition Similarity Principle requires that we check whether we could cure a fatal or nonfatal illness without there being conditions similar to the ones we aimed to cure occurring in the patient in any case. (The Condition Similarity Principle, however, will not correctly deal with a case in which we could successfully treat a *nonfatal* disease equally well in a disabled or a nondisabled candidate, but his disability will soon cause the disabled person *to die*. This is because while the soon-to-occur death should undercut the candidacy of the disabled person, this is not because a negative condition *like the one* we are trying to treat will occur in any case from a different cause. Further modification, which I shall forgo, could correct this problem.)

So far, I have discussed the role of linkage in making it permissible to deny a scarce resource to a disabled person, whether we are using the Treatment Aim Principle or other principles I have discussed. But linkage involves a disability having a causal relation to some other property relevant to allocation. The Condition Similarity Principle shows us a way in which the disability itself (i.e., the synchronic property) could sometimes be morally relevant to the allocation decision. Suppose a nonfatal disease will cause paraplegia and also pain; and we are interested in treating it in order to prevent both of these bad states. We can prevent the pain equally effectively in either a paraplegic or a nonparaplegic candidate, but the fact that we can successfully prevent the disease from attacking the nerves in either candidate results in the prevention of paraplegia only in the candidate who is not already a paraplegic. If avoiding paraplegia is the most important part of our aim, it could be morally correct that the disabled person not be a candidate for the treatment. Furthermore, this is not because of the further causal effects of his disability but simply because of (what I call) the role of disability as a *component of his life*. We have previously seen that the Condition Similarity Principle extends the limits of the Treatment Aim Principle. Now, we see that it also sets a limit to the Principle of Irrelevant Type Identity. It accounts for why it may sometimes be permissible to deny a scarce resource to someone who is disabled because he is disabled per se.

Consider again the Treatment Aim Principle. Arguably, a treatment can be considered just as successful if it achieves its aim even if it has bad side effects. Suppose that giving a scarce non-lifesaving treatment to a disabled person will result in a bad side effect caused by the interaction of the treatment with his disability. The bad effect is not so bad as to totally outweigh the good the treatment does him. A nondisabled person will get the same good effect without the bad side effects. The Treatment Aim Principle might be further modified to take account of side effects. Then it would imply that treatment with bad side effects is less effective, and so we should help the nondisabled person. The other principles I have discussed could imply the same only if the side effects were significant enough.

In the next section, I shall consider further the possible role of side effects of treatments, not necessarily due to a causal effect of disability or nondisability, on the allocation of scarce resources to the disabled versus the nondisabled.

D. FURTHER GROUNDS FOR SOMETIMES NOT IGNORING DISABILITY WHEN ALLOCATING SCARCE RESOURCES

Switch Cases and the Causative Principle

Suppose that the extended Principle of Irrelevant Goods (or another principle that supports it) implies that we should not prefer saving an unparalyzed person to saving a paraplegic person (other things equal). Then it would also imply that we should not prefer saving a paraplegic who, as a side effect of lifesaving treatment, will also be able to walk again to saving a paraplegic who will remain a paraplegic. That is, it would imply *no role* for such a quality difference in expected outcome among equally disabled candidates. It would also imply no role for such a difference in outcome between equally nondisabled candidates—so if one unparalyzed person would become paraplegic as a side effect of lifesaving treatment but another would not, this should make no difference to whom we choose to save. I call these cases in which the disability condition of a person changes as a result of lifesaving treatment the Switch Cases. Are these results correct?

These Switch Cases raise the following possibility: (1) Sometimes a sizable extra synchronic good (or bad) *that we can produce* in the outcome, if we treat one person rather than another, should be morally relevant in deciding whom to help with a lifesaving resource.[43] (2) Yet, if candidates for treatment who present themselves have this difference in good (or bad) between them, and this is why it shows up in the outcome, the extra good (or bad) should be morally irrelevant in deciding whom we help with a lifesaving resource. The Principle of Irrelevant Goods cannot account for the simultaneous truth of (1) and (2). I call this the Asymmetry Problem.

Proponents of the view involving both claims (1) and (2) need a principle that will explain why the fact that a person is and will be disabled to a certain degree should sometimes be irrelevant in deciding whose life to save, but the presence of the same disability in an outcome can sometimes be morally relevant and used in a nondiscriminatory fashion in deciding whose life to save. That principle would imply that a QALY evaluation could sometimes be relevant in making life-and-death choices, *depending on how the difference in quality comes about.* This implication differs from the position described in part II, which excluded a role for most quality-of-life evaluations in allocating scarce lifesaving resources.[44] It is still different from Singer's position, described in part III, which would generally require quality-of-life evaluation, other things equal.

There could also be Switch Cases and an Asymmetry Problem in non-life-and-death situations. For example, suppose that a scarce drug that prevents impending blindness will also cure the paraplegia in one candidate but not cure the paraplegia in the other. Alternatively, the same scarce drug could be imagined to prevent blindness in either nondisabled candidate but cause paraplegia as a bad side effect in only one candidate. These Switch Cases are meant to contrast with one in which we can prevent blindness in either someone who has recently become paraplegic and will remain so or in someone who will remain nondisabled. In these Switch Cases, the principles suggested earlier imply that either equal chances should be given or we should take into account that someone will have a much harder life if he will be both paraplegic and blind rather than just blind. The Principle of Irrelevant Goods and some other principles discussed earlier might be understood to imply that we should ignore the good and bad side effects in allocating the drug in non-life-and-death Switch Cases, at least on the supposition that blindness is a significantly worse fate than paraplegia.[45] Those who support claims comparable to (1) and (2) in non-life-and-death situations will also need a principle that makes them compatible.

Even someone who thought a difference in outcomes such as disability should not matter, regardless of how it comes about, might be interested in seeing if we can distinguish a *discrimination objection* to counting the difference from a more general objection to counting such a difference in outcome based on the Principle of Irrelevant Goods (or principles that support it). One claim about these Switch Cases might be that sometimes, even if we do wrong in violating the Principle of Irrelevant Goods in taking account of certain differences in outcomes, we would not be engaged in (invidious) discriminatory conduct. Our conduct might be wrong but not because it involved discrimination, given that we focus on how the difference in outcome came about.

(We have already seen that the Treatment Aim Principle, if modified, might suggest that when disability causes a worse outcome of treatment for another condition than the one we aim to treat, it is not discriminatory to select a nondisabled candidate. We also suggested that the Condition Similarity Principle implies that when the disability is another cause of the type of condition that we are aiming to treat, or is itself the type of condition we are aiming to treat, it is nondiscriminatory to allocate a drug to the nondisabled person. Nevertheless, favoring the nondisabled person in these cases may still be a mistake, if the differences in outcomes between candidates should be irrelevant goods.)

It is important to realize that the Asymmetry Problem raised by the Switch Cases does not depend on another issue I have discussed—that is, the fact that, prior to being disabled, people rate the disabled state as much worse than they do once they are disabled. It might be thought that it is because the disabled person who comes for treatment rates his life equal to the nondisabled person but the nondisabled person rates the same disability we will produce in his future as very bad that an Asymmetry Problem arises in the Switch Cases, at least when life-saving treatment would make a nondisabled candidate disabled.[46] But this is not so, because *I am holding constant the negative value of the disability in those already recently disabled and those who will be newly disabled due to treatment.* So, I am assuming that the life of the already-recently disabled is worse than the life of the nondisabled, other things equal—that is *the reason why* a new disability should be avoided—and yet it could still be wrong to treat differently two people just because one is nondisabled and the other is already recently disabled. Nevertheless, sometimes, though the continuation of the disability is as bad as its future occurrence, *our producing* the new disability might provide a reason to favor the candidate who will not be disabled as a result of our treatment.

It will be useful to present some cases and the judgments in each for which the new principle would try to account. Let "P" stand for paraplegia and "U" for unparaplegia in the following cases in which we must decide to whom to give a scarce lifesaving procedure. (See figure 21.4.)

Persons	Case 7		Case 8		Case 9	
	A	B	C	D	E	F
	P	U	U	U	P	P
	↓	↓	↓↓	↓	↓↓	↓
	P	U	P	U	U	P

FIGURE 21.4 Nonswitch and Switch Cases

In Case 7, a lifesaving procedure will save A or B, but not alter the recipient's initial status as paraplegic or not. I shall assume at this stage (given what was said in part IV, section B) that we should not favor B because a better outcome will thereby result (one with more QALYs).

In Case 8, we select between two nonparaplegic people, but only in the case of C will the lifesaving procedure also cause paraplegia. (The double arrow indicates causation as a result of what we do.) In this case, I believe some (who agree with the conclusion in Case 7) might decide it was permissible to save D on the basis of the fact that we would thereby get a better outcome because we would avoid harming someone. (This is so even if one could reasonably want to go on living just as much if one were to be in condition P as if one were to be in condition U.)

In Case 9, we select between two paraplegics, but only in the case of E will the lifesaving procedure have the additional good effect of curing her paraplegia. In this case, I believe some (who agree with the conclusion in Case 7) might think it permissible to choose to save E rather than F on the basis of the fact that we thereby get a better outcome by producing a cure for paralysis, as well as saving a life. (Differentiating between candidates in Case 8 may be less plausible than doing so in Case 9, I think. That is because the harm we would do to C is less than the harm that would befall him if he died.)

Notice that Case 8 differs from Case 10. (See figure 21.5.)

In Case 10, the single arrow leading from U is intended to symbolize the fact that person C*'s paraplegia is not caused by the lifesaving procedure, but rather by an independent cause that would have resulted in paraplegia so long as C* lived. It is possible that those who would save D rather than C in Case 8 would nevertheless see Case 10 as morally like Case 7: while the state of person C* when we treat him is unparalyzed, he is the sort of person who, independent of anything that we

Persons	C*	D*
	U	U
	↓	↓
	P	U

Case 10

FIGURE 21.5

Case 11

Persons	E*	F*
	P	P
	↓	↓
	U	P

FIGURE 21.6

do, will become paraplegic. I believe that, in this case, those whose judgments I am examining would say that we should *not* decide to save D* on the basis of his better outcome.

Similarly, Case 9 differs from Case 11. (See figure 21.6.)

In Case 11, the single arrow leading from P to U is intended to symbolize the fact that E*'s unparalyzed state is not caused by the lifesaving procedure or anything else we do, but rather by an independent cause that would have resulted in an end to E*'s paralysis, so long as he lived on. While the state of E* when we treat him is paraplegia, he is the sort of person who, independent of anything we do, will become nonparalyzed. I believe, in this sort of case, that those whose judgments I am considering might say we should *not* decide to save E* on the basis of his expected better outcome. That is, Cases 7 and 11 are morally alike. There should be no difference in how we decide to allocate a lifesaving resource just because one person is permanently paraplegic and the other is only temporarily paraplegic *in this way*. However, to be "temporarily paraplegic" because our lifesaving cure can also sometimes cure paraplegia has, it might be argued, different moral significance. (Cases analogous to 10 and 11 involving non-life-and-death situations could be constructed. For example, someone who will become paraplegic independent of what we do is competing for the drug to prevent blindness with someone who will remain nondisabled. And someone who will outgrow his paraplegia is competing for the drug to prevent blindness with someone who will remain paraplegic.[47])

A principle that can account for the responses I have described in the preceding cases can be referred to as the Causative Principle. It tells us that we may decide whom to help based, in part, on the synchronic difference we can make to a person's situation, not on the synchronic difference he brings to the situation. (By "we," I do not mean doctors in particular, but the health-care intervention system generally.) More particularly, the Causative Principle is concerned with the differential effect of our treatment in producing nondisability and our being entitled (though not obligated) to bring about a better outcome by using our skills in this way. The principle is also concerned with not causing disability. So it could distinguish between someone who was and remains P and someone whom our treatment causes to be P. It could also be concerned with causing someone to remain U who would otherwise change from U to P or causing someone to remain P who would otherwise change to U.

The Causative Principle tells us to ignore this difference in outcome when it arises in any other way, whether because the disability or nondisability inheres in the person or will arise because of what inheres in him, or even will arise from causes outside of him other than our treatment. (For example, if we know a criminal will do something to one nonparalyzed person to make him paraplegic if he lives, we should ignore this knowledge.) The Causative Principle is applied against a background in which the outcome that results is (i) still one that is a life worth living, and (ii) reasonable for someone to do a great deal to retain. I also continue to assume that one can permissibly compare outcomes regarding length of life for purposes of choosing whom to save, even when the difference in quantity of life is *not* caused by what we do (though it may follow on what we do). (The difference we *make* does not include every change that will occur in people's lives through other causes that will occur following what we do to them.)

For convenience, I will just say that the Causative Principle tells us to "ignore who the candidates are, as evidenced by the synchronic properties they have and will have, and look to what we do even with respect to synchronic properties." The Causative Principle can be combined with a limited use of the Principle of Irrelevant Goods, in that some differences we cause are still morally irrelevant if they are relatively too small.

In Case 7, we save life in the paraplegic person as much—by hypothesis, no more than and no less than in terms of length—as we save life in the nonparaplegic person, and we do not cause nonparaplegia in the nonparaplegic person. By contrast, in Case 9, we cause the additional large good of nonparaplegia in one patient. In doing this, we produce a nonparalyzed life *by saving a life and by making it unparalyzed*. In Case 7, when we save the life of a nonparalyzed person, we produce a nonparalyzed life *by saving a life that is nonparalyzed*; the synchronic outcome *piggybacks* on a property the person brings with him. We might say that this is the difference between doing what makes people unparalyzed and doing what makes unparalyzed people. (There is a comparable distinction between causing a paralysis, and paralysis in an outcome piggybacking on a synchronic property someone brings with him.)

In non-life-and-death cases, there is a comparable difference, for example, between (a) an outcome in which a person is nonparalyzed and not blind because we prevent blindness and piggyback on the person's nonparalysis, and (b) an outcome in which a person is nonparalyzed and not blind because we cure paralysis as well as prevent blindness.

One proposed justification of the Causative Principle is that when outcomes are affected by who a person is and/or by what we do, counting only what we do is consistent with the account of respect for different types of persons given above (in part IV, section B), at least so long as what we do is significant. Counting the qualitative differences that the people themselves bring, I have suggested, is not consistent with respect for different types of persons, except when the difference results in a life below a certain minimum (e.g., a life not worth living or not worth doing a lot to save), or there is significant conflict with the Treatment Aim Principle or the Condition Similarity Principle. However, we can reasonably value paraplegia less than nonparaplegia as a state, without this in itself showing disrespect for paraplegic people, and without treating a person who is or will be (through causes independent of us) in the state less well just because he is or will be in the state. But if we accept the Causative Principle, valuing the nonparaplegic state more than the paraplegic state can have a worse consequence for one person than for another. For suppose we use these values to choose whom to aid when we can, for example, do more good for one paralyzed person by making him nonparalyzed. Then the person who will not be cured of paraplegia will not be given the scarce lifesaving resource (and a person who will not be cured of paraplegia will not get the scarce blindness-preventing resource in our other case).

Notice that the Equal Respect Argument said that choosing whom to save based on how long each of the people will live is consistent with respect for different types of people, and it drew no distinction between extra life being (1) something we produced (e.g., by being able to do a certain type of procedure on one person but not another), and (2) something that results only from what the person brings with him (e.g., extra genetic hardiness). It is only in dealing with the synchronic properties that characterize the time a person lives and the type of person he is that, it is suggested, we should distinguish between producing and piggybacking in order to act consistently with equal respect for persons.

Here is an illustration of the Causative Principle on a large scale. Suppose there is a volcano erupting on an island. We could either save 100 people on the left side of the island or 100 on the right, but not both. In Case A, the people on the left are paraplegics, the people on the right are not paralyzed, and the groups are equal in all other respects. The claim is that we should choose randomly if we are not to invidiously discriminate. In Case B, the people on both sides are paraplegics, but because of the peculiar circumstances, if we save the people on the right, we will unparalyze them; if we save the people on the left, we will not unparalyze them. The Causative Principle implies both (a) that it is permissible to choose to save the people on the right because they will be unparalyzed by what we do, and (b) that, even if it were impermissible to do this, it would not be because it discriminates against paraplegics. (It might be impermissible because, for example, the Principle of Irrelevant Goods rules it out on the ground that, in a life-and-death contest, nonparaplegia is an irrelevant good.)

We could now re-examine the Islands Case (discussed above) to see whether our judgment there is really best explained by the Causative Principle rather than by the Principle of Irrelevant Goods. The test is to see whether our *correcting* the loss of a hand while saving someone's life could help determine which one of two people we save—one whose lost hand we could not correct and one whose lost hand we could correct in saving him. If such effectiveness should matter to our choice in this case, then *not* distinguishing between the people in the original Islands Case would only reflect the inappropriateness of distinguishing between people when we do not cause the difference between having a hand or not. By contrast, if the difference in what we can do would not be relevant to our choice, it is the moral irrelevance of the differential good that is crucial. I think the difference between having a hand or not is an irrelevant good in the Islands Case, even when we would correct its absence in one person, and so it is the Principle of Irrelevant Goods rather than the Causative Principle that accounts for our judgment in that case.

One concern about the Causative Principle is how it will deal with other quality-of-life differences. That is, suppose that of two people who have always been mentally dull, if we save the life of one person but not another, we can also make him intelligent. Should the fact that we can cause this difference make it permissible for us to choose to save one person rather than another, when all else is equal between them and each wants to live for the extra ten years each could have?

Treatment Aim Principle Modified

As a preface to introducing the Switch Cases, I noted that it is possible that a treatment could be considered more or less successful depending on whether it has bad side effects, even if it achieves the aim of treatment per se. This raises the possibility that the Treatment Aim Principle, if modified, might also be able to deal with the Asymmetry Problem raised by the Switch Cases.

Suppose that if we use a certain treatment for a deadly heart problem in one paralyzed person, but not if we use it in another, it also cures his paralysis. This was not our original aim. For this reason, the Treatment Aim Principle might seem to be equally satisfied whichever paralyzed person is treated. However, it might be argued that once we know that the drug can treat two conditions (heart failure and paralysis), we could aim at treating them both. Since we cannot achieve both our aims by treating the person who remains paralyzed, this would imply that we do not violate the Treatment Aim Principle in not giving him a chance for treatment of his heart condition. (Another way of looking at this case involves the Condition Similarity Principle: the person who remains paralyzed has a condition that is like the one we are trying to treat with the dual-aim drug. This could be true if the cause of paralysis in the two people differs.)

But how would the Treatment Aim Principle modified in this way justify, in a different case, treating the unparalyzed person who will not become paralyzed rather than the one we will paralyze? It might simply be said that successfully treating someone is a function not only of achieving the treatment's aim but also of avoiding bad side effects of treatment. I am not certain that this modification is consistent with the spirit of the Treatment Aim Principle. This is because, in this case, the bad side effects in one person will not be as bad as the death she will otherwise face, and ordinarily one would not refuse to treat the more serious problem just because a less serious side effect will occur. It is only the fact that someone else will not have the bad side effect that tempts us not to treat where the side effect would occur.

However, if these (and earlier suggested) modifications were successful, then what I shall call the Treatment Aim Principle Modified would result. It may overlap, at least in part, with the Causative Principle. And both have to be constrained by the Principle of Irrelevant Goods, I believe; for minor differences that we cause in treating or achieving the aims of treatment may be morally irrelevant when what is at stake is a chance for a great good that could be had by either patient.

The Treatment Aim Principle Modified could also apply in non-life-and-death cases. Either we turn the additional large, good side effect into a further aim, or we judge a treatment to be more successful if it avoids a significant bad side effect.

Switch-and-Reduce Cases: Can Causation Affect the Role of Intrapersonal Quality and Quantity Tradeoffs in Interpersonal Allocation?

Now consider a further modification of the Switch Cases. Suppose that in a modified version of Case 9, G and H have a disability giving them a QALY rating of 0.25. We can save G and also render him nondisabled by using a scarce resource in a particular way that would reduce the number of years he can live to five. He has the option of going through such a procedure or of going through a different lifesaving procedure. The latter is the only procedure open to H, and it uses the scarce resource so that either G or H could live for twenty years but remain disabled (0.25). If G chooses the latter nonswitch option, we should give him and H equal chances for the procedure using the scarce resource. However, it is not unreasonable for G to trade some extra years of life for improved quality of life. If it were true that the disability reduced the QALY rating of a life to 0.25, then it would not be unreasonable for G to take the switch option with slightly more than five years of life.[48] Suppose he takes (what I shall call) this Switch-and-Reduce Option. Should we then continue to give him an equal chance to receive the lifesaving resource because it makes it possible for us to cause in him as much good from his point of view (though in a different form, combining quality and quantity in a different way)? This will involve giving weight to U that we cause but also *interpersonally* granting that a given length of life has greater significance when it comes to someone who is U than when it comes to someone who is P. This seems inconsistent with a nondiscrimatory attitude to disabled and nondisabled.

Suppose, for argument's sake, it were permissible to give G and H equal chances when G takes the Switch-and-Reduce Option. This would be consistent with still *not* giving equal chances to H and B' in a modified version of Case 7, when H will be paralyzed but live for twenty years and B', who is and continues to be *un*paralyzed, would live for only five years. Hence, even though G has the same outcome as B', when G chooses the Switch-and-Reduce Option, G would be given an equal chance to be saved relative to H, but B' would not be given an equal chance relative to H. These options are represented in Case 12, in figure 21.7.

This difference in the relation of B' and G to H, if it were correct, would imply that there is a way in which an aggregation of quality and quantity that makes

Case 12

Persons	G	H	B′
	P	P	U
↙ ᵥ	↓↓	↓	↓
20P	5U	20P	5U

FIGURE 21.7 Switch and Reduce Cases

sense in an intrapersonal choice could bear on interpersonal choice. In the case we have considered, when a person chooses a certain quality/quantity tradeoff that we can produce, the higher quality would be allowed to compensate for the reduction in quantity. By contrast, the higher quality would not be allowed to compensate for the lower quantity when the quality is due to piggybacking.

What if G had no choice to make between five and twenty years because we could only save him by using the scarce resource in a way that makes him nondisabled (i.e., he goes from 0.25 to 1) and gives him only five years of life? If G should have an equal chance relative to H, this would mean that it is not just respect for someone's choosing one option over another and giving up longer life that justifies allowing intrapersonal aggregation of quality and quantity to affect interpersonal allocation.

There are also Switch-and-Reduce Cases in non-life-and-death contexts, and they might have different implications than those in life-and-death contexts. For example, suppose that one of two paraplegic candidates for a scarce resource that could permanently prevent blindness also has a further option: If we deliver the drug in a certain way, it will also cure his paralysis but at the cost of less prolonged retention of vision (e.g., he will have only half the years of sightedness that the other candidate would). It might well make sense for someone to trade off some vision for some years of free mobility. Each of the candidates should have had an equal chance for the resource if both would remain paralyzed and have as lengthy prevention of blindness. If a candidate chooses to produce a balance between two aims that makes intrapersonal sense, should he lose his equal chance for the resource? If someone who was all along not paralyzed could be saved from blindness only half as long as a paralyzed candidate for the blindness cure, the principles we considered earlier suggest that he should not get an equal chance for the scarce resource. Should this outcome that is a result of piggybacking on nonparalysis be treated differently from the outcome in which nonparalysis is caused?

What conclusions would the Treatment Aim Principle Modified yield if producing nonparalysis became a second aim of the treatment for blindness? It would be considered invidiously discriminatory to give a blindness treatment to a nondisabled person that turns out to last much longer in a disabled person, other things equal. Is it also invidiously discriminatory to give a treatment to a disabled person because we can count the change we will cause in his disability status to nondisabled as another aim of treatment that compensates for the reduced length of his cure from blindness relative to that cure in another disabled person?

The Switch Cases and the Causative Principle opened the way for QALYs to be used in allocating scarce lifesaving and non-lifesaving resources interpersonally, even though candidates' expected life years (and achievement of the original treatment aim) were the same, because we *could cause a significantly improved quality of life* (from disabled to nondisabled) in one candidate. Depending on how they are decided, the life-and-death Switch-and-Reduce Cases might open the way for QALYs to be used in allocating lifesaving and non-lifesaving scarce resources interpersonally when candidates' expected life years (and achievement of the original treatment aim) are different, if each candidate's outcome *is equivalent according to the intrapersonal quantity/quality* tradeoff test.[49]

Switch-and-Reduce Cases and the Nonconstant Role Principle

Consideration of the Switch-and-Reduce Cases also suggests another way of dealing with large quality differences that does not depend on the Causative Principle and that may capture some people's intuitions about cases. Suppose that someone who will continue to be U (unparalyzed) can be saved for only five years, whereas someone who will continue to be P (paralyzed) can be saved for twenty years. (We play no causative role in their quality of life per se.) It might be suggested that someone's piggybacking as P or U should make no difference when other significant factors (such as length of life) are the same, but that even piggyback U can compensate for a deficiency in other factors in a way that P cannot. U can do this to the degree represented by an intrapersonal equivalence point between U with fewer years of life and P with more years of life. The intrapersonal equivalence of two outcomes implies that a given person would get as much out of U for five years as he would get out of P (rated at 0.25) for twenty years. The interpersonal implication of this, according to the new way of dealing with quality differences that I am now exploring, is that even if someone will piggyback on U for five more years, he should get an equal chance relative to another person who is P (0.25) and will live for twenty years. This conclusion differs from what the Causative Principle implies for such a case because the Causative Principle provides no reason not to favor a person who is P and will live for twenty years over someone who piggybacks as U and will live for five years.

In a sense, this new proposal envisions *a nonconstant* role for U, at least as a piggyback property: It cannot add any positive weight for interpersonal allocative purposes in order to move us away from equal chances when all other relevant factors besides piggyback properties U and P are equal between candidates; it can only sometimes lead us to "forgive" the absence of other positive factors in a person and so maintain equal chances. The absence of comparable positive factors would not be "forgiven" if P were present instead of U. Hence, if a candidate with P could live for only five years, he should not be given an equal chance relative to a candidate with U, who can live for twenty years, according to this proposal. If the

U candidate can live for twenty-two years, *intra*personally this is preferable to P (0.25) for even eighty years. That is, (1)(22) is greater than (0.25)(80). Nevertheless, *inter*personally, a person with piggyback U for twenty-two years shows up as having only a two-year difference by comparison with a person with piggyback P who can live for twenty years. This is because each can have at least twenty years, and U's positive weight is not being called on to compensate for any deficiency in respect to years of life expected in the U person. Because the proposal envisions a nonconstant role for at least piggyback U (and perhaps certain other positive properties), I shall call it the Nonconstant Role Principle.

Here is an analogy (though it is not intended to support the permissibility of using the Nonconstant Role Principle): If a man and a woman have the same skills, they should be treated alike. If a man lacks a certain skill, this should not be held against him in a contest with a more skilled woman, but if a woman lacks the skill, this should be held against her. In this case, if we assume that there is nothing intrinsically better about being a man or a woman, we would say that the nonconstant role for the property of maleness is wrong. But if we assume that U (being unparalyzed) is truly preferable to P (being paralyzed), the question then is whether it can be coherent and morally permissible to have such a nonconstant role for U (whether we cause U or not). We would certainly be favoring piggyback U over P, in the sense that a U person gets to retain equal chances in circumstances where a P person would not; a P person is held to a higher standard than a piggyback U. However, the latter is never allowed to win in a contest merely because he is U; the most he gets on account of U per se is sometimes retaining an equal chance and so avoiding an immediate loss.[50] (And, of course, in an intratype context, a U person who will live for five years would lose to a U person who will live for twenty, even though relative to a P person who will live for twenty years, each U person would have equal chances.[51] This is explained by the different factors present in the three pairwise comparisons.)

Consideration of the Switch-and-Reduce Cases raised the possibility of the Nonconstant Role Principle. I shall, however, set it aside for now and focus on principles that emphasize our causative role. To recap before we proceed: We have now considered principles that suggest how calculating QALYs should sometimes play a role in life-and-death and non-life-and-death decisions (as shown in the Switch Cases, where we cause a change in QALYs). We have also considered whether intrapersonal aggregation of quality and quantity could bear on interpersonal allocation choices (as in the Switch-and-Reduce Cases, in life-and-death and non-life-and-death contexts).

A Problem for the Causative Principle

Now consider a problem for the Causative Principle. (See figure 21.8.)

Case 13 is one in which if we save person I, we will also cure his paralysis, whereas if we save J, we will just save his life, there being no paralysis to cure. Here the outcomes are assumed to be the same in quality and quantity, but *we produce* a

Case 13

Persons	I	J
	P	U
	↓↓	↓
	U	U

FIGURE 21.8

significantly larger difference if we treat person I than if we treat J. Therefore, the Causative Principle, as presented above, says that it is permissible to save the paralyzed person rather than the unparalyzed. However, I think that this is the wrong conclusion and that there is no good reason for favoring one over the other.

When the same outcome (U) will come about in the case of the other candidate (J), albeit not because of our causative power, the benefit of having U as an outcome can be achieved no matter which person we choose. This is what seems morally important, not whether we causally contribute to U. What motivates the Causative Principle is not pride in our causing more good, but permission to seek a better outcome for someone when we can cause U because we then (supposedly) do not violate moral side-constraints.[52]

Though we achieve the lifesaving aim of treatment equally in both candidates, suppose we acquire an additional treatment aim once we learn of the additional effect that can be achieved in one patient. Do we then also satisfy the Treatment Aim Principle Modified better if we treat the paralyzed person? If so, the Treatment Aim Principle Modified faces the same problem with Case 13 as the Causative Principle because, strictly speaking, our treatment does achieve more in the paralyzed than in the unparalyzed person.

Now, consider Case 14. (See figure 21.9.)

In this case, we would do harm in the life of an unparalyzed person by causing her to be paraplegic when we save her and cause no additional harm to an already paraplegic person in saving him. The Causative Principle here tells us to favor treating the paralyzed person, but I think there is no moral reason to do this, since the final outcomes are the same.

Case 14

Persons	K	L
	U	P
	↓↓	↓
	P	P

FIGURE 21.9

Does a similar problem arise for the Treatment Aim Principle Modified? It seeks not to produce bad side effects in treatment and this may imply giving greater weight to paralysis that is a side effect we cause than to the paralysis that remains unchanged with treatment. But one could think that this implication is wrong, for an aim of avoiding paralysis is equally poorly achieved whoever is treated in Case 14. However, suppose we allow bad states that we do not strictly produce to count equally with those that result from our treatment. Then in our original Case 7, where we must choose between saving a paralyzed and an unparalyzed person who would each remain so, it might be said that we fail to achieve our aim of unparalyzed people if we save the paralyzed person. But it was assumed that favoring the unparalyzed person in Case 7 would be (invidiously) discriminatory. Hence, the Treatment Aim Principle Modified has to distinguish between caused and not-caused states if it is to distinguish Case 7 from Cases 8 and 9, and this is what leads to a problem with Case 14.

Similar results hold for a non-life-and-death case. If we can prevent someone from going blind and also cure his paralysis, the Causative Principle and the Treatment Aim Principle Modified seem to imply that we should help him rather than prevent an unparalyzed person from going blind. However, I think there is no good reason to favor one over the other. (In addition, if we can prevent a paralyzed person or an unparalyzed person from going blind, but the cure will cause paralysis in the unparalyzed person, the two principles suggest that we should avoid the treatment that has the worse side effect. Yet given that both will wind up paralyzed, I think there is no good reason to favor the paralyzed person over the unparalyzed one.)

The Principle of Irrelevant Type Identity

Suppose we accept the implications that the Causative Principle has for some cases (such as Case 9) but reject its implications for others (such as Case 13). Then we will have to find a principle to account for both sets of judgments. Here is a suggestion: The important point of the Causative Principle is that who the person is (consisting not only in what characteristics he has now but in what characteristics he would come to have due to causes independent of us if he survives) should not determine whether he is helped, so long as the outcome that can come about through helping him is significant (e.g., a life for which it is reasonable to take important risks, rather than saving someone already in a permanent coma). This does not mean that the quality of outcome does not matter per se, only that we do not let the differences in who the person is (independent of the change we make) make a difference to whom we choose to help. This has two implications. When the synchronic outcomes expected in different individuals are different, to pay attention to anything but the causative difference we make would be to make the difference in them affect our decision of whom to aid. Hence, we can abstract from who they are by attending solely to the causative component. Or, alternatively, we can imaginatively add to his outcome the good synchronic property that one party is missing (or imaginatively subtract from his outcome the good property that the other party has). But when the synchronic outcome we expect in different individuals is the same, the decision to attend only to the causative difference we make (from how they were or would have been independent of us) results in the differences in who they are (independent of our action) playing a role in our decision regarding whom to treat.

That is, when the bottom line is the same, paying attention to the difference we make is an indirect way of treating people differently on the basis of who they are. Showing that we need to do less to reach a given bottom line (outcome) implies that the person had more to begin with, and thus the Causative Principle would imply, for example, that we should not give an equal chance to someone who had and would retain better characteristics to begin with.[53] The principle would hold his nondisabledness against the person who is nondisabled, since this is what accounts for our making less of a difference in his being alive and nondisabled. If we do not want who the person is to count against him (or for him) when outcomes are the same, we could imaginatively add (in our calculation) the disability condition to one person who actually lacks it or take it away from the other who actually has it. Then the causative difference we make would be the same in each person's case. But we achieve the same result by just attending to the fact that the outcomes are the same.

Notice, however, that our cases are consistent with "who the person is" still making a difference, for example, to how each of two people compare with a third. For example, in Case 7, person B (who remains unparalyzed) will not be favored for the scarce resource over A (who remains paralyzed); but in Case 9, person E (whom we switch from paralyzed to unparalyzed) can be favored over someone identical to A. The person who remains U has the same outcome as the person who switches to U, but according to the Causative Principle, he has different prospects relative to someone who starts and remains P. This means that it is only the identity a person brings to the circumstances—whether someone starts as U or starts as P—that determines his differing chances relative to someone who remains paralyzed.[54] This has the result that in "within-type" contests—for example, between two people who are both paralyzed to begin with—certain factors (such as being unparalyzed in the outcome) can sometimes count in favor of a candidate that cannot count in "between-type" contests—for example, between a paralyzed and an unparalyzed person. Hence, if we say that "we do not want who the person is to count against him (or for him) when the outcomes would be the same," we must mean "when the outcomes would be the same for the contestants for the resource in a pairwise contest."

Similarly, recall that in the Switch-and-Reduce Case 12, person B′ had the same outcome (U for five years) as G (U for five years). Yet the question was whether they might fare differently relative to H (with an outcome of P for twenty years), with B′ disfavored and G possibly treated equally, if we use the Causative Principle. This is because of their starting points. Yet, suppose what I have said about Case 13 is correct. Then if we had to decide whether B′ or G gets the scarce

Case 15

Persons	B	F	E
	U	P	P
	↓	↓	↓↓
	U	P	U

FIGURE 21.10

resource, each should be given an equal chance, for their bottom lines are the same. One difference that Case 12 introduces is the possibility that when the quality property is something we cause, it can aggregate with quantity to determine the outcome that is relevant to an interpersonal allocation. This is what might account for equal chances between G and H, even though their outcomes are not alike except in QALY terms.

What if the three types of people found in Cases 7 and 9 are all present at once? For example, consider Case 15, where each person we might save would live equally long in the future. (See figure 21.10.)

It would seem that E may be chosen over F on grounds that we cause a better outcome without either one's type identity counting for or against him. Then it is a toss-up between B and E, because we would hold the type identity of B against him if we were to favor E. If B wins this fair toss-up, F cannot complain about the lack of an equal chance with B, because there is sufficient reason for his elimination from the contest by E. Why do we choose this way of proceeding rather than the following way—start with a toss-up between B and E, which B might win, and then have a toss-up between F and B that F might win? I believe the answer to this question is important: We may decide on the basis of which path leads to the best outcome so long as doing so does not violate a moral side-constraint; for example, it does not hold anyone's type identity for or against him.[55] (I shall return to this point below.)

Hence, the dominant point of the discussion in this subsection is that we should treat persons so that who they are (their type-identity, but also, more generally, what type they will be independent of the change we make) does not count for or against them. This only sometimes commits us to the subsidiary Causative Principle. To capture this dominant point in a principle, I shall use the Principle of Irrelevant Type Identity, which I originally introduced in connection with the Equal Respect Argument. Note that we are concerned with abstracting from what people are independent of the change we make, though we are still concerned with achieving the best outcome. Usually, abstracting from characteristics people have and treating them equally is associated with theories of individual rights; such theories try to capture the idea that it is certain characteristics that all and only persons have which are sufficient for certain forms of treatment (whatever other characteristics a given person may have). But these theories of rights are also associated with ignoring potential outcomes entirely when deliberating about what to do. The limited form of abstraction from outcomes (i.e., abstraction from who people are, independent of what we do) that we are considering is interesting, in part, because of its contrast with these rights theories.

Indeed, the fact that we are still concerned with outcomes can help us place the point of the Principle of Irrelevant Type Identity in its proper context. One may put this as follows: (1) We aim at doing what results in the best outcome, (2) on the condition that we not hold someone's type identity for or against him. Failing in (2) will defeat our pursuing the aim in (1). What's more, (3) abiding by the Causative Principle is important when it defeats the charge that we have not met the condition in (2). That is, the Causative Principle defeats the defeater of (1), thereby allowing us to proceed with (1). However, (4) if we focus on the Causative Principle more than as a way of meeting (2), we will also violate (2) (e.g., in holding against U → U that he was not P to begin with). (Points 1 through 4 are reflected in the path that we took in deciding what to do in Case 15.) This all also implies (roughly) that rather than focusing on whether we *cause* a good or bad outcome, we should focus on whether we *cause* a (significantly) better (or worse) outcome than would otherwise exist among any of the candidates. If not, we should give all the candidates equal chances. (Determining whether we cause a better outcome might involve aggregation of quality and quantity, a possibility raised by the Switch-and-Reduce Cases.)

I have used life-and-death cases in trying to deal with problems raised by the Causative Principle, but the same points apply to non-life-and-death cases.

The Causal and Componential Role of Identity in Relation to the Principle of Irrelevant Type Identity

When I originally introduced the Principle of Irrelevant Type Identity in connection with the Equal Respect Argument, I pointed out that the principle did not rule out *linkage*; that is, it permitted counting relevant differences causally due to a person's type identity. This is quite independent of *our* causing differential effects. I also said that it was a permissible limit on the principle to take account of the noncausal, component role of who the person is in accordance with the Condition Similarity Principle. Let us review these points again, now that we have discussed how our causing the nondisabled or disabled conditions matters for allocation purposes.

Distinguishing between (a) who the person is and (b) what results we will produce (abstracted from who he is) should not, I believe, prevent our attending to results that occur *due to who he is*. If we wish not to discriminate invidiously against a person with a disability at the time of treatment, we should abstract from his disability as a *component of his life*, not from its *causal* role. Thus, for example, suppose that if we save a paraplegic he will remain a paraplegic and live for two years, but if we save a nonparaplegic he will remain a nonparaplegic and live for ten years. Assume the two candidates for treatment are alike in all other morally relevant respects. Even if the fewer years of life we can expect for the paraplegic are entirely due to his being a paraplegic, it need not be discriminatory to take them into account in the allocation decision. This is *linkage*. It takes account of paraplegia's effects (its causal role), for example, on quantity of life, but it is consistent with not attending to the synchronic properties of paraplegia in deciding how to allocate resources. (Such properties would include, e.g., not being able to walk, being in more pain, or whatever else are components of the life of the paraplegic in virtue of his paraplegia.) The causal effects could also include other disabilities. For example, suppose that the drug that could save life causes blindness in the disabled person but not in the nondisabled person, due to an interaction between the disability and the treatment. This difference in the outcome that we can produce in the two candidates might justify giving the scarce resource to one candidate rather than another, or at least not constitute invidious discrimination. This is so even though it involves making use of the value judgment that it is worse to be blind than not to be blind when judging the outcome we produce. (The Treatment Aim Principle Modified could also take account of bad side effects in deciding whom to treat.) Obviously, to make this account work, more would have to be done to distinguish the characteristics of a condition from its effects. One cannot just identify effects as those things not distinctive to that condition (e.g., not living long is an effect that has many causes), because characteristics not distinctive of a condition (i.e., occurring in other conditions, too) can be components of a condition.

The distinction between the purely causal role of paraplegia and its component role is also crucial in answering one potential objection to the Principle of Irrelevant Type Identity.[56] It may be said that if our treatment cures paraplegia in addition to saving a life only in one person and not in another, this must be because of some difference between the two people—for example, an allergic reaction in the second person that blocks a cure. Therefore, to let the difference in outcome count makes the difference between people count, and is that not contrary to the Principle of Irrelevant Type Identity? I would argue, however, that there can be a moral difference between counting against someone his allergy's synchronic properties as a *component* in his life and counting the allergy's *causal* effect. Only the former involves treating people differently because we dislike the allergy they have.

That we are not holding the disability that someone would have (independently of what we do) against him as a component of his life when we count its causal effects is further reinforced, I argued earlier, by considering something that improves a life when it is considered as a component. For example, suppose painfreeness adds positively as a component to a life, and yet painfreeness is uniquely carried by a protein that interacts badly with our lifesaving treatment and so causes paraplegia or much shorter life. Ignoring painfreeness as a good component and thus not discriminating in favor of the people who have it would be consistent with attending to its bad effect. Deciding not to help the person with painfreeness because of its causal effects would not constitute discrimination against him on grounds of his painfreeness.

I also suggested that there could be cases in which type identity as a component feature may permissibly count in selection because its properties are like ones the treatment in question aims to deal with. When type identity factors are used as a basis for selection for this reason, there may also be no invidious discrimination. Suppose that there are two patients who must be treated for fatal kidney disease—one patient who is weak and one who is hardy. The first patient's weakness is not due to the kidney disease. It has another cause that cannot be affected even by a kidney cure that reverses past effects of kidney disease. We can cure the kidney disease equally effectively in both, and this means that we can prevent the weakness *due to kidney disease* equally in both persons. The Principle of Irrelevant Type Identity would tell us to ignore the weakness that preexists from another cause in one of the patients. The Treatment Aim Principle and the Treatment Aim Principle Modified agree, the first because we cure kidney disease as well in each and the second because there are no differential good or bad side effects of our treatment in each.

However, the weakness that has another cause is *like* one of the effects of the disease that we are trying to treat. After all, it may be said, one of the reasons we treat kidney disease is to prevent not only death but continual weakness; we can prevent that state (by stopping the kidney disease) in one patient, but we cannot prevent that state in the other patient because it is overdetermined. (That is, we can stop weakness from kidney disease but not from the other cause.) The Condition Similarity Principle says that when we cannot prevent in a person a state that is like one that gives us a significant reason to try to treat a condition, it is not wrong to ignore the fact that the state is a type identity factor.

All these results should still be constrained by the Principle of Irrelevant Goods, so that at least small differences do not make a moral difference. It remains open that something like curing weakness in one person but not another is too small a difference to make a moral difference relative to avoiding death.

Now suppose, counterfactually, that paraplegia was one effect of kidney disease that we were interested in preventing. If one candidate were a paraplegic as a result of some other event in his life besides his kidney disease, then our treatment of his kidney disease would not cure or prevent his paraplegia the way it would cure or prevent the paraplegia of a second candidate. Suppose that, in our previous case, it would be permissible to treat the hardy candidate as opposed to a candidate who is weak due to causes other than his kidney disease, despite equal prospects for success in treating the effects of his kidney problem. Then it would also be permissible to treat the nonparaplegic patient rather than the paraplegic patient in the present example. The Condition Similarity Principle is here overriding the Treatment Aim Principle and the Treatment Aim Principle Modified. However, we cause the unparalyzed person to remain unparalyzed—not piggybacking on his initial unparalyzed state—and this is consistent with the Principle of Irrelevant Type Identity.

Views of Discrimination and a Decision Procedure

The previous discussion implicitly gestures toward *three possible understandings of (invidious) discriminatory conduct*. The *first* possible understanding tells us that acting in any way on the differential value attributed to being nondisabled or disabled is discriminatory. But this would imply that common surgeries undertaken to cure people of paraplegia are discriminatory conduct if we perform them because we think it is better to be unparalyzed than paralyzed. I believe we should reject this first suggestion. Rejecting it helps us see how the claim of discrimination against the disabled differs from the claim of racial discrimination. For a claim of racial discrimination could be supported just by showing that our act was undertaken because we believe it is better to be white than to be black per se (i.e., independent of any other factors, such as having to live with negative social attitudes toward blacks). Notice that a discriminatory attitude against blacks relative to whites could be present even if we were deciding *only between blacks* who should get a scarce resource. This would be true, for example, if we decided to give a scarce lifesaving resource to one black person rather than another because it had the side effect of turning him white. (This implies that the fact that we are only choosing between paraplegic people in Case 8 does not, by itself, settle the question of whether we would be engaged in discrimination by deciding to help the person who will stop being paraplegic.)

The *second* possible understanding of discriminatory conduct tells us that acting on the differential value attributed to being nondisabled or disabled when this makes the person who will be disabled worse off than he might otherwise have been (for example, losing a scarce resource he might have gotten on a coin toss) is discriminatory. This understanding of discrimination would rule out the Causative Principle and the Principle of Irrelevant Type Identity (in part because the latter permits attending to the best outcome (sometimes) the Condition Similarity Principle and the causal effects of one's type).

If we think this view of discrimination is wrong, we could endorse a *third* possible understanding of discrimination: It is discriminatory to act on the differential value attributed to being nondisabled or disabled as a component of someone's life if that component is not like the condition that we aim to treat and not a condition that we cause, when doing this makes the disabled person worse off than he might have been because of who he is or would be. It leaves open the possibility that the value of a component can sometimes count for or against someone if we cause that component (even if this further implies that those in whom we cause a component, for example, are favored relative to someone else when those who have the same component independently of what we do do not get favored in the same way).

Notice that the Treatment Aim and Condition Similarity Principles can lead to someone's being worse off than he would have been because of his disability, but not *directly* because his disability is *disvalued* per se relative to nondisability. For example, it was pointed out that a positively valued state (e.g., hardiness), as much as a disability, could reduce the effectiveness of our ability to treat an illness. And if a disability is another cause of a condition that it is our aim to treat, this could also be true of a positively valued state (e.g., hardiness). Whether the state is negatively or positively valued, the Treatment Aim and Condition Similarity Principles could prefer the individual without the trait that has these effects. However, the negative value of the disability could come up in deciding what condition we should aim to treat.

Can we summarize our discussion of principles as a decision procedure (for life-and-death and non-life-and-death cases) to decide if (the third view of) discrimination is involved? Here is one attempt:

1. Check the level of well-being (including, possibly, quantity modified by quality) to which you can bring someone relative to another;
2. Check to see if, in reaching this level, counting his starting point (or any factor independent of what we do), when it is not similar to a condition we are trying to treat, would make the starting point (or factor independent of what we do) work, as a component feature, in favor of or against someone relative to another in pairwise comparison;
3. If the answer to (2) is no, deciding whom to help by differences in the level of well-being to which you can bring someone will not involve invidious discrimination (on the third view of discrimination). If the answer to (2) is yes, deciding whom to help by differences in level of well-being to which you can bring someone will involve such discrimination; and
4. If avoiding such discrimination is all that should stand in the way of producing the best outcomes, then decide how to allocate by following (1), (2), and (3).

Steps (1) and (2) amount to saying that the outcome level matters *on condition* that making that level matter does not involve holding good or bad component features (per se and not produced by you) in favor of or against someone *on further condition* that the components are not like ones we are trying to treat.

This leaves it open that differences in outcome should not matter because they are morally irrelevant goods, even if attending to the goods would not involve the third view of discrimination. Indeed, my conclusion is that while it may be wrong to ignore the Principle of Irrelevant Goods, doing so need not involve inappropriate discrimination. Hence, some complaints on behalf of the disabled may have to appeal to the Principle of Irrelevant Goods, rather than to a claim of discrimination.

If we decide according to this four-step procedure, it is what we can do for someone (in the sense of the level of well-being at which our behavior will leave him) that will matter, at least so long as making this matter does not involve treating factors (that are unlike those we are trying to treat) beyond those we produce as component features in favor of or against some person relative to another.

It is important to remember that this conclusion implies something that may be hard to accept, namely that nondiscriminatory conduct involves treating P → U (i.e., independent of our efforts, he will become unparalyzed) no differently from P → P or P ⇒ U, but permits treating P ⇒ U differently from P → P because U is a better outcome and we produce it. (Analogous results will follow for switches to P.)

One problem with this decision procedure is that it just attends to our treatment of one person relative to another in deciding whether there is invidious discrimination. However, suppose we treat B correctly relative to A and B loses the scarce resource, but we do not treat C correctly relative to A (or D) in order that C not lose the scarce resource. Might not B complain that he is being discriminated against relative to C, for we are holding him to standards to which we do not hold C, and that is enough to support a claim of discrimination?[57] In order to avoid this problem, we might modify step (3) to: If the answer to (2) is no, and the procedure in steps (1) and (2) is applied pairwise generally (or impartially), deciding whom to help by differences in levels of well-being to which you can bring someone will not involve discrimination. If the answer to (2) is yes, or the procedures in steps (1) and (2) are not applied generally or impartially, deciding whom to help by differences in this level of well-being will involve discrimination.

In sum, I have argued that there are several ways in which interpersonal differences which we can produce (and sometimes even differences we will not produce) allow us to decide whom to treat without committing the wrong of invidious discrimination. But narrowing the ground on which one may complain of discrimination may only empower the Principle of Irrelevant Goods instead, for that principle may possibly be called on to prohibit actions that one might have thought could be ruled out on grounds of discrimination.[58]

What if there were cases where we see a role for both the Principle of Irrelevant Type Identity, which has a causative component, and the Nonconstant Role Principle, which does not have a causative restriction on counting U? Then the Principle of Irrelevant Type Identity might be modified to allow type identity—in the sense of quality properties that are present independent of what we do—to matter in order to preserve equal chances for those whose shorter lives would be as good for them as a longer life of lower quality.

Intransitivities

A problem that we must be prepared for in using the Causative Principle, the Principle of Irrelevant Type Identity, and their accompanying decision procedure is apparent intransitivity in choices. Let us consider this issue further. My discussion implies that it is nondiscriminatory to prefer a paraplegic candidate (P) who will become unparalyzed (U) as a result of what we do over one who will not. That is:

$$\begin{pmatrix} A \\ P \Rightarrow U \end{pmatrix} > \begin{pmatrix} B \\ P \rightarrow P \end{pmatrix}$$

Nondiscrimination requires giving equal chances to a paraplegic candidate who will remain that way in a contest with an unparalyzed candidate who will remain that way; that is:

$$\begin{pmatrix} B \\ P \rightarrow P \end{pmatrix} = \begin{pmatrix} C \\ U \rightarrow U \end{pmatrix}$$

It also requires not favoring a paralyzed candidate who will become unparalyzed over someone all along unparalyzed; that is:

$$-[\begin{pmatrix} A \\ P \Rightarrow U \end{pmatrix} > \begin{pmatrix} C \\ U \rightarrow U \end{pmatrix}]$$

In other words, it would be discriminatory to pick immediately A over C, even though it is nondiscriminatory to pick A over B, and B must be treated as equal to C. (That is, A > B, B = C, −(A > C).)

There is also a second possible intransitivity:

$$C > D \quad [(U \rightarrow U) > (U \Rightarrow P)]$$

$$D = B \quad [(U \Rightarrow P) = (P \rightarrow P)]$$

$$-(C > B) \quad -[(U \rightarrow U) > (P \rightarrow P)]$$

These apparent intransitivities, however, really raise no deep problem, as the choices are fully explicable on a pairwise basis. Because the pairwise options give rise to different factors that determine our choice in them, we should not expect transitivity. Still, the apparent intransitivities give rise to new questions.

Due to the first "intransitivity," it might be said that U has an incentive to paralyze himself prior to our choice since then if he could be made to recover from paralysis, his life will be favored over P, and not otherwise. Because of the second intransitivity, U has an incentive to paralyze himself if he knows the lifesaving procedure will paralyze him anyway, since then he will be on an equal footing with U who will remain U. In sum, the sort of distinctions involved in the Causative Principle and the Principle of Irrelevant Type Identity give perverse incentives to people. This, however, does not necessarily show them to be wrong. (If affirmative action gave one an incentive to change one's race and doing so were possible, would affirmative action be wrong for that reason?)

What should we do when the three people involved in each triplet present themselves to us at once? As I said above, in the first "intransitivity," my sense is that nondiscrimination requires us to toss a coin between (P ⇒ U) and (U → U), even though, if the coin favors (U → U), this will mean that he is selected over (P → P). This is nondiscriminatory in the context because (P → P) has been *eliminated* as a candidate already, not by (U → U) but by (P ⇒ U). There is no "money pump" phenomenon. (That is, having to move from selecting U → U to tossing a coin between U → U and P → P and then favoring P ⇒ U to him and onward.) This is because one option (P → P) has been eliminated. (Admittedly, the candidate who is eliminated is eliminated by someone who may not ultimately win the contest. Some may say that such phenomena violate Arrow's Principle of Independence of Irrelevant Alternatives, but I think such cases help show that the principle is either incorrect or its correct interpretation does not conflict with such a result.) In the second "intransitivity," we may select (U → U), even if this means he is selected over (P → P), just in case (P → P) loses a fair toss first with (U ⇒ P) and is thus eliminated.

E. AN INADEQUATE GROUND FOR CONSIDERING DISABILITY WHEN ALLOCATING SCARCE RESOURCES

Let us now consider the ex-ante choice behind a veil of ignorance as Singer envisions it in (S3), which results in all quality and quantity distinctions being relevant to interpersonal allocation decisions.[59] The argument might be criticized as follows: We will get the wrong result for a moral principle if we think, as Singer does, that ex-ante reasoning behind a veil of ignorance involves each person's thinking of himself as having a possibility of occupying each outcome-position—for example, disabled or nondisabled. Rather, the veil of ignorance should be understood as a device that leads each person to take seriously the fates of the separate persons who will actually occupy each of the outcome-positions, disabled and nondisabled. Thomas Scanlon makes this point in distinguishing his form of contractualism from that of John Harsanyi.[60]

Scanlon's basic objection to Harsanyi's approach is with its interpretation of impartiality—that is, what it means to choose principles that are not designed to favor one person over another and that one could accept independently of knowing what one's actual position is or will be. Scanlon agrees that it can be helpful in finding such principles for each person to imagine that he is in every other person's actual position in life (outside the veil of ignorance), having that person's perspective on things, in order to see whether each person in any actual position could reasonably approve (or not reasonably reject) a proposed principle governing relations between people. While Scanlon does not make use of a veil of ignorance, his interpretation of impartiality implies that (i) if no person in any position outside the veil could reasonably reject a principle on his own behalf, then (ii) any individual behind a veil of ignorance could agree to the principle. If someone from some position outside the veil could reasonably reject the principle, then it could not be agreed to by a person behind the veil of ignorance, because it is not a principle that one could agree to without knowing into which position one would fall. The reasonableness of rejection outside the veil is, according to Scanlon, a function of pairwise comparing the possible complaints of people in different generic positions.[61]

Scanlon rejects the alternative interpretation of impartiality that Harsanyi accepts and that Singer also seems to accept—that being impartial is best understood as deciding behind a veil of ignorance on the assumption that one has an equal probability of being in any person's position outside the veil. The assumption of equal chances of being in any position is supposed to ensure that one does not choose principles that favor one position over another. But there is still no requirement on this view that a decision-maker behind the veil first take account of whether each person occupying each generic position could beyond the veil reasonably reject a principle before he, behind the veil, decides to accept it. Rather, the order is the reverse of what it should be in Scanlon's view; namely, the order is: (i)′ if any individual behind the veil of ignorance would choose a principle on his own behalf, then (ii)′ no person in any position outside the veil could reasonably reject the principle. It is this Order Reversal, as I refer to it, that lies at the heart of Scanlon's disagreement with Harsanyi's approach and the approach Singer takes.

Scanlon also argues by example against the conclusion that what an individual would choose behind a veil of ignorance in order to maximize his *average* expected utility determines whether someone outside the veil can reasonably raise a moral complaint against a principle. Suppose one maximizes one's average utility by accepting a principle that allows many people to receive small benefits when only a few will be very badly off. Scanlon thinks that people who would be very badly off could reasonably reject the principle because no one of the many stands to gain much individually, while some others are very badly off, and there is an alternative principle that could greatly improve the worse off at a small cost to each of the many. It is the latter alternative that is preferable, although it reduces aggregate utility and hence is not what maximizes any individual's ex-ante average utility. Scanlon considers a principle from the perspective of each type of position that will actually be occupied by someone and compares its effects on a position pairwise with every other position in order to decide whether the principle should be adopted.[62] I believe that Scanlon's example shows that attending to the maximal sum of utilities, regardless of what distribution of these is involved, would not yield the right principle.

I suspect that emphasizing the distinction I drew in part IV, section A, between (1) caring more for (or to be in) one position rather than another and (2) caring equally about remaining alive in the less favorable position in which one winds up, when there is no possibility of moving to a better position, coincides (at least in part) with Scanlon's view. His approach, in telling us to focus on how someone will approach things from the position he will be in beyond the veil, is like (2), insofar as (2) implies what Singer denies, namely that a person can have as strong an interest in going on living, even when the objective good in his life is less than in someone else's life. It contrasts with considering someone's preferences when he thinks he has a chance to be in any of many positions, which is like (1).[63] Perspective (2), rather than perspective (1), is the relevant one to take even in an ex-ante thought experiment.[64] If we have policies that we know will leave some disabled people to die when they could otherwise be helped, simply because we can achieve some additional good if we help others instead, we must be able to give a justification to those who are actually threatened with death. We must be able to show them that the additional good is worth depriving them of an equal chance at life. Saying to them, "Agreeing to such a policy would have maximized your ex-ante chances of benefit because you might have been the nondisabled person" is not the right kind of justification.

This point is connected with the objection to Harsanyi's and Singer's use of the veil of ignorance—that it does not take the separateness of persons seriously. To make this objection, it is sometimes said that a person's willingness to risk *his* having a bad fate for the sake of maximizing *his own* expected average utility (intrapersonal risk) does not bear on whether he may endorse a principle that risks *someone else's* having a bad fate for the same goal (interpersonal risk). (Recall my earlier discussion [in part IV, section A] of the cases in which someone will either risk immediate death or arrange to abandon himself if a surgery does not render him nondisabled, in order to possibly be cured of a disability. It was supposed to show that intrapersonal risk could be permissible when interpersonal risk is not (although that discussion was put in terms of these people not necessarily being willing to die, if each was disabled, as a result of our choosing to help someone else live who was nondisabled.) We could also say that the fact that someone would exchange a certain quality and length of life for a better quality and length for himself does not mean that he would agree to a principle that involves his having the better life because someone else loses a chance to have the less good one, or vice versa.

In one sense, this objection to Singer and Harsanyi seems misplaced. For suppose it is the case that *any* individual—A or B—deprived of knowledge that distinguishes his eventual position from that of others would take the small risk of being in a bad position in order to maximize his own expected average utility. Then when A suffers a bad fate while B has a good fate, this does not straightforwardly mean that A suffers because *B decided to risk A's having a bad fate*, for A would have taken this risk for himself.

What must be emphasized in order to make the objection that Singer's and Harsanyi's use of the veil of ignorance ignores the separateness of persons when considering whether risk-taking is appropriate is the difference between (i) one's *actually* (beyond the veil, not behind it) losing out on something or running a risk of death in order to have some good and (ii) being willing to have someone else actually (beyond the veil, not behind it) lose out on something or run a risk of death as a result of one's having one's good. In order for this difference to come to the fore, one must not interpret one's "being willing to run a great risk to have one's good" as including a decision behind the veil of ignorance to run a great risk that one will be left to die (for example, if one turns out to be the person who is in the bad position) in order that one get to keep one's better life (if one turns out to be the *other* person who is in the good position). However, this is how reasoning behind the veil of ignorance in the Harsanyi/Singer manner works; hence, it tends to assimilate interpersonal to intrapersonal sacrifice, and one might object to it on this ground.

Thus, one could refuse, beyond the veil, to let something bad happen to another as a result of one's outright being chosen to benefit, although one is willing, beyond the veil, to let the same bad thing happen to oneself as a result of seeking one's own benefit. Notice that the difference between self and other that is retained here has nothing to do with whether each person behind the veil would or could reasonably agree to accept the same risks. They each may be willing to accept the same risks behind the veil and yet still distinguish between (1) the case where they actually (not behind the veil) run risks for which only they may have to pay (if they lose) and (2) the case where others run risks or suffer losses, including being left to certain death, so that one may have a good. This, I think, is the way to understand the point of the initial response that we considered to Harsanyi/Singer-style veil-of-ignorance reasoning—the response that said one might be willing to take on risks and suffer losses oneself for one's own benefit but not be willing to accept that others must outright do the same if one is to benefit or to accept that one must do the same if others are to benefit.

V. The Supererogation Argument

So far, I have dealt with The Problem by considering reasons to deny or accept Premise 3 in the argument supporting it. Now, I wish to consider a different type of argument that also denies the conclusion that we should help the nondisabled rather than the disabled with scarce resources. This argument raises concerns about Premises 1 and 2 in the argument leading to The Problem (and the parts of [S1] that contain similar ideas). Premise 1 says: "Disabilities make life worse for the person whose life it is, other things equal, and this is why we try to prevent or correct them." Embedded in this premise are a proposition and a claim that the proposition explains our behavior. The proposition is that disabilities make life worse for the person whose life it is, other things equal. The behavior it explains is that we try (presumably correctly) to prevent or correct such disabilities.

Premise 2 says, "Hence, we will get a worse state of affairs if we help a disabled person . . . rather than someone equal in all respects except that he lacks the disability."

An objection to deriving Premise 2 from Premise 1 is that there is an explanation of why we correctly try to prevent or correct disabilities that is consistent with the view that a disabled life is as good as or even better than a nondisabled life, and so if we help a disabled person we produce an even better state of affairs, other things equal. Further, the life of a disabled person could be as good or even better than the life of a nondisabled person, even if the proposition part of Premise 1 is true (i.e., the disability makes the life in some respect worse). This is because things may not be equal if there are sources of good in the disabled life not available or not typical in the nondisabled life. Of course, one may doubt that there are such great goods only in the disabled life. My point now is that, even if there were, we could still have reason, all things considered, to try to prevent or cure disabilities.

Our reason for trying to prevent or cure disabilities, as suggested by Premise 1, could be that a disability makes life harder and so worse *for someone*, even if it also makes him have a life that is no worse (or even better) than others have. Among those who have drawn a distinction relevant to this point are Shelly Kagan and Ronald Dworkin. Kagan, for example, distinguishes between how things are *going for me*—a matter of my well-being—and how my life is going, for example, as a matter of achievement. So my life could be going well but I might not be doing well.[65] Ronald Dworkin distinguishes between experiential and critical interests, so one's life could be experientially bad but one could still have an important and meaningful life.[66]

Thus, it could be supererogatory for someone to choose to live a hard life and wrong for us to force such a life on an unconsenting individual, even if it is a good life in terms of meaningfulness and achievement. Analogously, we could know that if someone were left to suffer a great deal of pain rather than be treated for it, he could become a great artist. This would be a better state of affairs and result in his having had a better life than the state of affairs that would result if he is treated. For then, he will not suffer pain and will live a life of only ordinary insight and achievement. It would be wrong of us (in the absence of his consent) not to treat his pain and also permissible for him to refuse to suffer the pain, even if he then misses out on an extraordinary life. Call this the Supererogation Argument for curing and preventing disability.[67]

The Supererogation Argument accepts Premise 1 but denies that Premise 1 makes Premise 2 relevant. That is, if the lives of the disabled were overall as good as or even better than the nondisabled lives (even if not *for them*) because other things were not equal, this would imply that we would not achieve a worse state of affairs if we helped a disabled person rather than a nondisabled person. This could be true even though Premise 2 is strictly correct, since the premise would just be made irrelevant by the fact that other things are not equal if extra goods occur in the life of the disabled that do not occur in other lives.

The Supererogation Argument may even apply within the realm of experiential goods alone. This is because, I believe, one need not go through a period of great pain even if this will make possible a future with enough experiential (let alone nonexperiential) goods to make one's life overall have positive value. Analogous to a moral prerogative one has not to make sacrifices to promote what is good for others, one may have a prerogative consistent with self-interested rationality not to do what maximizes one's own experiential good. For example, refusing to go through torture at t_1 in order to achieve subsequent pleasure that outweighs the pain does not seem unreasonable.[68]

If states of affairs could be as good or better if we help the disabled rather than the nondisabled, we can deny the view that we should help the nondisabled with scarce resources. (But, again, this would be because other things are not strictly equal between able and disabled people.) This conclusion is consistent with it being right to try to prevent or cure the disabilities, even if the lives with the disabilities would produce equal or better states of affairs. This is because, as the Supererogation Argument says, it would be supererogatory to choose to live such good lives and wrong for us to impose such good lives on people without their consent.

I think that the Supererogation Argument can help us better understand the debate between Peter Singer and the advocates for the disabled. Singer seems to accept that our preventing and curing disability is evidence for disability being a bad thing, other things equal. He also seems to believe that the fact that a disabled person would seek a cure is evidence that the disability does not lead to other goods that make his life equal to or better than a nondisabled life. As a consequentialist, Singer is interested in producing the best outcome. Therefore, he accepts that scarce resources should go to the nondisabled, other things equal. Some advocates for the disabled answer that their lives are as good as the lives of the nondisabled and hence will produce as good an outcome with a scarce resource. But how can they then explain someone's interest in being cured of the disability? The Supererogation Argument could account for the consistency of the advocates' argument and pinpoint an error in Singer's argument. It does this by saying that some people might not want to pay a price in difficulty for what is as good or even better.

Suppose the Supererogation Argument is valid. Is it sound? That is, is it true that a disabled life is as good as or even better than a nondisabled life, in virtue of special features typically lacking in a nondisabled life? I do not believe so. While I cannot here examine this question in great detail, I will consider one aspect of it. Suppose that the special feature is a form of courage or determination that is present when a disabled person accomplishes something with difficulty that a nondisabled person does easily. For example, there may be no special merit in a nondisabled person walking up stairs on his own, while there may be such a merit in a disabled person doing it. Suppose, however, that because basic tasks such as walking up stairs are done easily in the nondisabled life, courage and determination can be exercised in achieving more sophisticated and novel accomplishments. From the point of view of a human ideal, it seems better to exercise courage and determination in achieving nonbasic rather than basic goals. Indeed, it seems like a waste of courage and determination to have to apply them to tasks that could easily be accomplished by people without disabilities, at least on the supposition that these virtues would instead be developed in pursuit of intrinsically higher goals.

Hence, it could be true that if two individuals did no more than walk up stairs, the life of the disabled person who does this may be harder but still more worthwhile than the life of the nondisabled person because the former life exhibits virtues the latter does not. But it would be better still if people were free to do basic things without determination and courage, so that they are free to actually achieve higher goals and still exercise determination and courage in those other pursuits.[69]

VI. Conclusion

I have been discussing factors relevant to the allocation of lifesaving and non-lifesaving resources. I have suggested that it is important to consider need and not only outcome in deciding how to allocate such resources. In evaluating outcomes, the difference a resource can make to quantity of life in one person rather than another may be relevant. A difference in quality of life in one person's outcome rather than another's may be relevant when a large difference in quality between persons would be produced by our efforts (rather than when we save a person whose much better quality of life is not due to us) or when someone's unchangeable quality is like, or causally linked to, what we aim to treat. This difference in how quality and quantity should be treated conflicts with a general use of QALYs in allocating resources.

I have also argued that the fact that a person may generally trade off quantity and quality and take risks intrapersonally in order to achieve a better outcome (1) may not mean that he has less of an interest in retaining a worse outcome when this is all he can have, and (2) does not imply that the same tradeoffs and risks can be assigned interpersonally as intrapersonally. These two points conflict with premises in some arguments for the general use of QALYs in allocating resources. Nevertheless, if the use of QALYs is permissible when our efforts cause a large quality-of-life difference between persons, this could indicate that some use of QALYs in the allocation of lifesaving and non-lifesaving resources can be defended even if points (1) and (2) are correct.

On the basis of these conclusions, I distinguished different views of invidious discrimination against the disabled in allocating resources and suggested a decision procedure for allocating resources that would not involve invidious discrimination.

Finally, I considered how distinguishing between (1) the hardness of a life and (2) the goodness of a life might play a role in debates about disability.

Notes

1. This chapter is based on my (1) "Deciding Whom to Help, Health Adjusted Life-Years, and Disabilities," in *Public Health, Ethics and Equity*, eds. S. Anand, F. Peter, and A. Sen (New York: Oxford University Press, 2004); (2) "Disability, Discrimination, and Irrelevant Goods," in *Disability and Disadvantage*, eds. K. Brownlee and A. Cureton (New York: Oxford University Press, 2009); (3) "Aggregation, Allocating Scarce Resources, and the Disabled," *Social Philosophy and Policy* 26 (Winter 2009): 148–97; (4) three lectures I gave in May 2006, February 2007, and March 2007 in the Department of Philosophy and at the Program in Ethics and Health, Harvard University; and (5) "Should You Save This Child?: Gibbard on Intuition, Contractualism, and Strains of Commitment," a comment on Allan Gibbard's Tanner Lectures in *Reconciling our Aims* by Allan Gibbard (New York: Oxford University Press, 2008).

For comments on earlier versions of this chapter, I am grateful to audiences at the Kennedy School of Government, the Program in Ethics and Health, and the Law School at Harvard University. I also thank audiences at Amherst College, Georgetown University Law Center, NEH Summer Session on Disability, University of Southern California Law School, and the Pacific Division APA, March 2003. I received additional feedback from the members of Philamore and the WHO Fairness and Goodness Project, John Broome, Ruth Chang, James Griffin, Shelly Kagan, Eva Kittay, Jeff McMahan, James Lindeman Nelson, Andrei Marmor, Rosemary Quigley, Gideon Rosen, and Anita Silvers. I am grateful for further comments to the contributors and editors of *Social Philosophy and Policy* 26.

2. For example, in my *Morality, Mortality,* Vol. I: *Death and Whom to Save from It* (New York: Oxford University Press, 1993). All references in the text to my "earlier work" will refer to this volume unless otherwise noted. Some of my earlier work on allocation is also presented in chapters 18 and 20 this volume.

3. In *Morality, Mortality*, Vol. I, I called it the principle of Irrelevant Utilities and referred to irrelevant utilities.

4. I have said that all candidates are to be imagined as equal in respects other than expected life years due to the resource. It is still possible that if they are equally young, the value to each candidate of the additional years will vary from what it would be if they were all old, but still equal in age. At minimum, I only require one case in which the claim I have just described in the text holds—that is, the claim about the difference between the effect on interpersonal allocation of interpersonally aggregating (when we can give five years to G) versus intrapersonally aggregating (by giving five years to B). Notice that even if we thought that B should be given a somewhat higher chance of getting the resource than A, this would still differentiate the effect of the extra five years in Case 1 from its effect in Case 2, where I think it could reasonably mandate the outcome in which we help F and G.

5. Initially, the DALY does not seem to be a well-being measure but rather a record of a physical defect, whether or not compensation makes it have little impact on well-being. If this were true, it would raise concern about the use of the measure. For example, suppose one society decides to spend *x* amount to compensate for a disability and another society spends the same amount to cure the disability. Well-being levels might be the same in the two societies, but one society's DALY rating could be much higher than the other's. If this were the case, should the DALY rating be at all relevant for deciding whom to help? However, DALYs in the two societies may be the same because compensation functionally *enables* people, and so their DALYs could go down. I shall assume that higher DALY ratings reflect differences in well-being or other forms of goodness in a life.

6. For example, in Peter Singer, John McKie, Helga Kuhse, and Jeff Richardson, "Double Jeopardy and the Use of QALYs in Health Care Allocation," in *Unsanctifying Human Life: Essays on Ethics*, ed. Helga Kuhse (Oxford: Blackwell, 2002); first published in the *Journal of Medical Ethics* 21 (1995): 144–50. All references to Singer are to this essay.

7. Singer grants that other things—including the long-term effects on society of such a policy—may weigh against choosing a candidate who promises to have a better outcome. I shall return to this point below.

8. Singer et al., "Double Jeopardy," pp. 284–85.

9. I have modified the figures, but a discussion like this is present in Singer et al., p. 286.

10. Singer et al., "Double Jeopardy," pp. 289–90.

11. Carlos Soto, "Choosing Whom to Aid," unpublished paper.

12. He says this in his response to my "Faminine Ethics: Peter Singer's Ethical Theory," in *Singer and His Critics*, ed. D. Jamieson (Oxford: Blackwell, 1999).

13. Peter Singer, *Practical Ethics*, 2d ed. (Cambridge: Cambridge University Press, 1993), pp. 230–31.

14. I made these points in my "Faminine Ethics: Peter Singer's Ethical Theory," pp. 162–208.

15. Singer et al., "Double Jeopardy," p. 286. I have already noted that even someone who would take need into account might object to counting differences in past quality of life in deciding on need, if the past has been adequate conscious life.

16. Singer et al., "Double Jeopardy," p. 288.

17. The impulse to compensate the disabled person would be especially strong if quality of life were generally relevant to allocation decisions, when the disabled person would also be cured and live a normal life in the future. Yet Singer's forward-looking view also implies not giving preference to such a person in a contest with someone who had always led a normal life and would continue to do so. (But Carlos Soto raises other objections to "compensating" the nonrecently disabled in his "Choosing Whom to Aid.")

18. Singer et al., "Double Jeopardy," p. 292.

19. Singer et al., "Double Jeopardy," pp. 292–93.

20. Singer et al., "Double Jeopardy," p. 293.

21. Material in this section is based on, but adds new arguments to, a section of my essay, "Deciding Whom to Help, Health-Adjusted Life Years, and Disabilities," in *Public Health, Ethics, and Equity*, eds. Sudhir Anand, Fabienne Peter, and Amartya Sen (New York: Oxford University Press, 2004).

22. As noted earlier (note 5), it might seem that if we could only compensate for but not cure their disability, the DALY measure might still be as high as it would be without compensation. This is because the DALY measure might not seem to be a well-being measure but rather a record of a physical problem, independent of whether or not compensation makes the physical problem have little impact on well-being. If this were true, it would raise concern about the use of the measure. To repeat what was said above, suppose one society decides to spend x amount to compensate for a disability and another society spends the same amount to cure the disability. Well-being levels might be the same in the societies, but could one society's DALY rating could be much higher than the other's? However, DALYs in the two societies may actually be the same because compensation functionally *enables* people, and so their DALYs could go down. I shall assume that higher DALY (and lower QALY) ratings reflect differences in well-being or other forms of goodness in a life.

23. I thank Samuel Kerstein for helpful comments on the precise formulation of the argument.

24. A somewhat different view of this case stems from the claim that the badness of death as an event depends on how much good it deprives us of. Since the person who has not lost his hand is deprived of a slightly better future, it might be argued that death per se is slightly worse for him, though, of course, this is only because in his case the event of death itself imposes a total loss, one part of which (loss of a hand) the other person has already suffered. If the person who could have a hand suffers a worse fate in dying, then helping the person who would suffer the worst fate avoid it would lead us to help him. However, considering how big a loss of future goods someone will suffer in dying may be the wrong way to determine who would suffer the worst fate, though it would tell us who will benefit more from being saved.

25. The moral difference that distributing rather than concentrating the benefit can make was discussed in Cases 1 and 2 above.

26. I first discussed cases of this sort in arguing against Thomas Scanlon's view that it is only how the treatment we have to give bears on the problem it is meant for in each candidate that is relevant to its allocation, in my "Owing, Justifying, and Rejecting," *Mind* 111(442) (2002): 323–54. Different issues about whether to give priority to helping the worse-off person would arise if the person without the hand had lived without it for a long time in the past as well (or even instead). I shall not discuss these different issues in this chapter.

27. However, defending such a reason would require showing that it was consistent (a) not to hold someone's disability against him because it is irrelevant and (b) to hold his disability in his favor because it is a relevant burden. For if (a) is correct, why is it not also correct that the nondisabled person has an extra good that is irrelevant when it comes to choosing against him in the matter of preventing gastritis? I was prompted to think of the issue by Carlos Soto's work on the tension between compensating for past paraplegia but ignoring paraplegia in future outcomes in life-and-death cases. See his "Choosing Whom to Aid."

28. Presumably, we are not interested merely in creating perfect specimens, as this would commit us to curing minor conditions in the almost-well rather than making big differences to those who are very badly off though they will never be perfect.

29. This argument implies that when 0.5 by itself is compared with 0, it is worth some maximal sacrifice x, and when 1 by itself is compared with 0, it too is worth x. This suggests that by the measure of sacrifice, and relative to 0, 0.5 equals 1. But that does not mean that 0.5 is equivalent to 1 per se on all measures. For example, we could give up 0.5 for 1 and also risk going from 0.5 to 0 to get 1, but (obviously) not be willing to risk going from 1 to 0 to get 0.5. This argument could even be taken to generate an intransitivity, that is, 0.5 equals x, and 1 equals x, but 0.5 does not equal 1. But the supposed intransitivity is explicable because of the effects of different contexts, where different alternatives are available: 0.5 is worth x in a context where 0 is the only alternative; 1 is worth x in a context where 0 is the only alternative; 0.5 is not worth as much as 1 when both are alternatives to 0 for a given person.

30. I thank Susan Wolf, David Sussman, and other members of Philamore for discussion of this point. It is worth pointing out, as an analogy to someone's concern for his own life, a parent's concern for the life of his child. One child may have many more good traits than another. A parent could prefer that his child have better traits. He might even allow the child to take certain risks in order to become better, for the child's own good. But that does not mean that a parent would make greater sacrifices to save the life of the child when he has better traits than when he unavoidably has less good traits. And this may be due to love for the actual child, rather than from duty.

31. Singer et al., "Double Jeopardy," p. 286.

32. Though this view might be supported in other ways.

33. However, it is worth emphasizing a difference in the causal route in the intrapersonal and interpersonal cases. Intrapersonally, a person may give up, or risk giving up, something of his in order to get something better for himself. The exact parallel in the interpersonal context would be that someone gives up something, or risks giving it up, in order to *cause* someone else to get something. Here the "in order" involves a causal relation. Someone might object to a principle permitting the latter and yet distinguish it morally from what happens when we outright give a scarce resource to one person with *the result* that another person loses his life or loses a chance to keep it. In this case, the loss, or risk of

it, for the second person does not cause the gain to the first person. Without denying the moral significance of this difference, what I am discussing throughout this chapter is the possibility that one person could object to our concluding, on the basis of the reasonableness of his intrapersonal sacrifice of something (*x*), that it is permissible to outright give a scarce resource to another person when it results in the first person's losing, or risking the loss of, that same type of thing (*x*).

34. Note that the two intrapersonal cases are also different from a case in which someone must make the following decision for himself: He will have surgery that has an equal chance of curing and not curing a disability. It so happens that depending on his outcome, he *must* be taken to one of two different rooms that are far apart. Either way, lifesaving medicine will be needed after his surgery. Should he (1) put all the medicine in the room he goes to if he is nondisabled, thus raising the probability that he will survive if he is nondisabled to 1, but ensuring that he will be left to die if he is disabled, or (2) should he divide the lifesaving resource, giving him a 0.5 chance of survival, whatever the outcome is? In this case, like the second one in the text, death is not unavoidable if he remains disabled; it is only if he decides in a certain way that aid will be unavailable to him. In this respect, the second and third intrapersonal cases are more like the decision (either ex-post or ex-ante behind a veil of ignorance) in an interpersonal case to abandon the disabled in order to save the nondisabled. If it would not be irrational in this third *intra*personal case to split the resources, the decision in the intrapersonal case could clearly provide no support for a decision to automatically provide lifesaving resources to the nondisabled in the interpersonal case.

35. Both these notions are different from the idea of the worth of the person independent of the contents of her life.

36. This claim may be in tension with the view that the badness of death for someone is a function of the goods of which it deprives him.

37. Singer et al., "Double Jeopardy," pp. 289–90.

38. I owe this point to David Sussman.

39. This issue is discussed by Derek Parfit in his *Reasons and Persons* (New York: Oxford University Press, 1984) and by Ruth Chang and others in *Incommensurability, Incomparability, and Practical Reasoning*, ed. Ruth Chang (Cambridge, MA: Harvard University Press, 1997).

40. Ruth Chang has suggested (in conversation) that the separateness of persons serves as insulation in interpersonal allocation even when it is not reasonable for one person to care about his sufficiently good only option as much as another person cares about his better option. This is certainly true when we would have to take away from someone something that is his (e.g., his leg) in order to help someone else (e.g., save his life). I believe she is suggesting that it may be true even when we deny someone help, as in the cases we are discussing. This would mean that the explanation of the fact that an additional good that matters in the intrapersonal context does not matter in an interpersonal context could be independent of the distinction between "caring for" and "caring about" on which I have focused.

41. How long someone will live is not a quality of a life such that someone might say that we are discriminating against those who will not live long (or have the property of short-livedness), at least when we are deciding so as to determine whether there will be a long or a short life. A context in which we would be discriminating against those who will not live long

is, for example, when we refuse them admission to a park more than we refuse admission to those who will live a long time, even though both can make equally good use of the park.

42. This paragraph was added subsequent to the publication of the article on which this chapter is based.

43. This revises the view I presented in my *Morality, Mortality*, Vol. I.

44. Hence, this implication departs from the view I defended in *Morality, Mortality*, Vol. I, that in life-or-death situations, quality of life (above a certain minimal level) should not affect our decision about who gets a scarce lifesaving resource, given that each person wants the resource.

45. If this were not true, we might imagine that the drug prevents impending blindness and deafness on the supposition that these together are worse than paraplegia.

46. This explanation need not help with the case in which one paraplegic will become nonparalyzed.

47. I am using paraplegia in discussing the Switch Cases. But it is possible that only if we could cure a worse disability (e.g., quadriplegia) would it be appropriate to respond differently to cases in which a better outcome occurs as a result of our curing a disability as opposed to our saving a person who is not disabled. I am concerned only with whether such causation ever matters morally, not so much when it does.

48. In this case we would both be producing a quality increase and producing a quantity decrease. The Switch-and-Reduce Cases are derived from my initially considering a scenario in which a paralyzed person who will remain paralyzed and will live twenty years gets a lifesaving resource rather than someone who will remain unparalyzed but live for only five years, because we abide by one of the principles discussed in part IV, section B. After getting the resource, the paralyzed person opts for a separate surgery that he knows will cure his paralysis but reduce his life expectancy to five years. Would we want to rule out his intrapersonally reasonable choice of the surgery simply on the ground that he is opting for an end state identical to the one that resulted in someone else's being deprived of an equal chance for the scarce resource relative to him? This case seemed problematic to me.

49. For a negative view on this matter, see chapter 22 this volume.

50. Notice that the fact that piggyback U adds positive weight when the candidate will live five years cannot be accounted for by the U property's standing out in this particular context but not when a candidate can gain twenty years. For if a P candidate could also gain only five years, the Nonconstant Role Principle would recommend equal chances for a P candidate and a U candidate, with U adding no additional positive weight.

51. This was pointed out to me by Shelly Kagan.

52. Here is a way in which we should *not* explain our judgments about Case 13. We should not disaggregate interpersonally and turn the greater difference we make intrapersonally into a greater difference we make interpersonally. If we disaggregate, we claim that the two-person choice case is like the three-person choice case. That is, Case 13 is treated as though it were equivalent to the case shown in figure 21A.1:
In this disaggregated case, we choose between saving the life of an unparalyzed person or saving the life of a paraplegic (who remains such) and also curing paraplegia in a third person who does not need his life saved. In this case, where the additional good is distributed over a third person, I believe the extra good done could permissibly determine our choice of whom to help. But if this conclusion carried over to Case 13, it would imply that we should save I (who is paralyzed) rather than J (who is not), and I think this is wrong. (We

$$
\begin{array}{ccccc}
\text{U} & & \text{P1} & & \text{P2} \\[4pt]
\downarrow & \text{vs.} & \downarrow & + & \downarrow\downarrow \\[4pt]
\text{U} & & \text{P1} & & \text{U2}
\end{array}
$$

(cure of paralysis only)

FIGURE 21.A1

already saw in discussing Case 1 and Case 2 that turning a case of a concentrated aggregate of goods into a case of a distributed aggregate of goods need not lead to the same interpersonal allocation decision. In that set of cases, the outcome in the two-person case differed from what it was in the three-person case: A would live ten years and B fifteen years. In Case 13, the outcomes of I and J are the same.)

53. It is very important to repeat that I continue to imagine that the disabled person has (only recently) become disabled, and also that the nondisabled person has always been nondisabled. I do this in order to avoid the issue of one candidate's being needier than another because he will have lived a worse life if he is not aided, in having lived for a long time as disabled. If we were to give some priority to helping the person who will have been worse off if not aided, this might be a reason to hold someone's having lived a long time nondisabled against him in a choice between him and the disabled person (though not if only quantity-and not quality-of-life considerations should play a role in the evaluation of need in life-and-death choices). But I have constructed the cases so that this is not a factor.

54. I owe this point to Gideon Yaffe.

55. Notice the difference between this argument for deciding among the three contestants and the argument (in chapter 18 this volume) for how to stop the move (via a transitivity argument) from helping the person who will be worst off to helping many people each of whom will only suffer a headache. In the current argument, it is thought to be sufficient justification to say to $P \rightarrow P$ that even if he does not get an equal chance with $U \rightarrow U$ (and $U \rightarrow U$ wins the contest), this is permissible because there is a permissible intermediate step through which $P \rightarrow P$ is eliminated from the contest, namely by selecting $P \rightarrow U$ over $P \rightarrow P$. By contrast, in the discussion in chapter 18, it was argued that it is *not* a sufficient justification to say to the person who would die that even if many people, each of whom stands to lose much less, will be saved instead of him, this is permissible because he was eliminated from the contest by a large number of people, each of whom would suffer a loss that is not too much less than what *he* would suffer, and they in turn were eliminated by the many others whose loss was not too much less than theirs, though much less relative to that of the person who would die. Why is it that in one case, the possibility of helping the worst-off person (e.g., $P \rightarrow P$) does not rule out helping a much better-off person and, in the other case, it does?

Here is one possible answer: In the disability case, it was claimed only that $U \rightarrow U$ could not win the scarce resource outright in a contest with $P \rightarrow P$; there was to be equal chances and it is still true that if $U \rightarrow U$ wins over $P \rightarrow U$, that he has not won outright over $P \rightarrow P$ because he might have lost to $P \rightarrow U$. By contrast, in the earlier case, it may be said, those who stand to suffer the much smaller loss win outright over those with the intermediate-sized loss. But this response suggests that matters would be all right in the earlier case if there were *only a chance* that the great many with much smaller losses at stake would be selected over those with the intermediate-sized loss. That seems not to be true.

Here is another possible answer: The person who is the intermediate contestant in the disability case is someone who *was* as badly off as the worst-off person, namely he was paralyzed, though we can unparalyze him. So a representative of the worst-off group is, in a sense, still in the contest against U → U. By contrast, in our earlier case in chapter 18, where the worst-off person is someone who would die, no one in the group with intermediate losses will have been the worst-off person; they were always better off. So even if there was only a *chance* that the great many who stand to lose even less will be helped, there is no sense in which the worst-off person would still be in the contest.

56. The objection was raised by Douglas MacLean and John Broome.

57. I owe this point to James Lindemann Nelson.

58. Consider two interesting implications of what we have so far said. Considering the first implication involves examining two more cases (see figure 21A.2).

In Case A, the outcomes differ, and in addition to saving lives, we would make a positive difference in P and a negative difference in U. In this case, we may decide on the basis of the difference in outcomes since we produce these in both persons, but the fact that we cause an improvement in one person and a decline in another has no independent weight. That is, it is not the pride and shame a doctor might take in her/his work that should affect our decision but the differential outcome level to which we bring a person (on condition that we produce it). *Our producing it* is a side constraint on considering what is important, namely the differential outcome level. (This could also be said about Case 8, where harming U but not harming P is present, and yet a doctor's disappointment in causing harm should be irrelevant; also in Case 7, where improving P but not improving U takes place and a doctor's pride should be irrelevant.) We may take account of what we do, but not because it is reflecting well or ill on us. Now consider Case B (see figure 12A.3):

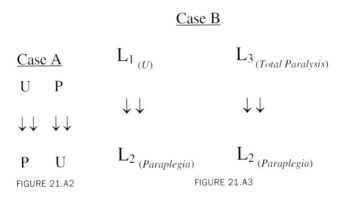

Case B

Case A

U   P

↓↓ ↓↓

P   U

FIGURE 21.A2

L_1 (U)

↓↓

L_2 (Paraplegia)

L_3 (Total Paralysis)

↓↓

L_2 (Paraplegia)

FIGURE 21.A3

In this case (where L stands for "level"), we would bring each person to the same level if we save him, but in one case by lowering and in the other case by raising; we also make the same difference to produce the same outcome, but in one case negative and in the other positive. These differences should not matter, given that the outcome is the same.

59. This section is based on a section of my published response to Allan Gibbard's Tanner Lectures, included in his *Reconciling Our Aims*; parts of it are also present in chapter 18 this volume.

60. See Thomas Scanlon, "Contractualism and Utilitarianism," in *Utilitarianism and Beyond*, eds. Amartya Sen and Bernard Williams (Cambridge: Cambridge University Press, 1982). Scanlon discusses John Harsanyi, "Cardinal Welfare, Individualistic Ethics, and Interpersonal Comparisons of Utility," *Journal of Political Economy* 63(4) (1955): 309–21. Singer's approach to the veil of ignorance seems like Harsanyi's.

61. See Thomas Scanlon, *What We Owe to Each Other* (Cambridge, MA: Harvard University Press, 1998), chapter 5.

62. Scanlon follows Thomas Nagel, who argues for pairwise comparison as coming closest to being the correct way to combine people's different interests in an outcome. See Nagel, "Equality," in his *Mortal Questions* (Cambridge: Cambridge University Press, 1995).

63. I shall have more to say below about what sort of "chances to be in any of many positions" are relevant to focusing on (1).

64. Indeed, Scanlon believes that forcing people to identify in this way with each person is why Rawls uses a thick veil of ignorance (excluding probability calculations). See Scanlon's "Contractualism and Utilitarianism." Singer, like Harsanyi, does not object to probability calculations, as can be seen in his discussion of the morality of slavery (Singer et al., "Double Jeopardy," p. 291).

65. See his "Me and My Life," *Proceedings of the Aristotelian Society* 94 (1994): 309–24.

66. See his *Life's Dominion* (New York: Knopf, 1993). I make a similar distinction in *Morality, Mortality*, Vol. I.

67. Perhaps another way to make this point is to say that we need not suffer harms for the sake of achieving benefits that consist in more than the avoidance of even greater harms. Some support for the view that others may not impose harms on us for the sake of such benefits is to be found in Seana Shiffrin's "Wrongful Life, Procreative Responsibility, and the Significance of Harm," *Legal Theory* 5 (June 1999): 117–48. I discuss some of her views in chapters 12, 15 and 16, this volume.

68. On this, see my *Morality, Mortality*, Vol. I.

69. One alternative objection to Premises 1 and 2 is that if a disabled life is better because other things are not equal, it will not be worse *for the disabled person*, even if it is harder for him. (This is a rejection of Premise 1.) It leaves it open that we could try to prevent disabilities, even though lives with them will be better *for* people with disabilities, because the lives are too hard.

A second alternative objection to Premises 1 and 2 and Singer's use of them assumes something close to the reverse of the assumption of the Supererogation Argument. That is, it assumes that experientially, the lives of the abled and disabled do not differ; due to adaptation, the disabled life is not harder. As Singer may be attracted to an analysis of a good life in terms of experiential states, this should lead him to rank their lives equally. However, from the point of view of perfections, or nonexperiential goods, having a disability could still make a life worse. It could be for this reason that we prevent or cure disabilities, and that these cures are desired, even by the disabled whose lives are not worse experientially in virtue of their disabilities. (Indeed, if we realize the happy disabled would want to be cured, this could be our grounds for preventing disability in someone who is not yet able to have an opinion, such as a child.) On this view, it is only if Singer accepted the nonexperiential measure of a good life that he could argue that we should prevent and cure the disabilities, and that we would get worse outcomes in aiding the disabled rather than nondisabled.

The second alternative is suggested by the results of psychologists. For example, Daniel Kahneman reports that, in terms of daily mood, the life of a severely disfigured person (after adaptation) does not differ from that of anyone else. Nevertheless, the same person wishes very much that he could get rid of his disability (independently of the belief that this would improve the experienced quality of his life). Reported by Kahneman in his third Mind, Brain, and Behavior Lecture, Harvard University, April 2008.

22

Rationing and the Disabled

SEVERAL PROPOSALS

In this chapter I will first critically examine some recently published views of Peter Singer about rationing scarce health care resources, in particular to the disabled. For purposes of comparison, I will then briefly summarize some alternative proposals about rationing and the disabled which I have made in greater detail in earlier work. This will lead me to also compare my proposals to some of those more recently made by Dan Brock. I hope that distilling the essence of my proposals will make them more accessible, and comparing them with other proposals will show the need for distinctions they draw. Finally, I shall point to some concerns raised by my proposals.[1] Throughout, the discussion focuses on resources that are not under personal control and that it is impermissible to distribute according to purely personal preferences. I shall be particularly concerned with whether favoring the nondisabled over the disabled in distributing scarce resources involves invidious discrimination, mistakenly focuses on maximizing health benefits, or exhibits no moral fault at all.

I. Singer

Singer is concerned with maximizing health benefits per dollar spent using a quality adjusted life year (QALY) measure.[2] For example, he thinks a teenager should be saved rather than an 85-year-old person because we can expect much more future life from the teenager than from the old person. In response, it should be pointed out that this is also true if we compare a teenager with a 50-year-old. If we think the 50-year-old should not be disfavored relative to the teenager, it may be because sometimes persons have a right to certain types of health care independent of whether this maximizes health benefits per dollar.

On the other hand, suppose that the teenager could be saved for fewer good years than the 85-year-old. It might be argued that we should still save the teenager because she would die having had much less life overall than the older person if she is not helped. Helping the person who if not aided will have had much less life overall so that she improves to some significant degree might also be relevant to how to allocate resources, not just maximizing expected health benefits per dollar. This is related to giving priority to the worst off.

Singer also considers how to compare the health benefit achieved in saving one person's life with the benefit achieved in curing a serious condition in another person that does not threaten that person's life (e.g., quadriplegia). He argues that the way to think about this question is to consider the tradeoff each person would reasonably make in his own life between years lived and quality of life. For example, if every person (already disabled or not) believed that living ten years as a quadriplegic or living five years nondisabled were equally good options, this would indicate that people take living as a quadriplegic to be half as good as living nondisabled. Singer thinks that such data would show that using our resources to cure two quadriplegics is just as good as saving someone else's life, provided the life expectancy of all three people if helped would be the same (for example, ten years).[3] His reasoning (which he does not spell out but which I shall now try to supply) seems to be that if someone would give up five out of ten years of his own life rather than be quadriplegic, that would justify curing one person's quadriplegia rather than saving someone else's life for five years. If there are two people whose quadriplegia we can cure, the combined benefit of curing both, he thinks, is equal to saving the life of another person who would live for ten years.

There are several problems with this conclusion and the reasoning that leads to it, I think. First, in the tradeoff between quality and quantity that a person might make in his own life, it is that person who benefits from the tradeoff. When we make tradeoffs between different people, the people who get the improved quality of life are not the same people who suffer the loss of more life years. Rather, we are doing what results in the loss of life for one person who does not benefit for the sake of benefiting others. This raises different moral issues than the tradeoff within one life, I think.[4]

Second, the conclusion that curing two quadriplegics who would live for ten years anyway is equal to saving someone else who would otherwise die so that he can live for ten additional years depends on weighing the aggregate (total) benefit to *two* people against the loss of the benefit to the third person. However, calculating total health benefits produced by aggregating smaller benefits to a greater number of people can be problematic. For example, suppose the tradeoff test within one person's life showed that a small disability (e.g., a damaged ankle) made life only 95 percent as good as a nondisabled life. Then a person would rather have 9.5 years without the small disability than ten years with it. On Singer's view, this implies both that we should cure one person's small disability rather than save someone who would otherwise die so he can live for an additional half year,[5] and that we should cure small disabilities in twenty-one people rather than save a single person who would otherwise die so that he could then live for ten years. This is the sort of reasoning that led to the discredited rationing plan in Oregon many years ago in which resources were to be allocated to cap many people's teeth rather than save a few people's lives. It can lead us to deny significant help to people who will be the worst off (and badly off in absolute terms) because they will die if they are not helped in order to help many who are disabled only in a small way and thus not very badly off.[6]

To see a third problem, notice that Singer's way of reasoning is independent of the particular values found through intrapersonal tradeoffs of quality and quantity of life. Suppose people who are severely paralyzed would trade off only a few days of life in order to live without their disability. This result in a tradeoff between quality and quantity of life would imply that their disability has only a slightly lower value than nondisability. Taking this data, Singer's method of reasoning implies that we simply need a much larger number of people who could be cured of severe paralysis in order to compensate for not saving the life of someone who would go on to live for ten years. A particular problem to which this case gives rise is that the conclusion to which Singer's method leads may now seem reasonable. That is, it may be said that curing thousands of severely paralyzed people *is* indeed to be preferred to saving one person so that he can go on to live for an additional ten years. Aggregating benefits across people seems to give the right answer here. However, if we agree with this conclusion, it is probably because we are assuming that severe paralysis makes for a type of life that is very bad for each person in contrast with nondisability and, hence, that someone would trade much more than a few days of life in order to be unparalyzed. But Singer's reasoning implies that such a low value need not be attached to the paralysis in order for curing the many paralyzed people to outweigh saving the life, and this is why his reasoning is problematic.

Finally, Singer argues that if we accept that disability can make a person's life less good healthwise, other things equal, and we want to maximize the health benefits we get with our resources, we should save the life of a nondisabled person rather than someone whose disability cannot be cured, other things equal. The only alternative to this, he says, is to deny that disability per se makes someone's life not as good healthwise, and to say *that* would have the unpalatable implication that there is no reason to allocate resources to cure or prevent disabilities.[7] (Notice, in Singer's defense, that saying that "a life is not as good with a disability" in the sense that the quality of life for the person goes down does not itself imply that the person herself is not as good as or not worth as much as a nondisabled person.)

I have argued that there is another alternative that does not deny that disability makes life significantly worse for a person, other things equal, and yet does not lead to Singer's conclusions about allocation: We should recognize that a consideration can give us a reason to do something in one context but not another. For example, having a paralyzed finger can make life not as good in a small way, holding other factors constant. This can give us some reason to try to cure this condition while also recognizing that, when it comes to deciding whose life to save, it is an irrelevant consideration that one person has a paralyzed finger and another person does not. The additional admitted good of a nonparalyzed finger in the life of one person is what I called an "irrelevant good" when deciding whose life to save, and so equal chances should be given to each. It is not necessarily irrelevant when deciding whether to spend dollars on a curative treatment for finger paralysis.[8]

This explanation suggests that it is not the judgment that disability can make an outcome worse that has to go; it is the judgment that we should always maximize health outcomes with our resources that has to go.

It may be clear that small differences in victims, like a paralyzed finger, should not affect who is chosen for a lifesaving resource. But what is the explanation of this irrelevance? Here is a possible explanation: In this two-person contest for a scarce lifesaving resource, either person would get the greater part of the best possible outcome that can be gotten by someone (i.e., a worthwhile life whether with or without a paralyzed finger). It is also the case that the alternative for each to being saved would be very bad (death), and each wants to be the one to survive. It is crucial to this explanation that we are dealing with separate persons and that we think that from a moral point of view their different perspectives on an outcome (viz. each cares who survives) should influence what we should do. Otherwise, it would be clear that we should maximize QALYs. This is what we would do if we had a choice with respect to one person of merely saving his life or saving his life and also unparalyzing his finger, holding costs constant.

But what of larger disabilities that bring down quality of life as far as 0.5 or somewhat below, so that it is not true that either person would get the greater part of the best possible outcome that can be gotten by someone? I have suggested at least two grounds for why we should still give equal chances for a lifesaving procedure to the disabled and nondisabled. Importantly, neither ground depends on the view that a disabled life is as good for someone as a nondisabled one, other things equal. First, each person can get what it is most important that people have, namely a worthwhile life, and each wants to be the one to survive. (Call this the Moral Importance Ground.) Second, when one's only option is to have a life at 0.5, it may be reasonable to *care about* keeping it as much as it would be reasonable to care about keeping a life rated at 1. (Call this the Only Option Ground.) Note that this is consistent with its being reasonable to *care to have* the life rated at 1 rather 0.5 and even its being reasonable to risk death to get it, were this possible. This implies that it could be reasonable to risk death to get a life at 1 about which it will not be reasonable to care more, once one has it, than one should care about the life one has now (at 0.5) were it one's only option. All this may seem puzzling, yet I think it is true. Neither of these grounds applies when quality of life rating falls very low (e.g., coma) and I will not consider such cases here.

But now imagine two nondisabled patients. One could live for *twenty* years if he had a scarce lifesaving surgery and the other could live for five years. The Moral Importance and Only Option Grounds also seem to imply that it would be wrong to favor the person who would live much longer. If we disagree, we will need an argument that allows significant differences in length of life, but not significant differences in quality of life, to count in rationing decisions. One suggestion I have made is that we distinguish between the "type" of person someone is, constituted by the qualitative features of his life, and how long any type of life goes on. Respect for persons might often require ignoring types when rationing but not big differences in how long any given type will persist.[9] (Call this the Respect Ground.)

In sum, using quality-of-life considerations and comparing and aggregating benefits across different people, at least in the manner Singer recommends, to determine how good a health outcome is often seems to be the wrong way to ration scarce resources. It is important to realize that we might be able to think seriously about how to allocate scarce resources among different people—and even be willing to endorse rationing sometimes—without necessarily reaching all of Singer's conclusions.

It is also worth pointing out that, in *cases not involving life-and-death* decisions (such as treating gastritis with a scarce resource),[10] arguably it need not matter whether we treat the disabled or nondisabled even if we, like Singer, were only concerned with how much good health there will be in an outcome overall. This is because if a scarce treatment for gastritis is equally effective in a disabled or a nondisabled person, both people will continue to exist and the same improvement in the gastritis will occur whomever we treat. Using abbreviation makes this clear, where C is "cure gastritis," P is "paralyzed person," and U is "unparalyzed person." If we treat P so that we have P(C), U is still alive (unlike in a case in which we do not treat his life-threatening illness in order to save P), albeit with gastritis, and prima facie P(C) + U(−C) contains as much good as P(−C) + U(C), only distributed differently. It is true that there is no "perfect specimen" in the outcome if the nondisabled person is not treated—no U(C)—but medicine is not concerned with producing perfect specimens. (Of course, it might be reasonable to give the cure for gastritis to someone who will already have the problem of paralysis to deal with, rather than treat someone who has no such additional problem. This concern for the person who would be worse off is, arguably, independent of concern for the amount of good in the outcome overall, unless we think there is diminishing marginal utility of a gastritis cure to the nondisabled, which seems unlikely. It may simply be that there is greater moral value in giving the same amount of physical good to someone who otherwise would have less physical good.)

II. Proposals for Counting Disability

Although I have provided some possible reasons for ignoring many quality-of-life differences in rationing, in earlier work I have also suggested additional reasons why taking account of such differences sometimes does not involve the particular problem of invidious discrimination. This is so even if taking account of the differences raises the *different* problem of giving too much weight to what should be irrelevant goods, and even if favoring the nondisabled over the disabled for scarce lifesaving resources sometimes does involve invidious discrimination. Consider some of the arguments for the view that there need not be invidious discrimination when deciding whether to treat someone just recently seriously paralyzed or, instead, some unparalyzed person.[11] One argument focuses on cases where there are multiple causes of a condition such as paralysis. This condition gives us a reason to treat a specific illness with a scarce resource. For example, suppose we are equally able to treat two patients for a specific illness that causes both paralysis and pain, but we are most concerned with the illness because it causes paralysis. However, there is another cause of paralysis in one of the patients that we cannot treat. We can refer to such cases as "condition similarity cases."[12] I argued that there would be good reason not to treat the patient who will still be paralyzed due to the other cause even though our treatment against the specific illness is equally effective in both patients. It seems that it is better to get rid of both pain and paralysis than to just get rid of the lesser problem of pain. Hence, it may be permissible to leave the unavoidably paralyzed person with pain and treat pain and paralysis in the other person.

I also argued that we should distinguish treating a person differently on the basis of (a) disability as a component of someone's life, making him a certain type of person, versus (b) disability as a cause of other bad effects in the person's life. So when the presence of a disability has the causal effect of interfering with treatment of another condition (e.g., we cannot perform heart surgery as well because of paralysis), there might be no objectionable discrimination in providing treatment to a nondisabled person instead.[13] (This is consistent with there possibly being objectionable failure to prioritize the worse off.) Also, counting differences in life expectancy caused by the disability in deciding whom to help need not involve invidious discrimination if it is permissible to count an otherwise-caused difference in life expectancy.[14] Similarly, it can be permissible and nondiscriminatory to take into account obstacles to treatment that arise from *not* having a disability (e.g., we cannot perform heart surgery as well because someone has two legs rather than one). Or if nondisability reduced life expectancy, this may be taken into account consistent with nondiscrimination. Hence, someone's undeserved disability can sometimes determine that he suffers a further loss (his life), without this involving objectionable discrimination. This is what I called "linkage."[15]

I further distinguished between (1) producing a better outcome in one patient than in another by (what I call) "piggybacking" on the good property a patient already has or *will have* but that we do not, per se, produce, and (2) producing a better outcome in one patient than in another by causally producing the additional good property. For example, I discussed what I called Switch Cases.[16] (See figure 22.1, where ⇒ signifies causing paralysis or nonparalysis and → signifies absence of such a causal role, all in cases in which we would cause the saving of the life of any person we treat.) In all three cases, two people compete for a scarce lifesaving treatment. The difference is only in the impact on paraplegia.

	Case 1	Case 2	Case 3
Person one	$P \Rightarrow U$	$U \Rightarrow P$	$P \rightarrow U$
Person two	$P \rightarrow P$	$U \rightarrow U$	$U \rightarrow P$

FIGURE 22.1 Switch Cases

In Case 1, two paraplegic people are up for a scarce lifesaving treatment but in the first person the treatment, as a side effect, will undo the paralysis (i.e., $P \Rightarrow U$). In Case 2, two unparalyzed people are up for a scarce lifesaving treatment but in the first person the treatment, as a side effect, will cause paraplegia (i.e., $U \Rightarrow P$). (Case 3 will be discussed later.) In Case 1, if we choose to save the paralyzed person whom we cause to become unparalyzed, we do not merely get a better outcome by saving an already unparalyzed person or one who will become unparalyzed independently of our treatment that cures paralysis. Rather, we get a better outcome by saving a person *and* unparalyzing him. I argued that this different causal route to *the same better* outcome might make a moral difference to whether it is permissible to decide not to save a person who will remain paralyzed. That is, it might be permissible not to give a person who will remain paralyzed an equal chance to be saved relative to another person whom we can save *and* unparalyze. This is so even if it is impermissible not to give a person who will remain paralyzed an equal chance relative to another person whom we can save but whose being unparalyzed, per se, is not due to our efforts. This moral difference is not taken into account by those who, like Singer, claim that all that matters is how good the outcome is (i.e., that the person we save be unparalyzed). Nor is it taken into account by those who claim that deciding whom to save on the basis of whether they will be disabled always involves objectionable discrimination. (This is so even if we assume, for the sake of argument, that favoring $U \rightarrow U$ over $P \rightarrow P$ involves invidious discrimination and not just giving too much importance to maximizing QALYs.) To capture these results, I described the following principle:

> *The Causative Principle:* It may be morally permissible to take account of large differences in QALYs if and only if we cause them.[17]

But how can we justify there being a difference between a better outcome *achieved* by piggybacking and one achieved by causing? Perhaps we have greater entitlement to decide on the grounds that a better outcome will come about (i.e., there will be a nonparalyzed person in existence rather than a different paralyzed person) if we cause the nonparalysis rather than piggyback on this property by saving a person already unparalyzed. This entitlement could weigh against other factors pulling in another direction. (Similarly, we might be entitled to avoid causing something bad like paralysis in $U \Rightarrow P$ rather than piggybacking on it as in $P \rightarrow P$, in Case 2.)

I argued that the Causative Principle could not simply be subsumed under what I called the Treatment Aim Principle.[18] The latter is the view that if our treatment for a particular problem would be equally effective in a narrow sense (e.g., cure heart failure) in either a disabled or nondisabled patient, each should have an equal chance for the treatment. This is a common justification for giving equal chances for a scarce lifesaving drug to a disabled and nondisabled person. However, the Treatment Aim Principle also implies that if the treatment outcome in a narrow sense would be different, we might permissibly decide to treat the patient who will get the better outcome. One reason I gave for not subsuming the Causative Principle under the Treatment Aim Principle is that if a treatment aimed at curing heart failure unexpectedly cures or causes paralysis, as in the Switch Cases, this would ordinarily be considered a side effect of treatment, not part of the narrow sense of effectiveness of the heart treatment. By contrast, the Switch Cases and the Causative Principle are intended to suggest that the good or bad *side effect* we cause might also be relevant to deciding how to allocate the scarce lifesaving resource. I did note that we might modify the Treatment Aim Principle so that it would take account of side effects in determining the effectiveness of treatments.[19] (However, this would be a wide rather than a narrow sense of equally effective treatment.) I also noted that if a drug's good side effect were consistently present in many patients, one might come to consider the drug as a treatment for two different problems, either together or alone (even though it was not developed with this in mind). If the drug were considered a treatment for two problems *at once*, its effectiveness might be judged, even in a narrow sense, by whether it cured both problems rather than just one.

The important point, I argued, is that sometimes having a causal role in making someone disabled or nondisabled might be a ground for deciding whether to treat someone with a scarce resource for a completely different problem, such as heart disease, without this involving objectionable discrimination. This could be true regardless of whether having this causal role means that our treatment is more effective for the different problem per se.

In sum, I argued that even those who disagree with Singer and think that picking U→U instead of P→P is objectionably discriminatory could agree with the following: There is no objectionable discrimination in taking disability into account when (1) our treatment causes or cures it, (2) the disability affects treatment, (3) the disability causes further bad effects such as reduced life span, or (4) the disability is similar to the effects of an illness we are specifically trying to treat.

However, even if these four reasons for distinguishing people do not involve objectionable discrimination, attending to them may involve giving too much weight from a moral point of view to differences in outcome. That is, some differences in outcome may still be "morally irrelevant goods" in certain contexts. For example, given that life itself is at stake for both candidates for the scarce resource and each wants to be the one to live, the fact that taking account of a minor difference in outcome that we cause did not involve objectionable discrimination per se need not show that taking account of it is morally permissible. Hence, I suggested, objections to not treating the disabled in many contexts may have to rest on violation of a Principle of Irrelevant Goods rather than a claim of improper discrimination.[20]

III. Brock on Equally Effective Treatment

The distinctions I drew between the Causative Principle and the Treatment Aim Principle are relevant to evaluating some views of Dan Brock's on rationing and the disabled. By contrast to Singer, Brock suggests that we accept a narrow notion of equally effective treatment. This is a "treatment specific" understanding of effectiveness (p. 41). He considers the case of heart surgery. Brock says that surgery that fixes heart valves can be equally successful in each of two people even though we can predict that one person will live for ten years and another will live for one year, because the second will be executed within the year (p. 41). The measure of the surgery's success on this account is how well the valves are fixed, independent of how long the person goes on to live. Similarly, he says, "specific medical treatments are developed for specific medical conditions and their effectiveness is determined by how well they correct that condition" (p. 41). This implies that if a treatment designed to remove an impairment does so entirely in one person (even for a limited time, e.g., before she is executed), but only partially in someone else, the treatment is more effective in the first person.

Given this narrow notion of treatment effectiveness, it is theoretically possible for a paralyzed person to have just as successful a heart surgery as a nonparalyzed person. Hence, contrary to what Singer suggests, Brock thinks that if surgery must be rationed, there is no reason to favor the nondisabled person. Indeed, it could be objectionably discriminatory not to give equal chances for surgery to each.

My concern is whether Brock's narrow notion of treatment effectiveness is consistent with some other claims that he goes on to make. This is where the discussion of my earlier work is relevant. *First*, in discussing a case of hip replacement, he says:

> . . . a pre-existing disability in effect often acts as a co-morbidity that makes treatment less effective in improving a patient's health-related quality of life. Patients with COPD [chronic obstructive pulmonary disease], for example, have substantial limitations in mobility and ability to carry out a variety of activities requiring physical exertion; this would reduce the benefit they would otherwise receive from an intervention like a hip replacement, which is also intended to restore mobility and ability to carry out physical activities. (p. 30)

If we were to decide not to treat the COPD patient for these reasons, Brock says it would be a "form of discrimination [that] seems less morally problematic because it is based on an arguably relevant and defensible difference in treatment effectiveness, although that difference in effectiveness is caused by a pre-existing disability" (pp. 41–42).

What Brock means here is *not* that the hip cannot be replaced as successfully because the COPD makes surgery more difficult. Rather, Brock is here considering that the disabled person *will get less out of what the new hip is meant to help provide* (e.g., mobility). But this does not seem to involve use of a narrow notion of treatment effectiveness because it considers what further benefits someone gets from a treatment in judging how effective the treatment is. This is a wider notion of treatment effectiveness. If we used this wider notion, then if one person got more out of heart valve surgery because he got more of what it is was supposed to provide than someone else (e.g., longer life), then the first person's heart treatment would be judged more effective. This seems contrary to what Brock originally claimed to be the correct understanding of surgery that would fix each person's heart to the same degree. (Brock's case is also like the Condition Similarity Case that I discussed earlier: We can treat one cause of absence of mobility equally well but only get mobility in one patient due to another cause of immobility in the other patient.)

Second, Brock considers a hypothetical case considered by a government agency using the Americans with Disabilities Act (ADA). In that case, two people are imagined to have sustained life-threatening injuries in a car accident that also left them unable to walk (p. 29). We can save each person's life but a cure for the disability only works in one of the people. The agency argued that automatically saving the person who could also be made nondisabled would be objectionable discrimination according to the ADA. One reason given for this conclusion was that judging an unparalyzed life to be better than a paralyzed life, other things equal, was itself discriminatory. This reason seems wrong for, as Singer noted, it is because we think an unparalyzed life is better for someone than a paralyzed life, other things equal, that we try to cure and prevent paralysis in cases where there is no conflict for a scarce resource. Doing so is not thought to involve an objectionable discriminatory judgment.[21] The agency also suggested that choosing to save the unparalyzed life implies that one thought the life of a paralyzed person was not worth as much. Brock thinks this complaint fails to distinguish between the equal worth of a person and the unequal worth of the contents of that person's life. Apparently, he thinks the latter can be relevant to allocation decisions consistent with respect for the equal worth of persons.

Brock's positive view about the hypothetical case considered by the government agency is that our treatment will be more effective if it both saves a life *and* cures a disability incurred in the accident. Therefore, it is not objectionable discrimination to save the person who will not be disabled.[22] Notice that we are probably considering this to be a case in which we are *aiming* to reverse all the damage—life threatening as well as disability causing—that has occurred in the accident. Hence, we are probably not conceiving of this as a case in which a treatment that is aimed only at saving someone's life also has *a foreseen but unusual side effect* of curing his disability, as in my Switch Cases.[23] Indeed, in the government's case there may be two treatments: one is life saving and will work on each person equally well in the narrow sense; another is a disability-curing treatment that will work on only one person. Suppose we are concerned not with whom we can treat most effectively (as Brock puts it), but with in whom *a treatment* will be most effective. Then the question becomes whether we should choose one of the patients to get a lifesaving treatment that works equally well in either patient simply because another treatment we have is effective at curing disability only in him. But loss of life is the most pressing concern (and length of the expected survival is not said to be different). So it seems that the narrow standard of treatment effectiveness implies, as it would imply in my Switch Cases, that we should ignore whether we can cure a disability in deciding whom to save.

Third, Brock says that if a treatment for an unrelated condition (such as heart disease) causes a disability (such as paralysis) in one person but not in another, as it did in my Switch Case 2, the treatment is less effective in the first person, other things equal.[24] However, the idea of unequal effectiveness that Brock employs here seems inconsistent with his original, narrower notion of treatment effectiveness: If the fact that it caused disability counted against a treatment's narrow effectiveness, so should the fact that it caused a reduced life span in one patient but not another. This limits the scope of Brock's view that we should not consider how long a patient survives after a lifesaving treatment in deciding on treatment effectiveness (p. 41). Further, if a drug for heart disease caused paralysis, on the narrow view of treatment effectiveness, we would presumably consider it a bad *side effect* of the drug, just as if it caused dandruff; causing a bad side effect is not an indication of a less effective treatment for heart disease. We might seek another drug that treated the heart disease *as effectively* but without the bad side effect, but we would not describe this as seeking a more effective treatment, in a narrow sense, for heart disease.

It is only if we adopt a wide notion of treatment effectiveness that good or bad side effects will speak against treatment being equally effective in different people. Hence, it does not seem that the narrow standard implies that we should prefer to save the person in whom the treatment does not produce or does cure a disability. (This issue arises, in part, because Brock introduces the narrow notion of treatment effectiveness in conjunction with the idea that "specific medical treatments are *developed* for specific medical conditions." So it seems that it is only the condition for which the treatment is developed that matters in deciding whether effective treatment is present. Focusing on development for specific medical conditions, if this means specific illnesses, will also raise problems if we consider cases in which "condition similarity" due to different illnesses (as described earlier) exists, or in which a patient will be treated successfully for heart disease but soon die of liver failure anyway.

Brock himself specifically qualifies his conclusions based on the narrow notion of treatment effectiveness, saying that they hold "unless attending to treatment effectiveness is ruled out on other moral grounds" (p. 42). Still, I think that Brock does not correctly draw out the implications of the narrow conception of treatment effectiveness that he favors. Furthermore, the correct implications of the conception are often inconsistent with what seem to be the correct views about possible nondiscriminatory handling of cases. Hence, we have reason not to always rely on such a narrow notion in deciding whether allocating scarce resources is or is not invidiously discriminatory.

IV. Problems with the Causative Principle and Ideas of Discrimination

Having distinguished the Causative Principle from a narrow treatment effective-ness view, I want to discuss some problems I have elsewhere raised for the Causa-tive Principle. The problems show that the principle fails, despite avoiding some of the problems raised by the narrow treatment-effectiveness view. Moreover, some of its failings involve (other) forms of invidious discrimination.

1.

Recall that the Causative Principle states that it is morally permissible to take ac-count of large differences in QALYs if and only if we cause them (rather than pig-gyback on them). Consider a case in which we must choose whether to give a lifesaving scarce drug to an unparalyzed person who will remain unparalyzed because we do not affect this property of his in any way (U→U) or, instead, to a recently paralyzed person in whom the lifesaving drug has the side effect of unpar-alyzing him (P⇒U), where ⇒ indicates our causal role in treating paralysis. (This case involves the second person in Case 2 and the first person in Case 1, figure 22.1 earlier.) In this case, our causal role is greater in the originally paralyzed person than in the originally unparalyzed person. Yet, I believe, it would be morally wrong and even invidiously discriminatory to make this factor relevant in deciding whom to help. This is because both people will be unparalyzed in the outcome and there is no difference in their past lives that would imply that one person will have lived a much worse life overall if he is not helped to live on. That is, suppose we endorse some morally acceptable role for the Causative Principle (on the basis of cases where the choice is between giving a scarce lifesaving drug to P who will remain P and P whom our treatment can make U, as in Case 1). Then we may make the wrong decision and, it seems, even an invidiously discriminating one, in some cases. This is so if we choose to aid the person on whom we have a much greater positive causal effect, in cases where the candidates' outcomes are the same. (Brock does not consider such cases and the problems they raise in his discussion of our greater impact on one patient than another. I shall comment on this further below. [25])

   In response to such same-outcome cases, I suggested that a mark of invidious discrimination may be that we hold it for or against someone in a contest for a scarce resource that he is disabled or nondisabled when we did not cause those states in him. In cases in which the outcomes for both patients would be U, if we count it in favor of one person that we would cause his being U, we will really be holding it *against* the other person that he would be U rather than P independently of anything we do. [26] This is because it is his being and remaining U that makes it true that we cannot have a causative role in producing U in him. Hence, sometimes if we want not to be engaged in invidious discrimination against either the disabled *or* the nondisabled, we should *not* attend to the causative role of our treatment.

(The same may hold when we must decide between saving U⇒P and P→P. The fact that our causative effect is negative in one person but not the other can be irrelevant if the outcome is the same. This is so even though we would be harming one of the people, especially since depriving him of a chance for the procedure that paralyzes him would result in a worse effect for him, namely death.) This is why I suggested that we should move beyond the simple Causative Principle (and also beyond seeing where our treatment narrowly construed is most causally effective). Hence, in deciding how to allocate a scarce resource, insofar as we are concerned with quality in outcome and assume that invidious discrimination can occur when we piggyback, we should focus on whether *we* would *cause a significantly better or worse* outcome in one patient than in another.[27]

This solution to the problem raised by the simple Causative Principle for same-outcome cases helps refine the idea of invidious discrimination.[28] As suggested by what I have said above, I do not think that judging paralysis to be worse than nonparalysis, other things equal, is itself an instance of an invidiously discriminatory value judgment. Now suppose it is sometimes not invidiously discriminatory to differentiate candidates for a scarce resource on the basis of the expected presence or absence of disabilities when our treatment for some other condition would cause or cure the disabilities. Then we also cannot conceive of invidious discrimination as taking account of someone's disability when this will lead to a worse outcome for him (e.g., he loses his chance for a scarce resource for another medical problem). But one sense of invidious discrimination seems to involve doing what holds someone's disabled or nondisabled state against or in favor of him just because our treatment does not cause the state *when outcomes are the same*. Finally, we have been supposing that someone believes that invidious discrimination occurs in attending to differences in outcome when they come about through piggybacking, yet he also thinks this is not true when the same difference is caused by us (as in the Switch Cases). Putting all this together, we get a conception of discrimination that seems to involve holding someone's nondisabled or disabled state against or in favor of him in a contest for a lifesaving resource when our treatment does not cause the difference (i.e., whether outcomes are different or the same). (One exception is when the disabled state is similar to the condition that gives us reason to try to treat an illness with our scarce resource.)

2.

Another problem with emphasizing whether our treatment causes or cures disability is the threat of intransitivities:[29] Suppose we may sometimes take account of how we causally affect disabilities when deciding how to allocate scarce resources. Then it may be morally permissible to treat P⇒U and U→U differently when they are each in contests for resources with someone who is P→P. That is, P⇒U may be preferred to P→P without invidious discrimination, but if we assume the view that taking account of piggybacked disability is wrongly discriminatory,

U→U may not be preferred to P→P. Yet, it was argued earlier that P⇒U and U→U should be treated as equals in a contest between them alone for a scarce resource. So individuals who are equals in a pairwise comparison fare differently when they are compared pairwise with a third party (P→P). This gives rise to the (apparent) threat of intransitivity and the problem of whom we should select when all three of these individuals are present at once. (It also implies that it is being held against someone that he was U without our assistance, since he fares worse relative to P than someone who began as P and whom we would *make* U. To avoid this problem, we could simply settle for avoiding invidious discrimination, as I described it above, in pairwise comparisons only.)

More specifically, the problem of (apparent) intransitivity can be put as follows, where > is "preferred without invidious discrimination": (1) P⇒U > P→P; (2) P→P = U→U; and yet (3) –(P⇒U > U→U).[30] Brock does not speak to this issue because, as I noted earlier, he does not deal with cases in which our causative role in helping (or harming) one person would lead to the same outcome for both patients. That is, Brock's discussion considers the comparisons in (1) and (2), but not the comparison involved in (3). This may be why he does not notice that (1) and (2) imply what seems to be untrue, namely that P⇒U > U→U.[31]

What should we do when all three individuals (i.e., P→P, U→U, and P⇒U) are in competition for the same scarce lifesaving resource? When all three are present, I suggested that it would not involve invidious discrimination to select one of the people who would have the best outcome.[32] We could reason in the following way: P→P could be eliminated from the contest by P⇒U, and so not have to be directly compared with U→U. Then we can give equal chances to P⇒U and U→U. (There will be no cycling.) The underlying view is that we are morally permitted to seek a significantly better outcome, and to follow a path in decision-making that leads us there, so long as our path to this end is not invidiously discriminatory and no other relevant moral principle is violated.[33]

3.

Let me present a third problem I have discussed. I think it is a problem for those opposed to taking account of disability and nondisability in allocating lifesaving scarce resources when P→P and U→U, but who nevertheless think that significant differences in life expectancy—whether they come about through our causation or piggybacking—*should* sometimes matter in allocation decisions. Suppose candidate A for a lifesaving treatment will live for one year and candidate B for six years, and this is a reason to select B. Suppose A is nondisabled and B was recently severely paralyzed. Other things equal, if we do not give the treatment to B, we would be holding his disability against him. Suppose B receives the treatment and subsequently wishes to take advantage of a new surgery that will unparalyze him, though it reduces his life expectancy to slightly over one year. (I called this a Switch-and-Reduce Case.) He wants to do this because, let us suppose, it is a reasonable *intra*personal tradeoff to exchange six years of severely paralyzed life for slightly more than one year of nondisabled life. In fact, it makes him better off. With the Switch-and-Reduce surgery, B would be almost identical to the way A was; the difference in length of life expected (one month) would presumably be morally irrelevant in an interpersonal choice of whose life to save. Had B's prospects earlier been nearly identical to A's, the objection we raised to the simple Causative Principle implies that we should have given them equal chances for the lifesaving resource. Even if at the time of allocating the scarce treatment we only knew that B would have the Switch-and-Reduce surgery were his life to be saved, it seems we should have given A and B equal chances.

Might it be that if we select B over A because he will live for six years, we should elicit a promise that he will not have the later surgery so that the five additional years of life that gave us a reason to deprive A of his chance will come about? Limiting B's options subsequent to his selection would imply that there are moral reasons for his having to make decisions only about his own life from the same perspective that led to him rather than someone else being alive. (This would be even clearer if A would have been preferred over B, with a life expectancy of slightly over one year, because A had a significantly longer life expectancy than one year—e.g., three years.)

Further, suppose that at the time of the choice with A we could have saved B in two different ways: (i) so that he will live for six years paralyzed or (ii) so that we switch him to being unparalyzed with a life span of slightly more than one year. Then if B chose the Switch-and-Reduce option (ii), it seems that equal chances should have been given to A and B. Hence, if at the time of selecting a candidate, B chose the lifesaving procedure (ii) that was better for him intrapersonally, he would eliminate the superior chances to live relative to A that he would have had if he chose to be P for six years.[34]

The problem in these cases arises because we are refusing to allow the same tradeoff between quality and quantity of life interpersonally that we (are assuming) is reasonable intrapersonally. Such a tradeoff interpersonally (we are assuming) would make six years P in B equal to one year U in A. One ground for not allowing quality/quantity tradeoffs interpersonally was suggested earlier: When all one can have is a life with severe P, it may be reasonable to care about one year with such a life as much as someone else cares about one year with U.[35] However, we are also allowing the reasonableness of bringing about the intrapersonal tradeoff between a long life with severe P and a shorter one with U when this can be done. That is, someone who reasonably cares maximally for a year with severe P, when it is all he can have, can consistently care to be U for even much less time when that is an option. As a result of these two moves, B's P life lasting for six years is judged better *interpersonally* than A's U life lasting for one, and yet B's U life for slightly more than one year, which would *intrapersonally* be better than the better *interpersonal* option, is not judged better *interpersonally* than A's year.

These cases may remind us of what Thomas Scanlon famously emphasized, that intrapersonal tradeoffs that are adequately reasonable for an individual to make can lack moral relevance from an interpersonal point of view. He described someone (call him Joe) who had a claim on us for food to meet his nutritional needs but for whom it was more important to build a monument to his god than to eat. Scanlon claimed that Joe would have no claim on us to provide him with funds to build the monument instead of spending the same amount for his food. Now suppose that our money is scarce and both Joe and Alice have an equal claim on us for food. The amount we can purchase is the minimum necessary for survival and so there is no point dividing it between them. Then if other things are equal between them, we should give each a maximal equal chance for food. However, if Joe will sell the food we give him to get supplies to build the monument to his god, then, presumably, he should lose his equal chance for the food. His not unreasonable intrapersonal tradeoff would not have a legitimate interpersonal role in his retaining an equal chance with Alice for food. This would be true even if Alice had the same preference ranking as Joe but would not be able to act on it with her food supply.[36]

Notes

1. My remarks on Singer are in response to his "Why We Must Ration Health Care," *New York Times Magazine*, July 19, 2009. All references to Singer are to that article, which he wrote while the Obama health-care proposals were being discussed. A short extract of my discussion of Singer was published as a Letter to the Editor of the *New York Times Magazine*, August 13, 2009. My remarks on Brock are in response to his "Cost-Effectiveness and Disability Discrimination," *Economics and Philosophy* 25 (2009): 27–47. All references to Brock are to this article. I am grateful for comments to audiences at the Conference on Rationing, Erasmus University, Rotterdam, December 2010, at the Bioethics Colloquium, New York University, April 2011, and at the Department of Clinical Bioethics, NIH June 2011. I am grateful for comments to the editors of *Rationing Health Care: Hard Choices and Unavoidable* Tradeoffs, eds. A den Exter and M. Buijsen (Apeldoorn, Netherlands: Maklu, 2012), in which this chapter also appears, and to the editors of Health *Inequality: Ethics, Measurement and Policy*, eds. N. Eyal, O. Norheim, S. A. Hurst, and D. Wikler (New York: Oxford University Press, forthcoming), in which this chapter will also appear.

2. The QALY, which multiplies years of life times quality, was invented by Richard Zeckhauser, who also thinks we should allocate health resources to maximize QALYs per dollar. It is not clear why Singer favors maximizing health benefits rather than all benefits. Prima facie, the latter standard could imply that we ought to save rich, beautiful, and productive people over those who lack such traits.

3. He says:

How can we compare saving a person's life with, say, making it possible for someone who was confined to bed to return to an active life. . . . One common method is to describe medical conditions to people—let's say being a quadriplegic—and tell them that they can choose between 10 years in that condition or a smaller number of years without it. . . . If most . . . have difficulty deciding between 5 years of nondisabled life or 10 years with quadriplegia, then they are, in effect, assessing life with quadriplegia as half as good as nondisabled life. . . . (These are hypothetical figures. . . .) If that judgment represents a rough average across the population, we might conclude that restoring to nondisabled life two people who would otherwise be quadriplegics is equivalent in value to saving the life of one person, provided the life expectancies of all involved are similar.

4. On why this might be so, see my "Should You Save This Child? Gibbard on Intuitions, Contractualism, and Strains of Commitment," a comment on Allan Gibbard's Tanner Lectures, in Gibbard's *Reconciling Our Aims* (New York: Oxford University Press, 2008).

5. Such a rescue is different from deciding when someone is, for example, 20, whether to allocate resources in such a way that he lives to 60.5 rather than to 60. I discuss this distinction briefly in "Aggregation, Allocating Scarce Resources, and the Disabled," *Social Philosophy and Policy* 26 (Winter 2009), and in chapter 21 this volume.

6. In general, Singer believes that it could be morally correct to aggregate small benefits to many people, each of whom is not badly off, and produce a large overall benefit, rather than to provide a significant benefit to prevent someone else from being much worse off. So although he is known for his views on the duty to save people from famine, his theoretical position actually implies that it could be morally preferable to save many from headaches rather than save a few from death. For this and other criticisms of Singer's views, see my "Faminine Ethics," in *Singer and His Critics*, ed. D. Jamieson (Oxford: Blackwell, 1999), which somewhat revised is also chapter 13 in my *Intricate Ethics* (New York: Oxford University Press, 2007).

7. It is sometimes argued that people who are not disabled mistakenly believe that becoming severely disabled is very bad. This is because, it is said, they are poor predictors of how unhappy they would be if they were disabled, as shown by the fact that the disabled are as happy as the nondisabled due to adaptation and various protective psychological mechanisms (even including self-deception). These points are made by Timothy Wilson in his *Strangers to Ourselves* (Cambridge, MA: Harvard University Press, 2004).

However, there are disturbing implications to basing rationing decisions on these findings, in addition to not allocating funds to cure disabilities. Suppose many people come to an emergency room with severe headaches that will last several hours. At the same time, someone else comes in with a spinal injury that will paralyze his legs if surgery is not done right away. Should we treat all the headaches or do the surgery if we cannot do both? Suppose that we can predict that someone will quickly adapt to paralysis but the people with severe headaches cannot adapt to them now. If experienced well-being were all that mattered, we should cure the headaches. This is the wrong conclusion, I believe. This is an indication that experienced well-being and accurate predictions about it are not all that matters in rationing decisions. The fact that people can adapt to, and deceive themselves about, a bad condition does not mean that we should not prevent the bad condition. (In this connection, it is interesting to note that Daniel Kahneman, who reports that disfigured people's "daily mood" is the same as nondisfigured people's, also reports that the disfigured people themselves want to have the disfigurement removed (mentioned in his "Evolving Notions of Well-Being," a lecture in the Mind, Brain, and Behavior Distinguished Lecture Series, Harvard University, April 17, 2008).

8. This explanation and others I am about to describe are presented in greater detail in my "Deciding Whom to Help, the Principle of Irrelevant Goods and Health-Adjusted Life Years," (1999), unpublished but circulated as a working paper of the Center for Population Studies, Harvard University; "Deciding Whom to Help, Health-Adjusted Life Years, and Disabilities," a revision of the working paper, in *Public Health, Ethics, and Equity*, eds. S. Anand, F. Peter, and A. Sen (New York: Oxford University Press, 2004); "Aggregation, Allocating Scarce Resources, and the Disabled" and a slightly different, longer version, "Disability, Discrimination, and Irrelevant Goods," in *Disability and Disadvantage*, eds. K. Brownlee and A. Cureton (New York: Oxford University Press, 2009. (Chapter 21 this volume consists of a combination of these papers.) I discussed the Principle of Irrelevant Goods in my *Morality, Mortality*, Vol. I (New York: Oxford University Press, 1993).

9. For more on this issue, see chapter 21 this volume.

10. See my "Aggregation, Allocating Scarce Resources, and the Disabled," pp. 160, 169–70.

11. I deal with the recently paralyzed to factor out the relevance for rationing decisions of one candidate having had a worse life in the past than another candidate. See my *Morality, Mortality*, Vol. I, for a theory of rationing that takes into account different pasts in candidates for a scarce resources. See also chapters 18 and 20 this volume.

12. See my "Aggregation, Allocating Scarce Resources, and the Disabled," p. 172. There I called it Treatment Similarity. See also chapter 21 this volume.

13. See my "Disability, Discrimination, and Irrelevant Goods."

14. See my "Deciding Whom to Help, Health-Adjusted Life Years, and Disabilities," p. 240.

15. Brock refers to "Kamm's Nonlinkage Principle" (p. 35) to describe the view that linkage might be morally objectionable in general, but he does not note that I specifically rejected this view. See "Deciding Whom to Help, Health-Adjusted Life Years, and Disabilities," p. 240. I discuss this further in "Aggregation, Allocating Scarce Resources, and the Disabled," pp. 171–72.

16. See my "Deciding Whom to Help: The Principle of Irrelevant Goods and Health-Adjusted Life Years."

17. I first discussed the Switch Cases and the Causative Principle in "Deciding Whom to Help: The Principle of Irrelevant Goods and Health-Adjusted Life Years," and again in "Deciding Whom to Help, Health-Adjusted Life Years, and Disabilities," p. 238.

18. In "Aggregation, Allocating Scarce Resources, and the Disabled," p. 178.

19. In "Aggregation, Allocating Scarce Resources, and the Disabled," p. 179.

20. In "Deciding Whom to Help, Health-Adjusted Life Years, and Disabilities," p. 242.

21. It is possible that there is a different reason, in general, for trying to cure and prevent paralysis, namely a life with the disability is harder even if not less good. It could be supererogatory for people to lead the harder life even if it were no less good. But it is also not objectionably discriminatory to judge that the paralyzed life is harder. For the "supererogation argument," see my "Disability, Discrimination, and Irrelevant Goods" and chapter 21 this volume.

22. He says, "The fifth form of discrimination is where a particular treatment is less effective in some kinds of patients than in another kind, leaving the first kind disabled, but not due to any background conditions of pre-existing disability. This case seems simply to be a difference in treatment effectiveness, with disability entering the picture for some

patients but not others only as a result of the treatment" (p. 41). This quote probably applies to both cases in which treatment does not cure disability acquired in an accident (as in the text) and where it actually causes a disability (as in my second Switch Case).

23. In my Switch Case that involves life saving and a cure of disability in one patient but not another, the disability was recently acquired in both patients, but independently of the life-threatening illness. When I first wrote about the Switch Case in "Deciding Whom to Help: The Principle of Irrelevant Goods and Health-Adjusted Life Years," I did not know about the hypothetical case considered by the government agency and its analysis of the case. Indeed, Brock informed me of it as a way of criticizing my conclusion that curing disability could matter morally in the Switch Cases. He seems to have changed his position on this.

24. Although Brock cites "Deciding Whom to Help, Health-Adjusted life Years, and Disabilities" in his article, he does not mention the discussion in that article of the Switch Cases.

25. I raised this issue in "Deciding Whom to Help, Health-Adjusted Life Years, and Disabilities," pp. 239–40.

26. A full discussion of this point would have to consider as an exception the idea of giving priority to a worse-off paralyzed person because her past and the past of the unparalyzed persons are very different. I owe this point to Carlos Soto.

27. For a more detailed discussion of this, see my "Aggregation, Allocating Scarce Resources, and the Disabled." In moving beyond the simple Causative Principle, I introduced another principle, the Principle of Irrelevant Type Identity. I omit discussion of it here to avoid unnecessarily complicating matters. Elizabeth Pike has suggested that in same outcome cases not involving life and death, we *should* attend to our causative role. For example, suppose that we could treat either P or U for gastritis. U would remain U if he is treated, but the drug for gastritis would also have the side effect of making P unparalyzed. Surely, she says, we should give the drug to P, for then the person who remains U will still be alive and U, albeit with gastritis, and we will both cure gastritis in someone and produce another unparalyzed person. I agree that in this case we should give the treatment to P. However, this case shows that it is not enough to focus on just the outcomes for the competitors for a scarce resource in order to know whether we will have produced the same outcome whomever we treat. Because if we treat U instead of P, we will have a world in which there is still a paralyzed person (P), whereas if we treat P we will reduce the number of paralyzed people and cure the same amount of gastritis. Hence our *overall* outcome will be *different* depending on whom we treat.

28. I discuss this in "Deciding Whom to Help, Health-Adjusted Life Years, and Disabilities," pp. 238–39.

29. This was discussed in "Deciding Whom to Help, Health-Adjusted Life Years, and Disabilities," p. 242, note 13. Further discussion of this is in "Aggregation, Allocating Scarce Resources, and the Disabled."

30. Also, $P{\Rightarrow}U = U{\rightarrow}U$, and $U{\rightarrow}U = P{\rightarrow}P$, yet $-(P{\Rightarrow}U = P{\rightarrow}P)$.

31. Perhaps there is another reason for his not seeing this problem. It is possible that a treatment that did more for one patient than another should, as in (3), still be considered equally effective in a wide sense in both, and so not grounds for permissibly preferring one patient. This is because the treatment equally deals with *all* the problems each patient had, even if the nondisabled patient has fewer problems. It would be just as *effective* in a wide sense although it did not literally *affect* as much.

32. In "Deciding Whom to Help, Health-Adjusted Life Years, and Disabilities."

33. A round-robin procedure would lead to the same result, according to Peter Graham.

34. A similar issue arises if B who would be P for six years confronts C who would be P for six years, when only B has the option of another lifesaving treatment that would result in his being U for one and one-eighth years. Suppose the latter is his intrapersonally preferable option. Should B be deprived of his equal chance simply because he selects a better intrapersonal option that we would cause? It at least seems so, because giving him an equal chance with A would involve counting the length of someone's life differently depending on whether she was U or P. An earlier discussion of this issue is in chapter 21 this volume.

35. I discuss this in "Deciding Whom to Help, Health-Adjusted Life Years, and Disabilities," "Aggregation, Allocating Scarce Resources, and the Disabled," and in chapter 21 this volume.

36. For Scanlon's case, see his "Preference and Urgency," *Journal of Philosophy* 72(19): 655–69. Thomas Nagel reminded me of the relevance of Scanlon's case for my discussion of the Switch-and-Reduce Cases. Suppose, however, that Joe used money of his own on monument building when he could have used it for food, and this (foreseeably) left him without money for his food. Would Scanlon think that Joe now had no claim on us to provide him with food? Would he think that Joe had at least a weaker claim on food than someone else whose hunger was not the result of having spent his money on this other project? This case raises many interesting issues about the specificity of the use of our aid (after all, Joe will eat the food we give him) and also about responsibility for one's condition.

23

Learning from Bioethics

MORAL ISSUES IN RATIONING MEDICAL AND *NONMEDICAL* SCARCE RESOURCES

This chapter is an attempt to survey some basic issues in the morality of rationing in relation to nonmedical resources.[1] The morality of rationing involves determining priorities in allocating goods (to which potential recipients have no prior property rights) in conditions of scarcity. (Sometimes, the term "priority setting" is used instead of "rationing." This can be misleading because we can still set priorities when there is no scarcity—i.e., we decide who will be helped first and who will be helped last to the full extent of his need. "Rationing" implies that not everyone can be helped to the full extent.) This topic is of importance in a wide number of areas—such as medicine, education, and legal services—where restrictions on funding mean that not everyone who could be benefited can be helped to the fullest extent. Sometimes scarcity is the result of injustices, but it need not be. For example, restrictions on funding could be the result of justice for a world where not everything is possible. And then we must decide who shall get what.

It is only recently that rationing has been discussed in some detail in the area of medicine. In education, legal services, and other areas where providers may have to choose whom to serve, basic issues in the morality of rationing have yet to gain currency. My aim is to extend the subject of rationing into these areas, hoping that we can learn from rationing theory in bioethics. I will not propose solutions so much as survey some types of issues that arise, some types of factors that are important to consider from a moral point of view, and possible principles of allocation for application to cases.[2]

I. What Is Allocated?

A fundamental issue is whether we should think that we are allocating resources or, rather, the benefits that may come of resources. (In "benefit," I include prevention of harms.) We can have conflicting intuitive judgments about this issue. For example, suppose we thought that an equal allocation was correct in some circumstances. If we

506

distributed educational resources equally, some who are strong learners would achieve much more with their share of resources than some who are weak learners. The latter might need more resources in order to attain the same level as the strong learners. In this situation, we may think that equal concern for all people and treatment of them as equally important persons requires giving unequal resources because our aim should be the equal attainment of some level of knowledge or skill in each person. In other cases, however, if resources are distributed equally despite different outcomes for some recipients, there may be no complaint. An example is the allocation of an equal number of textbooks to each school child, even though the more imaginative children will get more out of each reading. In what follows, I assume that we are concerned with the allocation of resources, though as we shall see, sometimes concern for benefits that come of the resources must come into the picture.

Sometimes, when we do not have enough resources to help everyone, some of our resources will go to waste if we help some people rather than others. For example, suppose a country has many schoolbooks but not enough for everyone who needs them, and far fewer teachers than it needs. If each child who gets a book goes to class, all the book resources will be used up but low levels of education will be achieved because there are more students per teacher and this inhibits high levels of achievement. Alternatively, if class sizes are kept small to allow the students to achieve the highest possible level of education, many books will be left unused. The argument for educating the greater number of children cannot be merely that it wastes no books. Hence, the best allocation of a scarce resource is not necessarily the one that uses up all of the available scarce resource.

II. In What Context Are the Resources Allocated?

It is important to establish a rationing decision as either microallocation or macroallocation. Microallocation is a question of deciding between individuals here and now by persons who have certain professional responsibilities for the resources; for example, a teacher deciding who receives textbooks when she has more students than available books. By contrast, macroallocation can be a question of how much to invest so that certain resources will or will not be available for populations in existence now or to come. What factors it is permissible or obligatory to consider may vary with the context.[3]

III. Some Factors to Consider When Allocating Resources

A. DIFFERENTIAL NEED FOR THE RESOURCE BY DIFFERENT PEOPLE

Some may already have a lot of the resource that we have to distribute and others may have little of it. The latter are thought of as needier with respect to the resource. There are at least two ways of looking at this. In the first, we consider present and (expected) future access to the resource: Some now have or will have more of the resource than others, independent of our allocation. In the second, we consider not only present and future but also *past* access to the resource: Some have had more of the resource than others have had, independent of our allocation. On the first perspective, someone who does not have and will not have any books has greater need for books than someone who has and will have many books. On the second perspective, someone who has had many books in the past, though she now has none and will have none in the future, does not necessarily have a greater need for books now than someone who has and will have some but not many books in the future but had none in the past (other things equal between them). It seems reasonable to think that past access to the resource should affect our decision about neediness. Hence, I shall assume in what follows the second perspective: that need is determined based on past, present, and future access to the resource, independent of our allocation—in other words, how well off, resource wise, the person will have been overall. It is possible that not all differences in need are morally relevant. For example, considering two people who each need to learn English, the person who has had one English lesson is slightly less needy of English lessons than someone who has had none, for he can already say a few words in English. But this difference seems irrelevant in the specific context where we are deciding who should go to a full English course.

Another important issue in thinking about someone's need for a particular resource A is whether that need should be affected by how much he has had of another resource B. For example, suppose two people are in competition for a health resource and one but not the other has had a great deal of educational resources. Is the need of one person for the health resource less because he has had another good that the other person has not? It seems odd to think so. Nevertheless, might it be just to provide the health resources to those who have not had other resources before we provide health resources to those who benefit resource-wise on some other important dimension? The issue here is whether how we allocate will be determined according to separate spheres (health, education, etc.) or by taking into account all the resources that a person will have had. An in-between position is to consider how important it is to provide someone with resource A by also considering how much he will have had of resource B, even if we do not consider how he fares with respect to another resource C. For example, suppose that among a set of people who all need literature books is a subset of people who have more math books than the others, and who are also healthier than the others. Perhaps the fact that this subset has math books is relevant to the question of who should get the literature books, even if the fact that the subset is healthier is not relevant. I think the question as to what approach to take on this issue remains but to simplify, I shall assume the separate spheres view, which does not exclude considering different aspects of one sphere (e.g., education).

B. POSSIBLE BENEFIT

"Possible benefit" refers to the differential outcome *with* the resource versus *without* it. Even if someone is in greater need of education, he may not be smart enough to achieve a great increase in his abilities per unit of resources. By contrast, someone who does not have as great a need may produce a much better outcome per unit of resources. (Of course, these predictions are subject to error, so they are really views about expected benefit. I shall ignore this complication, but it could be relevant to allocation that we are more certain of outcomes in one group than in another, even though the latter has the potential to achieve better outcomes.) Sometimes, differential outcome should be relevant to allocating, I believe.

But in dealing with outcome, should only the benefit to the direct recipient of the resource be considered, or also the effects on others who may benefit indirectly? For example, suppose each of two women needs an education and one has children while the other does not. If we can only provide the education to one of the women, should the indirect beneficial effects on the children matter? If we think that each person has a right to an education, it may be that this by itself excludes consideration of the effects on others as a ground for deciding between the two of them. (The right is then treated as what is known as an exclusionary reason, which excludes consideration of the children.) This is even clearer when property rights are involved. For example, suppose people have paid a company—using money justly distributed or earned—to produce educational materials for them. However, there is a shortage in production, and we must decide who will get the materials when all cannot get them. It seems wrong to think that the beneficial effects on people who did not pay for the resource (nonowners) should affect the decision as to who will benefit among those who have already paid (owners). The property right serves as an exclusionary reason, excluding consideration of the nonowners.

If this analogy is relevant, we will have to decide, in working out what outcomes are morally relevant to allocation decisions, whether we think someone has some sort of (nonproperty) right to the scarce resource or if it is merely something we wish to provide. In macroallocation contexts where we consider persons to have rights against society to healthcare, education resources, and legal services, perhaps how much we will invest in each should be affected by the degree and type of indirect benefits to people other than potential recipients of these services. Different indirect benefits will result from different investment patterns, even when the indirect beneficiaries have no rights at stake. (For example, how will potential employers of those who need the services be affected by one pattern of investment rather than another?) In what follows, for simplicity's sake, I shall (for the most part) abstract from the issue of indirect benefits to others, but it is an important issue to resolve.

As was true with need, it may be that some differences in even direct outcomes are not morally relevant. For example, if we have only enough funds to send one of two people to school, that one will wind up scoring 95 percent in English and the other 93 percent seems to be a morally irrelevant difference in outcome. That is, it is not an adequate reason to justify depriving one person of her chance to go to school in order to be able to send the other person. So sometimes when other things are equal, a difference does not decide the matter, because each of the candidates can still achieve the most important part of what should be achieved, the alternative for each if he does not get that important part is very bad, and each wants to be the one to be educated. However, whether an outcome difference is morally irrelevant can depend on the neediness of the candidates. For if both people are very well educated and we are distributing resources for higher education, the fact that one will get a 95 score and the other a 93 in an advanced course may now be a reason to choose one candidate over the other. Though each here achieves the most important part of what is to be achieved from the course, and each wants to be the one to get the education, the alternative each faces without the course is not very bad; this may affect whether we should search for the absolutely best candidate instead of distributing resources impartially.

C. URGENCY

How soon someone will suffer a harm if we do not help him is a common notion of urgency.[4] It might be thought that how we allocate a scarce resource should depend on urgency in this sense. But if a resource is truly scarce, the less urgent person will never be helped. So, why should it matter that he could wait longer to be helped by contrast to the more urgent individual? Where life is at stake, being able to wait for treatment means that one will get more life than someone else will, even without our help. But where goods other than time alive are at stake, the less urgent person, if not helped, can wind up just as deprived as the more urgent person. For example, if one person must get training by age 5 or else never be trainable and another will remain trainable until age 6, the latter will be just as badly off as the former if never trained at all. On the other hand, if the less urgent person will eventually be helped, there is only temporary scarcity, not real scarcity. Hence, I shall ignore urgency (in the sense of how soon someone must be helped) in what follows.

D. RESPONSIBILITY

What if some are causally and morally responsible for being in need or for the fact that they will have a poor outcome if given resources? Typically, one thinks of such cases as involving some moral defect, such as failure to take precautions or self-indulgence. But someone may be needy or unable to generate a good outcome because of having fulfilled a duty (e.g., used her money for her children's education and hence have none for her own) or having done some supererogatory act. Furthermore (as Scanlon has emphasized),[5] there is a difference between the sense of moral responsibility that involves attributing a problem to someone's failure and the sense of moral responsibility that involves his having to bear the costs of the problem. (The latter Scanlon calls "substantive responsibility.") One possible cost is being at a disadvantage when others must choose whom to aid with a scarce resource. If someone is negligent in a minor way and the need that results is very great, it seems that his having to bear the cost in the form of being at a great disadvantage relative to other, equally needy candidates for a scarce resource is not commensurate with his negligence and should not be used as a tie-breaker between him and others. However, this leaves it open that being placed at a slight disadvantage in distribution decisions—what form this takes depends on the principle of allocation one decides upon—is not inappropriate. For example, if educational funding were scarce, someone who had failed to register for school in time might be made to walk further rather than have an equal chance to go to the school closer to his home.

No doubt there are many more factors than the four outlined above that may be relevant in deciding how to allocate scarce resources. I have just tried to open the issue of what such factors might be. In doing this, however, it must be remembered that deciding that it is morally required or permissible to select candidates for scarce resources on the basis of need, outcome, or responsibility does not mean that any of the candidates is not worthy of being helped if there is no scarcity.

IV. Principles for Allocation

Now let us consider various principles for allocation and some of the contexts in which they may apply. The principles, in part, attempt to relate to each other the factors we have been discussing. (I shall ignore the issue of responsibility in discussing these principles.)

A. EQUAL NUMBERS WITH DIFFERENT CHARACTERISTICS

First, let us look at principles for allocation where the choice affects an equal number of people whatever we do, and where all the people in any given nonoverlapping group in competition for resources are relevantly identical in need and outcome, but the groups differ from one another in these respects. (For example, each group has five people, but one group's members are all needier than another group's members.)

(1)

If the resources in question are divisible between groups, we do not have to choose to give to some and not to others, for we can give a small amount to everyone (in accordance with need, for example). Divisibility, however, should be constrained at least by producing some good outcome in each person, even if it is minimal. The decision that it is morally better to produce more in some people than an absolutely minimal benefit in everyone may be based on the significance of *indirect benefits to the very people who would be deprived of more of the resource in question.* For example, in a very poor country, instead of making sure everyone can simply write his name, we might leave some people completely illiterate, if this is necessary, so that others can read and write at a high school level. This is because if some have greater skills, this will improve economic development and even those without any education may benefit more than if all people had absolutely minimal literacy. (This is a different sort of indirect benefit from that considered above. For here, it is the very same people who were eligible to have received the original good who benefit as a side effect from another good.) However, suppose we abstract from such indirect effects in a different (e.g., economic) sphere from the one within which the resource we are allocating lies, and just consider the greater benefits to the direct beneficiaries of the resource. Deciding not to divide the divisible good to the point of minimal benefits represents a concern for outcome in each person as an individual. That is, even if the very minimal benefits in everyone when aggregated would create an enormous sum of benefits, this might not be as morally important as some individuals getting substantial changes in their lives.

(2)

Suppose a resource is not divisible between the two groups or, for the reasons given in (1), we decide against divisibility between groups on moral grounds. A possible principle of allocation is random selection, giving each side maximal equal chances. This means that we ignore differential neediness and outcome where they exist. This choice denies the moral relevance of those factors. It implies that giving scarce educational resources to those who already have a lot of such resources and who also get very little benefit from them is as morally important as giving the resources to those who have fewer resources and/or can produce better outcomes. This seems implausible.

(3)

An alternative principle is to allocate the resources on the basis of which side produces a significantly better expected outcome, so that we maximize total good. But suppose that individuals on that side are already much better off in the way the resource can make them than individuals on the other side are. Even taking into account diminishing marginal utility of resources, they may produce a better outcome, but still, might it not be morally more valuable to significantly improve the worse off group, though their expected outcome is not as great?

(4)

This question suggests that another possible principle is to allocate resources to those who need them most, regardless of degree of outcome, so long as some significant good will accrue to the persons helped. Such a principle might still consider small differences in need morally irrelevant, not distinguishing, for example, between those who have never had English lessons and those who have had two English lessons when the goal is to enable people to have basic skills in English. (Recall that if we take need into account, we must decide whether we will measure need on one dimension [i.e., the one directly relevant to the resource we are allocating] or whether we will measure need by considering whether people are compensated for need on one dimension by being less needy on other dimensions.) A principle that takes account only of need and considers that there is more moral value in giving to the neediest regardless of the size of the benefit so long as it is a significant benefit is close to a Maximin Allocation Principle.

Is the underlying idea behind maximin the attempt to achieve equality between persons by raising up the worst off before giving anything more to those who already have more? Not necessarily, because it is possible that if a resource is not divisible, by helping the worst off, we will wind up making him better off in resources (and possibly in outcome) than the person who was originally better off, even introducing more inequality than existed before. In such a case, however, even though there is as much or more inequality than originally, the person helped is better off in absolute terms than he was and the other person has not been made worse off in absolute terms. To get more equality, sometimes we would have to "level down"—that is, make someone worse off without making anyone better off—and this is not required by maximin. If we should not level down, it may be either because equality is of no intrinsic value or because it is of intrinsic value but it can be overridden in favor of simply making someone who is badly off in absolute terms better off without making anyone else worse off.[6]

Furthermore, concern about taking care of the neediest first (even if we only give them priority to a moderate degree), unlike concern for equality, need not be based on a comparative judgment—that is, how one person fares relative to another. Rather, it can be decided that giving resources to someone has greater moral value the worse off in absolute terms she is. She could be in this absolute condition even if there were no one else in the world with whom to compare her. In that case, giving to her would still have the same value even though it did nothing for equality.[7]

If we do not give absolute priority to helping the neediest, as long as they get some significant benefit, this may be because they are already at a quite high absolute level of resources. Hence, a principle of giving absolute priority to the worst off may have a threshold: below the threshold, they get absolute priority (given some significant benefit); above it, they may get different degrees of priority but we do not automatically favor them over people who are less needy to a morally relevant degree, but who can, for example, get more benefit out of the resources. We can call this a Threshold Principle.

(5)

If we do not give absolute priority to the neediest, no matter how badly off they are (i.e., there is no threshold below which they always win the resource for a significant outcome), then we should always compare the benefits that would be produced by helping the neediest or the less needy. We could still give the neediest some, if not absolute, priority. This means multiplying the outcome we can produce in the neediest by a factor proportionate to their absolute level of need so that a unit of benefit in them is worth more morally than a unit of benefit in someone less needy. Given a big enough benefit, giving resources to someone less needy could take precedence over giving it to the neediest, on this view. I call this an Outcome Modification Principle, as the significance of helping the worst off shows up in the multiplication of their outcome. The idea is to maximize the weighted benefit produced. Alternatively, we can think of the loss of benefit that would be sustained by individuals if they are not helped relative to what they would have if helped, and try to minimize the maximum weighted loss (i.e., the loss multiplied by a factor for need). This is called a Minimax Weighted Loss Principle.

(6)

Might it be true that sometimes (morally relevant) differences in outcome independent of any consideration of need should determine allocation? Some have argued that no matter how needy one is, if a benefit is small enough, this is a reason all by itself to provide a bigger benefit to someone else, even if this other person is much less needy. According to this view, unlike minimax weighted loss, we need not even multiply the small benefit by the factor of neediness; the larger benefit per person automatically wins—we simply ignore need altogether. Here is an example from medicine:[8] Someone who is already blind can be prevented from suffering a week of pain. Someone else who has suffered only a week of pain in his life can be prevented from losing a hand. Let us assume that the people are equal in all other respects, that it is worse to be blind than to lose a hand, and that it is a significant benefit to avoid a week of pain. This implies that the blind person will be significantly worse off if we do not help him than the other person will be. Yet we can do very little to make a difference to the worse-off person. We cannot alleviate in any way the primary cause of his being worse off (his blindness). By contrast, we can do a great deal to help the other person. It seems clear that we should prevent the loss of a hand. (Larry Temkin has argued for a view that implies that even if there were very many such blind people in competition with the single person facing the loss of a hand, it would be morally wrong to help the many who will be much worse off if not aided. He points out that this is true even if the total aggregated good of many people avoiding a week of pain were greater than the good done in preventing the single lost hand. Hence, he says, the principle that justifies such an allocation of resources would be in conflict with principles favoring maximizing total good, maximin, and equality.[9])

Notice that whether it is true that a big outcome always wins over a much smaller one could depend on *how* allocation makes it the case that the neediest lose out on a very small benefit. Ordinarily, we think that it is our allocation to the neediest that would provide them with the small benefit, and in helping someone else, the neediest lose out. But suppose that our allocating assistance to someone else caused those who are very needy not to get the small benefit that someone else would have given them. Or suppose we indirectly reduced future resources they would have had independently of us by the small amount, due to the increased productivity of the better-off in whom we produce a great benefit. Then, our allo-cating to the better-off actually indirectly makes the neediest worse off to a small degree rather than merely not helping them. When this is true, sometimes (though not necessarily always) the loss of a small good could be morally significant when it is occurring to the neediest, especially if they are very much needier than those we would aid. Hence, we may have to be aware of the *causal route* by which our allocating to one party results in the absence of a small benefit to another party before we can ignore the level of need of each party, I think.

B. DIFFERENT NUMBERS OF PEOPLE

Here we look at principles of allocation for situations in which the only difference between nonoverlapping groups of people is the number of individuals whom we can help in each. The different groups in competition for a scarce resource do not differ in terms of the need of their members or the benefit each is expected to get if aided, though individuals within each group may differ from one another in these respects.

(1)

It seems completely unproblematic to most people to allow numbers to count in deciding whom to help, yet it is surprisingly difficult to justify doing this on some ethical views. Hence, I shall give considerable attention to whether and how we can justify the very basic principle of allocation that tells us to do what helps the greater number of otherwise relevantly similar people.

Some (e.g., Taurek) have argued that the number of individuals should not count.[10] For example, rather than automatically helping the greater number when all are equally needy and stand to benefit as much, if we wish to show equal concern and regard for people, we should give each person an equal chance by, for example, toss-ing a coin between competing groups. His reasons for this are (a) no one in the larger group will suffer a greater loss or benefit to a greater degree than will anyone in the smaller group, and (b) it is not true that it is a better outcome if the greater number are helped; it is only better for them and worse for those in the smaller group.

Taurek's first claim depends on a common nonconsequentialist procedure of reasoning called "pairwise comparison." This procedure requires that when de-ciding whom to help, we should look to see how each person as an individual will fare if helped and/or not helped, rather than aggregating by adding the benefits to all people. So, we compare each person in one group with each person in the other group, checking for neediness of each and also, on some (but not all) views of pairwise comparison, how much each stands to gain (i.e., to what degree the need of each can be relieved). Concern to pairwise compare suggests that if each mem-ber of a large group of people is less needy and will benefit to a lesser degree than one person in another group, then the claim of the latter person to be aided could be greater than the claims of any and all of the people in the larger group.

Taurek's second claim, however, is to some degree in conflict with this conclusion. The second claim suggests that Taurek believes only in relative goodness (i.e., something can only be good-for-someone, rather than simply good). But suppose that an individual will lose a year in his PhD education unless he is helped and another individual will lose out on even a basic high school education unless he is helped: it is still worse *for the first individual* who will suffer the lesser loss that he suffers his loss, than that another person suffers the greater loss. Yet the procedure of pairwise comparison suggests that we should often help the person who would suffer the greater loss.

Hence, deciding to help the worse-off person in a pairwise comparison seems to depend on reasoning from some point of view outside that of any individual's subjective perspective—that is, from some impartial perspective. Could we extend the use of the impartial perspective further and argue that it is better from the impartial perspective if many are helped than if fewer are helped when we cannot help everyone? Consider what I call the Argument for Best Outcomes. First, it is better if B and C are provided education than if B alone is. This is simple Pareto optimality: someone is improved and no one is made worse off, so there is no conflict between one person's interest and another's. In this sense, numbers can count even to those who reject counting numbers when groups are in conflict over resources. Second, from an impartial perspective, it is morally just as good for A to receive an education as for B to receive one, even if it is not just as good from the perspectives of A and B. This moral equivalence of A or B being educated allows us to substitute A for B into the first step in our argument and to conclude that it is better if A and C are provided with an education than if B alone is. Hence, it is better if we educate a greater number of people of equal need who will benefit equally than if we educate fewer different people.

However, at least from the point of view of nonconsequentialist ethical theory, it is not always permissible to bring about the better state of affairs if this would involve unfairness or injustice to some. (For example, we may not kill B in order to save A and C from being killed, even if this would produce the best state of affairs.) Is it unfair not to give B a chance to be educated merely to educate the greater number, assuming equal need and benefit to each person? Not if we can argue that we are not unfair to anyone if we give him what he is owed, and that what each is owed is to be pairwise compared with individuals in an opposing group in a way that allows us sometimes to balance equal and opposite individuals and then to decide what group to aid based on counting the remaining unbalanced individuals. (This is a further interpretation of what it means to engage in pairwise comparison. I have said that pairwise comparison is a common nonconsequentialist form of reasoning. But it is not often noticed that there are different variants.)

Imagine a group of 1,000 individuals who are in competition with another group of 900 individuals for an education, where all are equally needy and capable of equally good outcomes. We pair off 900 of the 1,000 with each of the 900 on the other side. Because there are people on one side with no matches on the other, each as needy and capable of benefit as the original 900, we balance the two sets of 900 individuals and break the tie between them not by tossing a coin but by doing what, in addition to saving the 900 on one side, will also help 100 additional people. Notice that in this way of doing pairwise comparison, we allow ourselves to be aware of the context in which equal sets of individuals are situated. That is, we are aware that there are further people as well, and this leads us to balance the members of a set. Balancing "silences" the people balanced: they are not further compared with any other individuals. This Balancing Argument is intended to justify counting numbers independently of producing the best outcome.

Contrast this with what, I believe, is another interpretation of how to do pairwise comparison. We take one individual from one side, call him A, and pairwise compare him with someone on the other side, but we do so "with blinders on" as to the context of these individuals. If they are equal in all morally relevant respects, we would see no reason yet not to toss a coin between them. We then take the blinders off before tossing the coin, and if we find another individual on the side opposite to A's with whom to compare A, we compare the two again with blinders on as to the context. If they are equal in all morally relevant respects, we see no reason not to toss a coin. We follow this procedure until A is compared with all individuals on the opposite side. A is not balanced and silenced by having met his match. (He would only be silenced by meeting more than his match—that is, someone needier or perhaps likely to produce a better outcome.) Then, we compare anyone else on A's side with all the same individuals on the opposite side in the same way, pulling blinders on and off. This way of doing pairwise comparison would eventually result in our having to toss a coin between a smaller group and a larger group of persons of equal need and outcome, because each person on one side would be owed an equal chance against any number of other individuals on the other side.[11]

A balancing that silences can result from a pairwise comparison match only when we are aware of a context in which there are other individuals who could be helped on the side of some who would be balanced. By contrast, suppose we could either help (1) one group of 900 people, or (2) another group of 900 people, or (3) another group of only 100 people. (They are all in separate communities.) It would be a mistake to think that the first two groups of 900 balance and silence each other and that we should therefore educate the group of 100. Even if the third group had 900 people instead of 100, it would be a mistake to think that the first two groups balance and silence each other, and that therefore we should help the third group. Rather, in the latter case, we should give each group a maximal equal chance (e.g., pick one group using the three straws method). It is only when the additional 100 people will be educated along with one group of 900 that balancing (which "silences" those balanced) is allowed to occur.

But does this mean that the balancing argument for counting numbers is circular? That is, does the balancing argument for counting additional people simply assume that other people being helped *as well* should make a difference? My answer is as follows: Pairwise comparison combined with an impartial perspective on the individuals implies that there is equal moral value in helping either person who is equal in morally relevant respects. Hence, we can treat 900 on one side as morally equivalent to 900 on the other side. (This was a premise also made use of in the earlier Argument for Best Outcomes.) This implies that at the point where we consider that people will be helped *in addition* to one set of 900, the counting of numbers is no more controversial than the claim that it is better to save B and C rather than B alone. So, the Balancing Argument for counting numbers does not depend on the claim that numbers count in the controversial sense that in conflict situations we should help the greater number. It tries to prove this, and it is the use of an impartial perspective that implies there is equal value in helping equal persons that is bearing most of the weight of the argument.

(2)

But imagine a new case in which, in addition to 900 individuals in each community who are in great need of education and can be benefited greatly by having it, there is one person in the second community who is already educationally advanced but who would get a bit of pleasure out of attending courses that would become available for the general population in his community. Have we given all that we owe the 900 in the first community by balancing them against the second group of 900 and then allowing the interests of this one person to determine that we help the second community? If all that we owe the first 900 is that they be pairwise compared with equal and opposite numbers and be balanced, then they would have no complaint. But I think that they would have a complaint if that small additional good on the other side deprived them of an equal chance to be educated. The good seems to be a *morally irrelevant* good in this context. This means that it would not be appropriate to treat the two groups of 900 as balanced and silenced. Rather, taking seriously that each community wants to be the one to receive the education, and even has a right to the education, might require that we use a random decision procedure to decide between them. This means that whether we balance and silence rather than toss a coin between the groups depends not only on pairwise comparing equals but also on how strong or weak the needs and rights of the additional individuals on one side are.

Now, consider a further variant on this case. Suppose that, in addition to the 900 people in the second community in need of basic education, there are a few people who already have a grade school education but who could benefit by going to high school as well. In this case, although the needs of these additional people are not as great as the needs of the sets of 900 people in either community who need basic education, it does not seem unreasonable to allow the benefit to them that we could also achieve to determine the outcome between the two communities. Here the significant need of the additional individuals for, or even the right to, a high school education can determine that we should balance and silence the sets of 900 rather than decide between the sets by a random decision procedure. This is so even though the needs or rights of the additional individuals are not equal in strength to the needs or rights of those evenly matched.

These cases suggest that we owe each individual something in addition to pairwise matching, namely to balance and silence them only when the nature of the need of the additional persons is serious enough relative to their own need. This really means that we should balance and silence them only when *the additional people on one side would themselves have a complaint if their need were not taken into account*, given the context. This is one reason why I think it is misleading to describe the balancing argument I have described as a tiebreaking argument (as Thomas Scanlon does), for when we must break a tie our focus is on the individuals tied, not on how the refusal to use someone else's need or right as a tiebreaker will wrong the tiebreaking individual.

C. HELPING A FEW OF THE NEEDIEST GREATLY OR MANY OF THEM TO A LESSER DEGREE

We discuss here principles for allocation for situations in which everyone's need is the same but we can either help a few who will benefit greatly or many others who will benefit significantly less (though still to a significant degree in absolute terms). A case of this sort involves a choice between (a) a few people who have no education but are extremely smart and will, if helped now, go on to achieve (on their own) higher education, and (b) many people who have no education but who will, if helped by us now, achieve only grade school education. If we only face a choice between one person of each type, it seems that significant differences in outcome should lead us to conclude that there is no match between the two and we should help the one who will achieve much more. But even if there is no such match, it might still be true that we should sometimes give priority to helping many needy people who will achieve less rather than helping a few equally needy who will achieve much more. (I am now ignoring indirect benefits that come to the less smart themselves in having some others more highly educated.) One way of reaching this conclusion is to emphasize total good produced: the sum of the lesser good produced in many people might be greater than the sum of the greater good produced in a few people. But what seems morally important is how much each person is affected rather than what total is produced. Similarly, it would be better to produce ten years of good in each of ten people rather than one minute of good in each of a trillion equally needy people, even if the total in the latter case is greater than that in the former.

Another way of thinking about whether to help a few of the neediest greatly or many others of the neediest to a lesser degree that retains some idea of pairwise comparison may be to employ what I call the method of "virtual divisibility."[12] That is, imagine (counterfactually) that we could divide our resource to some degree. We can then imagine that we could either give to the smarter people what makes them achieve a grade school education or else give to an equal number of the less smart people what gives them a grade school education. To decide what to do, we could break this tie between them either by helping other equally needy people to also achieve a grade school education or by helping the smarter people to achieve even more higher education. If we should choose the former way of breaking the tie, it is because it is of equal moral value to give either group of the same number of people a grade school education, and we next give priority to helping additional equally needy people achieve a basic level of education before benefiting further those who would already have such an education.

Sometimes, it is true that smaller benefits to each of many people should not be aggregated so as to outweigh a big benefit to each of a few. The case we have just considered reminds us that this need not be true when the smaller benefits are sufficiently great and would come to people who are as needy as the few who would get the bigger benefit.[13]

What of cases where the many, who are as needy as a few others, would get only a very small benefit by comparison to the few? For example, suppose we could educate one person for ten years or each of ten thousand people for one week. It seems clear that it would be better to do the former, if this is a one-time decision.[14] But, as Larry Temkin has argued, often allocation decisions are repeated (iterated) and at least some of the same people can be affected in multiple allocations.[15] So, suppose that in each of many cases we can either educate one person—a different one in each case—for ten years or the *same* ten thousand people for one week. On each occasion, when we have to choose between preventing ten years of no education in one person or one week of no education in many others, it seems to make sense to take care of the one person. But the result of making 520 such individual decisions is that we will have educated 520 individuals for ten years each when we could have educated ten thousand people for ten years instead.

Temkin draws the following conclusion from his discussion of such cases:

> [O]rganizations are often in a position to trade off between helping or burdening a few people a lot, or many people a little. When this occurs, such organizations must pay close attention to the nature and possibility of iterations. If an organization can help a few people a lot, or many people a little, it makes a great difference whether they will face similar choices many times, and also whether it will be the same or different people who are affected each time. If the choice-situation is rare, it may be morally imperative to help the few a lot. Similarly, if the choice-situation is frequent, but different people will be involved each time, it may again be morally imperative to choose on each occasion, so as to help the few a lot, rather than the many a little. But if the choice-situation is frequent enough, and the opportunity obtains to help the *same* large group on each occasion, then it may be imperative to help the large group repeatedly, even if one is only helping the members of that group a little each time. In such a case, one must look at the *combined* effects of one's actions as a *complete set*, as in fact, one would then be helping a large group of people a lot, over time.[16]

D. HELPING A FEW VERY NEEDY OR MANY LESS NEEDY

Here we consider principles of allocation for situations in which the choice is between helping a few who are worse off to achieve significant benefits, or helping many in a nonoverlapping group who are significantly less needy to achieve smaller individual benefits.

These sorts of cases pose an even larger challenge to the procedure of pairwise comparison in allocation decisions. For those in the larger group may be both less needy and achieve less benefit than members of the smaller group. There is no overall match between persons in the larger and smaller groups, and no equal or greater need on the part of those in the larger group relative to those in the smaller group. Could the fact that there are more of these people mean that we should help them rather than members of the smaller group? Would this imply that we should allocate resources to help an enormous number of people who are all very well educated to read another book rather than to help a far smaller number of people get a significant basic education? This is the analogue to the threat in bioethics of being committed to curing a headache in each of a trillion people who are otherwise fine rather than saving a few lives.

Indeed, the following argument can make more precise how this threat could arise. Suppose we ought to allocate so as (a) to help many people in group B, who are relevantly less needy but not extremely so, to achieve a lesser but significant educational gain, rather than (b) to help a much smaller group A, composed of needier people, to get a significant basic education. (Suppose the total expected good—the product of the number of people multiplied by each person's gain—in group B is not greater than the total expected good in group A. It may still be morally appropriate to help the greater number in B. Total benefit produced may even be less, and yet there could be moral value simply in affecting a greater number of lives significantly.) Now suppose we face that choice between helping group B and helping an even larger group C whose members, relative to B's, are less needy but not extremely so, to achieve a lesser but significant gain. It may that we ought to allocate so as to help C. The same argument type can repeat for C and D, D and E, and so on. If transitivity of "ought to allocate to" holds, we would be committed to allocating to group Z, each of whose members is very well off, in order to help each improve in a very small way, rather than to helping the members of the very needy smaller group A to each achieve a very significant gain.

One response to this argument is to deny the transitivity of "ought to allocate to" on the grounds that what we should do can change depending on the alternatives we face. So, when we could help A, it is permissible to go so far as to help B instead, as its members are not extremely less needy and will achieve a gain that is not very much less than what people in A would achieve. These claims may not be true of the people in group C, D, and so on, relative to A. However, if we did not have the option of helping A, and the choice was between B and C, it would be appropriate to help C. Hence, on this view, we cannot know whether we ought to allocate to B or instead to C until we know whether we are in a situation where we would be *denying* A assistance. The idea is that it is wrong to prefer to help more people whose need and potential benefit are too distant from those of fewer other people who are worse off and could be helped more even if we will not actually decide to help those people (e.g., in A) rather than other people (e.g., in B).[17]

E. A MORE COMPLICATED TYPE OF CASE

Finally, let us look at principles of allocation for situations in which groups of different numbers of individuals unequally contain individuals who are diverse in their need and potential for benefit. This is the most complicated situation that I will consider. It is illustrated as follows. Suppose group A contains more people who are very educationally needy than group B does, although all these people can equally achieve high school education. Group A also contains quite a few people who are educationally advanced, and who could he helped to achieve higher education. Group B, however, contains a great many people significantly less educationally needy than the neediest in A and B, but also more needy than the most educationally advanced people in A. Each person in this subgroup of B can also achieve high school level education, if helped. What procedure might we use to decide to which group to allocate if we cannot allocate to both groups or to individuals independently of groups (because money must go to a local school system)?

We might proceed to "segment" the population as follows: First, balance out the neediest members of the two groups as far as possible. Then, see if helping the number of less needy people in B who will benefit less (but reach the same high school level) should outweigh taking care of the remaining neediest in A. Suppose it should. If A contained the neediest only, this might decide matters. But A also contains a sizable number of educationally advanced individuals who could achieve higher education. Hence we must finally consider whether helping the less needy in B outweighs taking care of both the remaining neediest in A and the educationally advanced in A.

Notes

1. This chapter is a revised version of my "Moral Issues in Rationing Scarce Resources," in *Contemporary Debates in Social Philosophy*, ed. L. Thomas (Oxford: Blackwell, 2007). In addition to those I cite below, the following works informed my original essay: Derek Parfit, *Climbing the Mountain*, unpublished manuscript; John Taurek, "Should the Numbers Count?" *Philosophy & Public Affairs* 6 (1977): 293–316; and Larry Temkin, "A 'New' Principle of Aggregation," *Philosophical Issues* 15 (2005): 218–34.

2. I have dealt in some detail with problems of rationing in the medical scenario elsewhere (*Morality, Mortality*, Vol. I [New York: Oxford University Press, 1993]). Here I shall try to use hypothetical examples from nonmedical areas where scarcity drives us to think about rationing. See also chapters 18–22 this volume.

3. In *Morality, Mortality*, Vol. I, I suggested there might also be different principles of allocation for different contexts. Dan Brock's discussion of this issue argues that different factors might be relevant in micro and macro contexts (e.g., benefits to people other than the potential direct recipients of the scarce resource might sometimes be relevant in macro but not micro contexts). See his "Fairness and Health," in *Summary Measures of Population Health*, eds. C. J. L. Murray et al. (Geneva: World Health Organization, 2002).

4. This conception of urgency differs from the one in *Morality, Mortality*, Vol. I. There I took it to mean (atypically) how badly off someone will be and I contrasted it with how badly off someone will have been overall (need). In this chapter, how badly off someone will be is included under need.

5. Thomas Scanlon, *What We Owe to Each Other* (Cambridge, MA: Harvard University Press, 1998); also in his "Blame" (unpublished).

6. For more on these issues, see: Derek Parfit, "Equality or Priority?" The Lindley Lecture (Lawrence, KS: University Press of Kansas (1991), pp. 1–42: article of same title is also in *The Ideal of Equality*, eds. M. Clayton and A. Williams (London/New York: Macmillan and St. Martin's Press, 2000), pp. 81–125; and Larry Temkin, "Equality, Priority, and the Levelling Down Objection," in *The Ideal of Equality*, eds. M. Clayton and A. Williams (London/New York: Macmillan and St. Martin's Press, 2000), pp. 1–38 (2000).

7. Derek Parfit emphasized these points in "Equality or Priority?," note 6.

8. Constructed on the model of cases presented by Derek Parfit in his "Innumerate Ethics," *Philosophy & Public Affairs* 7 (Summer 1978): 285–301.

9. Temkin, "A 'New' Principle of Aggregation."

10. Taurek, "Should the Numbers Count?"

11. I argue elsewhere ("Aggregation and Two Moral Methods," *Utilitas* 17 [March 2005]: 1–23; *Intricate Ethics* [New York: Oxford University Press, 2007], chapter 2), that the first way of doing pairwise comparison is assumed by Kamm ("Equal Treatment and Equal Chances," *Philosophy & Public Affairs*, 1985; *Morality, Mortality*, Vol. I note 2) and Scanlon (*What We Owe To Each Other*), and the second way is adopted in Michael Otsuka's criticism of Scanlon and Kamm ("Scanlon and the Claims of the Many Versus the One," *Analysis* 60 [2000]: 288–93).

12. See my "Aggregation and Two Moral Methods," and *Intricate Ethics*, chapter 2.

13. Derek Parfit has emphasized this point in his *On What Matters* (Oxford: Oxford University Press, 2011).

14. As noted above, Larry Temkin has argued that we should produce the bigger benefit for an individual, even if the one person was not as needy as each of the greater number of people who would get the very small benefit.

15. The following case I discuss in the text is a variation on ones discussed by Temkin in which the many are needier than the one.

16. Temkin, "A 'New' Principle of Aggregation," p. 225.

17. Suppose we have already denied A assistance in order to help B, and it is no longer possible to help A. This does not mean we are forced to choose to help C rather than B. The reason A is no longer available to be compared with C is that he was eliminated in order to help B, and it is wrong to ignore this history in deciding what to do, I believe.

PART FIVE

Methodology

24

The Philosopher as Insider and Outsider

HOW TO ADVISE, COMPROMISE, AND CRITICIZE

Philosophers, and in particular those who specialize in ethics, now often participate in the public realm—for example, as members of government commissions or as consultants to commissions dealing with issues that raise ethical questions.[1] The "insiders," as I shall refer to them, have been said to face certain ethical dilemmas in their roles. Other philosophers, the "outsiders" who evaluate the results of these commissions—recommendations to legislatures or public reports—may face other ethical dilemmas.

In this chapter I will first consider some insider problems discussed in the very useful writings of Dan Brock, Alan Weisbard, and Mary Warnock. I shall structure my discussion of these problems around the following questions: How ought a philosopher who is a member of the staff of a commission that is dealing with ethically important issues handle each of the following different situations?

1. All members of the commission and the philosopher agree on a bottom-line position, but the philosopher and commission members disagree on the reasons for that bottom line.
2. There is what I shall call unstable agreement on a bottom line, and the philosopher and the commission members disagree on the reasons for the bottom line.
3. There is disagreement among commission members on a bottom line.

Among my major conclusions is the claim that the insider philosopher's primary duties should be to clarify and inform as well as to philosophize with the commissioners and help them stay on a course in which moral considerations are given their proper weight. Fulfilling these duties means that the philosopher will sometimes have to help produce a weaker intellectual document than he would prefer, or lose a chance to directly promote the public good. The insider philosopher will also have to consider whether it is appropriate for a policy from a commission to differ from much current government policy, and how morally appropriate compromise can be reached among commissioners.

Given an outsider philosopher's understanding of how an insider philosopher should function and how commission reports are constructed, I claim that the outsider philosopher can comment both on how close a report comes to being a perfect example of its type, and how far short of an ideal philosophical analysis even a perfect government report is. It may be appropriate for her to give greater weight to the public good, if her comments are very likely to affect it, than the insider philosopher should.

Examples for discussion of these claims are drawn from government reports on organ transplantation, embryo research, terminating care, and compensation for research subjects.

I. Advising: Disagreement Over Reasons

Dan Brock has argued that the virtues of philosophers in the academy are to follow the truth wherever it leads regardless of consequences and to leave no assumptions unchallenged, but that these are not the virtues of philosophers in the public realm.[2] (One might note that even in the academy, sometimes consequences should count and it would be wrong to ignore them. For example, scientists in Nazi Germany ought not to have done research that would have directly led to a Nazi atomic weapon. Furthermore, the image of Neurath's Raft reminds us that academic philosophers do not challenge all assumptions at once, though they have the liberty, which philosophers in the public realm may lack, to pick the time at which they will attack any given assumption.)

To illustrate his point, Brock presents a particular problem case which he confronted as a staff philosopher to a government commission.[3] I shall discuss this case with the addition of some of my own assumptions for the purpose of creating a situation of a certain type. Therefore, one should not assume that the philosopher I describe is Brock.

Suppose commission members agree with the philosopher that it is permissible for life sustaining treatment sometimes to be terminated, but they think this is so because it is a case of letting someone die. The philosopher thinks that there is often no moral difference between killing and letting die, and that terminating treatment is (often) a case of justified killing.[4] He decides not to *mention* his views about reasons to the commissioners, and not to *argue* with them about theirs, for fear that if they became convinced that terminating care is a killing, they would think it unjustified. That is, they would cease to hold what he thinks is the wrong view—that terminating treatment is always letting die—but not accept the argument that terminating treatment can be permissible even if it is a killing. Hence, they would not come to the right conclusion about the permissibility of terminating treatment. Furthermore, we might add, if they came to believe that letting die and killing are often morally equivalent, they might think that more lettings die were unjustified and refuse to allow the omission of treatment to begin with.

The philosopher thinks both that the consequences of this for the public in terms of suffering and loss of self-determination would be very bad and that it is the insider philosopher's responsibility to act in the light of these consequences. However, the philosopher also believes that in acting as he does, he has betrayed the truth and been manipulative toward the commission members.[5]

A problem with a similar structure arises when discussing the acquisition of organs from the deceased for transplantation. There is a shortage of organs for transplantation, in part because individuals whose organs they are do not donate enough. Allowing families to donate organs rather than just relying on the person whose organs they are may increase the supply, but it is not clear how the family can, morally speaking, have a right to donate. Arguments can be given for the permissibility of society taking the organs through its agent the State. The State in turn may delegate its power to the family, and in this *indirect* way the family can be shown to have a right to take organs. However, most are more willing to believe the correctness of a direct argument for the family's right to donate than to believe the correctness of an argument for the State's right to take. Therefore, if we successfully dispute the argument for a direct family right, and do not get agreement on the argument for an indirect right, we may lose public support for a family's right to donate. This could reduce the number of organs acquired.[6]

Brock's discussion suggests a general argument that can be used to defend the philosopher's refusal to mention his reasons for endorsing terminating care:[7]

a. The reason philosophers join public commissions is that they want to help effect good consequences for the public.
b. Therefore, they must shift their primary commitment from knowledge and truth to the policy consequences of what they do.

But this argument as it stands seems fallacious. One reason is that the desire to have a good effect on the public, which prompts some philosophers to join the public process, does not by itself mean that they should attend more to the consequences of their acts than to truth, since they may have entered the public realm believing that attending to knowledge and truth will be beneficial for the public. If it turns out that it is not, they may decide to leave a commission. Hence, premise (a) does not imply premise (b).

To see a second reason why the argument is inadequate as it stands, consider why the philosopher in Brock's case feels manipulative. Suppose premise (a) is true, and the philosopher enters the public realm because of the opportunity to have a good effect on the public. This desire to have a good effect on the public does not mean that, as an insider with the opportunity to effect good for the public, the philosopher has a duty (or even a permission) to do so. That is, the combination of *desire* and *opportunity* does not imply that he has a *duty* (or even a permission) to act directly for the public good. After all, his desire to do good for the public has led him to a particular role of staff philosopher, and his (most direct) duty in this role may not be to the public at all, but to the commission members.

He may, of course, hope to achieve his goal of helping the public by carrying out his duties to the commission. However, if there is a conflict between his role as staff philosopher and promoting the public good, the former may have precedence (though not necessarily absolute precedence). Even if he believed speaking the truth would harm the public, he might have a duty in his role as staff philosopher to speak the truth as he sees it to commissioners.

Whether he has such a duty depends on how we conceive of his role. There are at least two ways of doing this: (1) consider an actual contract for his services and determine his duties from this contract; (2) provide a normative account of what a contract should be. I am concerned with the latter. I suggest that the philosopher's primary duties should include helping point out problems with and implications of the commissioners' own views, giving the commission his considered judgment on what a bottom line should be and his reasons for it, and informing the commissioners of reasonable philosophical views held by others when these differ from his own. The first and last duties derive from a normative theory of why we have a commission; namely, we select certain individuals to become better informed about issues so that they may reach a better conclusion. The second duty—actually to philosophize—is consistent with another aspect of the normative conception of a commission. For the sake of public credibility, a commission may include representatives of various views present in the community, but these individuals should engage in reflection and reason giving, not merely voting and compromising. A philosopher should be able to guide them in certain respects in trying to reach a conclusion by his own reflection and reason-giving. That is, he should develop a view on an issue rather than being merely an "ambassador" reporting the views of other philosophers or an aide in helping the commissioners understand their own views clearly.

If an insider philosopher had (at least) these special duties, this would account for the philosopher in our example feeling that he was manipulative in concealing his views. For if one had no special duty to point out problems with the commissioners' views or to reveal one's views, one would not be obligated to do either of these things or to argue for one's own reasons for a bottom line with which everyone already agrees, especially if one were not a commissioner. So in the absence of a duty to inform and reveal, concealing need not be manipulative. (Of course, if reasons are not revealed and examined, there is some chance that no one's reasons are any good and the wrong bottom line has been chosen.)

Suppose the philosopher has these duties (to discuss commissioners' views, mention his own views, and give arguments of other philosophers which diverge from his). He may still have no duty to get the commissioners' agreement on the same reason for a bottom line, since the report is not intended to be a scholarly document. A commission report might list the commissioners' various reasons for that bottom line, explaining them in some detail. There is then a significant chance that among the various reasons in the report, a correct argument for the bottom line is present. (Explaining why some philosophers are prepared to justify terminating assistance even if it is a killing might serve as a stronger fallback position for future public discussion.) Of course, the chances of the correct argument appearing somewhere in the text are greater if there *is* intense scrutiny of reasons for a bottom line.

Two fears may be associated with the philosopher's *mentioning* different reasons for a bottom line. (For the sake of this discussion, I emphasize the distinction between merely mentioning a reason and trying to convince commissioners of its correctness.) First, those who are to act on the report (e.g., Congress) may not feel compelled to follow the expert opinion of a commission if disagreement over reasons (as evidenced by multiple and conflicting ones) is revealed. A possible response is that Congress might be more impressed by unanimity on a bottom line if it could be the conclusion of many different arguments. Further, the fact that there is this disagreement need not reduce the sense that the commission represents expert opinion, where "expert" means someone who is better informed, more skilled, or more creative at certain ways of reasoning. Such a person need not have a decision procedure that yields a unique argument with which all will agree. (Even if different *bottom lines* were suggested by different philosophers or commissioners, this should not lead one to revoke the title of expert from someone who recommends one particular bottom line.[8])

A second fear associated with merely mentioning different reasons for the bottom line is one contained in our case description, namely if commissioners hear that some hold an argument with which they disagree and which is inconsistent with their argument for a bottom line, they will change their position on the bottom line with bad consequences for the public.

As I have described the particular case we are considering, this may not be a great worry, in part because it is quite possible for the philosopher to report truthfully that other philosophers agree with the commissioners that a doctor terminating treatment is a letting die. Furthermore, some of those philosophers who believe terminating is a killing would think it a fine point rather than a major revision to call it this rather than a letting die. In addition, I believe we should consider the possibility that the commissioners are firmly wedded to their conclusion, and that they may well believe that terminating treatment is a letting die just because they are so firmly convinced of the bottom line. That is, instead of thinking terminating treatment is a letting die and therefore permissible, they think terminating treatment is clearly permissible and therefore it must be a letting die. (They do this because they think that if it were a killing, it would be impermissible.) This form of reasoning seems incorrect, since it confuses a descriptive judgment about what a termination of treatment is (a killing or a letting die) with an evaluative judgment about the permissibility of terminating treatment, but it may nevertheless be the way they reasoned.[9]

If the mere mention of an alternative reason *would* raise moral doubt and lead a commissioner to change his mind on a bottom line, that is something the philosopher will have to live with, I believe.[10]

It might be suggested that one's duty as staff philosopher is to get only good reasons into a commission report (rather than listing a variety of supposed reasons), and this will require *arguing* with commissioners about their reasons. Here again, there may be no outcome problem if the commissioners are firmly committed to the correct bottom line. But if the document is not intended as a scholarly work, is there such a duty to argue for the best reasons, and how far must one carry it?

If a commissioner, having heard of a different reason from his own, wishes to engage in detailed argument with the philosopher concerning reasons, I believe the duties of the *philosopher as educator-on-call* to the commission require him to engage in such a discussion (e.g., showing him that some philosophers believe killings to terminate aid are permissible, or even trying to convince the commissioner that some such killings are permissible, should that be his own view).

If the result of that argument is that the commissioner changes his mind about the bottom line, that is also something the philosopher will have to live with. One can only hope that, on balance, more informed discussion will lead to better outcomes.

If philosophically informed public commissions do not produce better outcomes on the whole, then philosophers might do well to avoid serving on commissions, or we might decide not to have commissions (as I have described them). That is, commissions and the specific role of philosophers serving on them are thought to be justified by their promoting the public good. Once in his role, the philosopher should carry out his obligations even if they conflict on occasion with the public good, since he is involved in a primary commitment to the commission. But if this role was for the most part contrary to the public good, it might be wise to eliminate it.[11]

II. Unstable Agreement on a Bottom Line

Alan Weisbard discusses a case in which there was only what I shall call unstable agreement on a bottom line.[12] All individuals on the commission, he reports, agreed initially that compensation for volunteers injured in research experiments was required on the basis of fairness. (Call this the fairness reason.) However, he also suggests that some the scientist commission members wished this conclusion were not true, because they thought its being true conflicted with their interests in running experiments. This makes for the "unstable" nature of the agreement. Unlike the members of the commission I have described in part I, we are here dealing with some individuals looking for a way out of their moral response for reasons of scientific progress. To this background is added the fact that there is a libertarian argument against requiring compensation. This argument is based on the (supposed) legitimacy of an agreement for no compensation to which the volunteer consented. (Call this the consent reason that leads to a different conclusion.) The philosopher believed reasons of fairness and consent were both wrong, and that a better argument was available for a bottom line to award compensation. This better argument was still in a broad sense about fairness, but instead of considering the particular context in which a person decides to volunteer and what is fair in that context, it derives a characterization of fair institutions from a general theory of a just society. (Call this the justice reason.) However, the commissioners could not be convinced of the justice reason, and the force of fairness was already weakened by the presence of the consent reason plus the philosopher's view that the fairness reason was not quite right. In the midst of division, the (supposed) interests of science determined the outcome and compensation was not recommended.

What could have been done in this situation? I have suggested that the philosopher has a direct, primary duty to express his own view of the best bottom line and reasons for it, as well as to mention seriously held opposing views. This implies that reasons of justice, consent, and fairness should be mentioned. In this case, however, it seems that we are dealing with some *commissioners* who want only scientific interests to determine an outcome. Seeing this, the philosopher may think that a morally acceptable course which attempts to reinforce the moral best of which these individuals are capable would be as follows: He should investigate thoroughly whether a system of compensation would, indeed, seriously hamper scientific progress. (Weisbard suggests the scientists' case was weak, since they claimed both that compensation was not necessary, as few would need it, and that compensation was burdensome, since so many would need it!) When mentioning consent and the libertarian solution as a seriously held option, the philosopher could argue that sometimes consent does not legitimate agreements, that we may not be released from duties we have to treat people in certain ways even if they waive their rights. Most importantly, he should point out that the implications of the consent argument are inconsistent with the way much current government policy deals with other problems, and it might be unwise to support a radical departure from the reasoning behind other government policies on the basis of a view which is also in much dispute in philosophical circles. If the commissioners would *not* accept the consent reason generally, and would otherwise avoid sharp breaks with the views underlying other government policies, the consent reason should not play a role in determining an outcome in this case.

(Suppose the consent reason was not in fact foreign to much extant government policy. If mentioning it would move the commission away from compensation as a bottom line, despite the philosopher's arguments against it, he would, I believe, have to tolerate this result.)

Furthermore, if fairness is an imperfect treatment of a point of view best expressed by justice, the philosopher might in good conscience settle for fairness without even mentioning justice, or else emphasize the positive connections between the two reasons. Again, the commission report is not a philosophical treatise where we strive for perfection. It may be best to think of nonphilosophers on a commission as in some ways like students—meant in a completely nonpatronizing way—who are not ready to deal with the best arguments or positions available, but whose approximations to truth should be encouraged by the philosopher-as-educator. (In addition, concern for a "publicity condition"—i.e., that proposals on the moral direction of public policy be understandable to the public—may limit the drive to philosophical accuracy.[13])

However, if fairness were an argument of a totally wrong type, the philosopher should *mention* his opinion that justice is the correct reason, despite the effect of his doing this on the commissioners.

(For the same reasons, an incomplete argument might permissibly be given for a conclusion in the area of acquiring organs. It could include the true step that the family sometimes has a right to donate organs without including the steps from which this might be thought to be derived; i.e., society has a right to take by using the State and the State has a right to delegate its power to the family.)

It is important to note, however, that settling for fairness as an argument and incorporating it into a report without mentioning justice raises the danger that a strictly speaking inadequate argument will set a precedent, and be referred to and used in other government decision-making which depends on the commission's work. (This is what seems to have happened with the argument given for funding an adequate level of health care, in the report of the President's Commission for the Study of Ethical Problems in Medicine and Biomedical and Behavioral Research. I shall discuss this example in more detail below.) This is a danger whenever "compromise" arguments for bottom-line positions are constructed.

In our current case as described, the consent reason is opposed by the philosopher. What of the case in which the philosopher would like to recommend policies that could only be based on views that represent a big departure from the philosophical underpinnings of current government policy, views that are also in much dispute in the philosophical literature? Weisbard suggests that only reasoning which is consistent with other established parts of national policy should be allowed weight in commission deliberations, as opposed to introducing philosophical theories radically different from what is consistent with much current national policy. This would suggest that there is another duty of the insider philosopher: *not* to recommend policies based on views that are big departures from the philosophical underpinnings of current government policy. Because he is working on this *government's report* and not a scholarly paper, he can accept less than perfect arguments, and because he is working on *this government's* report, he should accept the intellectual foundations of this government (to the extent that they are clear). (This, of course, leaves it open that different interpretations are available of what these foundations are. On this account, only philosophical criticism which is "internal" to the governmental system and strives for consistency and coherence is allowed; "external" criticism is excluded.)

But suppose the commission were willing to accept the views that the consent reason represents and implies quite generally, and recommend a radical break with current reasons for government policies. I believe that if the commission is fully aware that it is making this break and open about it, it may do so if it believes the correct conclusion could not be reached in any other way. Then a philosopher should also be free to argue for a radically different view if he believes the correct bottom line can be derived in no other way.[14] In deciding that it is morally correct to recommend such a radical shift, the philosopher, like the commission, will have had to take into account that this is a radical shift and weigh the value of integrity—continuity with extant policy or with the theory commonly thought to underlie extant policy[15]—against it. If his view is also philosophically radical, he will have had to consider that he is isolated among his philosophical colleagues and deal with any uncertainty about his position which this generates.

Questions about skepticism and democratic procedure arise in this connection. The skeptical question is: If the philosopher stands alone in his views, how can he rely on his own judgment before the commission; *how* does he know what is right? A possible answer is that he can only do his best, and he must be careful to point out in presenting his views that both government tradition and other philosophers disagree with him. Commissioners may find this good grounds for not heeding his advice. The democratic question is: *Who is he* to recommend when others disagree? A possible answer is that the insider philosopher is not the representative of other philosophers but should present reasons as best he can for what he thinks is correct. So, while he may be bound to inform about others' views, he is not others' agent. Of course, if commissioners heed his radical advice, they may reduce their chances of having their policy accepted by a democratic representative legislature. The opposite worry, that a philosopher-influenced commission may succeed in undemocratically imposing a radical view on the public, is reduced if a representative legislature must approve any policy the commission recommends.[16] (Even if a report recommending radical policy is ultimately rejected, it might be intellectually most respectable and set the stage for future public reflection.)

To summarize, in the compensation case, as in the terminating aid case, I construe the philosopher's desire to achieve a good bottom line for the public and to produce an intellectually commendable document as constrained by his primary duty to serve and inform the commission itself. But his duty to the commission does include helping it act on the appropriate types of reasons (broadly, principled moral ones which may conflict with self-interest or other socially important goals). When there is an agreed bottom line, he need not press for agreement on reasons, though he should mention his own views. When the correct bottom line requires a particular reason, he should introduce it and argue for it. However, he may present an approximation to what he thinks is the best reason and best bottom line, and should consider their fit with existing government policy. In the compensation case, the duty to maintain the integrity of the commission and not allow moral considerations to be swamped by scientific expedience seems to weigh even more than the philosopher's duty to inform the commission of his own view on justice.

In short, the two cases I have discussed so far suggest that the primary duties of an insider philosopher are not to achieve good consequences for the public or to produce the philosophically best public document, but to serve as educator and guide to the commission he serves.

I have discussed these two particular cases in some detail, in part because I believe that sensitivity to the particulars of the situation he is in is important in an insider philosopher. This means that the insider philosopher must not only have technical expertise and knowledge, he must also have the ability to judge correctly in particular settings what is morally appropriate conduct given his general duties.

Now it is worth considering Weisbard's *general* criticism of philosophers in the public process.[17] He makes four points:

1. Philosophers' advice is likely to be too universalistic rather than stemming from the particular commitments of the community.
2. The philosopher's standard of justification is too high, seeking policies that all philosophical theories could support.
3. Analogical reasoning avoids these problems. It, rather than philosophical justification, is needed, leading to results in new and problematic cases that are in keeping with other existing legislation.
4. Philosophers qua philosophers do not have the much-needed skill of hammering out compromise positions that a policy expert has.

How might a philosopher respond to these criticisms? *First*, some philosophers are defenders of "common-sense morality." They try to describe in detail the principles which underlie our ordinary moral views and concepts and try to show the further implications of views which are typically held by the average person. They avoid the most abstract philosophical justifications of morality. They focus instead on the principles and concepts that they think inhere in common-sense morality, becoming more sensitive than others to its character.[18] Most of these philosophers are still "universalists," in the sense that they are not moral relativists. They think it is worth analyzing pre-theoretical moral responses common in the community and tracing their underlying principles and further implications because they believe these responses can be justified and are objectively correct, not merely correct relative to a system under which we happen to live.

Another group, attracted to the Rawlsian idea of reflective equilibrium, will modify common-sense judgments of individual cases on the basis of abstract theory (as well as modify theory on the basis of common-sense judgments), but they do so tentatively, in a balancing process. Very few philosophers—though they will argue they are correct in doing so—only move down from abstract theory to responses sanctioned by that theory about real-life cases.

Second, it is true that few social policies are in accord with all possible philosophical theories—right answers are usually in conflict with wrong theories. But philosophers do not decide a policy is right by seeing whether it is implied by or consistent with all theories; arguments are presented for particular policies and also for the merits of some theories over others. Commissioners should be made to understand that. And while there may be other, high standards for philosophical justification, I have already suggested that the argumentative rigor typical of the best philosophical discussions is not a necessary standard for government reports. Many social policies could be justified by what, at a given time, a large part of the philosophical community takes to be the best theory. But we must also remember that no theory underlying our extant policies may yield an answer to radically new questions—for example, in areas of biomedical research. Indeed, we may find ourselves using these new cases to revise the theories underlying past policy.

Third, the analogical reasoning which Weisbard recommends is frequently used by philosophers. However, its use by anyone will not necessarily have unitary or conservative implications. The capacity of creative analogical reasoners to find in extant policy different relevant similarities to a case at hand, similarities not noticed by most others, is what is most interesting in the use of analogy. (For example, Judith Thomson found a relevant analogy to some abortions, not in the way we currently treat children, but in the way we would treat a violinist hooked up to someone else's body against the latter's will.[19])

Finally, it is wrong to hold that philosophers qua philosophers are irrelevant to the process of real-life compromise, for they can play an important role in seeing to it that compromise is of the morally appropriate sort. That is, the sort of policy analysis practiced by policy experts that Weisbard recommends may allow a compromise to be influenced by the relative threat position of the disputing parties, their ability to bluff (e.g., pretend to hold a more extreme view than they in fact do, so that a compromise will fall closer to the position they actually hold), the ability of a party to hold out longer, differences in who needs agreement more (because the status quo without an agreement on a government policy favors one view rather than another), and so on.

By contrast, a *moralized compromise procedure* would filter out such factors in the search for compromise. The use of such a procedure is part of the answer to what I have called the general problem of applying applied ethics;[20] that is, what we should do if we think we have the correct solution to a problem in applied ethics but others disagree and it is morally wrong to force compliance. One specific approach to achieving morally appropriate compromise that might be suggested is contractualist in spirit. For example, we might try using the model which Thomas Scanlon describes (in arguing for a contractualist account of "morally wrong"). We seek solutions that:

> . . . would not be disallowed by any system of rules for the general regulation of behavior which no one could reasonably reject as a basis for informed, unforced general agreement. . . . The intended force of . . . "reasonably" . . . is to exclude rejections that would be unreasonable *given* the aim of finding principles which could be the basis of informed, unforced general agreement. Given this aim, it would unreasonable, for example, to reject a principle because it imposed a burden on you when every alternative principle would

impose much greater burdens on others. . . . The only relevant pressure for agreement comes from the desire to find and agree on principles which no one who had this desire could reasonably reject.[21]

In this scheme everyone has a desire to reach agreement on principles which no one could reasonably reject given a desire to reach unforced agreement based on full information. We search for principles that all can live with, so that there is something akin to consent of all. Whether this is the correct procedure for reaching compromise about practical matters or not, the point is that one duty of the insider philosopher is also to philosophize about—rather than have committee members merely vote on—how to reach agreement when there is disagreement. (A theory of morally appropriate compromise should also tell us when it would be wrong to compromise or to expect others to compromise.)

The importance of a moralized compromise procedure can be viewed most clearly when there is true, principled disagreement on a bottom-line position, rather than just disagreement over reasons for a common bottom line (as in our first case in part I) or unstable-agreement on a bottom line (as in our second case in part II). We turn to such a case now.

III. Compromising: Bottom-Line Moral Conflicts

As an example of principled conflict over a bottom line, we can consider the problem that the Warnock Commission faced in deciding about research on the embryo.[22] Mary Warnock emphasizes that commissions must represent diverse constituencies and views in order to have credibility, but it is just this that makes it hard for them to reach a unanimous decision. Yet sometimes, at least, unanimity is important: all want some public policy, law must be uniform, and a legislature will not act without a unanimous commission decision. (A different reason for seeking unanimity, which she does not endorse, is to conceal differences of opinion and give the impression that there never was any disagreement.)

In a case of principled disagreement on a bottom line, an insider philosopher should first examine the various proposals and offer an alternative proposal. But let us suppose no bottom line proposed by the philosopher is accepted by all (even if it is right). It is tempting to analyze the remaining conflict between different proposed bottom lines on the model of conflicts within an individual.[23] Let us consider such conflicts first.

INTRAPERSONAL CONFLICT

In some cases of intrapersonal conflict, a single individual decides on one course of action concerning either himself or others because the value it represents dominates, though there remains, as it is said, a "negative residue" from the conflicting values left unsatisfied.[24] This description of conflict and its resolution coheres with the theory of value Thomas Nagel presents.[25] Nagel argues that there are multiple values which are not reducible to any common unit; when we "weigh" them against each other, there is no single scale of value on which we weigh them. Yet, he insists, the choice among such values can be rational. The most general way in which conflict is generated, he claims, is through the clash of the objective and subjective perspectives. In his view, the former is represented (roughly) by a consequentialist calculation, the latter by deontological restrictions on intending harm. Morality, he thinks, has these two irreducible components. Even if we disagree with Nagel's characterization of the deontological restrictions and their source,[26] we can agree with the idea of fragmented value and the deontological/consequentialist distinction he describes.

Suppose we side with maximizing utility on some occasion when it conflicts with deontological restrictions (e.g., torturing one innocent person to save many). The negative residue (due to the torture) indicates that we continue to evaluate the bottom-line decision from the perspective of the deontological component of morality. It is not simply a factor that gets outweighed in the consequentialist calculation; it is a perspective that remains on the bottom line.[27]

One test for the presence of a residue may be that the victim in the case can claim that no adequate justification has been provided to him for what is done to him; he has the right not to be tortured even to save many, yet it is permissible for us to act. By contrast, in cases in which there is simple outweighing of one factor by another with no residue, the victim should feel only that he has been made to carry his fair share of a socially necessary burden.

Sometimes in an *intra*personal conflict between the parts of fragmented value, one side is not chosen over another. Rather, a bottom line is constructed which in some way incorporates conflicting values. This procedure represents the construction of more complex and refined values or principles, which limit or specify more general values or principles in the light of apparent exceptions to them.[28]

INTERPERSONAL CONFLICT

It seems that it is inappropriate to call *either* the construction of complex and refined principles which give proper weight to different relevant factors *or* the dominance of one value with a negative residue a "compromise" between the different factors. This is because a compromise connotes some bottom line that does *not* represent the complex truth, but gives weight to conflicting factors *despite* the fact that doing so does not lead to the truth. So a person's search for the truth about how conflicting values relate in the intrapersonal conflict case differs in this way from compromise in the interpersonal case. There are other differences as well.

For example, some cases of *inter*personal conflict are like intrapersonal conflict, in that some value in each person's position is recognized by every other person and compromise is sought (rather than allowing one value to dominate or providing a true refined principle). However, some cases of interpersonal conflict are unlike intrapersonal conflict, in that while multiple values or principles *must* be recognized as having some validity for there to be conflict between them in one person's mind, in the interpersonal case, someone's bottom-line position may not be recognized by anyone else as representing anything of real value. (Or it may be recognized as representing a true value that is easily outweighed with no negative residue.) For example, no one else may agree with a single commission member who believes that the embryo has some moral significance; all other commissioners may think the embryo has no moral significance.

These points about interpersonal compromise also affect the use of a contractualist model for seeking agreement. Scanlon's procedure (described above) is meant to reach ideal agreement on true, complex principles. Furthermore, in his system a reasonable objection to a proposal can be made only by someone who has a truly greater complaint to a proposal than anyone else would have to other proposals. (So, an ideal rational judge would find the complaint greater.) If a position is correctly assessed as presenting no valid objection to a proposal, the ideal contractualist would refuse to give it any weight.

In a real-life compromise situation, a contractualist account (that remains moralized rather than merely pragmatic) may have to be modified. Not only will it have to take account of the fact that those who judge someone else's position may assess its soundness incorrectly, but it may have to give some weight to positions out of proportion to their objective merit merely out of respect for the persons who hold the positions.[29]

Within this modified contractualism, one specific approach (Compromise Type A) says that mutual respect requires us to behave as if we did see as much value in the other's position as he sees in it himself. That is, we pretend our situation is like intrapersonal conflict, and give full weight to a position we really believe has no merit. "Full" weight need not mean equal weight. For suppose side one is concerned with kindness (which the other side does not see as at issue at all), and side two is concerned with justice (which the other side does not see as at issue at all). Even given its full weight, kindness might not be a consideration with as much weight as justice.

The second approach (Compromise Type B) would involve giving others' views some weight, insofar as they are seriously held moral views. However, we and they both recognize that we need not behave as though their view represents a real opposing value. This is because everyone, including those who hold the apparently opposing value, can agree that the argument for their view is not completely convincing; a reasonable person could reject it.[30] (This may not be true of everyone's position equally. For example, the possible benefits of research on the embryo, though not the moral status of the embryo, are widely agreed upon.) Furthermore, it may be that as the number of people (e.g., commission members) who agree on a certain bottom line increases, the more weight that bottom line should be given in a compromise position, even though its value escapes others. Weighting would then be aggregative to some degree.

To receive consideration in either approaches A or B, a point of view must at least be a moral one. That is, what is expressed must be more than a mere sentiment or preference. This is in keeping with the idea that moral positions are the sorts of things for which reasons could be given, and in particular, given to others even if those others cannot reasonably be expected to be convinced and would not be unreasonable to not be convinced.[31] Furthermore, since a commission is concerned with formulating policy for the general public, restricting moral views to those that can be backed by reasons that are publicly recognized as having weight (even if not determinative weight) seems appropriate. (This could also be seen as part of respect for each member of the commission, since it prevents their being bound to policies in virtue of factors they cannot begin to see as reasons.) This means that the content of purely religious reasons for restricting research on the embryo need not be shown "argumentative respect" for purposes of getting a compromise bottom line.[32] This leaves it open that religious reasons can be publicly recognized as important to those who hold them, and on *this ground* the religious views are given weight. Secular reasoning that is believed ultimately inadequate by some but is nevertheless part of public reason *is* shown argumentative respect.

The two approaches to moralized compromise can yield very different outcomes. To see this, consider what Compromise Type A, according to which we should behave as though all conflicting positions had the sort of full (if not equal) value they would have in a conflict intrapersonally, would have yielded as bottom line for the Warnock Commission on embryo research. Let us make the (untrue, simplifying) assumption that there were no strict utilitarians on the commission, but rather that all the members subscribed to a pluralistic value system like the one Nagel describes. This means that those who believed the embryo has moral status disagreed with others on the ontological status of the embryo rather than on basic moral issues.

Many who hold such a pluralistic value system give priority to deontological restrictions on producing good consequences. For example, they would not kill someone in order to save many other lives. They may sometimes violate a restriction for consequentialist reasons with an ensuing negative residue, but the circumstances in which this occurs tend to be special. For example, it is not merely that very much good could be done by torturing someone that makes the pluralist I have in mind decide to torture; the victim must have a particular involvement in the circumstances (e.g., be a political supporter of terrorism) and it must be for the sake of avoiding a particular sort of disaster (e.g., deaths caused by the terrorist activity he supports). That is, qualitative as well as quantitative factors are relevant.

Suppose also that it is reasonable for someone to reject a compromise that demanded a more significant sacrifice from him than another compromise would demand from someone else. Then it may seem wrong to ask those who oppose embryo research on grounds of a deontological restriction on killing persons to compromise their position rather than to ask those concerned with good consequences of such research to compromise theirs. The idea that morally appropriate compromise requires each side to give up something may be out of place in this analysis using Compromise Type A. If the model of intrapersonal conflict between deontological and consequentialist factors is applicable in interpersonal conflict, it seems that we should expect that it would be just as wrong to ask opponents of research to agree to a compromise in which one embryo is deliberately killed per year to save many lives, as to ask a deontological/consequentalist value pluralist to agree to a compromise in which one adult person is killed in research per year to save many lives.[33]

One problem with this description of the implications of Compromise Type A is that it is not clear that it is represents the correct way of giving full weight to both positions on the status of the embryo. Perhaps using Compromise Type A for interpersonal conflict entails imagining an intrapersonal conflict in which one person sometimes thinks the embryo is a person and sometimes thinks it is not a person. Suppose each of those different views on ontological status must be represented in the conflict. Then the question may be whether deontological restrictions imply not taking a 50 percent chance of killing a person in deliberately killing an embryo in order to save people's lives.[34]

Yet the Warnock Commission's bottom line did require the anti-research position to compromise. It did not compromise by limiting the number of occasions when embryos could be used, but it suggested what seemed to be a principled distinction between using embryos in the time before and after the primitive streak appears in the embryo. This compromise could be accounted for if the second approach to compromise (Type B) that I have described was (implicitly) employed. That is, we are not required to behave as though all views have full weight but that are in conflict with each other; rather, we require holders of a disputed view to recognize that others could reasonably reject the view even as a contender.

The compromise on developmental lines, rather than a compromise on the numbers of occasions when any embryo is used, corresponds to the distinction between principled and checkerboard compromise which Ronald Dworkin describes.[35] The compromise is, it is thought, principled insofar as we use some factor (i.e., primitive streak) which all sides can see as a possible ground for a moral distinction, even if they do not believe it is correct. The principled compromise aims to make it less likely from the point of view of those who believe the embryo has moral significance that a morally significant entity will be used for research.[36] It also appeals to a factor that even those who think the embryo has no significance might see as in the logical territory of justification: the older the embryo, the more value it would have. (These points are usefully clarified by the case of capital punishment that Dworkin describes: Consider those who believe capital punishment is not justified even for the most heinous crimes. They could still more easily understand imposing capital punishment for triple murder than for triple parking.[37]) In addition, the compromise on developmental lines might be seen to give what is *most* significant to those who want to use embryos (i.e., at least some period of use) by sacrificing what is *least* significant to those opposed to the use (i.e., early versus late use). The method of sacrificing what is of least significance to one side for what is of most significance to the other is better than sacrificing what is of moderate significance to give what is of only moderate significance or sacrificing what is of greatest significance to give what is of least significance.[38]

Seeking unanimity by compromise on a bottom line has its dangers. As noted above, it is often morally inappropriate to cover up the fact that many on the commission are (or everyone is) dissatisfied with the bottom line, finding objectionable features in it. (I distinguish this from dissatisfaction with a bottom line because it is only a part of what one would like—i.e., everything it contains is unobjectionable; only what it lacks makes it nonideal.) The danger with compromise reasons is present in the compromise bottom line as well: that an imperfect item, announced as a unanimous decision, will be taken for a perfect product and passed along for use in other documents.[39]

The alternative to concealing the imperfections of a compromise need not be a mere listing of possible bottom lines, though sometimes this may be unavoidable. If one has assembled a group of especially varied, informed, and creative individuals, their chances of achieving a high-quality compromise may be greater than a legislature's, to whom the task would otherwise fall. Having reached a compromise, however, the commission should lay out its reasoning, including the costs to various views that have been required to get the agreement, and intrinsic negatives of the bottom line as seen by those holding various views.[40] Outsiders will then have a better idea of both the mechanics of achieving high-quality compromise and what changes in the future might remedy some of the defects, having been told in what sense the outcome is nonideal to different parties. (In cases where legislation is not immediately required, the need for a unanimous bottom line is diminished. Then the description of bottom lines that would be recommended by those with different views, with reasons for them, may be sufficient and helpful. A good model of this might be the usefulness of majority and separate minority dissenting opinions in Supreme Court cases.[41])

To summarize, a philosopher may have a duty to consider the meta-question of moralized compromise procedures. These may be contractualist in spirit, aiming to defend different views in accord with public reason, but also requiring compromise out of respect for individuals who represent views in the community.

IV. Criticizing: The Outsider

Philosophers in the academy are outsiders relative to any reports or processes of a commission which they do not serve. These same philosophers may well be insiders to other commissions or institutions, of course, where their behavior should have insider characteristics. This is to say that while some philosophers may be *essential* outsiders—Socrates portrayed himself in this way in the *Apology*—others can adopt insider and outsider roles on different occasions if society permits it. (Society may not permit it, if it refuses to allow a philosopher who plays the outsider on occasion to assume the insider's role. Or vice versa, if an insider were not allowed back in the academy.)

A problem for an outsider philosopher is how to deal with a commission report. One general danger is raised by a slippery-slope argument against criticism, such as the following: If the insider philosopher should pay more attention to consequences than to truth lest he harm the public,[42] then an outsider philosopher whose criticisms of a report might weaken its effectiveness and so harm the public should not criticize the report. This is especially true since she should understand how the report was constructed—no one should criticize it as if it were an attempt to arrive at truth with philosophical rigor.

(Most outsider philosophers are impotent to affect the public by their criticisms, but the point is that power to affect the public is not necessarily limited to, nor always greatest in, those with official insider positions.[43])

In discussing the insider philosopher, I have suggested that the first premise in this slippery-slope argument is incorrect, and that the insider's concern with consequences should not be as great as some have suggested. Hence, the premise does not imply the conclusion. (Of course, this does not show that the outsider's concerns with consequences should not be great.)

Furthermore, insiders may not always perfectly carry out their role obligations. It seems that the outsider (as well as other insiders) should then feel free to criticize this failure to meet the ideal. For example, a report may use an inadequate argument that is not even in the general area of the correct argument, or employ a "manifesto sentiment" from one report as a premise for an argument in another report.[44]

There is the additional possibility that the commission and staff philosopher have done their jobs perfectly, given their constraints, but the arguments and/or bottom line, considered independent of the context that produced them, are not as good as they ideally could be. For philosophers not to criticize or offer alternatives would give the impression that the correct solution and correct reasons had been found, and that further philosophical discussion is beside the point. For outsider philosophers to stop criticizing imperfect arguments and conclusions encourages the view that the activity of the outsider philosopher is unnecessary, whereas in fact outsiders make us conscious of what we should be striving for, in what way a context for producing a report is imperfect, and how it could be altered to make possible better products.

Outsider philosophers will often be critical. Tolerance for the whole practice of criticism varies among different groups of nonphilosophers. If there is extreme intolerance of rational criticism or a misunderstanding of the spirit in which a philosopher undertakes it, it is possible that the quality of insider philosophers' contributions will drop. One reason is that there will be no desire to anticipate criticism. Another is that one-time outsiders will be excluded from insider roles.

What should be done in the rare (hardly imaginable) circumstance in which an outsider philosopher's criticism could damage truly worthwhile policies? One might think the responsible critic could solve his problem by making no criticism without offering a positive solution in its stead. But, we are told, it may be that no one will believe the positive solution, only the criticism. If there is truly a very high probability—and less is not enough, I think—of criticism greatly harming very important justified policies, then possibly the outsider may be in a better position than the insider to attend to the duty he has, simply as a person, not to cause unjustified harm. After all, he does not have the same role-related duty as a staff philosopher to inform the commission, and his general duty to pursue truth can be carried out in many other ways.

V. Conclusion

The insider philosopher who serves a commission should think of his primary duties as informing and philosophizing with the commissioners, rather than producing a perfect philosophical document or acting directly for the public good. The insider philosopher's duty may include considering the meta-question of moralized compromise procedures. The outsider philosopher should understand constraints on the production of reports, but can still criticize and present more ideal alternatives. Since the outsider lacks a strong duty to inform the public about any particular document, it is possible he might give more weight to the public's good than the insider philosopher should in deciding what he will do.

Notes

1. This chapter is a combination of my "The Philosopher as Insider and Outsider," *Journal of Medicine and Philosophy* 15 (1990): 347–74; and "The Philosopher as Insider and Outsider: How to Advise, Compromise, and Criticize," *Business & Professional Ethics Journal* 9 (1990): 7–20. The first article was written while I was a Fellow in the Program in Ethics and the Professions at Harvard University. I thank the members of the Seminar on Ethics and the Professions at the Kennedy School for their help in discussing the topics of this article. For reading and commenting on an earlier draft of this article, I thank Arthur Applbaum, Sisella Bok, Baruch Brody, Amelie Rorty, Dennis Thompson, Alan Wertheimer, David Wilkins, Ken Winston, and Peter Yeager. I especially thank Baruch Brody for his initial suggestion that I write this article and for his support of my efforts. I thank Jane Marsh for her research and copy-editing assistance.

2. D. Brock, "Truth or Consequences: The Role of Philosophers in Policymaking," *Ethics* 97: 786–91, 786.

3. Brock, "Truth or Consequences," pp. 788–89.

4. In chapter 2 this volume, I have discussed and disagreed with Brock's argument that terminating treatment is killing.

5. One effect of the insider eventually publishing a description of his manipulative behavior is that his directive to others to do likewise is less likely to be acted on successfully. This is because the next commission may have access to the publication and be forewarned of the possibility of such behavior; they will trust their philosopher less. Whether behavior of the insider philosopher should be revealed in philosophical journals could fall under the topic of "outsider problems" discussed below.

6. For detailed discussion of this series of arguments and related issues in the acquisition and distribution of organs, see F. Kamm, "The Report of the U.S. Task Force on Organ Transplantation: Criticisms and Alternatives," *The Mount Sinai Journal of Medicine* 56: 207–20; and F. Kamm, *Morality, Mortality*, Vol. I (New York: Oxford University Press, 1993).

7. Reconstruction of Brock, "Truth or Consequences," p. 787.

8. I was reminded by John Rawls that when different economists offer conflicting advice to Congress *on bottom lines*, no one doubts they are all experts, though Congress may be confused about whose advice to rely on.

9. This sort of commitment to a bottom line based on an initial response to a type of case, a commitment that precedes reasons and is maintained in the face of opposing argument, is something which, I believe, we often encounter even in morally good people. Some bad people, however, exhibit the same sort of commitment. For example, the prejudiced person who is not swayed by an argument is like this. What is the difference between him and the committed good person, aside from one having the incorrect view and the other the correct one? Perhaps, the bad person refuses really to listen to counterarguments—he closes his mind—but the good person listens to arguments against his own position and truly permits himself to be open to change. If he is not swayed by the counterarguments, he retains his commitment even if he is not clear about the reasons for doing so, hoping the reasons will eventually become clear.

10. As Peter Yeager pointed out to me, this conclusion may vary with how disastrous an outcome would result. In personal correspondence received after the article was written, Brock informed me of what he did not make clear in his article: He argued vigorously in meeting with commissioners for his view on the killing/letting die issue and its relation to life-sustaining treatment. By and large, the bad effect he was concerned about did not occur, in part because commissioners remained adamant that killing was worse than letting die.

11. A rule consequentialist could accommodate these positions: desire for public good drives creation of the role and a philosopher's seeking the role, but on the occasion of action the duty is to carry out the role obligations rather than to promote the value that led to the role, even if this is sometimes contrary to that value.

12. A. Weisbard, "The Role of Philosophers in the Public Policy Process: A View from the President's Commission," *Ethics* 97: 776–86.

13. I owe this point to Dennis Thompson.

14. Bernard Williams (in conversation) noted that, given the established discourse in England, unlike America, it would have been inappropriate to give rights-based rather than utilitarian arguments in government reports, *except* if getting much closer to the correct bottom line required it.

15. On this idea of integrity in law, see Ronald Dworkin, *Law's Empire* (Cambridge, MA: Harvard University Press, 1986).

16. I have been helped in constructing these views (as distinct from the more conservative position that a philosopher has a duty not to recommend policies inconsistent with most extant government policy) by Arthur Applbaum and David Wilkins. The problems of undemocratic control, skepticism, and meeting the publicity condition are also raised by judicial decision-making. It is claimed by some—generally in the work of John Rawls, and by Thomas Nagel ("Moral Conflict and Political Legitimacy," *Philosophy & Public Affairs* 16 [1987]: 215–40)—that certain crucial parts of public deliberation must be undertaken in the language of "public reason." That is, only reasons that could be accepted as having some (if not determinative) weight by all should be appealed to in political discussion. However, as an extension of this view, it has also been argued (by Dworkin, *Law's Empire*) that in hard cases where past decisions and tradition do not determine an outcome, a judge may introduce her own moral views if they are not inconsistent with a plausible interpretation of our tradition, and extend it by way of publicly acceptable reasons. This leaves it open that she may engage in complex philosophical argumentation such as might appear in a professional philosophy journal, and have her decision become law without further discussion by either legislators or other philosophers.

17. Weisbard, "The Role of Philosophers in the Public Policy Process," p. 782.

18. To some degree they embody the practical recommendation on how to do ethical theory which Bernard Williams makes in *Ethics and the Limits of Philosophy* (Cambridge: Cambridge University Press, 1985).

19. J. Thomson, "A Defense of Abortion," *Philosophy & Public Affairs* 1: 47–56.

20. F. Kamm, "Ethics, Applied Ethics, Applying Applied Ethics," in *Applied Ethics and Ethical Theory*, eds. D. Rosenthal and F. Shehadi (Salt Lake City: University of Utah Press, 1988), pp. 162–87. See also chapter 26 this volume.

21. T. M. Scanlon, "Contractualism and Utilitarianism," in *Utilitarianism and Beyond*, eds. A. Sen and B. Williams (Cambridge: Cambridge University Press, 1982), pp. 103–28. (Since the article on which this chapter is based was written, Scanlon has expanded on his theory in his *What We Owe to Each Other* [Cambridge, MA: Harvard University Press, 1998].)

22. M. Warnock, "Moral Thinking and Government Policy: The Warnock Committee on Human Embryology," *Milbank Quarterly* 63: 504–21. I was prompted to think about this case by reading a draft of Martin Benjamin's article, "Philosophical Integrity and Policy Development in Bioethics," *Journal of Medicine and Philosophy* 15 (1990): 345–89.

23. For discussion of moral conflicts that individuals face, see articles in *Moral Dilemmas*, ed. C. Gowans (New York: Oxford University Press, 1987).

24. Conflicting values are not a necessary condition for a conflict; a single-valued system can lead to dilemmas, as when two promises conflict.

25. T. Nagel, "The Fragmentation of Value," in *Moral Dilemmas*, ed. C. Gowans (New York: Oxford University Press, 1987), pp. 174–87.

26. For an alternative characterization, see F. Kamm, "Harming Some to Save Others," *Philosophical Studies* 57: 227–60, and *Morality, Mortality*, Vol. II (New York: Oxford University Press, 1996).

27. For an alternative view of torturing the guilty, see my *Ethics for Enemies: Terror, Torture, and War* (Oxford: Oxford University Press, 2011), chapter 1, written after the articles on which this chapter is based.

28. So, for example, we may begin with the principle that not killing takes precedence over not letting die. This is consistent with our not taking organs from one live person to

save the lives of five, but it is inconsistent with the permissibility of a mere bystander turning a trolley to save five though it will then kill an innocent bystander. To account for both cases we would have to construct a more complex principle. I briefly note the way in which general factors can be formed into specific principles, rather than just intuitively held in mind together, in "Ethics, Applied Ethics, and Applying Applied Ethics." Henry Richardson discusses the specification of principles in detail in his paper, "Specifying Norms as a Way to Resolve Concrete Ethical Problems," *Philosophy & Public Affairs* 19 (1990): 279–310.

29. Scanlon warned me, in a general way, to distinguish the contractualist procedure for achieving ideal results from a procedure used in reaching actual compromise even if the latter is morally sensitive. These specific suggestions, however, are my own and should not be put at his doorstep. (Giving things weight out of proportion to their objective merit is also typically described as a characteristic of the subjective perspective but here it is functioning differently.)

30. As Nagel notes in "Moral Conflict and Political Legitimacy," there is an outside point of view from which what one believes to be true is seen as just one's belief rather than as a truth, though as people's beliefs (rather than as truths) they are given some weight in the compromise process.

31. Warnock, by contrast, seems willing to give moral weight to any strong sentiment. This could stem from a Humean theory that moral views are sentiments not defensible by reasons. Such a position about moral views seems to lead to the incorrect conception that Lord Devlin had of what counts as the morality of a community (in his *The Enforcement of Morals* [Oxford: Oxford University Press, 1965]).

32. These views about reasons are related to Rawls's idea of public reason. See his "Public Reason Revisited," in his *Political Liberalism* (expanded ed.) (New York: Columbia University Press, 2005).

33. That is, many supporters of a pluralistic moral view that includes a concern for good consequences would not accept a compromise that calls for a full-grown person to be sacrificed to save many lives just once a year rather than whenever it would be useful. Since a pure consequentialist does not accept the validity of this pluralistic view (from within which deontological considerations have some sort of priority over consequentialist ones), he cannot sympathize with this pluralist's refusal to compromise.

34. This last paragraph was added after publication of the original article on which this chapter is based.

35. See Dworkin, *Law's Empire*.

36. However, it might be argued that the possibility of harming a significant entity is the same whether we (a) multiply a small probability of its being a significant entity times frequent use or (b) multiply a high probability of its being a significant entity times infrequent use. I believe this reasoning is incorrect.

37. See Dworkin, *Law's Empire*, p. 436.

38. This analysis was added after publication of the original articles on which this chapter is based. For further discussion of views on using embryos for stem cell research, see chapters 9–10 this volume.

39. For example, a government report may treat a mere "manifesto sentiment" from another government report as a premise in an argument. The latter occurs in the *Report of the U.S. Task Force on Organ Transplantation*. Three separate arguments are offered for a government duty to fund transplants. The first two are based on the duty the government

has assumed to provide equal access to adequate health care. (This duty seems to be a manifesto sentiment. Its existence was treated as an assumption in the earlier report on *Securing Access to Health Care* by the President's Commission for the Study of Ethical Problems in Medicine and Biomedical and Behavioral Research, without, however, acknowledging a right to health care or granting that the government's assuming the duty was inescapable, or making clear what such a duty entailed.) These arguments are: (1) A duty has been assumed to provide equal access to an adequate level of health care. Transplants are part of an adequate level of health care. Therefore they are covered. (2) There is no relevant way to distinguish between procedures necessary for adequate health care already funded and new ones, so all must be funded. (3) That donors give organs to use for free implies that they are a national resource, and we have a duty to distribute them for free (and hence we must fund the procedures).

Each of these arguments seems unsound, in part because the "manifesto sentiment" is too weak to carry the weight of the argument. Even if transplants are (always) part of adequate health care—and an argument is needed for this—it is hard to believe that any duty to provide equal access to adequate levels of health care which was assumed would come without an upper limit on the price tag. This means that the duty does not involve a commitment to fund all procedures. Further, if different procedures are truly indistinguishable from the point of view of their role in adequate health care, this does not mean they must all be funded. A fair random-decision procedure might be the way to choose between them. Finally, we cannot be put under an obligation to expend funds to distribute something just because someone has freely given it to us hoping we will do so. Charities typically *sell* donated goods. (For detailed consideration of these and other issues in the distribution of organs and other scarce resources, see F. Kamm, "The Report of the U.S. Task Forces on Organ Transplantation," and *Morality, Mortality*, Vol. I.)

These criticisms do not mean that there is no government duty to fund transplants. What they suggest is that a stronger premise than that a government has assumed a duty to aid is necessary to yield a conclusion. A right on the part of citizens to, or an inescapable duty on the part of government to provide, health care where the dollar limit is set by reference to (a) how important alternative uses of public funds are in comparison with transplants, and (b) how much justice permits us to tax citizens, is minimally necessary to support an argument for funding certain procedures. If the argument necessary to support such a right or duty, or an argument sufficiently close to the correct one, cannot be agreed to by a commission, then the manifesto sentiment to which the commission can agree should be recognized for what it is, and not be used to support conclusions in other reports. (The issue of a compromise argument for a conclusion or a compromise conclusion spreading through a system (like a computer virus) is raised in the law as well. For example, the decision in *Brown* v. *Board of Education* has been said to be an example of compromising on reasons when unanimity was necessary, with ultimate bad effects on subsequent court decisions.)

40. I owe this point to Dennis Thompson.

41. This was first suggested to me by members of the Fellows at the Center for Ethics and the Professions. Yet another issue arises when the commissioners agree on a bottom line and the reasons for it, but realize that this proposal would conflict with what society could accept. This might occur even though representatives of different views in society are on the commission. The Warnock Commission was very sensitive to this factor, even to the

point of accepting what seem like mere emotional responses of society as unopposable barriers. Such a position is suspect since it might lead to the refusal to recommend rights for blacks or women in racist or sexist societies, even when the theories underlying past government policies (or conservative extensions thereof) would support such rights. This topic is large and I will not discuss it here.

42. This was the first premise in the version of Brock's argument.

43. This point was emphasized to me by Alan Wertheimer. A related argument meant to stem criticism claims it is unfair to judge insider philosophers qua philosophers, as though they were free to produce the best document they could.

44. As described in note 39.

25

Theory and Analogy in Law and Philosophy

I. Introduction

In his essay "In Praise of Theory," Ronald Dworkin defends his views about the role of theory in legal reasoning.[1,2] He contrasts his views with those of Cass Sunstein.[3] In this chapter, I shall argue that analogy and, in general, the use of case-based reasoning has an important role to play in adjudication. Indeed, I hope to show Dworkin's own arguments employ such reasoning, and that there are reasons to limit the role of deduction from theory in the law. I first lay out Dworkin's position as I understand it, and then address several arguments presented by Dworkin and his opponents.

II. Dworkin's View

When presented with a problematic case (e.g., should a company that produces drugs be held liable for damage that we cannot prove it caused?), Dworkin claims that we should proceed by finding a principle that best explains or coheres with other principles that explain not only the case at hand but also other settled cases in different areas of law or, at the limit, of all law. He argues that this process always involves a possibility of *justificatory ascent*—that is, judges must be prepared to reconcile the case at hand with other areas of law and/or find deeper principles and theoretical (philosophical) justification for those principles. There is no a priori way to rule out justificatory ascent, though it will not always be necessary to embark upon such a climb in order to decide a case.

Dworkin describes justificatory ascent by considering its mirror image: the descent that his fictional Judge Hercules makes to decide a case. Whereas we decide cases from the inside out (or bottom up), Hercules decides cases outside in (or top down):

> Before Hercules sits on his first case, he could build a gigantic, "over-arching" theory good for all seasons. He could decide all outstanding issues of metaphysics, epistemology, and ethics, and also of morality, including political morality. He could decide what there is in the universe, and why he is justified in

thinking that is what there is; what justice and fairness require; what freedom of speech, best understood, means; and whether and why it is a freedom particularly worth protecting . . . weave all that and everything else into a marvelously architectonic system. When a new case arises, he would be very well prepared.[4]

The descent to a case decision thus proceeds from more abstract principles (including metaphysics and epistemology) to less abstract ones, and also can involve complete empirical knowledge. According to Dworkin, the justificatory ascent that judges must be prepared to make is the analog of Hercules's descent to a case decision. Consequently, we cannot rule out a priori the possibility that judges may have to deal with epistemology, metaphysics, and other issues of a theoretical nature, and also decide what there is in the universe.

Because adjudication of certain issues may require this ascent, whoever has the jurisdiction or authority to adjudicate—whether the courts or the people themselves—must carry out the ascent when necessary, even if they cannot do so with assurance, and perhaps even if they cannot do it well. Dworkin says:

> At one point Sunstein . . . says that, "Judges should adopt a more complete theory for an area of law only if they are very sure that it is correct." . . . But he cannot really mean this, because . . . some cases cannot be decided at all, and others cannot be decided well, without introducing theory, which means that judges will often have to make theoretical judgments that bring conviction . . . even when this falls short of certainty.[5]

I shall call this the Principle of Imperfect Competence.

Finally, Dworkin defends justificatory ascent, and its concomitant need to find unifying principles, based on the essentially moral proposition that citizens in one case should not be governed by principles that we reject in other cases.[6] Dworkin believes that to do otherwise would be objectionable in a community committed to equal government.[7]

III. Theory and Analogy

In the last section of his essay, Dworkin discusses what he understands to be Cass Sunstein's proposal to replace an ascent to theory with analogical reasoning. Two major issues arise from Dworkin's discussion: (1) the merits of the use of analogy, and (2) the possibility of knowing a priori that justificatory ascent must stop at a certain point. I shall deal with these questions in turn.[8]

A. ANALOGY

Sunstein, according to Dworkin, says, "[J]udges should decide hard cases not by turning to more abstract levels of theory but in a more lawyer-like way—by analogy."[9] Dworkin replies that "[a]n analogy is a way of stating a conclusion, not a way of reaching one."[10] Analogy without theory is blind, he says. We need a theory to explain why case A is really more like case B than case C.

I first wish to ask: Is analogy more *lawyer-like?* Some time after I published *Creation and Abortion,*[11] a professor of law at McGill University compared it with Dworkin's *Life's Dominion*[12] in the following way: He found it interesting that I, a philosopher, had written a very detailed example of legal reasoning, whereas Dworkin, a lawyer, had written a work of philosophy! Why did he think my work more lawyer-like than Dworkin's? He probably thought so because *Creation and Abortion* begins by arguing from several cases—such as the violinist case originally introduced by Judith Thomson[13]—to the abortion case, noting similarities (and differences) between cases by referring to features that made them analogous, occasionally also employing principles, without aspiring to great generality. At a certain point in my examination of the abortion issue, however, I found it necessary to abandon the use solely of what seemed like analogous cases, and to develop additionally a theory of responsibly creating persons. Here is where my argument by reference to *analogous cases* ended. This is not to say, however, that the use of *cases* ended, for a theory may be tested and rejected by considering its implications for cases, and judgments in cases may be used as evidence in support of a theory. But using a case to verify a theory is not the same as deciding a case on the basis of comparison with another case.

In *Life's Dominion,* Dworkin, by contrast, focused on the question of the intrinsic value of life in his discussion of abortion. He moved beyond analyzing abortion in terms of rights based on interests, instead analyzing it in terms of respect for what he calls nonincremental intrinsic value, or the sacred.

I suspect that my approach in *Creation and Abortion* might exemplify some of what Sunstein recommends. When faced with a problematic case, first find an analogous case that provides a fixed or settled point: a judgment about a particular case which we can assume is shared and for which we therefore do not need to give a deep theoretical justification. Dworkin would not object to this method, presumably, so long as the questions of whether the case is a fixed point and whether it is like the disputed one do not arise. But, he asks, is abortion more like infanticide or appendicitis? He thinks we need a theory about the fetus to decide.

However, an alternative approach is to find a third case (other than infanticide or appendicitis) that is analogous to abortion in certain respects and about which our judgments are clear, though they do not depend on a theory about the nature of the fetus. If such a case exists, the settled position in that case, if it is sufficiently analogous, may suggest the correct result about an abortion case. It also furthers our task if any differences between the case that is analogous in some respects and the abortion case would only make it *harder* to justify action in the analogous case. Then we need not fear that a positive answer in the analogous case does not determine one in the abortion case. Thomson's violinist case is meant to be like this, since she assumes for the sake of argument that the fetus is a person. The idea is that if we may kill a person, then it should be easier to justify killing a fetus. Of course, this approach might not always work because there may be other differences that make it harder to kill a fetus than the violinist. However, the approach can provide a starting point for the resolution of an issue that does not require deep theoretical justification: it shows that in order to defeat the permissibility of abortion in some cases, we must point to some other difference between the violinist and a fetus that would make it harder to justify killing the fetus than to kill the violinist.[14]

This all bears on whether analogy is a way of stating a conclusion or a way of reaching one. On the basis of my own experience, I disagree with Dworkin when he says analogy is only a way of stating conclusions. Analogy can be a way of reaching a conclusion. The relevance of another case to the initial problematic one can be clear, even if one does not have a theory that links the analogous case and the original case, and even if one is initially uncertain about what one may permissibly do in the analogous case, so that what one may do in *that* case is also a conclusion for which one searches. While we may sometimes need a theory to *explain* why case A is more like case B than like case C, without deep theoretical justification we may still see that case A is more like B than like C and use that conclusion to help us find a solution to case A. Indeed, sometimes one reaches a conclusion about a case by way of an analogous case and one still cannot provide an adequate theoretical justification of one's position in either case. This does not (or should not) necessarily lead one to reject one's conclusion.[15]

By contrast, when someone states a conclusion by the use of an analogy and says that a theory leads us to see that one case is like another (Dworkin's view), I may challenge the theory by presenting a third case that demonstrates that the theory is incomplete because it incorrectly groups this third case with the others. The theory may imply that the three cases are analogous in virtue of some properties, but it may ignore other significant differences. For example, in the abortion case, consider a theory that focused only on the nature of the fetus and then analogized abortion to appendectomy because the theory explains why the fetus is like an unimportant appendix. Such a theory might fail to give adequate weight to the nature of the relationship between the fetus and the woman's body—specifically, that the fetus is dependent on that body for life. This theory could fail to predict that I might have no right to destroy something that is not very valuable (like an appendix) in another case in which it is independent of my body, but have a right to destroy something of comparable (or greater value) when it is dependent on my body.[16] In other words, a case that the theory picks out as analogous to abortion may show the theory to be an incomplete basis for generating a conclusion in an abortion case.

If analogy is a way of reaching a conclusion, does this mean we must also reject Dworkin's views that analogy without theory is blind and that we need a theory to explain why case A is really more like case B than case C? Not necessarily, since needing a theory to explain an analogy is consistent with analogy being a way of reaching a conclusion.[17] Analogy can be a way of reaching a conclusion, and because it does this, it can help us build theories that identify and explain the factors present in cases that have moral or legal significance. In fact, it might be that theory without analogy is blind, since we should test a theory by seeing whether it correctly predicts that one case is analogous to another (as I described above).

Dworkin et al. rely on both cases and theory in their amicus brief on physician-assisted suicide.[18] The case-based portion of their argument asserts that if current law allows us to terminate treatment intending the patient's death, it follows that—when all other factors are the same—we may kill intending the patient's death. We are encouraged to proceed from an assumed-to-be-acceptable starting point (termination of treatment is generally accepted as proper even when one intends death so long as a patient consents) to a conclusion that physician-assisted suicide (which involves actively causing death) is acceptable. Dworkin et al. support this leap by way of *another* case-based argument, which they claim demonstrates that killing and terminating aid are not, in themselves, morally distinguishable. They assert that when killing is wrong, it is only because intending death is wrong. (They argue in this way even though in assisted suicide, by contrast to euthanasia, the doctor does not kill anyone per se but helps a patient kill himself.)

For example, Dworkin et al. first discuss cases in which doctors take an action that fails to effectuate their patients' desires to live. They agree that a doctor, when faced with two patients in need of and desiring an organ transplant, may permissibly deny an organ to one patient in order to give it to another. But they also agree that a doctor may *not* kill a patient to recover an organ for the use of another. The explanation of the moral difference between these cases, they argue, is *not* that in the first case the doctor lets the patient die versus actively killing him. Rather, Dworkin et al. argue that the cases are morally different because in the first case the doctor only foresees death, whereas in the second case he wrongly intends death. Hence, they conclude that when intending death is acceptable, killing or letting die are equally acceptable. Is this an argument by analogy? Not quite, since the case-based argument (for the claim that there is no moral distinction between killing and letting die per se) is not itself based on an analogy. Still, the focus is on using cases rather than theory in this argument.

I do not think that the preceding argument is a good case-based argument, however. For, if it did demonstrate that killing per se does not make a moral difference, it would also imply that it is permissible for a doctor to use a chemical that is necessary to transplant organs into several dying patients though he *foresees* it will seep into the next room and kill an immovable patient. In this case, the doctor does not intend to kill the patient in the next room, but only foresees his death. Presumably, however, the doctor's behavior is both wrong and a killing. This case demonstrates that, contrary to what Dworkin et al. argue, killing can be wrong when we merely foresee death, even if letting die in a comparable case when we merely foresee death is not wrong (as when the doctor must operate on several dying patients and so has no time to treat a dying patient in the next room). Since their case-based argument does not show that killing per se makes no difference, without further argument they cannot conclude that killing (or assisting killing) with the intention to bring about death is permissible if terminating aid with the intention to bring about death is permissible.[19]

Relying on cases, I have constructed a different argument in favor of assisted suicide. It also moves from what is assumed to be a fixed point in patient care—the permissibility of sometimes giving morphine for pain relief, foreseeing that the morphine will cause death, when death is a lesser evil and pain relief is a greater good—to the permissibility of helping someone kill himself while intending death, when death is a lesser evil and pain relief a greater good. Thus, I argue from the permissibility of one type of killing (in administering morphine for pain relief) to the permissibility of assisting in another type of killing. (By contrast, Dworkin et al. argue from the permissibility of letting die to the permissibility of assisting in killing.) There is a second premise linking the first premise in my argument to the conclusion and it is an argument from *analogy*: If it is permissible for a doctor to intend a lesser evil which is *not* death (such as blindness in a patient) to achieve a greater good for that patient (save his life), why is it not permissible to intend death when *it* is a lesser evil for a patient to achieve a greater good (pain relief) for him?[20]

These case-based arguments—whether employing analogy or not—also contrast with the more theoretical arguments that Dworkin et al. make in favor of physician-assisted suicide. Dworkin et al. adopt the view proposed in *Planned Parenthood* v. *Casey*[21]—that a person has a right to self-determination in the most intimate and important matters in his life—and from that view deduce a right to determine the time and manner of death. But does their theory then endorse the conclusion that a person has a right to assisted suicide from a willing doctor if he decides that his medical treatment is consuming too much of his family's finances or if he wishes to give up his life for some noble cause? Seeing the implication of the theory for new cases is one way of testing it and recourse to analogy is one way of helping determine what our views about these new cases should be. For example, one might argue that: (a) giving morphine for pain, foreseeing that this causes certain death, stands to (b) assisted killing while intending death in order to stop pain as (c) treating an illness by giving a less costly drug though we foresee it causes death stands to (d) assisted killing while intending death in order to save money on treating with costly drugs. Do we approve of (c)? If not, why should we approve of (d)? By contrast, we sometimes do approve of (a), so why not (b)?

My point is that theory not refined by consideration of cases can be overly broad and therefore problematic. This is exemplified by the U.S. Supreme Court's attempt to be theoretical in *Casey*, focusing on the right to self-determination in the most intimate and important matters in his life. Further, in both *Roe* v. *Wade*[22] and *Cruzan* v. *Missouri Department of Health*,[23] the members of the Court may have grasped at the wrong theories because they did not consider a wide range of hypothetical cases on which their theory would bear. In *Roe*, they focused on privacy rather than on bodily autonomy, and in *Cruzan*, they focused on the importance of life-and-death decisions rather than on a prima facie right against having one's body invaded against one's will. If the Court had considered more hypothetical cases it might have theorized differently and more narrowly, accepting the least broad theory necessary to defend abortion rights and rights to terminate treatment. Then it would not later have been in the position of having either to accept all implications of, for example, the *Casey* theory or to deny those implications, thereby threatening to undermine the theory's defense of abortion and termination of treatment. Given the route it actually took, the Court could use the assisted-suicide issue to *refine* the *Casey* theory. This would be useful. However, this does not imply it should be a matter of general practice to generate a theory that is more general than is necessary for a particular case at hand and then wait for future cases to refine it.

Mine is not an argument against employing theory and for merely relying on cases. It is an argument for doing theory well, so that we do not generate an overly broad theory that carries with it unforeseen and *incorrect* implications for other cases. We should generate theory that explains and justifies correct case judgment. In the context of the real judicial world, it may also be an argument for not choosing broad theories whose morally *correct* implications will be difficult to affirm. However, mine is also an argument for doing case reasoning well. Can we share Sunstein's confidence that judges are in fact more adept at case reasoning than at the use of theory? Let me only say that arguing well by using cases can be very difficult. I have already noted one possible difficulty with the use of cases in Dworkin et al.'s amicus brief on physician-assisted suicide. I will now try to show that judicial case-based reasoning is also not always done well.[24]

For example, in *Compassion in Dying* v. *Washington*, the majority judges suggested that they could not distinguish morally or legally between what is already permitted—here, terminating treatment while intending death and giving morphine foreseeing death—and assisting killing with the intention to cause death.[25] In other words, their strategy is to triangulate between two legally permissible practices to a conclusion about assisting suicide. Let us consider whether this strategy works or whether assisting in killing someone while intending his death could be morally different from the two practices they cite. By pointing to the permissibility of giving morphine they are at once saying that we allow some cases of causing death and also, implicitly, narrowing their focus to cases where death is assumed to be a lesser evil by comparison to the greater good of relief from pain. In pointing to terminating treatment intending death, they may think they show that there is no objection to intending death per se, and so it is permissible to add such an intention to cases of causing death when death is a lesser evil. However, if a competent patient wishes to terminate treatment, we must permit it even when he (or his physician) does so with the intention that his own death occur simply because the alternative is forcing contin-ued treatment on someone, which we must not do unless public safety requires it. Hence, permitting termination with an intention to cause death does not show that intending death is per se unobjectionable. By contrast, the alternative to assisting killing by providing lethal pills is leaving the patient alone; it does not involve forcing treatment on someone. Hence, we could prohibit assisting killing (but not termi-nating aid) when it is accompanied by the intention to cause death without raising the problem of forcing treatment on a competent patient against his will.[26] The upshot is that assisting in killing someone while intending his death could be mor-ally distinguished from the permissible practices cited by the Court.

This, of course, does not mean assisting killing cannot be justified. I have already tried to do so by arguing from the permissibility of intentionally bringing about other lesser evils. This is, I think, the crucial missing step in the Court's ar-gument (absent a theoretical argument to the effect that intentions cannot affect the permissibility of acts). But notice that my argument also justifies the doctor killing the patient in euthanasia rather than merely assisting killing. The argu-ments given by the judges in *Compassion in Dying* v. *Washington*, to the effect that they cannot distinguish between giving morphine foreseeing death, terminating treatment while intending death, and assisting suicide while intending death, also imply that they should distinguish morally and legally between giving morphine foreseeing death and a doctor committing active euthanasia. Yet it is not clear that they would have accepted this implication.

Notice also that the *Compassion in Dying* court was concerned to limit the doctor's right to assist in killing to cases where the patient's life is going to end shortly anyway and death is not against his interests.[27] However, the scope of the right to refuse treatment and to have treatment terminated is broader. A mentally competent patient may legally refuse treatment, intending to die, even when it is not in his best interest to do so and, on many occasions, even when he could be cured. Presumably, in many cases, the competent patient could also insist on ter-minating treatment, even if his intention is to die when it is not in his interest to die. Furthermore, even if the doctor in these cases improperly intends that the patient die, the treatment must be terminated. *This is because the alternative to letting the patient die is forcing treatment on him.* We think that a competent patient's right not to be physically invaded against his will is typically stronger than our interest in his well-being (though this right is, to be sure, not absolute and can sometimes be overridden by considerations of public safety). But if the patient asks for assistance in killing himself when it is not in his interest to be killed, it might well be morally impermissible to help him. If, however, the distinction between providing lethal pills to a person who is not on life support and termi-nating life-sustaining treatment as such makes no moral or legal difference, then terminating treatment should be permitted no more broadly than is assisting killing.[28] That is, moving from permissibility causing or helping to cause death *only* when death is a lesser evil without taking note of the difference between what we do to a patient if we fail to kill him, in contrast to what we do to him if we fail to terminate treatment, could lead to *reducing* the right to terminate treatment.

The judges in *Compassion in Dying* also disagreed with the claims that terminating aid is less active than assisting killing and that terminating aid involves letting "nature" be the cause of death.[29] Let us consider these two claims. While terminating aid is active, it is often a letting die rather than a killing. That is, acting to stop aid that one (or the agency one is authorized to represent) is providing to another is a letting die, not a killing.[30] It is true that this act of letting die is a partial cause of death,[31] but what is the other partial cause? The answer is: the patient's underlying physical condition. If the patient dies of starvation because food is stopped, this does not mean—contrary to what the judges in *Compassion in Dying* claim—that we do not let nature take its course. It is the nature of the body to die when not fed. If the patient dies of asphyxiation when the respirator is stopped, this is because his illness (his nature) prevents his breathing on his own. This contrasts with providing a drug that interferes with the patient's own life-sustaining bodily processes and thus induces death.

Finally, it is worth noting in this discussion of analogy that while some (e.g., Sunstein) may support the use of analogical reasoning merely because it avoids commitment to controversial theories, I recommend it primarily because it may be an epistemically privileged way to reach right answers in cases and even to build theories. Along with theory, legal education should include practice in the imaginative and precise formulation of analogies and use of cases, which are techniques that characterize some contemporary moral theorizing.

B. A PRIORI LIMITS ON JUSTIFICATORY ASCENT

If there were limits to the necessity of justificatory ascent, this would be another way in which the need to use theory would be reduced. Let us now consider this issue. As previously described, Dworkin's fictional Judge Hercules could begin each case by deciding:

> . . . all outstanding issues of metaphysics, epistemology, and ethics. . . . He could decide what there is in the universe, and why he is justified in thinking that is what there is. . . . From outside—beginning, perhaps, in the intergalactic stretches of his wonderful intellectual creation—he could work steadily in towards the problem at hand: finding the best available justification for law in general, for American legal and constitutional practice as a species of law, for constitutional interpretation, for tort, and then, finally, for the poor woman who took too many pills.[32]

Since Hercules's descent would be the reverse of an ordinary judge's ascent, there being no a priori limit to an ascent means that there is no reason, a priori, to deny that a judge might have to "decide all outstanding issues of metaphysics, epistemology, and ethics . . . decide what there is in the universe, and why he is justified in thinking that is what there is."[33]

Is this claim true? If it were known, a priori, that the answers to some of the questions Hercules could answer were irrelevant to deciding a particular issue of political morality or law, then the position one takes on these irrelevant questions could not affect one's position on the legal issue at hand. Thus, an ordinary judge would not have to "decide all outstanding issues." The fact that Hercules could deduce the answer to a legal question, given the *true* position on those irrelevant questions, need not imply that one could not deduce the same answer even if one held a false position on an irrelevant issue. Presumably, Hercules would also know this. If this were so, then if Hercules did more than he needed to do (by addressing the irrelevant issue), Hercules's actual route down would not bear on whether there was, a priori, a limit on how far a judge had to ascend. She would, a priori, have to ascend no further than the last level that was relevant to deciding the issue.

Can we know a priori whether any of the questions that Hercules might answer are irrelevant to deciding legal cases? In what circumstance (to choose an example) would the question of whether meson particles in fact exist be relevant to a legal decision? In a case where the controlling moral/legal principle told us to award damages to the person who knows the most arcane facts, the truth of that assertion could be relevant to the outcome of the case. But, I believe, this is not the way in which a theory about the universe is supposed to figure in justificatory ascent. The ascent makes possible a deduction; that is, a lower-order claim *about principles* is justified (and distinguished from another claim which is not justified) by a higher-order claim, which in turn is justified by even higher-order claims, and so on.

So the question is whether there is any level of argument or type of knowledge that Hercules could master that we could know, a priori, is irrelevant to deriving any *principle* ever needed to decide a legal case. (1) It seems that I can know a priori that whether there is one more or one less meson in the universe, or whether objects are really colored as opposed to just appearing colored to humans, is irrelevant to which legal or moral principles are correct. (2) If it could be shown a priori that one can know that a normative theory is correct without first knowing which metaethical theory is correct, then one could know a priori that metaethics will be irrelevant to legal decision-making. (3) If "ought" cannot be derived from "is," then no theory about actual behavior can be relevant to a deduction of principles of political morality. (Of course, a moral principle might say that consequences are morally significant, and one might need to know physical or psychological behavior to figure out consequences and thereby determine what is right to do in the situation. Still, this does not place the physical or psychological knowledge in an *ascent*, as it is not justifying lower-level *principles*.)

If it is correct that these are examples of what we could know a priori to be irrelevant to resolving legal disputes, then some of the things Hercules could know, our judge would not need to ascend to know *in order to deduce principles* with which to decide a case. Her ascent up would only mirror Hercules's *most direct* descent down (that is, that descent which avoids all irrelevant issues).

Is there a second way in which some ascents might be blocked a priori? Suppose that Hercules could prove (or knew) that God exists, or that Christianity is the true religion, or that love is the most important component in a good life, and from this knowledge he could deduce answers to legal cases. If bottom-up investigation were to reveal that the foundation of our legal system is liberal, then our judges might be committed to acting as though the truth of certain of these claims is not known. This is because in a liberal system citizens have a right to decide such matters for themselves and to have the government be neutral with respect to different views about religion and the good life. Hence, though the judges could deduce the answer to a case by ascending to these truths, they might deliberately behave as if they have no access to such truths (or as if those truths do not determine an outcome). Hercules himself, however, might be able to deduce the principles of a liberal legal system using these premises as well as in other ways. To do so, he might reason in any of the following ways: (a) such truths as "God exists" and "Christianity is correct" themselves imply that our political morality should be liberalism (i.e., those religious truths would then dictate that they themselves be irrelevant to any further legal decision-making); (b) ordinary mortals should construct legal systems within the limits of their uncontentious beliefs, and the truth of God's existence and Christianity's correctness are not uncontentious for them; or (c) some other argument for liberalism requires us to ignore religious truths in legal decision-making. If the best justification of liberalism were via (a), this is presumably how Hercules would come to justify a liberal system of government if he simply started from the top and worked down. But judges in a liberal society cannot offer such a justification of our liberalism, since given a liberal way of thinking the premises in (a) upon which Hercules relies must be treated as though they are unavailable. Hence, assuming a liberal foundation for our government, it seems that we could know a priori that certain sorts of truths and ascents cannot serve as the basis for an ordinary judge's deeper justification of decisions, though they still might be Hercules's reasonably preferred route down. The best ascent could fail to mirror the best descent.

A third way in which limits on ascent might be set is connected to what I above termed the Principle of Imperfect Competence. If I understand him correctly, Dworkin argues that his model of adjudication would be required even if the judge cannot apply it well. Of course, he concedes that the jurisdiction of judges could be limited so that they do not attempt fully to adjudicate issues that are beyond their abilities; other agents more competent at certain tasks might undertake the more crucial or difficult issues. But if adjudication is left only to judges, they must do the best they can.

Sunstein says that "[j]udges should adopt a more complete theory for an area of law only if they are very sure that it is correct," implying that they should refrain from developing a theory when they are not sure they will do a good job.[34] Dworkin responds that:

... Judges will often have to make theoretical judgments that bring conviction,[35] or at least greater conviction than their rivals, even when this falls
short of certainty. When, after all, is a judge right to think that he confronts a
case that can't be decided "at all" or "well" without some theoretical reflection?
Isn't it enough, to satisfy that standard, that without reflection, the judge lacks
conviction as to which answer is the one that, all things considered, best com-
ports with his responsibilities? And isn't it then sensible for him to carry his
theoretical reflection to the point at which conviction is reached?[36]

But if a judge finds conviction in an answer to a case through justificatory
ascent, does this always mean that it is reasonable for him to act on the case answer
he reaches? If not, then in some cases, the judge's decision to ascend to theory may
have been unreasonable. The question is, then: Is it ever unreasonable for a judge
to act on an answer derived from a justificatory ascent? Apparently, Sunstein
would require a certain degree of conviction (say, x degree) in a theory before one
reasonably relies on that theory to resolve a case. Dworkin sets no bottom limit on
the degree of conviction required in a theory (i.e., it can be x-n degree) so long as
it yields either (1) a case answer one finds convincing, or (2) a case answer one
finds more convincing than any of the alternatives yielded by other theories. In
either situation, resolving the case on the basis of the theory is appropriate.

It is possible that the degree of conviction in a case answer reached under
Dworkin's standard (1) might be as high as Sunstein's desired x degree for conviction in a theory. On the other hand, the degree of conviction in a case answer
reached under standard (2) could have no bottom limit. For example, if presented
with a case where there are several alternative positions, and we have twice as
much conviction in case answer A as in any of the other answers, it is possible for
us (under Dworkin's theory) to adjudicate A even if our degree of conviction in it
is very low in absolute terms.

Suppose that we combine low conviction in a theory (that yields a case
answer) with proposal (2), which only requires that the selected result be comparatively the most convincing. If Dworkin allows a judge to make a major change in
a legal system on the basis of such a combination of beliefs, he allows action on
the basis of very weak belief-preference (both concerning theory and concerning
case answer). Suppose that a judge has greater conviction in answer A than in B,
but the least good outcome if A is wrong is much worse than the least good outcome if B is pursued. Wouldn't Sunstein say that it would be unreasonable to
select answer A?

Suppose that we use Dworkin's standard (1), which requires that we find an
answer to a case to be convincing (to an unspecified degree). Suppose that a judge
confronts a case that requires an ascent to theory, and when he pursues the deeper
issues involved in ascent, he reaches a case answer with the conviction required by
(1). He now believes that answer A is right, but he recognizes that his belief (unlike Hercules's) may be erroneous. Indeed, is it possible that his confidence in his

treatment of the deeper issue is so weak that he believes that even if the result for a case seems right to him, there is a great chance of its being wrong? Perhaps this is not possible. I can then make my point by supposing that *we* know about a judge who has a case conviction that, given his imperfect competence at deeper theory, he is as likely to be wrong as right, even when he thinks he is right. It might be best to have such a judge refuse to decide the case on the basis of his conviction, at least when the worst outcome if his favored conviction is wrong is much worse than the worst outcome if an alternative is pursued.

Here is a possible analogy: A good parent is someone who makes the right decisions in child rearing. These decisions may require complete information about child development, psychoanalysis, a theory of the good life, and so on. As a result, there may be very few good parents. However, we should not change our theory of good parenting just because few can do it. Perhaps the better approach is for parents to get consultants for the tasks they cannot do well (e.g., seek the advice of teachers and psychologists rather than figure out these disciplines for themselves). But sometimes even these experts are unsure of their theories, and sometimes there are no experts. Suppose that the parents or experts find themselves with convictions about child rearing, but they also have a second-order view, perhaps based on past experience, that the theory which seems correct to them may well be incorrect. Should they act on the answer that they believe is correct, as implied by the theory that seems best at the time? Or might they conclude that they will likely do less damage by not relying on the theory? In that case, the parents leave more up to luck (or to the children themselves) than they would if they were certain they had the right answer. This does not mean that they think the best theory of parenting leaves children to luck or to their own devices; indeed, it may be known that neither of these can be the best theory. Rather, these parents know that the risk of damage is great if they act on their favored theory and it is wrong, and the risk of damage is much less if the alternative "hands-off" policy is used. Hence, the latter may be the better course of action under the circumstances.[37] For these reasons, the government agency in charge of child welfare may even prevent parents from acting on the theories and case answers of which they are convinced.

It may be asked, however: If the judge discussed above pursues B over A, is he not acting in the light of a theory that states that we should act to avoid the worst possible outcome in uncertain circumstances? But this response obscures the fact that the judge still has conviction in A, or at least greater conviction in A than in B. This response also diminishes the distinction between Dworkin's and Sunstein's views, since it allows that sometimes one should act on one's conviction in A only if one is sure the theory is correct. And this is only what Sunstein is claiming, according to Dworkin's presentation of his views.

I will consider one final wrinkle in this discussion of competence and conviction. The possibility that a judge, through the process of justificatory ascent, may be convinced that he should not deal with a certain question seems quite compatible with Dworkin's ascent theory. For example, in the abortion context, a judge may become convinced that the question of the true nature of the fetus is not appropriately decided by the courts, but should be left to philosophers, scientists, or individual citizens.[38] But what if the Court were to conclude that justice demanded that it answer the question of the fetus's nature? Suppose its members deliberated but there was a division of opinion in the Court regarding the status of the fetus or a serious concern that the one view of which they were all convinced might be wrong. In either situation, it might be correct for the Court to bypass taking one side on the issue, even though it believes that it is its job to decide the question. Instead, the Court might take one of several routes: (i) a compromise position, giving something on the regulation of abortion to each side holding alternative accounts of the fetus, in accordance with differing degrees of confidence in the answers implied by alternative accounts; (ii) allowing state-by-state, or citizen-by-citizen, policies; or (iii) adopting the view that overriding the recognized liberty interests of women at all requires it to be *firmly* convinced of a position on the status of the fetus that no reasonable person could reject.[39] (A fourth possibility is to show that whatever the nature of the fetus is, abortion would still be permissible or impermissible.[40]) Sometimes, finding the right decision when conviction on a first-order theoretical problem (such as the nature of the fetus) is not sufficiently great might require taking a course of action that does not depend on a solution to this first-order problem. This is so, even if it would be appropriate to decide the first-order problem if one could do so with the right degree of conviction. Principles of decision-making under uncertainty then become relevant.

It seems then that imperfect competence could be a reason for limiting ascent to theory in deciding a case. If we could determine what degree of conviction is too weak to justify action, in what circumstances, we might decide a priori when ascent (that would lead to no more than that degree of conviction) is not reasonable.[41]

Notes

1. This chapter is a revised version of parts of my "Theory and Analogy in Law," *Arizona State Law Journal* 29 (1997). I include these parts in this volume because they bear on the use of hypothetical cases and analogy in bioethical reasoning, methods I have employed throughout this volume, by contrast to the use of moral theory. Another reason for including parts of the article is that many of the issues we have discussed in other chapters raise questions dealt with by courts (e.g., abortion, assisted suicide). Hence, some discussion of legal reasoning employed in discussing such questions is relevant.

2. Ronald Dworkin, "In Praise of Theory," *Arizona State Law Journal* 29 (1997): 357–60.

3. In the original article on which this chapter is based, I also discuss how he contrasts his own view with that of Richard Posner.

4. Dworkin, "In Praise of Theory," p. 358. Dworkin says that Hercules "could" do all this, as though this were optional, but he may mean that Hercules *does* do this—it is the nature of the figure Hercules to do so.

5. Dworkin, "In Praise of Theory," p. 374.

6. Dworkin, "In Praise of Theory," pp. 357–76.

7. Is it possible that citizens are treated equally (Dworkin's concern) even if principle *a* governs class of cases *x* and principle *not-a* governs class of cases *y*, as long as all citizens in a particular class of cases are treated in the same way—even if the distinction drawn between cases *x* and *y* is arbitrary (for example, if *x* involves blue cars and *y* involves red cars)? A complaint of arbitrariness seems distinct from one that citizens are not being treated equally.

8. The original first section of part III (of the article on which this chapter is based) deals with a debate between Dworkin and Richard Posner). It has been omitted, as it did not seem directly relevant to the issues discussed in this book.

9. Dworkin, "In Praise of Theory," p. 371.

10. Dworkin, "In Praise of Theory."

11. F. M. Kamm, *Creation and Abortion: A Study in Moral and Legal Philosophy* (New York: Oxford University Press, 1992). For a condensed version of arguments in that book, see chapter 12 this volume.

12. Ronald Dworkin, *Life's Dominion: An Argument about Abortion, Euthanasia, and Individual Freedom* (New York: Knopf, 1993).

13. Judith Jarvis Thomson imagined a case in which someone is kidnapped in order to attach a famous but dying violinist to his body to provide the violinist with life support. This is analogous, Thomson thinks, to pregnancy as a result of rape. See Judith Jarvis Thomson, "A Defense of Abortion," *Philosophy & Public Affairs* 1 (1971): 47.

14. In his response to the article on which this chapter is based ("Reply," *Arizona State Law Journal* 29: 431–56), Dworkin says:

> Kamm thinks that this analogy is helpful because it is obvious that the violinist is a person, and that once it is accepted that the woman linked to him has no duty not to detach herself, even though he will die, it must follow that the rape victim has no duty not to abort even if a fetus is a person. But that does follow only of there are no other differences of principle between the two situations, and, as the literature makes plain, that assumption is itself very controversial. The question immediately arises, for example, whether the rape victim has a duty the linked woman does not—a natural duty owed by all parents to persons who are their children, whether or not the former have consented to become parents. Kamm may think it is obvious that parents have no such duties, but she finds the analogy natural and helpful only because she does take that view of a crucial matter of principle. The example seems to me to help confirm, not undermine, my view that analogies are not independent sources of moral argument."

I think Dworkin's response is wrong on several counts. First, one can think that an analogy is helpful and so a source rather than a conclusion of moral argument, even if one does not think a conclusion "must" follow from it. It can situate the debate on a new question that was not previously thought to be important, such as whether parental duties rather than the impermissibility of killing are what stand in the way of abortion. Hence, it is not true that I found the violinist analogy helpful because I assumed a principle, namely that parents have no duties to support their offspring in their bodies. Indeed, I did not assume the principle. In *Creation and Abortion* (p. 83), I raised the very issue of parental duties and thought it useful in thinking about this issue to consider another case that immediately strikes one as analogous to abortion, once we abstract from the issue of killing the fetus and focus on parental duties. I said, "Imagine that someone has stolen your genetic material and is growing a fetus from it in a lab. He knew that at a crucial point it would be physically required for further development of the fetus that it be transferred into your womb. Are you obligated to let the fetus be placed in your womb? I think not." I believe this set of cases (and others one might construct) are useful in making one aware of factors that might be relevant to a final decision and in testing them. Hence, Dworkin's view of whether analogy is helpful as a source of moral argument seems to be wrong.

15. It has been noted that people can distinguish and group cases by responding to complex factors they cannot consciously formulate. I now find support for this view in what Timothy Wilson says about "implicit learning" by the adaptive unconscious. In discussing a demonstration of implicit learning in his *Strangers to Ourselves* (Cambridge, MA: Harvard University Press, 2004), p. 28, he says:

> The participants' task was to watch a computer screen that was divided into four quadrants. On each trial, the letter X appeared in one of the four quadrants, and the participant pressed one of four buttons to indicate which one. Unbeknownst to the participant, the presentations of the Xs were divided into blocks of 12 that followed a complex rule. . . . Although the exact rules were complicated, participants appeared to learn them. As time went by their performance steadily improved. . . . None of the participants, however, could verbalize what the rules were or even that they had learned anything. They learned the complex rules nonconsciously.

In this case, the formula that explained the placement of Xs in the grid was never made conscious.

16. On this as one criticism of Dworkin's approach to abortion, see chapter 11 this volume.

17. I owe this point to Lawrence Sager. It is also one of the points made in note 14 above.

18. See Brief for Ronald Dworkin et al. as Amici Curiae, *Washington v. Glucksberg*, 117 S. Ct. 2258 (1997), reprinted as Ronald Dworkin et al., "Assisted Suicide: The Philosophers' Brief," *New York Review of Books* 44 (March 27, 1997), p. 41.

19. This is one of several criticisms I make of Dworkin et al.'s amicus brief. For a complete discussion, see generally chapter 3 this volume.

20. F. M. Kamm, "A Right to Choose Death," *Boston Review*, Summer 1997 (among other places), and chapter 4 this volume.

21. *Planned Parenthood v. Casey*, 505 U.S. 833, 851 (1992).

22. *Roe v. Wade*, 410 U.S. 113 (1973).

23. *Cruzan v. Missouri Department of Health*, 497 U.S. 261 (1980).

24. The following discussion repeats some points made in chapter 4 this volume.

25. See *Compassion in Dying v. Washington*, 79 F.3d 790, 823 (9th Cir. 1996), *rev'd sub nom. Washing v. Glucksberg*, 117 S. Ct. 2258 (1997).

26. I believe that Dworkin et al. also fail to appreciate this in their amicus brief.

27. See *Compassion in Dying*, 79 F.3d at 834.

28. Dworkin et al. also miss this point, I believe, about the scope of the different rights. Contrary to what Dworkin et al. say, a doctor might in some cases be permitted (and even required) to turn off a respirator, but not permitted to provide pills.

29. *Compassion in Dying*, 79 F.3d at 822, 823.

30. By contrast, terminating aid that *another* (whom one does not represent) is providing may be a killing.

31. This contrasts with a situation in which one never began providing aid and, therefore, may not cause death in letting die.

32. Dworkin, "In Praise of Theory," p. 358.

33. Dworkin, "In Praise of Theory." I want to emphasize that my discussion of Hercules is limited to the description Dworkin gives of him in this article, rather than in Ronald Dworkin, *Law's Empire* (Cambridge, MA: Harvard University Press, 1986), and Ronald Dworkin, "Hard Cases," in his *Taking Rights Seriously* (Cambridge, MA: Harvard University Press, 1977), p. 81.

34. Dworkin, "In Praise of Theory," p. 374, quoting Cass R. Sunstein, *Legal Reasoning and Political Conflict* (New York: Oxford University Press, 1996), p. 57.

35. I assume he means conviction in a case decision.

36. Dworkin, "In Praise of Theory," p. 374.

37. Many years after writing the article on which this chapter is based, I learned of Derek Parfit's three-option mine shaft example that also seems to imply that we sometimes should do what we know *cannot* be the solution we would choose with perfect information. See his *On What Matters* (Oxford: Oxford University Press, 2011), pp. 159–61.

38. Lawrence Sager emphasized this to me, and I believe it is at least partially Dworkin's own view. See generally Dworkin, *Life's Dominion*. The Court in *Roe* said that it was not competent to decide the question of whether the fetus is a person in the philosophical sense. See *Roe v. Wade*, at 159. This is an argument from incompetence, not from the view that the question is, in principle, not for the Court to decide. The Court said that it could decide whether the fetus is a person within the meaning of the Constitution, however. To do this, the Court made reference to prior legal decisions concerning fetuses, noting that fetuses had never been treated as constitutional persons and concluding that birth was the point at which constitutional persons existed. See *Roe v. Wade*, at 158–62. But this legal conclusion is less than satisfying as a philosophical theory, since newborn infants and late-term fetuses probably do not differ in any characteristic a philosopher deems relevant to determining moral personhood. If the Court nevertheless distinguishes the fetus and the infant, this is probably because it is not aiming to settle the question of personhood as a philosophical issue. See Dworkin, *Life's Dominion*, pp. 15, 18, 20–21. Dworkin also thinks that some mental life is one philosophical criterion for personhood. So at least the early fetus is not a person in the philosophical sense, whatever else it may be; Dworkin, *Life's Dominion*, p. 23. Does he believe that the Court in *Roe* should have at least dealt with the philosophical issue of personhood of the early fetus—though it thought that it was not competent to deal with the issue—even if it should not settle other questions about the fetus's nature?

39. I suggested the latter position in "Abortion and the Value of Life: A Discussion of *Life's Dominion*," *Columbia Law Review* 95 (1995): 160–221; see also chapter 11 this volume; and Judith Jarvis Thomson argues for it in "Abortion," *The Boston Review*, Summer 1995, p. 11.

40. This is Thomson's approach in her "A Defense of Abortion." I examine the approach at length in my *Creation and Abortion*, a short version of which is chapter 12 this volume.

41. Thanks to Lewis Kornhauser, Liam Murphy, Lawrence Sager, Seana Shiffrin, and the editors of the *Arizona State Law Journal* for help with earlier drafts of the entire article of which this chapter is a revised part.

26

Types of Relations between Theory and Practice

HIGH THEORY, LOW THEORY, AND APPLYING APPLIED ETHICS

My basic concern in this chapter is with various ways of understanding the relation and contrast between theory and practice.[1] In particular, I am concerned with high theory, with what I call low theory, and with the actual (acted-out) application of these in the real world. By "high" theory I mean ethical theories such as utilitarianism, Kantianism, and contractarianism, but also one in which plausible principles concerned with several factors may have to be balanced or refined in light of each other. (This is what some refer to simply as "ethics.") By "low" theory I mean the theory of practical moral problems, such as whether affirmative action should be prohibited and what sorts of rules of war there should be. (This is what some refer to as "applied ethics." In using "low" I do not mean to imply inferior. Low theory in ethics need be no more inferior to high theory than designing Bauhaus utensils or art nouveau architecture is inferior to painting in the same styles. It is only closer to the "ground" of bottom-line production or action.) The real-world application of a solution to a moral problem I call "applying applied ethics."

I

When people discuss the relation between theory and practice, there are several different things they may have in mind. I will consider eight.

A.

People may ask about the relation between theory and practice when they really mean to speak about the relation between doing high theory and doing low theory. One relation between high and low theory I have noticed in my own work is the straightforward application of high-theory principles to cases. I emphasize this because some have said that this straightforward application never occurs. For example, in theoretical discussion of the possible moral distinction between killing and letting die, I emphasized that the two could differ morally per se, in virtue of their different definitional properties, and yet this need not lead to moral differences in certain cases. This was because some of the definitional properties of letting die (properties that made it morally different from killing) could occur in cases of killing, thereby compensating for the per se difference. I focused on one definitional property of letting die: that the person we let die loses only a life he would have had due to our aid, not a life he would have had independently of us. I argued that cases in which we kill someone who is already receiving life support from us are morally more like letting-die cases than are other cases of killing, because they share this definitional property of letting die. This principle finds a direct application in low theory on abortion, where we focus on killing a fetus that is dependent for life support on a woman.

Here is a second example: In theoretical work on the distribution of scarce resources, I argued for a Principle of Irrelevant Goods, according to which small differences in goods achievable by saving one person's life rather than another's do not constitute a reason for depriving either party of the equal chance to survive. This principle was (almost) directly applicable to decision making about who should get an organ transplant when the outcome of one patient differed only slightly from that of another. (I say "almost" because applying the Principle of Irrelevant Goods required us to reflect on the distinction between an extra good being concentrated in the same person getting the major benefit of life and being distributed in someone else.)

These two examples indicate that a case may offer the opportunity for a straightforward application of a theory or principle. The second example shows that variations in cases may lead to recharacterization of a theoretical principle (e.g., distinguishing concentration versus dispersal of benefits).

But sometimes, in order to do low theory, I found that one had actually to do *new* theory at the lower case level. Furthermore, this was not the sort of new theory that merely led one to refine one's original principle. For example, in the case of abortion one could not get a result on the question of the permissibility of abortion from applying the principle about killing to terminate life support without also considering whether the fetus is worse off for having lived a short life in the womb and then dying than it would be if it had never lived at all. This is because, in its general formulation, the principle that defines the significance of killing in cases that have the definitional property of letting die implies that it is permissible to kill only if the person killed is no worse off for having been supported and killed than he would have been if he had never been supported. So we cannot tell whether abortion is, in a morally important sense, even an instance of the general principle concerning killing and letting die until we deal with whether being created and dying at an early age is worse than never being created. Doing this requires the consideration of the specifics of creation and abortion. I believe that this involves doing nonderivative low theory.

It may be useful to employ the terms "topic-neutral" and "topic-specific" in discussing some relations of high and low theory. Straightforward direct application of a general, topic-neutral principle does not involve dealing with distinguishing factors in the case at hand. By contrast, theorizing directly at the low level (perhaps to see whether the case presents an instance of a general principle) is heavily involved with the significance of particular factors of the case. I call this topic-specific theory. Low theory that is topic-specific rather than topic-neutral can be just as deep as high theory, only it arises from and is designed to deal with a particular problem. Hence it is not as likely as topic-neutral theory to have implications for other problems that are more than analogies.[2] The distinction is one of breadth, not depth. Of course, new advances in topic-neutral higher theory can arise in the course of working on a particular low-theory issue as well as on a particular practical problem.[3]

To some people, it seems disappointing if we can solve problems using topic-neutral theory; it seems much more exciting to require topic-specific theory, for then, in a sense, every problem is a new problem. But it is also exciting to find that a problem yields to perfectly general concepts. A good example of this is Philippa Foot's discussion of euthanasia, in which the distinction between negative and positive rights is applied to anything that is one's own (and only as an instance to one's own life in particular).[4] Furthermore, in the same discussion, the general distinction between injustice, in taking away what belongs to someone without his or her consent, and uncharitableness, in showing no concern for what happens to what belongs to another, goes far toward solving problems. An analysis peculiar to euthanasia itself is called for only near the end of Foot's discussion, in order to deal with a slippery-slope problem that may be serious because life, rather than something else, is at stake.

B.

A second idea that people may have in mind when they discuss the relation between theory and practice is the view that the correctness of a theory can be tested, and a theory be changed, by seeing its implications for cases. I believe that theories *should* be tested, at least in part, in this way. (But notice that insofar as discussion of cases changes one's view of high theory, it may be through topic-specific, low theorizing). It is possible to test a theory in this way because judgments about cases are often intuitive and not theory driven.

C.

Change may also go in the other direction than described in (B), from high theory to a change in judgment about cases. This is one reason to think theory is related to practice in a third way; namely, it can lead us to change our mind about what to do in practical cases from our pretheoretical judgment. Stephen Toulmin argued that so long as we all agree on cases we need not worry about theoretical justification. One danger in this position is that we may all agree on the wrong answer to a case.[5] Doing theory can help us discover our mistakes and make us change our minds about cases. Furthermore, depending on what identity conditions we have for decisions, we may classify many more decisions as "different from what they would otherwise have been" in virtue of doing high theory. For example, suppose someone would have been in favor of constructing a weapon system before and after philosophical reflection. But before reflection he was in favor of it as a way of starting a war, and after reflection he is in favor of it as a way of avoiding a war. To say that philosophical reflection made no difference to what he decided was right to do conceals a lot.

D.

There are also dangers in emphasizing only the way theory can lead to change in case judgments (or vice versa). Often we are interested in theory even though we are quite certain of the correctness of our case judgments. Indeed, we are more certain of these judgments than we could be of the correctness of any theory. In such instances, we could be interested in a theory because it gives us hope of understanding our case judgments and practice in a deeper and more penetrating way.[6] This is a fourth sense of the relation between theory and practice.

E.

A fifth notion, emphasizing a theory/practice distinction, is invoked sometimes when people say that things are true in theory but not in practice. What they usually mean is that there are conditions in the "real" world that make it impossible to fulfill an "ideal." (I shall examine this interpretation more fully in [H].) On the other hand, "true in theory but not in practice" may signal that although theory would predict a moral problem because of a theoretical distinction, in practice there is no problem because events correct or compensate for the expected difference. For example, it is possible that killing and letting die differ morally per se (i.e., in virtue of differing conceptual properties) and yet a particular killing is no worse than a particular letting die, because, as described above, in our descriptions we have equalized the cases so that the killing case has a property not usually true of killing cases but definitionally true of letting die. Some will describe this as illustrating the fact that killing and letting die differ morally in theory but need not in practice; but really it should be described as their exhibiting a per se difference that may not show up in some real or even hypothetical cases.

F.

A sixth interpretation of the theory/practice question is suggested by Rawls's view (as described, for example, in *Political Liberalism*) on the relation between theory and practice for us as citizens.[7] He claims that in justifying public policy on constitutional issues and the basics of justice, we may not need theoretically correct or true positions but rather politically acceptable reasons. One understanding of politically acceptable reason, or "public reason" as Rawls calls it, is that it is reason for certain important practical purposes rather than for theoretical purposes. It makes reference only to factors that we could reasonably expect other reasonable persons to also accept as reasons. On Rawls's view, the theoretical arguments are given by comprehensive views (such as philosophical or religious systems), many of which are held by members of a democratic society but to which we cannot expect all to adhere. These arguments are not usually used in public justification of a position, except insofar as their terms overlap with those of public reason. Rawls's position is different from an anti-theorist such as Toulmin, since public reason provides some publicly accepted values (e.g., those inherent to constitutional democracy) that all should be expected to share as justifications for policies; we are not asked merely to accept agreement on policies for cases without justification at all.

Nevertheless, Rawls's view may give rise to the same sort of discomfort that we can feel with Toulmin's. That is, as holders of comprehensive views outside public reason, we may feel discomfort at being restrained in certain public contexts from offering what we conceive of as the most complete, deep, and true justifications for a position, and also uncomfortable if we find that those with comprehensive views with which we disagree reach the same conclusions on cases. From a practical (political) point of view we should be happy that there is an overlapping consensus on a position as well as a justification for it in the language of public reason. We may also be pleased that we are not required to discuss and justify our comprehensive doctrines in cases where public reasons coincide with these, nor have to convert others to our views. Yet we may want to know how it is that very different theories lead to the same conclusion, and we may want to judge between the comprehensive views. One can feel uncomfortable in the company of those who support the same actions one does but, at a level deeper than public reason, for what one considers the wrong reasons.[8]

G.

Consider now the seventh notion of the relation of theory and practice. It seems to me that a meaningful question about the relation between theory and practice is whether people will or should reasonably be expected to use a theory in deliberation about what to do, as a decision procedure. This question raises the possibility that a theory is *self-effacing*; that is, even though the theory is true, the results it demands would be better achieved if no one believed it or used it in deliberation. Utilitarianism may be such a theory. Sidgwick thought that nonconsequentialist theories should be used in deliberation but that consequentialism was the ultimate truth about morality; one simply achieved the best consequences more often if most people did not know the truth.[9] However, not all theories are self-effacing.

Self-effacement may tell against using one theory in practice but not against using theory in general.

Stuart Hampshire raises a more general objection to a role for theory in moral decision making.[10] He says that, for evolutionary reasons, it would not be surprising if most people could unconsciously and rapidly weigh factors correctly and yet not be able explicitly to give their reasons for deciding as they do. There are good evolutionary (survival) reasons for our being creatures who can make right decisions quickly and, he says, no good survival reasons for being able to give reasons.

In rebuttal of Hampshire, but arguing within his own framework, one might suggest that the ability to justify one's judgments to others might well have survival value. Furthermore, the innate capacity for moral judgment may well be at a disadvantage in trying to deal with complex problems that arise as a result of technology and social changes, changes that proceed more rapidly than biological evolution, and theorizing could help here. Furthermore, the thesis that any moral judging due to evolution should be left untouched conflicts with the idea that morality goes beyond any biologically/culturally given dispositions and it should be used to evaluate them.

It seems clearly false that all (theory-innocent) persons make equally good moral judgments, let alone act equally well. While variation in performance is consistent with an evolutionary account such as Hampshire's,[11] variation in judgment may still imply that some people need to have their attention directed to principles and general factors in order to judge and act well.[12]

The sort of rapid judgment Hampshire admires may sometimes be made possible by prior explicit acquaintance with concepts and principles, which then seep back to form the unconscious background of a person's thought. Ideally, all instruction in general theories, concepts, and principles should come to be internalized, allowing for the rapid perception of the moral character of a situation. So there is no necessary conflict between improving in judgment through acquaintance with general conceptions, first consciously introduced, and quick intuitive judging.

H.

The eighth notion of the theory/practice relation concerns the obstacles to acting on the known right answer to a practical quandary. This is the problem of applying applied ethics. Partiality on one's own behalf is often thought of as the primary obstacle to acting correctly (for example, recognizing that a scarce organ should go to someone with greatest need, but using one's influence to acquire it for oneself instead).[13] However, in *Equality and Partiality*, Thomas Nagel argues that high moral theory about right and wrong conduct does not imply complete impartiality, but itself endorses a certain range of decision making and behavior stemming from a partial point of view.[14] This is because morality must, he thinks, take into account the sort of creature it is for, and humans value many things out of proportion to their value from an impartial perspective. They are creatures with both an impartial and a partial perspective. Nagel thinks we should take the partial perspective into account in deciding what the demands of morality are, not merely because morality would not be a practical success if we did not do this, but because he thinks creatures with the partial point of view have good reason to reject totally impartial morality. However, Nagel also says that as rational beings, we are capable of developing new motives, besides desires or commitments we already have, if we are convinced that there is reason (including impartial reasons) for us to do so.

Samuel Scheffler presents a similar view. He says, "morality is addressed from the outset to human beings as they are. It affords them the prospect of integrating two different motivational tendencies [by which he means the partial and impartial], and it has no 'prior' content that must be 'reduced' or 'modified' when it is brought into contact with human nature."[15]

If there were reason to take a partial perspective into account in framing moral demands, this would mean that within a certain range, preferences for the self or partialist values are not really an obstacle to acting as morality requires. However, this is consistent with morality still requiring impartiality in the sense that if action and motivation from a partial point of view are permissible, they must be and be recognized to be equally permissible for all persons.

When the partial point of view is being accommodated, either by formulating a theory to reflect its weight or by giving in to it as an obstacle to implementing a true result in applied ethics, at least someone's good is being pursued. But arguably the worst obstacles to a theory or to its implications being applied in practice are such vices as envy, avarice, meanness, and competitiveness as an end in itself. With these often no one's good is being served, and there may be reason to believe that these are very widespread motives.

Developing a moral theory to deal with obstacles to applying morality is extremely difficult. It cannot merely be a matter of recommending actions so that we come out as close as possible to the end state we would have been in with perfect compliance to morality. Arranging things in this manner (e.g., checking up on hypocrisy or harassment) may itself involve doing something morally wrong. Further, it can seem artificial to distinguish between applied ethics and moral recommendations for applying applied ethics, since if we should take into account real-life obstacles to applying ethics, we will merely be theorizing again about what we should morally do in a certain situation (i.e., one where there are obstacles to an ideal applied ethics solution). This is a new part of applied theory, making it more complete, rather than anything separate from it. For example, often the "obstacle" to actually applying an ideal solution to a practical problem is another moral value or right such as patient autonomy. We may reason to the morally correct solution about whether a particular pregnancy should be ended, but if the pregnant woman does not agree to the abortion, respect for her autonomy implies that it would be morally wrong to require the "ideal" abortion. Nevertheless, I believe it pays to distinguish ideal high and low theory from theory that includes all real-world factors. First, we want to be sure we recognize certain real-world factors as obstacles which we might prefer to change rather than deal with, if we could. It is by the standards of ideal high and low theory that we can see their removal as desirable even if not possible. Second, in the case where the obstacles are other values or rights (such as autonomy or democratic decision making), we want to be able to retain the idea of someone's making a better or worse autonomous or democratic choice, based on evaluation of the content of that decision. We also want to be able to offer what reason shows is the best content as a possible option for the person to consider and accept or reject.

What both high and low theory would continue to do—even if not actually applied and heeded in action—is show people what the truth is. For example, they might teach persons what their true status is, what they continue to be and are entitled to, even if this status were not respected. Doing theory and inculcating it in others can also habituate people to high standards that make them dissatisfied with the inadequacies they and others exhibit in practice. This dissatisfaction is worthwhile in its own right, I believe, even if it has no further consequences, for at least we then evaluate ourselves and our failings correctly. But this dissatisfaction may also lead to a desire for improvement, and may at least lead to admiration for the few whose behavior is morally correct. These are indirect practical effects which the high and low theories could have even if they did not motivate much action directly.

Notes

1. This chapter is based on sections of my "High Theory, Low Theory, and the Demands of Morality," in *Theory and Practice*, eds. I. Shapiro and J. W. DeCew, NOMOS 37 (1995). The article was written at a time when there was much debate about whether those who taught classes on practical moral problems should spend any time in those classes teaching ethical theory. There was also debate about whether teaching practical ethics would have any effect on actual conduct. These debates continue to this day. I am grateful to the editors of this NOMOS volume, to Leigh Cauman, Sigrun Svavarsdottir, Julia Driver, and to the faculty and students at the University of Rochester Philosophy Department and at the Harvard Program in Ethics and the Professions for help with this article. It is a sequel to my "Ethics, Applied Ethics, and Applying Applied Ethics," (from which I have incorporated some points) in *Applied Ethics and Ethical Theory*, eds. D. Rosenthal and F. Shehadi (Salt Lake City: University of Utah Press, 1988).

2. After writing the article on which this chapter is based, I read Ronald Dworkin's endorsement in *Life's Dominion* (New York: Knopf, 1993) of creating theory explicitly for a practical problem. He writes:

> When we reason from the outside in, a practical issue must shop from among ready-made theories on the racks to see which theory asks and tries to answer questions that best fit its own dimensions. When we reason from the inside out, theories are bespoke,

made for the occasion, Savile Row not Seventh Avenue. Theories homemade in that way, rather than wholesaled or imported, may be more likely to succeed in the political forum. They may be better suited to the academy, too. (p. 29)

3. Then the danger is that the advances in high theory will be buried in the low-theory literature, when they could be of more general use. The philosopher may have a responsibility to re-present his or her general results in a more general context.

4. Philippa Foot, "Euthanasia," *Philosophy & Public Affairs* 6(2) (Winter 1977): 85–112.

5. Stephen Toulmin, "The Tyranny of Principles," *Hastings Center Report* 11(6) (December 1981): 31–39.

6. On how this gives us a form of self-knowledge, see chapter 27 this volume.

7. John Rawls, *Political Liberalism* (expanded ed.) (New York: Columbia University Press, 2005).

8. Ronald Dworkin does not share Rawls's views on the bracketing of comprehensive philosophical doctrines in public political debate of constitutional fundamentals. Nevertheless, in his recent work on abortion and euthanasia, he follows a different route which has the same effect of limiting discussion of certain theoretical issues for practical purposes: He classifies much of what seems to be philosophical argumentation about the meaning of life as religious, and so not eligible to be part of legal justification, on grounds of separation of Church and State. For details, see chapter 11 this volume.

9. Henry Sidgwick, *The Methods of Ethics* (7th ed.) (Indianapolis: Hackett, 1981).

10. Stuard Hampshire, *Two Theories of Morality* (Oxford: Oxford University Press/British Academy, 1976).

11. As Sigrun Svavarsdottir pointed out.

12. It may be worth noting that if *evolution* were responsible for implanting ethical judgments, one would expect such good judgments to lead more uniformly than they in fact do to good behavior. For would it be evolutionarily sound for judgments not to lead to acts?

13. Kant called making an exception of oneself "radical evil" (the root of all evil). See his *Religion Within the Limits of Reason Alone* (New York: Harper Torchbooks, 1793/1960).

14. Thomas Nagel, *Equality and Partiality* (New York: Oxford University Press, 1991).

15. He argues that morality is best presented as offering an Ideal of Humanity that is about the integration of partial and impartial points of view. However, I consider some possible problems with this view (given that supererogatory action might also be thought of an Ideal), in "Rationality and Morality," *Noûs* 29(4) (1995): 544–55.

27

Understanding, Justifying, and Finding Oneself

This chapter tries to explain some ways in which we can come to know about ourselves, in particular about what we think. It also tries to distinguish what we are and think from what we ought to be and think.[1]

I. Deciding versus Discovering

To begin, it is important to distinguish two different senses of coming to know what we think. The first sense is that of "making up your mind" about an issue: for instance, this is generally what someone wants you to do when they ask, "What do you think now about the invasion of Iraq?" This requires you to consider the facts and values in favor of and against the invasion and come to a conclusion about its merits. It does not usually involve your trying to introspect (or to use some more sophisticated way of gaining knowledge about your mental states) in order to find out what settled beliefs you already have about the Iraq War.[2] The same can be true if you are asked about a moral issue—for instance, what you think about the morality of capital punishment.

These questions are also asking you to come to a conclusion about what you believe is *true* about the invasion and about capital punishment. They ask you to form a true opinion not about yourself but about a form of action undertaken by others. This does not mean that what you think *is* true (your opinion might be wrong), but you are being asked to attempt to get at a truth about something other than yourself. This is so, even though the question asks about what you think.

This chapter is primarily concerned not with how we come to know what we think in the sense of making up our mind, but with the acquisition of self-knowledge in the sense of discovering things about ourselves that hold true independently of our now making up our mind.

II. Explaining Oneself

A. INFERENCE AND THE METHOD OF HYPOTHETICAL CASES

It is said by some psychologists (such as Timothy Wilson) that we often do not understand why we do or believe certain things because it is our "adaptive unconscious" that is in control.[3] Yet when asked why we have done or believe certain things, we nevertheless often confidently give answers that are, in fact, incorrect explanations. Wilson refers to these as "confabulations." For example, suppose there is a person who has been hypnotized to open a window at a certain time and does so. He may claim he did so because the room got hot even though there was no change in room temperature. Such events suggest that, at least sometimes, we have no privileged access to ourselves. That is, we do not know ourselves better than we know others and, in fact, others may know why we do or believe things better than we do.

As a philosopher, I might be expected to disagree with this claim. However, I am inclined to agree that in many cases with which I have dealt, it is hard for someone to know why he believes something and yet he may often offer an incorrect explanation of his beliefs, and others may know better than he does why he believes certain things.

Consider the so-called Trolley Problem.[4] In one case that exhibits one version of the problem, an out-of-control trolley is headed toward killing five immovable people on a track. If and only if a bystander presses a switch near to him will the trolley be directed away from the five onto another track. Unfortunately, there is a different immovable individual on that other track who, it is foreseen, will be killed by the redirected trolley (Redirect Case). Many people intuitively judge that it is permissible to turn the trolley, thus saving five and killing one. However, there is another variation of the Trolley Problem in which the trolley headed to the five can only be stopped if a bystander pushes a very heavy person from where that heavy person stands on a bridge over the track. The heavy person's falling in front of the trolley would stop it but kill him (Bridge Case). The same people who think it is permissible to divert the trolley in the first case usually intuitively judge that it is impermissible to push the man from the bridge. This is so even though in both cases five people will be saved and one will die.

While people have these responses consciously and with conviction, they do not consciously reason their way to them. That is why these responses are called intuitive judgments. Often people may not know how to explain why they respond as they do. Some have proposed that the reason many people respond differently to the two trolley cases is that the first case involves pressing a switch that leads to someone's death, whereas in the second case one must be "up close and personal" in pushing the person to his death.[5] (Those who have proposed this see it as a "debunking" explanation, in that the mere fact that one kills someone up close and personally could not actually make a moral difference between the cases, even if people react as though it does.) The question is whether this simple explanation of why people respond differently to the two cases is a "confabulation" or, as I would put it, a wrong conjecture. I am tempted to distinguish between a confabulation and a wrong conjecture because it might be thought that a confabulation should refer only to an explanation about his own responses that a person makes up quickly and of which he feels confident. Since not all wrong conjectures (even about one's own responses) are like this, not all wrong conjectures would be confabulations.[6]

I believe that we can test our conjectures about why people make certain conscious intuitive moral judgments by using what I call the Method of Hypothetical Cases.[7] Just as the two previous trolley cases did not occur in reality but were hypothetical cases, we may create other hypothetical cases that vary in certain ways from these and they can help us decide whether people are responding to the factor pointed to in the conjecture. For example, using this method allows us to mentally remove the factor of "up close and personal" pushing, creating another case that holds everything else constant as it was in the Bridge Case. So suppose a bystander needs only to press a switch that will activate a machine that will push the heavy person off the bridge. Will people who judged it impermissible to push the person off the bridge now think it permissible to press the switch? If not, then it is not being "up close and personal" per se that accounts for the differing views about the Redirect and Bridge Cases. The conjecture would be shown to be wrong. (It would also help to test the conjecture to imagine another hypothetical case that also involves "up close and personal" pushing of someone into a threat but was nevertheless judged permissible, due to our varying some other factor in the Bridge Case.[8])

Scientists use experiments in which they can change one variable at a time, holding everything else constant, in order to see if that variable is crucial to an explanation of a phenomenon. The Method of Hypothetical Cases is the use of thought experiments, which often seem bizarre because we can imagine a factor being present or absent, holding constant all other factors, though this could not happen in reality. But just as artificially controlled conditions in a lab can lead to results that are applicable to real life, the results of artificial thought experiments might help us explain intuitive responses in "messier" cases closer to real life or in real life.

Using the Method of Hypothetical Cases to explain one's own intuitive judgments about cases does not involve unaided introspective knowledge. It is more like inferring what drives one's responses by a process of testing and eliminating conjectures. Wilson himself says that we can have inferential knowledge of what is going on in our adaptive unconscious (which underlies our conscious awareness of a judgment). He says: "Many human judgments, emotions, thoughts, and behaviors are produced by the adaptive unconscious. Because people do not have conscious access to the adaptive unconscious, their conscious selves confabulate reasons why they responded the way we did. . . . In other words, to the extent that people's responses are caused by the adaptive unconscious, they do not have privileged access to the causes and must infer them."[9]

Daniel Kahnemann has said that when a philosopher offers explanations of his intuitive judgments he is like the hypnotized person who offers a confabulation (i.e., "the room got hotter") to explain his opening a window.[10] But when philosophers consider a wide range of cases in order to find out what factor may account for their judgments, they are trying to avoid the problem raised by the case of the hypnotized person. The hypnotized person's explanation could be determined to be a confabulation by the method of hypothetical cases, for if we kept all factors constant except that we made the room colder, we know that the person would still feel compelled to open the window, thus showing that his own explanation was wrong. By testing their conjectures on multiple cases, philosophers seek to identify an explanation that cannot be eliminated in this way. [11]

B. SELF AND OTHERS

The fact that we may acquire knowledge about ourselves through inference suggests that we may also understand others better than they understand themselves, and others may understand us better than we understand ourselves. This is because any given person may not have the ability to isolate a factor underlying his views that is only discoverable through consideration of many judgments about different cases. Someone else who has the ability may infer the factor that is leading another person to make judgments better than that other person could. Furthermore, if one does have the ability to come to understand what is underlying one's own judgments, then one may be able to understand others' similar judgments better than they can. So, if I were able to understand my responses to the cases exhibiting the Trolley Problem and your responses were like mine, I might have a true conjecture about what underlies your responses, even if you do not.

C. COMPLEX EXPLANATIONS

Suppose one uses the Method of Hypothetical Cases. The factor that one ultimately uncovers that seems to account for intuitive judgments may be complex or at least unexpected; it could be very hard to consciously formulate the factor and it might be a factor that does not ordinarily play a part in conscious thought. Does this mean that it could not really causally underlie people's judgments? I have argued that our ethics may be "intricate," and that complex factors may account for our responses without our ordinarily being capable of consciously formulating the factors or principles containing them.[12] Sometimes support is drawn for this view from the theory of innate grammar, in that complex unconscious principles seem to guide our understanding and production of language.[13] I now find support in what Wilson says about "implicit learning" by the adaptive unconscious. He says about a demonstration of implicit learning:

> The participants' task was to watch a computer screen that was divided into four quadrants. On each trial, the letter X appeared in one of the four quadrants, and the participant pressed one of four buttons to indicate which one. Unbeknownst to the participant, the presentations of the Xs were divided

into blocks of 12 that followed a complex rule. . . . Although the exact rules were complicated, participants appeared to learn them. As time went by their performance steadily improved. . . . None of the participants, however, could verbalize what the rules were or even that they had learned anything. They learned the complex rules nonconsciously.[14]

In this case, the formula that explained the placement of Xs in the grid, the grasp of which explained the ultimate behavior of participants, was never consciously recognized by them. I have suggested that the Method of Hypothetical Cases could help us make conscious the principle underlying certain moral judgments.

III. Beyond Explanation to Justification

Moral philosophers aim to go beyond finding out to what factors one is responding in cases. Moral philosophy is *normative*: it is concerned with the factors to which one should respond and, in general, with what one should think and do rather than with what one (or even everyone) actually thinks and does. So, if one uncovers factors or principles that explain one's responses, one has to reflect on whether those factors or principles also justify one's responses. That is, do they really represent or are they connected with reasons, considerations that have moral significance? (One part of Kahnemann's sense that true moral judgments could not be the result of complex factors uncovered via the Method of Hypothetical Cases is his sense that such complex factors or principles are unlikely to be inherently morally significant reasons, even if they do underlie our judgments. I suspect that he thinks this because he favors some form of utilitarianism [i.e., maximizing overall good understood as well being], and he cannot see the moral merit in various kinds of constraints on maximizing the good that prohibit bringing about the good in one way but not another.[15]) Notice that doing mere surveys of others' intuitive responses does not play a role in justifying or undermining one's intuitive judgments. Doing surveys gives the impression that one takes intuitive responses—one's own or others'—to be data that support or undermine a judgment. But intuitive responses are themselves judgments about correctness or incorrectness that may or may not be justified by reason. They are not data for judgments. (Consider that when a scientist collects data, she then forms a judgment about what the data show. She does not treat her judgment as itself a small piece of data in support of a judgment about the data. This is shown by the fact that she does not do a survey of the views of other scientists about her data and then form a judgment about the original data set based on the survey.)

Suppose the factors or principles uncovered do have moral significance. Indeed, suppose that a factor that explains different responses to different cases provides a sufficient reason for responding differently to the cases. Then it justifies the differential responses. Furthermore, given that one responded to a sufficient reason in having the intuitive judgment, even though the intuitive judgment was not reached by consciously considering such a reason, the judgment can be considered a reasonable (or rational) intuitive judgment. It is not merely a feeling that one tries to "rationalize" (in the sense of providing a confabulation for it after the fact[16]).

If factors or principles sufficiently justify responses they cause, they can become the basis for requirements on everyone's conduct, should they face situations in reality like those presented in hypothetical cases, and standards against which to measure the correctness of anyone's intuitive moral judgments. One way of putting this is that taking account of the justifying factors or principles is objectively correct and provides universalizable standards (i.e., they apply to everyone). If this is the case, self-knowledge that shows particularities about oneself that others do not share need not be relevant to whether one should judge or act in the way others should judge and act. Consider an analogy from another area: Suppose an art critic judges one work of art to be better than another. He is not just saying that he, in virtue of his particular history and characteristics, responds more favorably to one work than another. He is claiming to make a universalizable judgment. This is a judgment that everyone who is concerned with artistic merit should make, regardless of the particular personal characteristics that might distinguish him from the art critic and that might lead him to favor one work over another on grounds other than artistic merit (e.g., it reminds him of his parent).

The fact of normativity opens up the possibility that how one ought to judge or behave can differ from how one is revealed to actually judge and behave. Objective and universalizable truths about morality (and other things) open up the possibility that one could know what one should or should not do, or how one should judge, independently of knowing much about one's distinctive personal psychology. This possibility is one ground on which to be skeptical of the importance of self-knowledge, for finding out about oneself leaves one with the normative question of whether to endorse or reject what one finds in oneself. For example, if one finds that one has a strong desire to harm people, one may wish to be different and try to change, or at least to not give vent to the desire. People often wonder whether many things true of them are due to nature or nurture, but regardless of the origin of traits, the question remains of evaluating them either positively or negatively and deciding what to do about them. The fact that something is due to nature rather than to nurture does not mean it should be endorsed.

However, it might be argued that one's true self (knowledge of which is in question) is the part of oneself that evaluates other parts, since one identifies with it,[17] giving it an authoritative standing in relation to one's thoughts, desires, and actions. For example, it has been said, a drug addict may crave drugs and all the while judge that the craving is one he does not want to have because it is bad to have. These are not just two equal and conflicting "parts" of the self pulling in opposite directions. The person could, for example, identify with the negative judgment of his craving and ultimately want to get rid of the craving. This gives the judging part authority. The question is whether this means that the part of oneself that craves the drug is any less one's true self for being rejected. In any case, notice that knowing where one ultimately stands on the issue of craving for drugs—pro or con—is (often) a matter of making up one's mind rather than merely discovering where one already stands. This brings us back to the very first distinction we discussed in part I, between making up one's mind and discovering it.

There is another reason for being skeptical about the importance of a person acquiring knowledge of himself. Discovering things about oneself and even deciding what about oneself to endorse or reject may be less important than just quite unreflectively being a good self. And if one is already a good self—doing and thinking correctly—then one will presumably consider whether acquiring knowledge about oneself is the right thing to do by contrast with doing other things; for example, acquiring knowledge about how to cure cancer. Acquiring self-knowledge may be the right thing to do only if it is a means to making oneself or some other aspect of reality better. Indeed, the self-knowledge that people usually seek involves "finding oneself" in the sense of finding what one can do in life that is both worthwhile and authentic (true to one's interests and capacities).[18] Notice also that acquiring knowledge about oneself is to be contrasted with acquiring knowledge about self-knowledge. The latter is an inquiry into people's acquisition of knowledge of themselves, not the acquisition of knowledge of oneself in particular. Thus, inquiring into the acquisition of self-knowledge could be important even when acquiring self-knowledge is not itself important in particular cases.

Notes

1. The essay that forms this chapter was written in conjunction with (but after) the panel discussion on "Who Am I? Beyond 'I Think, Therefore I Am,'" at the New York Academy of Sciences (NYAS), May 24, 2011. As this chapter is short, none of the topics are dealt with thoroughly.

2. The distinction between making up one's mind and discovering one's mind was emphasized by Richard Moran in his *Authority and Estrangement: An Essay on Self-Knowledge* (Princeton, NJ: Princeton University Press, 2001).

3. In his *Strangers to Ourselves* (Cambridge, MA: Harvard University Press, 2005). Wilson was a fellow member of the NYAS panel.

4. Based on cases presented in Philippa Foot's "The Problem of Abortion and the Doctrine of Double Effect," reprinted in her *Virtues and Vices and Other Essays* (Berkeley: University of California Press, 1978), and in Judith Thomson's "Killing, Let Die, and the Trolley Problem," *The Monist* 59 (1976): 204–17. I discuss the problem in my *Morality, Mortality*, Vol. II (New York: Oxford University Press, 1996) and in my *Intricate Ethics* (New York: Oxford University Press, 2007), among other places.

5. This was suggested by the philosopher/psychologist Joshua Greene. See, for example, Joshua D. Greene et al., "An fMRI Investigation of Emotional Engagement in Moral Judgment," *Science* 293 (2001): 2105–8. I have discussed Greene's views on moral judgment in my "Neuroscience and Moral Reasoning: A Note on Recent Research," *Philosophy & Public Affairs* 37(4): 330–45.

6. On the other hand, in considering some of my proposals for explaining my own different responses to different Trolley Cases, the psychologist Daniel Kahnemann compared me to a person who confabulates. See his remarks in chapter 3 of *Conversations on Ethics* by Alex Voorhoeve (Oxford: Oxford University Press, 2009). This was so even though it should have been clear that my conjectures are the result of considering many variants on Trolley Cases and rejecting different possible explanations of responses to them. Thus my ultimate conjectures about what underlies my responses to cases were not immediate responses or held with complete confidence, yet he thought of them as confabulations. It is for this reason that he may also conclude that Professor Greene's proposal is a confabulation, if it turns out to be a false explanation of responses (at least if Greene intuitively also has these responses). I am not sure if Professor Wilson would assent to such a broad notion of "confabulation."

7. I make heavy use of this method in my work, as do many other contemporary philosophers.

8. I tried to do this in constructing what I call the Lazy Susan Case. In this case we cannot redirect a trolley from five people but only redirect the people seated on a swivel table away from the trolley, with the result that one other person on the other side of the table is pushed into the trolley. See *Morality, Mortality*, Vol. II, and *Intricate Ethics*.

9. Wilson, *Strangers to Ourselves*, p. 104.

10. As I noted in note 6 above.

11. The fact that one is conscious of intuitive judgments before becoming conscious of the (supposed) explanation for them does not mean that the explanation cannot point to factors that caused the judgment. The factors, while unconscious, could have caused the judgment.

12. Though I have also noted that heuristics—approximations to a complex principle—might be causally operative, I here wish to consider whether the complex principle might itself be causally operative. See my *Intricate Ethics*, chapter 14, among other places.

13. I referred to this example in the introduction of my *Creation and Abortion* (New York: Oxford University Press, 1992).

14. Wilson, *Strangers to Ourselves*, p. 28.

15. See his remarks in chapter 3 in Voorhoeve's *Conversations on Ethics*. For example, he says: "So I find it hard to believe that the two cases [of pushing the fat man in front of the trolley and of diverting the trolley onto the man on the side track] differ in morally relevant ways." I have discussed earlier work by Kahnemann related to moral theory in my "Moral Intuitions, Cognitive Psychology, and the Harming/Not Aiding Distinction," reprinted as chapter 14 in my *Intricate Ethics*.

16. This is contrary to the view of psychologist Jonathan Haidt. See his "The Emotional Dog and Its Rational Tail: A Social Intuitionist Approach to Moral Judgments," *Psychological Review* 108(4): 814–34. I also discuss Haidt in my "Should You Save This Child? Gibbard on Intuitions, Contractualism, and the Strains of Commitment," which is my response to Allan Gibbard's Tanner Lectures (published with them) in his *Reconciling Our Aims* (New York: Oxford University Press, 2008).

17. Perhaps this view could be supported by the views of Harry Frankfurt in "Freedom of the Will and the Concept of a Person," *Journal of Philosophy* 68(1): 5–20, and Gary Watson in "Free Agency," *Mind* 96(382) (April 1987).

18. It may be that certain fairly mechanical techniques (such as mantra meditation) can help with this task.

INDEX

CPSIA information can be obtained at www.ICGtesting.com
Printed in the USA
BVOW01s2320120916

461718BV00005B/7/P